Diabetes in Old Age

THIRD EDITION

Other titles in the Wiley Diabetes in Practice Series

Diabetes in Old Age

THIRD EDITION

Editor

Alan J. Sinclair

*Bedfordshire & Hertfordshire Postgraduate Medical School,
University of Bedfordshire, UK*

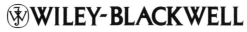

A John Wiley & Sons, Ltd., Publication

ISBN: 978-0-470-06562-4 (H/B)

A catalogue record for this book is available from the British Library.

Typeset in 9.75/11.75 Times Roman by Laserwords Private Limited, Chennai, India
Printed and bound in Great Britain by CPI Antony Rowe, Chippenham, Wilts
First Impression   2009

Contents

SECTION VI   OPTIMIZING DIABETES CARE IN OLDER PEOPLE

Foreword

The cognoscenti, the small cadre of experts on diabetes in the elderly, will skip this foreword and dive right into the individual chapters. There they will find many treasures related to clinical science and clinical care, as well as historical vignettes and current controversies related to diabetes in the older patient.

You, by reading this foreword in a book on diabetes in the elderly patient, are marking yourselves as non-expert but you are clearly ahead of your medical colleagues. You are recognizing that the excellent textbooks on diabetes and excellent textbooks on geriatric medicine, though they cover medical care of the older patient, typically fall short in dealing with the older patient with diabetes.

These textbooks mirror the state of affairs in medical care today. When I was a young physician, I was impressed that excellent internists provided excellent care for their patients, including very good diabetes management. My impression now is that very good internists continue to provide very good care, except for diabetes where the care often is only mediocre. Many endocrinologists, formerly excellent in diabetes, are also falling further and further back from the cutting edge of diabetes care. This is especially sad because we now know more than ever the importance of good management and have better tools with which to approach the desired goals. The gap between "excellent" and "actual" widens as the patient's age increases.

In this essay, I plan to inspire you, to help guide you into a highly satisfying professional path, a path that will please you, as well as enhance your value to your patients and to your medical community. The rest of this book is filled with instructional material that you will find very useful. My goal is to provide an overarching view from the top of the mountain.

Nourishing the soul

Champions seek new challenges, set new goals. For mountain climbers and cellists, surgeons and swimmers, dancers and authors, striving for excellence channels energies and rejuvenates the self. The physician who adopts the mindset of a champion helps his or her patients, helps other health care professionals with their patients and nourishes his or her own soul. At this time in medicine, when physician burnout is epidemic, nourishment for the soul can be life-saving. In the USA, where the pension systems are in disarray and large debts have been piled up to pay for schooling, physicians will be working many years past the hallowed 65. The best preparation for the long journey is passion in one's professional pursuit. As an internist, or endocrinologist, or geriatrician, join me in exploring the attractions of becoming skilled in the care of diabetes in the elderly.

When I entered the profession fifty years ago, antibiotics were routing many infectious diseases. The ancient aphorism "If you know syphilis, you know all of medicine" was being re-modelled; syphilis was replaced by diabetes.

I propose a new model: "If you know diabetes in the elderly, you know all of medicine".

The challenge for the profession

Increasingly, medicine in general is benefiting from the introduction of protocols and algorithms. While improving care, these also shrink the intellectual distance between the physician, the physician's assistant and the nurse. I am guessing that a 37-year-old professor of computer science with type 1 diabetes can probably manage well with a little help from a diabetes educator and an occasional visit to a physician. Recall the World War II pharmacist's mate who in the pre-antibiotic area successfully removed an inflamed appendix from a crew member of his submarine submerged beneath the waters of the Pacific.

Advancing age brings growing complexity. Elderly patients with diabetes need continuous input from skilled physicians. For these physicians, protocols and algorithms are the starting point but the real plan needs multiple modifications, surveillance, balancing of competing priorities, and skilled navigation of poorly charted waters. It demands professional skills at their best.

Interpreting data

Multi-centre trials, the foundation of therapeutics today, are typically performed on younger patients. With the basic and clinical science in the background, the data from widely heralded multi-centre trials (with patients who are typically younger and less complicated) provide a basis but not a recipe for care of the elderly patient. Advanced age and other exclusionary criteria, including medications, make extrapolations to the elderly more tenuous. The loud "microphones" supported by pharmaceutical company coffers often fill the air with information that is misleading for older patients.

Laboratory standards are based on younger populations. Data in the elderly are much sparser. Even when the mean and median for a lab test remain unchanged, the splay typically increases so that higher and lower values that are "normal" for an older patient are easily labelled as pathological.

New medications are largely tested on younger, less complicated patients. Data among older patients are sparse. Many side effects of drugs emerge gradually in the years after their introduction. The catalogue of side effects among older complex patients emerge more slowly. The sparseness of data dictates that new drugs should be avoided in older patients, except on the very rare occasion when the new drug is a very substantial advance and other drugs cannot meet the need.

Adverse drug interactions between two drugs are identified slowly. Many remain undetected. Typical elderly patients take many medications, exponentially increasing the likelihood of adverse drug interactions and, equally, making their detection most difficult.

Depression

Advancing age as well as medications and multiple medical conditions are associated with depression. The link between diabetes and depression has received a lot of attention recently. Growing evidence that depression impacts negatively on physical health mandates that depression, so common in the elderly, be detected and treated energetically.

In dealing with depression, especially in the older patient, recall that

(i) depression without sadness is easy to miss.

(ii) Screening instruments are helpful.

(iii) Personalized rationalizations ("If I was 82 and living alone, I would also feel that way ... ") can obscure the correct diagnosis and management.

(iv) Drugs as well as endocrine diseases and other disorders are common aetiologies of depression that is reversible.

(v) When medication and psychotherapy fail, ECT (electroconvulsive therapy), is an excellent therapeutic choice to consider.

(vi) With ageing, suicide rates rise sharply, especially among white males.

Demographics and disease

The population is being enriched progressively with patients who are over 65. They are living longer. The so-called old-old are a rapidly growing group. Objective data to guide the physician require ever longer lines of extrapolation, demanding more of the physician's judgment. The incidence and prevalence of diabetes increases with age. Ageing brings out diabetes, and diabetes accelerates biological ageing and onset of other pathology. Both processes corrode cognition.

Ageing in our Society: The universal reverence, or at least respect, for the elderly that held sway worldwide since the beginning of human memory, has been replaced in the industrialized world of today with a wide range of negative attitudes, mostly undeserved. In their care for the elderly, physicians and their teammates in care will be energized by recalling the widely appreciated positive features of a majority of the elderly:

(i) Every elderly patient can be improved in some way by an encounter with a professional.

(ii) Typically, the elderly are appreciative of the care and express their appreciation.

(iii) Their expectations for improvement are realistically tempered.

(iv) They are individually "more unique".

"More unique" is a phrase that will galvanize to action legions of amateur grammarians all over the English-speaking world. They will reflexly remind me that unique indicates one-of-a-kind and therefore no comparator is permitted. Biology and I will prove them wrong. Let's start with a fertilized egg that is just dividing to generate a pair of monozygotic twins. They are not identical and progressively diverge, distancing one biological self from the other. All humans do the same. The extremely similar looking zygotes, and highly similar looking newborns progressively diverge, biologically, sociologically and medically, to the delight and amazement of the skilled physician and other health care providers. Like snowflakes, Rembrandt paintings, precious gemstones, and leaves from a single tree, blessedly, there are no sames.

Valediction

With a little luck, it is likely that you, in your lifetime, will never lack for food for your body. Much more at risk, and therefore more to be guarded, is the supply of nourishment for your professional soul.

Jesse Roth MD
Feinstein Institute for Medical Research,
North Shore-LIJ Health System and
Albert Einstein College of Medicine,
Yeshiva University
New York

Preface

In this Third Edition, I have assembled an international set of distinguished authors from a range of medical disciplines to provide insight and expertise in the complex environment of the management of older people with diabetes. As before, this book should provide up-to-date knowledge and guidance in effective clinical decision-making both for the generalist as well as for the specialist. Unlike other books about geriatric medical practice, our authors have designed their individual chapters around the unique characteristics of older people with diabetes rather than merely adding one or two specific paragraphs at the end of a more general chapter.

It is increasingly recognised that very elderly people with diabetes pose considerable challenges to the diabetes care team, and in this book we offer direction in good clinical practice and a template for assessment and further care. We hope that this book will continue to stimulate interest in geriatric diabetes and that, with the publication of further large clinical trials in this area, the evidence base will be enriched.

Acknowledgements

This book is dedicated to all those who strive to enhance the quality of diabetes care for older people.

Very special thanks to my family and to many helpful colleagues at John Wiley.

Alan J Sinclair
March 2009

List of Contributors

Ahmed H. Abdelhafiz
Department of Elderly Medicine
Rotherham General Hospital
Moorgate Road
Rotherham
S60 2UD
United Kingdom

Koula G. Asimakopoulou
King's College London
Dental Institute
Oral Health Services Research and Dental Public
   Health
Denmark Hill
London SE5 9RW
United Kingdom

Terry Aspray
Sunderland Royal Hospital
Kayll Road
Sunderland SR4 7TP

and

Newcastle University
Campus for Ageing and Vitality
Newcastle upon Tyne NE4 5PL
United Kingdom

Michelangela Barbieri
Department of Geriatric Medicine and
   Metabolic Diseases
Second University of Naples (SUN)
Piazza Miraglia
2 80138 Naples
Italy

Antony Bayer
Department of Geriatric Medicine
Academic Centre
Cardiff University
Llandough Hospital
Penarth
Vale of Glamorgan CF64 2XX
United Kingdom

Susan Benbow
Department of Diabetes and Endocrinology
Aintree University Hospitals
Liverpool L9 1AE
United Kingdom

Caroline S. Blaum
Department of Internal Medicine
University of Michigan
Ann Arbor
Michigan 48109
USA

and

Ann Arbor VA Healthcare System
GRECC
Michigan 48109
USA

Andrew J. M. Boulton
Manchester Royal Infirmary
Oxford Road
Manchester M13 9WL
United Kingdom

Isabelle Bourdel-Marchasson
Geriatric Department
Hôpital Xavier Arnozan
CHU of Bordeaux
33604 Pessac cedex
UMR 5536 CNRS/Université Victor Segalen
   Bordeaux 2
146 rue Léo Saignat
33000 Bordeaux
France

Cristina Alonso Bouzon
Servicio de Geriatría
Hospital Universitario de Getafe
Ctra. de Toledo, Km. 12,5.
28905-Getafe
Madrid
Spain

Joe M. Chehade
Division of Endocrinology, Diabetes and Metabolism
University of Florida College of Medicine
Jacksonville
FL 32209
USA

Jay Chillala
Trafford General Hospital
Moorside Road
Davyhulme
Manchester M41 5SL
United Kingdom

Christine T. Cigolle
Department of Family Medicine
University of Michigan
Ann Arbor
Michigan 48109
USA

and

Ann Arbor VA Healthcare System
GRECC
Michigan 48109
USA

Stephen Colagiuri
Institute of Obesity Nutrition and Exercise
K25 - Medical Foundation Building
The University of Sydney
NSW 2006
Australia

Simon Croxson
United Bristol Healthcare NHS Trust
Bristol General Hospital
Bristol BS1 6SY
United Kingdom

Daniel Davies
Institute of Obesity Nutrition and Exercise
K25 - Medical Foundation Building
The University of Sydney
NSW 2006
Australia

Peter Fasching
3rd International Department PH,
Baumgarten,
A-1140 Vienna
Austria

Charles Fox
Diabetes Centre
Northampton General Hospital
51 The Avenue
Northampton NN1 5BT
United Kingdom

Brian M. Frier
Department of Diabetes
Royal Infirmary
51 Little France Crescent
Edinburgh EH16 4SA
United Kingdom

Roger Gadsby
Warwick Medical School
University of Warwick
Gibbet Hill Road
Coventry CV4 7AL
United Kingdom

Linda Geiss
Division of Diabetes Translation
Centers for Disease Control and Prevention
4770 Buford Highway
N.E. Mailstop K-10
Atlanta GA
USA

Geoffrey Gill
Department of Diabetes and Endocrinology
Aintree University Hospitals
Liverpool L9 1AE
United Kingdom

Christopher S. Gray
Department of Geriatric Medicine
University of Newcastle
Newcastle on Tyne
United Kingdom

Edward W. Gregg
Division of Diabetes Translation
Centers for Disease Control and Prevention
4770 Buford Highway
N.E. Mailstop K-10
Atlanta GA
USA

Timothy J. Hendra
Department of Geriatric Medicine
Robert Hadfield Wing
Northern General Hospital

Herries Road
Sheffield S5 7AU
United Kingdom

Peter Kempler
I. Department of Medicine
Semmelweis University
Budapest
Hungary

Anne Kilvert
Diabetes Centre
Northampton General Hospital
51 The Avenue
Northampton NN1 5BT
United Kingdom

Leocadio Rodríguez Mañas
Servicio de Geriatría
Hospital Universitario de Getafe
Ctra. de Toledo, Km. 12,5.
28905-Getafe
Madrid
Spain

Raffaele Marfella
Department of Geriatric and Metabolic Disease
Second University Naples
Piazza Miraglia
2 80138 Naples
Italy

Vincent McAulay
Department of Diabetes
Crosshouse Hospital
Kilmarnock KA2 0BE
United Kingdom

Marg McGill
Diabetes Centre
Royal Prince Alfred Hospital
Missenden Road
Camperdown
New South Wales
Australia

Graydon S. Meneilly
Division of Geriatric Medicine
Department of Medicine
The University of British Columbia
Vancouver BC
Canada

Begoña Molina
Servicio de Endocrinología y Nutrición
Hospital Universitario de Getafe
Carretera de Toledo Km 12,500
28905-Getafe
Madrid
Spain

Arshag D. Mooradian
Division of Endocrinology, Diabetes and
  Metabolism
University of Florida College of
  Medicine
Jacksonville
FL 32209
USA

John E. Morley
GRECC
VA Medical Center and Division of Geriatric
  Medicine
Saint Louis University School of Medicine
1402 S. Grand Blvd
M238 St Louis
MO 63104
USA

Latana A. Munang
Liberton Hospital
113 Lasswade Road
Edinburgh EH16 6UB
United Kingdom

Arie Nouwen
School of Psychology
University of Birmingham
Edgbaston, Birmingham
B15 2TT
United Kingdom

Janice E. O'Connell
Sunderland Royal Hospital
Kayll Road
Sunderland SR4 7TP
United Kingdom

Jan R. Oyebode
School of Psychology
University of Birmingham
Edgbaston, Birmingham
B15 2TT
United Kingdom

Giuseppe Paolisso
Department of Geriatric Medicine and Metabolic
    Diseases
Second University of Naples (SUN)
Piazza Miraglia
2 80138 Naples
Italy

Gurch Randhawa
Institute for Health Research
University of Bedfordshire
Putteridge Bury
Luton LU2 8LE
United Kingdom

Marta Castro Rodríguez
Servicio de Geriatría
Hospital Universitario de Getafe
Ctra. de Toledo, Km. 12,5.
28905-Getafe
Madrid
Spain

Alan J. Sinclair
Bedfordshire & Hertfordshire Postgraduate
    Medical School
Putteridge Bury campus
Hitchin Road
Luton LU2 8LE
United Kingdom

John M. Starr
Royal Victoria Hospital
Craigleith Road
Edinburgh EH4 2DN
United Kingdom

Carolin D. Taylor
Department of Geriatric Medicine
Robert Hadfield Wing
Northern General Hospital
Herries Road
Sheffield S5 7AU
United Kingdom

Solomon Tesfaye
Royal Hallamshire Hospital
Sheffield Teaching Hospitals NHS Foundation Trust
Glossop Road
Sheffield, S10 2JF
United Kingdom

Nina Tumosa
Geriatrics Research, Education, and Clinical Center
St. Louis VA

and

Division of Geriatrics
Saint Louis University
St Louis
MO 63125
USA

Tamás Várkonyi
Department of Medicine
University of Szeged
Szeged
Hungary

Jeremy D. Walston
Johns Hopkins University School of Medicine
5501 Hopkins Bayview Circle
21224 Baltimore
Maryland
USA

Matthew J. Young
Edinburgh Royal Infirmary
51 Little France Crescent
Dalkeith Road
Edinburgh EH16 4SA
United Kingdom

Dennis Yue
Diabetes Centre
Royal Prince Alfred Hospital
Missenden Road
Camperdown
New South Wales
Australia

Andrej Zeyfang
Bethesda Hospital Stuttgart
Department of internal medicine and geriatrics
Hohenheimer Strasse 21
70184 Stuttgart
Germany

SECTION I
Epidemiology and Pathophysiology

1

Pathophysiology of Diabetes In The Elderly

Graydon S. Meneilly

Division of Geriatric Medicine, Department of Medicine, The University of British Columbia, Vancouver BC, Canada

Key messages

- Lifestyle factors play a major role in diabetes in the elderly.
- Diabetes in the elderly is metabolically distinct.
- Elderly patients with diabetes have an increase incidence of severe or fatal hypoglycemia.

1.1 Introduction

In the past, numerous studies have been conducted to investigate the pathogenesis of type 2 diabetes [1]. Although, unfortunately, elderly patients were systematically excluded from these studies, we have more recently started to study, in systematic fashion, the pathophysiological alterations that occur in elderly patients with diabetes. These studies, the details of which will be reviewed in the following sections, suggest that there are many ways in which diabetes in the elderly is unique. Some of the factors that contribute to the high prevalence diabetes in the elderly are shown schematically in Figure 1.1.

1.1.1 Genetic factors

There are several lines of evidence which suggest that there is a strong genetic component to diabetes in the

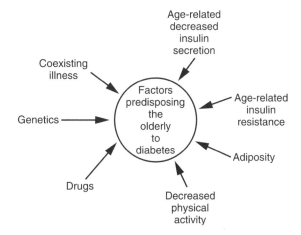

Figure 1.1 Factors that contribute to the high prevalence of diabetes in the elderly. Reproduced with permission from Halter, J.B., Carbohydrate metabolism, in: E.J. Masoro (ed.), *Handbook of Physiology, Volume on Aging*. New York, Oxford University Press Inc., 1995, p. 119.

elderly, although the specific genes responsible have yet to be defined [2]. If you have a family history of type 2 diabetes, you are much more likely to develop the disease as you age [3]. Diabetes is much more common in the elderly in certain ethnic groups [4], while the likelihood that an elderly identical twin will develop diabetes if their sibling is affected is over 80%.

Diabetes in Old Age. Third Edition. Edited by Alan J. Sinclair
© 2009 John Wiley & Sons, Ltd

Even in elderly identical twins discordant for type 2 diabetes, the unaffected siblings clearly have evidence of abnormal glucose metabolism [5].

1.1.2 Age-related changes in carbohydrate metabolism

The progressive alterations in glucose metabolism that occur with age explain why genetically susceptible older individuals may not develop diabetes until late in life. Pathogenic mechanisms which contribute to the glucose intolerance of aging include alterations in glucose-induced insulin release and resistance to insulin-mediated glucose disposal [6]. The results of early investigations suggested that glucose-induced insulin release was normal in the elderly. However, more recent studies enrolling large numbers of carefully characterized healthy young and old subjects have demonstrated definable alterations in glucose-induced insulin release in the aged [6, 7]. Of note, the magnitude of the decrement in insulin secretion is more apparent in response to oral than to intravenous glucose [6]. This may be due, in part, to a decreased beta cell response to the incretin hormones (see below). As with many hormones, insulin is secreted in a pulsatile fashion. Normal aging is also associated with subtle alterations in pulsatile insulin release, which further contribute to age-related changes in glucose metabolism [8]. Elevated levels of proinsulin, which suggest disordered insulin processing, predict the subsequent development of type 2 diabetes in elderly subjects [9]. Thus, it is clear that alterations in glucose-induced insulin release are an important component of the changes in carbohydrate metabolism with aging. However, the most important pathogenic mechanism underlying the glucose intolerance of aging is resistance to insulin-mediated glucose disposal [6, 10]. Debate persists as to whether the insulin resistance of the elderly is intrinsic to the aging process itself, or is the result of lifestyle factors commonly associated with aging. The consensus of opinion is that the aging process itself is the most important cause of insulin resistance, although lifestyle changes (see below), are clearly an important contributing factor.

1.1.3 Lifestyle and environmental factors

Despite the strong genetic component, it is abundantly clear that various environmental and lifestyle factors can increase or decrease the likelihood that a genetically susceptible individual will develop the disease in old age. Many older people have coexisting illnesses and take multiple drugs (e.g., thiazide diuretics), which can allow a latent abnormality in glucose metabolism to develop into full-blown diabetes [11, 12]. Obesity, especially with a central distribution of body fat, and a reduction in physical activity occur progressively with aging, and both of these factors are associated with abnormal carbohydrate metabolism [12–17].

The above information suggests that lifestyle modifications may be of value in the prevention of type 2 diabetes in the elderly, even in patients with a strong family history of the disease. Indeed, the Diabetes Prevention Program found that a combined lifestyle intervention consisting of weight loss and increased physical activity was effective in reducing the incidence of diabetes in elderly patients with impaired glucose tolerance [18].

1.2 Diet and diabetes in the elderly

The results of large epidemiologic studies have shown that diabetes is more likely to develop in older patients who have a diet that is high in saturated fats and simple sugars and low in complex carbohydrates [13, 19–21]. Moderate alcohol consumption may protect against diabetes in elderly women [22]. It has been suggested that deficiencies of trace elements or vitamins may contribute to the development or progression of diabetes in younger subjects, and it is increasingly recognized that the same may be true in the elderly [12, 21]. Elderly patients with diabetes have exaggerated free radical production, and administration of the antioxidant vitamins C and E to these patients improves both insulin action and metabolic control [23, 24]. Many elderly patients with diabetes are deficient in magnesium and zinc, and supplements of zinc and magnesium can improve glucose metabolism in these patients [25, 26]. Increased dietary iron may be associated with an increased risk of diabetes in aged individuals [20, 27]. Although chromium deficiency has been shown to cause abnormalities in glucose metabolism in animals and younger patients, there is no evidence to date that chromium supplements will improve glucose tolerance in the elderly. In summary, there is increasing evidence to suggest that dietary abnormalities may contribute to the pathogenesis of diabetes in the elderly, and that dietary modifications may be of therapeutic benefit in these patients.

1.3 Other factors

The presence of inflammation, as evidenced by levels of proinflammatory cytokines such as tumour necrosis factor-α (TNF-α) and C-reactive protein (CRP), is associated with an increased risk of diabetes in the elderly [28–31]. Higher levels of adiponectin (an adipocytokine that increases insulin sensitivity) are associated with a reduced incidence of diabetes in the aged [29, 32]. Sex steroid hormone levels also appear to be related to the development of diabetes in the elderly [33, 34]. In particular, higher testosterone levels in women and lower levels in men appear to be associated with an increased incidence of diabetes.

1.4 Metabolic alterations

The metabolic alterations which occur in middle-aged subjects with type 2 diabetes have been extensively characterized [1]. When compared to age- and weight-matched controls, both lean and obese middle-aged subjects have elevated fasting hepatic glucose production, a marked resistance to insulin-mediated glucose disposal, and a profound impairment in glucose-induced pancreatic insulin release.

Recently, metabolic factors have been characterized in lean and obese elderly patients with diabetes [35–38]. These studies have demonstrated some surprising differences in the metabolic profile between middle-aged and elderly subjects. In contrast to younger subjects, fasting hepatic glucose production is normal in both lean and obese elderly subjects (Figure 1.2). Similar to younger subjects, lean elderly patients have a profound impairment in pancreatic insulin secretion but, in contrast to the young, these patients have minimal resistance to insulin-mediated glucose disposal (Figures 1.3 and 1.4). In contradistinction to the young, obese elderly subjects have relatively preserved glucose-induced insulin secretion (see Figure 1.3), although pulsatile insulin secretion is clearly altered [8]. Similar to the young however, these patients have a marked resistance to insulin-mediated glucose disposal (Figure 1.4). In summary, the principal defect in lean elderly subjects is impaired glucose-induced insulin release, while the principal defect in obese patients is resistance to insulin-mediated glucose disposal.

One of the most interesting findings of these studies was that the ability of insulin to enhance blood flow

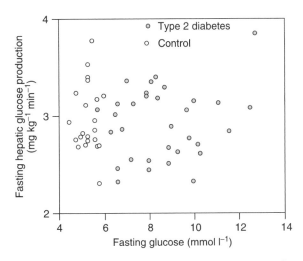

Figure 1.2 Fasting hepatic glucose production in relation to fasting glucose levels in healthy elderly controls and elderly patients with diabetes. Hepatic glucose production was measured by infusing radioactive glucose tracers.

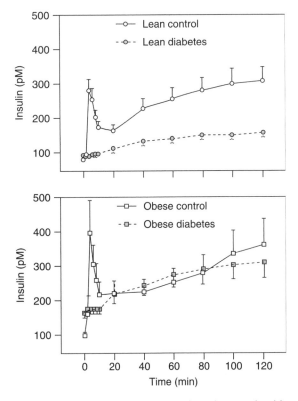

Figure 1.3 Glucose-induced insulin release in healthy elderly controls and elderly patients with diabetes. Insulin values were measured at glucose levels approximately 5 mmol l^{-1} above fasting levels.

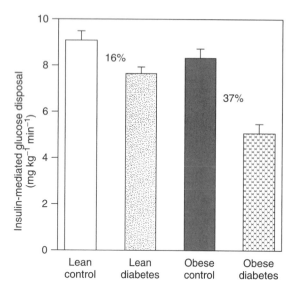

Figure 1.4 Insulin-mediated glucose disposal rates in healthy elderly controls and elderly patients with diabetes. Glucose disposal rates were measured utilizing the euglycaemic clamp technique. In this technique, insulin is infused to achieve levels occurring after a meal, and glucose is infused simultaneously to prevent hypoglycaemia.

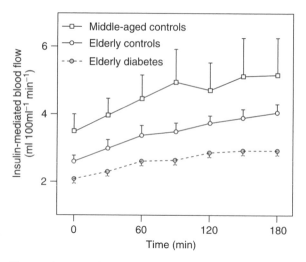

Figure 1.5 Insulin-mediated blood flow in obese middle-aged controls and obese elderly controls and patients with diabetes. Blood flow was measured in the calf during euglycaemic clamp studies utilizing venous occlusion plethysmography.

was markedly reduced in obese, insulin-resistant older patients (Figure 1.5) [37]. Insulin-mediated vasodilation is thought to account for about 30% of normal glucose disposal, presumably because it increases the delivery of insulin and glucose to muscle tissue. Indeed, it has been demonstrated that angiotensin-converting enzyme (ACE) inhibitors may improve insulin sensitivity in elderly patients with diabetes and hypertension [39]. This suggests that drugs which enhance muscle blood flow may prove to be valuable adjuncts in the future for the therapy of elderly patients with diabetes.

It has been known for a number of years that autoimmune phenomena play a pivotal role in the beta-cell failure that occurs in patients with type 1 diabetes [40]. It is also increasingly recognized that a subset of middle-aged patients with type 2 diabetes have a form of diabetes that is characterized by beta-cell failure, and these patients often have high titres of islet cell antibodies and antibodies to glutamic acid decarboxylase (GAD), similar to younger patients with type 1 diabetes. These patients have been said to have LADA (latent autoimmune diabetes in adults) [41–47]. It is tempting to speculate that autoimmune phenomena contribute to the profound impairment in

glucose-induced insulin secretion seen in lean older patients with type 2 diabetes. However, the clinical significance of elevated antibodies in the elderly is less certain. Some studies have found that elderly patients with diabetes who are positive for GAD have impaired beta-cell function relative to controls without these antibodies, but others have not [41, 48]. It has been suggested that screening for these auto-antibodies should be performed in elderly patients with impaired glucose tolerance (IGT) and newly diagnosed diabetes, in order to help predict which patients will develop islet cell failure. Although this is a compelling idea, we should only begin widespread screening when randomized studies have demonstrated that early intervention will protect the beta cells and reduce the need for insulin therapy [45–47]. Thus, it is unclear at present whether the measurement of auto-immune parameters can be used to predict future insulin requirements in the aged, or whether elderly patients with these abnormalities should be treated with therapies designed to modify autoimmune destruction of the pancreas.

Based on the above information, it is believed that the therapeutic approach to diabetes in the elderly should be different. In middle-aged patients, many endocrinologists recommend that patients be treated with drugs that both stimulate insulin secretion and improve insulin sensitivity, on the assumption that most patients have multiple metabolic problems. However, in lean elderly subjects, the principal defect is an impairment in glucose-induced insulin secretion, and the main approach should be to administer secretogogues to stimulate insulin secretion, or to administer exogenous insulin. In obese elderly patients, the principal defect is insulin resistance; hence, patients should be treated initially with drugs that enhance insulin-mediated glucose disposal, such as metformin.

1.4.1 The incretin pathway

The enteroinsular axis refers to hormones released from the gut in response to nutrient ingestion that result in enhanced glucose-induced insulin release, known as the 'incretin effect'. The most important incretin hormones are glucose-dependent insulinotropic polypeptide (GIP) and glucagon-like peptide 1 (GLP-1). Although, both basal and glucose-stimulated GIP and GLP-1 levels have been found to be unchanged or to be increased in healthy elderly subjects when compared to young controls, GIP and GLP-1 secretion is clearly enhanced in the elderly patient with diabetes [49, 50]. In addition, the levels of dipeptidyl peptidase IV (DPIV), the enzyme that breaks down GIP and GLP-1, is progressively reduced with aging and diabetes. Beta-cell responses to GIP are reduced in normal elderly subjects and are absent in elderly patients with diabetes [51, 52]. In contrast, beta-cell responses to GLP-1 are preserved in the elderly patient with diabetes [53]. These data suggest that GLP-1 and its analogues may prove to be useful therapeutic options in the elderly, but that agents which prevent the breakdown of GLP-1, such as DPIV inhibitors, may be less effective.

1.4.2 Glucose effectiveness or non-insulin-mediated glucose uptake

It has been recognized for many decades that insulin is an important hormone involved in the uptake of glucose into cells. It has been demonstrated that glucose can stimulate its own uptake in the absence of insulin [54], an effect which is known as 'glucose effectiveness' or non-insulin-mediated glucose uptake (NIMGU). Under fasting conditions, approximately 70% of glucose uptake occurs via glucose effectiveness, primarily in the central nervous system. After a meal, approximately 50% of glucose uptake in normal subjects occurs via NIMGU, with the bulk occurring in skeletal muscle. Because many middle-aged subjects with diabetes are insulin-resistant, it has been

suggested that up to 80% of postprandial glucose uptake in these patients may occur via glucose effectiveness. At the present time it is uncertain whether defects in NIMGU contribute to elevated glucose levels in middle-aged patients with diabetes, as studies which have evaluated this parameter in these patients have provided inconsistent results.

It has been shown previously in healthy elderly subjects that glucose effectiveness is impaired during fasting, but is normal during hyperglycaemia [55]. Recently, it was demonstrated that elderly patients with diabetes have an even greater impairment in glucose effectiveness than healthy elderly subjects (Figure 1.6) [56]. Although the cause of this abnormality is uncertain, it may relate to a decreased ability of glucose to recruit glucose transporters to the cell surface in these patients.

In the future, this metabolic abnormality may prove to be of great therapeutic relevance to the elderly. In younger patients, exercise, anabolic steroids and a reduction in free fatty acid levels have been shown to enhance glucose effectiveness [54]. Since we have shown that the incretin hormone GLP-1 may enhance NIMGU in elderly patients with diabetes [57], it is possible that future therapies for the elderly may be directed not only at increasing insulin secretion and reversing insulin resistance, but also at enhancing glucose effectiveness.

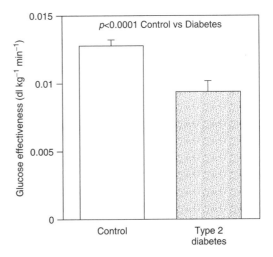

Figure 1.6 Glucose effectiveness in elderly controls and patients with diabetes. During these studies, insulin secretion was suppressed by infusing the somatostatin analogue octreotide. Glucose was then infused to assess glucose disposal in the absence of insulin.

1.5   Molecular biology studies

At present, there is very little information available regarding molecular biological abnormalities that may be present in elderly patients with diabetes. The glucokinase gene controls the glucose sensor for the beta cell, and defects in this gene could lead to the impairment in glucose-induced insulin secretion that is present in lean elderly patients with diabetes. To date, evidence for mutations in this gene in elderly patients is conflicting [58, 59].

In skeletal muscle, insulin binds to its receptor, resulting in activation of the insulin receptor tyrosine kinase. Activation of this enzyme sets in motion a cascade of intracellular events which although at present is incompletely understood, results in the translocation of glucose transporters to the cell surface. In theory, a defect in any of these pathways could lead to insulin resistance. To date, these intracellular processes have been incompletely studied in elderly patients with diabetes, but the preliminary information suggests that while insulin receptor numbers and affinity are normal, the insulin receptor kinase activity may be defective [60]. Recent data have suggested that mitochondrial dysfunction contributes to insulin resistance in middle-aged patients with diabetes, and potentially also to impairments in glucose-induced insulin release [61]. Although normal aging is characterized by progressive mitochondrial dysfunction, to date no studies have been performed to assess mitochondrial function in elderly patients with diabetes [62–64]. Clearly, further studies are required to elucidate the subcellular defects that cause abnormal glucose metabolism in the elderly patient with diabetes.

1.6   Glucose counter-regulation

Numerous studies have demonstrated that elderly patients with diabetes, when compared to younger patients, have an increased frequency of severe or fatal hypoglycaemia [12, 65, 66]. Recently, several studies have evaluated glucose counter-regulation in elderly subjects in an attempt to determine the cause of the increased frequency of hypoglycaemia, and a number of important observations have emerged. It appears that many elderly patients with diabetes have not been educated about the warning symptoms of hypoglycaemia and, as a consequence, do not

know how to interpret these symptoms when they occur [67].

The most important hormone in the defence against hypoglycaemia in normal subjects is glucagon. If glucagon responses are deficient, epinephrine becomes important, and growth hormone and cortisol come into play if hypoglycaemia is prolonged for several hours. The responses of both glucagon and growth hormone to hypoglycaemia are impaired in healthy elderly subjects, and to an even greater extent in older patients with diabetes (Figure 1.7) [68]. Yet, even when they are educated about the symptoms of hypoglycaemia, the elderly have a reduced awareness of the autonomic warning symptoms (sweating, palpitations, etc.) at glucose levels that would elicit a marked response in younger subjects. Consequently, the first symptoms of hypoglycaemia in the elderly are often neuroglycopenic. Finally, elderly patients have an impaired psychomotor performance during

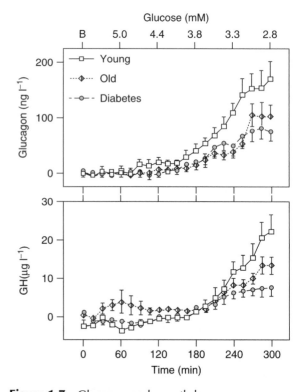

Figure 1.7 Glucagon and growth hormone responses to hypoglycaemia in healthy young, healthy old and elderly patients with diabetes. Controlled hypoglycaemia was induced using the glucose clamp technique. Glucose values at which hormone levels were measured are shown on the top x-axis.

hypoglycaemia, which would prevent them from taking steps to return the blood glucose value to normal, even if they were aware that it was low. Thus, the increased frequency of hypoglycaemia in the elderly is due to a constellation of abnormalities, including a reduced knowledge and awareness of the warning symptoms, a decreased counter-regulatory hormone secretion, and an altered psychomotor performance.

The levels of pancreatic polypeptide (PP) are elevated during hypoglycaemia, and this response is mediated by the vagus nerve. The role of PP in normal glucose counter-regulation is uncertain, but in younger patients with diabetes a reduced PP response to hypoglycaemia is an early marker of autonomic insufficiency. Recently, it was found that although elderly patients with diabetes often have evidence of autonomic dysfunction, their PP responses to hypoglycaemia are normal [69]. Thus, PP responses to hypoglycaemia cannot be used to predict autonomic function in elderly patients.

Based on the above information, there are a number of interventions that can be proposed to prevent hypoglycaemic events in the elderly. First, it would seem prudent to educate elderly patients about the warning symptoms of hypoglycaemia so that they can appreciate them when they occur. Second, consideration should be given to the use of oral agents or insulin preparations that are associated with a lower frequency of hypoglycaemic events in the elderly.

1.7 Conclusions

In summary, diabetes in the elderly is caused by a combination of genetic and environmental factors superimposed on the normal age-related changes in carbohydrate metabolism. The metabolic alterations that occur in elderly patients with diabetes appear to be distinct from those that occur in younger patients. As we gain a greater appreciation of the pathophysiological abnormalities that occur in the elderly, we hope to be able to develop a more focused approach to therapy in this age group. It is only in this way that we will be able to better cope with the epidemic of diabetes in the elderly which will befall us in the coming decades.

Acknowledgments

The studies described in this chapter were supported by grants from the Canadian Institutes of Health Research and the Canadian Diabetes Association. I gratefully acknowledge the support of the Allan McGavin Geriatric Endowment at the University of British Columbia, and the Jack Bell Geriatric Endowment Fund at Vancouver Hospital and Health Science Centre.

I am especially indebted to my longstanding collaborators in this work, particularly Dr Dariush Elahi at Johns Hopkins Medical School and Dr Daniel Tessier at the University of Sherbrooke. I thank Rosemarie Torressani, Eugene Mar, Gail Chin and Christine Lockhart for technical assistance in conducting these studies.

References

1. DeFronzo, R.A. (1988) Lilly Lecture 1987. The triumvirate: β-cell, muscle, liver. A collusion responsible for NIDDM. Diabetes, **37**, 667–87.
2. Kahn, C.R. (1984) Banting Lecture. Insulin action, diabetogenes, and the cause of type II diabetes. Diabetes, **43**, 1066–84.
3. Morris, R.D. and Rimm, A.A. (1991) Association of waist to hip ratio and family history with the prevalence of NIDDM among 25,272 adult, white females. Am. J. Public Health, **81**, 507–9.
4. Lipton, R.B., Liao, Y., Cao, G., Cooper, R.S. and McGee, D. (1993) Determinants of incident non-insulin-dependent diabetes mellitus among blacks and whites in a national sample. The NHANES 1 epidemiologic follow-up study. Am. J. Epidemiol., **138**, 826–39.
5. Vaag, A., Henriksen, J.E., Madsbad, S., Holm, N. and Beck-Nielsen, H. (1995) Insulin secretion, insulin action, and hepatic glucose production in identical twins discordant for non-insulin-dependent diabetes mellitus. J. Clin. Invest., **95**, 690–8.
6. Muller, D.C. Elahi, D., Tobin, J.D. and Andres, R. (1996) The effect of age on insulin resistance and secretion: a review. Semin Nephrol., **16**, 289–98.
7. Iozzo, P., Beck-Nielsen, J., Laakso, M., Smith, U., Yki-Jarvinen, H. and Ferrannini, E. (1999) Independent influence of age on basal insulin secretion in non-diabetic humans. European group for the study of insulin resistance. Journal of Clinical Endocrinology and Metabolism, **84**, 863–8.
8. Meneilly, G.S., Veldhuis, J.D. and Elahi, D. (2005) Deconvolution analysis of rapid insulin pulses before and after six weeks of continuous subcutaneous administration of GLP-1 in elderly patients with type 2 diabetes. Journal of Clinical Endocrinology and Metabolism, **90**, 6251–6.

9. Zethelius, B., Lithell, H.O., Hales, C.N. and Berne, C. (2004) Insulin resistance, impaired early insulin response, and insulin propeptides as predictors of the development of type 2 diabetes. Diabetes Care, **27**, 1433–8.

10. Ferrannini, E. and the European Group for the Study of Insulin Resistance. (1996) Insulin action and age. Diabetes, **45**, 949.

11. Pandit, M.K., Burke, J., Gustafson, A.B., Minocha, A. and Peiris, A.N. (1993) Drug-induced disorders of glucose tolerance. Ann. Intern. Med., **118**, 529–39.

12. Meneilly, G.S. and Tessier, D. (2001) Diabetes in elderly adults. J. Gerontol., **56A**, M5–13.

13. van Dam, R.M., Rimm, E.B., Willett, W.C. *et al.* (2002) Dietary patterns and risk for Type 2 diabetes mellitus in U.S. men. Ann. Intern. Med., **136**, 201–9.

14. The DECODE-DECODA Study Group, on behalf of the European Diabetes Epidemiology Group and the International Diabetes Epidemiology Group. (2003) Age, body mass index and Type 2 diabetes - associations modified by ethnicity. Diabetologia, **48**, 1063–70.

15. Goodpaster, B.H., Krishnaswami, S., Resnick, H. *et al.* (2003) Association between regional adipose tissue distribution and both Type 2 diabetes and impaired glucose tolerance in elderly men and women. Diabetes Care, **26**, 372–9.

16. Meigs, J.B., Muller, D.C., Nathan, D.M. *et al.* (2003) The natural history of progression from normal glucose tolerance to Type 2 diabetes in the Baltimore longitudinal study of aging. Diabetes, **52**, 1475–84.

17. Cassano, P.A., Rosner, B., Vokonas, P.S. and Weiss, S.T. (1992) Obesity and body fat distribution in relation to the incidence of non-insulin-dependent diabetes mellitus. American Journal of Epidemiology, **136**, 1474–86.

18. Diabetes Prevention Program Research Group. (2002) Reduction in the incidence of Type 2 diabetes with lifestyle intervention or metformin. N. Engl. J. Med., **346**, 393–403.

19. Feskens, E.J.M., Virtanen, S.M., Rasanen, L., Tuomilehto, J., Stengard, J., Pekkanen, J., Nissinen, A. and Kromhout, D. (1995) Dietary factors determining diabetes and impaired glucose tolerance. Diabetes Care, **18**, 1104–12.

20. Song, Y., Manson, J.E., Buring, J.E. *et al.* (2004) A prospective study of red meat consumption and Type 2 diabetes in middle-aged and elderly women. Diabetes Care, **27**, 2108–15.

21. Meyer, K.A., Kushi, L.H., Jacobs, D.R. *et al.* (2000) Carbohydrates, dietary fiber, and incident type 2 diabetes in older women. Am. J. Clin. Nutr., **71**, 921–30.

22. Beulens, J.W.J., Stolk, R.P., Van der Schouw, Y.T., Grobbee, D.E., Hendriks, H.F.J. and Bots, M.L. (2005) Alcohol consumption and risk of type 2 diabetes among older women. Diabetes Care, **28**, 2933–8.

23. Paolisso, G., D'Amore, A., Galzerano, D., Balbi, V., Giugliano, D., Varricchio, M. and D'Onofrio, F. (1993) Daily vitamin E supplements improve metabolic control but not insulin secretion in elderly type II diabetic patients. Diabetes Care, **16**, 1433–7.

24. Paolisso, G., D'Amore, A., Balbi, V., Volpe, C., Galzerano, D., Giugliano, D., Sgambato, S., Varricchio, M. and D'Onofrio, F. (1994) Plasma vitamin C affects glucose homeostasis in healthy subjects and in non-insulin-dependent diabetics. Am. J. Physiol., **266**, E261–8.

25. Paolisso, G., Scheen, A., Cozzolino, D. *et al.* (1994) Changes in glucose turnover parameters and improvement of glucose oxidation after 4-week magnesium administration in elderly non-insulin-dependent (type II) diabetic patients. Journal of Clinical Endocrinology and Metabolism, **78**, 1510–15.

26. Song, M.K., Rosenthal, M.J., Naliboff, B.D., Phanumas, L. and Kang, K.W. (1998) Effects of bovine prostate powder on zinc, glucose and insulin metabolism in old patients with non-insulin-dependent diabetes mellitus. Metabolism, **47**, 39–43.

27. Lee, D.H., Folsom, A.R. and Jacobs, D.R. (2004) Dietary iron intake and Type 2 diabetes incidence in postmenopausal women: the Iowa Women's Health Study. Diabetologia, **47**, 185–94.

28. Barzilay, J.I., Abraham, L., Heckbert, S. *et al.* (2001) The relation of markers of inflammation to the development of glucose disorders in the elderly. Diabetes, **50**, 2384–9.

29. Kanaya, A.M., Harris, T., Goodpaster, B.H. *et al.* (2004) Adipocytokines attenuate the association between visceral adiposity and diabetes in older adults. Diabetes Care, **27**, 1375–80.

30. Lechleitner, M., Herold, M., Dzien-Bischinger, C., Hoppichlert, F. and Dzien, A. (2002) Tumour necrosis factor-alpha plasma levels in elderly patients with Type 2 diabetes mellitus - observations over 2 years. Diabetic Medicine, **19**, 949–53.

31. de Rekeneire, N., Peila, R., Ding, J., Kritchevsky, S.B., Colbert, L.H., Visser, M., Shorr, R.I., Kuller, L.H., Strotmeyer, E.S., Schwartz, A.V., Vellas, B. and Harris, T.B. (2006) Diabetes, hyperglycemia, and inflammation in older individuals. Diabetes Care, **29**, 1902–8.

32. Snijder, M.B., Seidell, J.C., Heine, R.J., Bouter, L.M., Nijpels, G., Stehouwer, C.D.A., Funahashi, T., Matsuzawa, Y., Shimomura, I. and Dekker, J.M. (2006) Associations of adiponectin levels with incident impaired glucose metabolism and type 2 diabetes in older men and women. Diabetes Care, **29**, 2498–503.

33. Oh, J.-Y., Barrett-Connor, E., Wedick, N.M. *et al.* (2002) Endogenous sex hormones and the development

of Type 2 diabetes in older men and women: the Rancho Bernardo Study. Diabetes Care, **25**, 55–60.

34. Golden, S.H., Dobs, A.S., Vaidya, D., Szklo, M., Gapstur, S., Kopp, P., Liu, K, and Ouyang, P. (2007) Endogenous sex hormones and glucose tolerance status in postmenopausal women. Journal of Clinical Endocrinology and Metabolism, **92** (4), 1289–95.

35. Arner, P., Pollare, T. and Lithell, H. (1991) Different aetiologies of type 2 (non-insulin-dependent) diabetes mellitus in obese and non-obese subjects. Diabetologia, **34**, 483–7.

36. Meneilly, G.S., Hards, L., Tessier, D., Elliott, T. and Tildesley, H. (1996) NIDDM in the elderly. Diabetes Care, **19**, 1320–75.

37. Meneilly, G.S. and Elliott, T. (1999) Metabolic alterations in middle-aged and elderly obese patients with type 2 diabetes. Diabetes Care, **22**, 112–18.

38. Meneilly, G.S. and Elahi, D. (2005) Metabolic alterations in middle-aged and elderly lean patients with Type 2 diabetes. Diabetes Care, **28**, 1498–9.

39. Paolisso, G., Gambardella, A., Verza, M., D'Amora, A., Sgambato, S. and Varricchio, M. (1992) ACE-inhibition improves insulin-sensitivity in age insulin-resistant hypertensive patients. J. Hum. Hypertens., **6**, 175–9.

40. Zimmet, P.Z. (1999) Diabetes epidemiology as a tool to trigger diabetes research and care. Diabetologia, **42**, 499–518.

41. Monge, L., Brunot, G., Pinach, S., et al. (2004) A clinically orientated approach increases the efficiency of screening for latent autoimmune diabetes in adults (LADA) in a large clinic-based cohort of patients with diabetes onset over 50 years. Diabetic Medicine, **21**, 456–9.

42. Barinas-Mitchell, E., Pietropaolo, S., Zhang, Y.-J. et al. (2004) Islet cell autoimmunity in a triethnic adult population of the Third National Health and Nutrition Examination Survey. Diabetes, **53**, 1293–302.

43. Zinman, B., Kahn, S.E., Haffner, S.M. et al. (2004) Phenotypic characteristics of GAD antibody-positive recently diagnosed patients with Type 2 diabetes in North America and Europe. Diabetes, **53**, 3193–200.

44. Pozzilli, P. and Di Mario, U. (2001) Autoimmune diabetes not requiring insulin at diagnosis (Latent autoimmune diabetes of the adult). Diabetes Care, **24**, 1460–7.

45. Gale, E.A.M. (2005) Latent autoimmune diabetes in adults: a guide for perplexed. Diabetologia, **48**, 2195–9.

46. Fourlanos, S., Dotta, F., Greenbaum, C.J., Palmer, J.P., Rolandsson, O., Colman, P.G. and Harrison, L.C. (2005) Latent autoimmune diabetes in adults (LADA) should be less latent. Diabetologia, **48**, 2206–12.

47. Leslie, R.D.G., Williams, R. and Pozzilli, P. (2006) Clinical review: type 1 diabetes and latent autoimmune diabetes in adults: One end of the rainbow. Journal of Clinical Endocrinology and Metabolism, **91**, 1654–9.

48. Meneilly, G.S., Tildesley, H., Elliott, T., Palmer, J.P. and Juneja, R. (2000) Significance of GAD positivity in elderly patients with diabetes. Diabetic Medicine, **17**, 247–8.

49. Meneilly, G.S., Demuth, H.-U., McIntosh, C.H.S. and Pederson, R.A. (2000) Effect of ageing and diabetes on glucose-dependent insulinotropic polypeptide and dipeptidyl peptidase IV responses to oral glucose. Diabetic Medicine, **17**, 346–50.

50. Korosi, J., McIntosh, C.H.S., Pederson, R.A., Demuth, H.-U., Habener, J.F., Gingerich, R., Egan, J.M., Elahi, D. and Meneilly, G.S. (2001) Effect of aging and diabetes on the enteroinsular axis. Journal of Gerontology, **56A**, M575–9.

51. Meneilly, G.S., Ryan, A.S., Minaker, K.L. and Elahi, D. (1998) The effect of age and glycemic level on the response of the α-cell to glucose-dependent insulinotropic polypeptide and peripheral tissue sensitivity to endogenously released insulin. Journal of Clinical Endocrinology and Metabolism, **83**, 2925–31.

52. Elahi, D., McAloon-Dyke, M., Fukagawa, N.K., Meneilly, G.S., Sclater, A.L., Minaker, K.L., Habener, J.F. and Andersen, D.K. (1994) The insulinotropic actions of glucose-dependent insulinotropic polypeptide (GIP) and glucagon-like peptide-1 (7-37) in normal and diabetic subjects. Regul. Pept., **51**, 63–74.

53. Meneilly, G.S., McIntosh, C.H., Pederson, R.A., Habener, J.F., Gingerich, R., Egan, J.M. and Elahi, D. (2001) Glucagon-like peptide-1 (7-37) augments insulin release in elderly patients with diabetes. Diabetes Care, **24**, 964–5.

54. Best, J.D., Kahn, S.E., Ader, M., Watanabe, R.M., Ni, T.C. and Bergman, R.N. (1996) Role of glucose effectiveness in the determination of glucose tolerance. Diabetes Care, **19**, 1018–30.

55. Meneilly, G.S., Elahi, D., Minaker, K.L., Sclater, A.L. and Rowe, J.W. (1989) Impairment of noninsulin-mediated glucose disposal in the elderly. Journal of Clinical Endocrinology and Metabolism, **63**, 566–71.

56. Forbes, A., Elliott, T., Tildesley, H., Finegood, D. and Meneilly, G.S. (1998) Alterations in non-insulin-mediated glucose uptake in the elderly patient with diabetes. Diabetes, **47**, 1915–19.

57. Meneilly, G.S., McIntosh, C.H., Pederson, R.A., Habener, J.F., Gingerich, R., Egan, J.M., Finegood, D.T. and Elahi, D. (2001) Effect of glucagon-like peptide 1 on non-insulin-mediated glucose uptake in the elderly patient with diabetes. Diabetes Care, **24**, 1951–6.

58. Laakso, M., Malkki, M., Kekalainen, P., Kuusisto, J., Mykkanen, L. and Deeb, S.S. (1995) Glucokinase gene variants in subjects with late-onset NIDDM and impaired glucose tolerance. Diabetes Care, **18**, 398–400.

59. McCarthy, M.I., Hitman, G.A., Hitchins, M. *et al.* (1993) Glucokinase gene polymorphisms; a genetic marker for glucose intolerance in cohort of elderly Finnish men. Diabetic Med., **10**, 198–204.

60. Obermajer-Kusser, B., White, M.F., Pongratz, D.E. *et al.* (1989) A defective intramolecular autoactivation cascade may cause the reduced kinase activity of the skeletal muscle insulin receptor from patients with non-insulin-dependent diabetes mellitus. J. Biol. Chem., **264**, 9497–504.

61. Hawley, J.A. and Lessard, S.J. (2007) Mitochondrial function: use it or lose it. Diabetologia, **50**, 699–702.

62. Barazzoni, R. (2004) Skeletal muscle mitochondrial protein metabolism and function in ageing and type 2 diabetes. Current Opinion in Clinical Nutrition and Metabolic Care, **7**, 97–102.

63. Petersen, K.F., Befroy, D., Dufour, S., Dziura, J., Ariyan, C., Rothman, D.L., DiPietro, L., Cline, G.W. and Shulman, G.I. (2003) Mitochondrial dysfunction in the elderly: possible role in insulin resistance. Science, **300**, 1140–2.

64. Ritz, P. and Berrut, G. (2005) Mitochondrial function, energy expenditure, aging and insulin resistance. Diabetes Metab., **31**, 5S67–5S73.

65. Stepka, M., Rogala, H. and Czyzyk, A. (1993) Hypoglycemia; a major problem in the management of diabetes in the elderly. Aging, **5**, 117–21.

66. Lassmann-Vague, L. (2005) Hypoglycemia in elderly diabetic patients. Diabetes Metab., **31**, 5S53–5S57.

67. Thomson, F.J., Masson, E.A., Leeming, J.T. and Boulton, A.J. (1991) Lack of knowledge of symptoms of hypoglycaemia by elderly diabetic patients. Age and Aging, **20**, 404–6.

68. Meneilly, G.S., Cheung, E. and Tuokko, H. (1994) Counterregulatory hormone responses to hypoglycemia in the elderly patient with diabetes. Diabetes, **43**, 403–10.

69. Meneilly, G.S. (1996) Pancreatic polypeptide responses to hypoglycemia in aging and diabetes. Diabetes Care, **19**, 544–6.

2

Diabetes-Related Risk Factors In Older People

Stephen Colagiuri and Daniel Davies

The University of Sydney, Institute of Obesity Nutrition and Exercise, Medical Foundation Building, NSW, Australia

Key messages

- Older people with undiagnosed type 2 diabetes often have easily identifiable risk factors for this condition.
- The presence of cardiovascular or cerebrovascular disease in an older individual should be a prompt for the detection of diabetes.
- Specific risk factor studies in older people with type 2 diabetes are lacking; this emphasizes the importance of further research in this area.

2.1 Introduction

There are a number of well-established and emerging risk factors which are associated with undiagnosed type 2 diabetes, and which predict the future development of this condition. Most people with undiagnosed type 2 diabetes have easily identifiable risk factors, and these form the basis for the targeted testing of high-risk groups, not only to diagnose the condition but also to facilitate its earlier treatment. Similar risk factors can be used to screen for individuals at high risk of the future development of diabetes, who can be targeted for diabetes-prevention programs.

While few studies have specifically examined the risk factors for diabetes in the elderly, in this chapter we review the established risk factors, with particular emphasis on older people.

2.2 Age

Populations worldwide continue to show a consistent increase in the prevalence of diagnosed and undiagnosed type 2 diabetes with increasing age, with values reaching a plateau or even declining slightly in the very old. For example, in Australia among the 25–34 year age group, 0.2% of the subjects have diagnosed and 0.1% undiagnosed diabetes, these values increasing respectively to 9.4% and 8.5% among 65–74 year olds and to 10.9% and 12.1% for those aged 75 years and more [1]. In the US, among the age groups of 70–74, 75–79, 80–84 and ≥85 years, the prevalence of diabetes was shown to be 20.0, 21.1, 20.2 and 17.3%, respectively [2].

In the DECODE study, the data analyzed from nine European countries indicated a prevalence of type 2 diabetes of <10% among people aged <60 years, and of 10–20% in those aged 60–79 years [3]. The findings of the DECODA study in 11 Asian cohorts were similar, with the overall prevalence of diabetes (both known and undiagnosed) increasing with age, peaking at 70–89 years in Chinese and Japanese subjects and at 60–69 years, followed by a decline beyond 70 years, in Indian subjects [4].

Diabetes in Old Age. Third Edition. Edited by Alan J. Sinclair
© 2009 John Wiley & Sons, Ltd

2.3 Impaired glucose tolerance (IGT) and impaired fasting glucose (IFG)

The prevalence of IGT and IFG increases with age. For example, in the NHANES III study [5], the prevalence of IGT increased from 11.1% in people aged 40–49 years to 20.9% in those aged 60–74 years.

Both IGT and IFG are important risk factors for the development of future diabetes, increasing the risk between 10- and 20-fold compared to those subjects with normal glucose tolerance [6]. This increased risk does not seem to vary with age, however. In the US Diabetes Prevention Program, the incidence of type 2 diabetes was 11.0 cases per 100 person-years in the placebo group overall, compared to 10.8 cases per 100 person-years in those aged 60 and above [7].

Several studies have shown that progression to diabetes can be either prevented or delayed in people with IGT [7, 8]. In the US Diabetes Prevention Program, lifestyle modification achieved a 58% reduction in terms of diabetes progression, compared to a 31% reduction achieved with metformin treatment. The effect of lifestyle modification was greatest in people aged ≥60 years, whereas the effect of metformin was not significant in this age group [7].

2.4 Body weight

An increasing body weight is associated with undiagnosed diabetes, and is also a risk factor for future diabetes. A body mass index (BMI) of ≥30 kg m^{-2} increases the absolute risk of type 2 diabetes by approximately twofold, but up to 20-fold, relative to a normal BMI.

The association between obesity and type 2 diabetes is also observed in older people from different regions of the world. In a French study of people aged ≥60 years, the prevalence of type 2 diabetes was threefold higher in the upper quartile of BMI compared to the lowest quartile in both men and women [9]. In a Taiwanese study of people with a mean age of 72.8 years, a 2.5-fold increased risk of type 2 diabetes was observed with increasing BMI [10].

2.5 Ethnicity

It is well documented that the prevalence of diabetes varies among different ethnic groups [11], and this difference is also evident in older people living in the same country. McBean and colleagues [2] analyzed a random sample of US Medicare beneficiaries to examine the prevalence of diabetes in people aged ≥67 years from different racial/ethnic groups. Although the prevalence of diabetes was high in all groups, it was significantly higher among Hispanics (33.4%) than among blacks (29.6%), Asians (24.3%) and whites (18.4%, p < 0.0001).

2.6 Gestational diabetes mellitus (GDM)

Many studies have reported that women with a previous history of GDM are at increased risk of developing type 2 diabetes.

In a systematic review of 28 studies which examined the incidence of type 2 diabetes following GDM [12], the cumulative incidence ranged from 2.6% to 70%, with the follow-up period ranging from 6 weeks to 28 years postpartum. The cumulative incidence increased substantially during the first 5 years after delivery, but then increased more slowly after 10 years. However, as so few studies have been reported with long-term follow up, it is difficult to draw firm conclusions regarding the influence of previous GDM on diabetes risk during old age.

2.7 Family history

Individuals with a family history of type 2 diabetes are at an increased risk for the disease. The lifetime risk of developing type 2 diabetes is estimated at 40% if one parent has type 2 diabetes [13]. Although most studies have reported that the effect is not gender-specific, there have been some exceptions. For example, Mooy et al. [14] reported a positive effect only in males, and Sugimori and coworkers [15] only in females.

The effect of family history is seen across age groups. For example, when Costa et al. [16] studied 205 non-diabetic siblings of people with type 2 diabetes, compared to the general population – and within any age group – type 2 diabetes was more common among those people with a family history of the condition.

2.8 Hypertension

A number of studies have shown that hypertension is associated with an approximate twofold increase in undiagnosed type 2 diabetes [17–21]. This increase appears to be uniform across age groups; for example, when Bog-Hansen *et al.* [22] examined a community-based population with hypertension for the presence of undiagnosed type 2 diabetes, the overall prevalence of the previously undiagnosed condition ranged from 17% to 26% in those aged <70 years, and 31% in people aged ≥70 years.

2.9 Cardiovascular and cerebrovascular disease

Diabetes, whether diagnosed or undiagnosed, is common in people with cardiovascular and cerebrovascular disease. Consequently, testing for undiagnosed diabetes is routinely recommended in all people with macrovascular disease, including the elderly.

A number of studies have reported a high prevalence of undiagnosed diabetes among individuals with an acute myocardial infarction. Among 4961 subjects (median age 66 years) from 25 European countries, all of whom had coronary artery disease (CAD), type 2 diabetes had been previously diagnosed in 29% of cases. Among 1920 subjects without known diabetes who underwent an oral glucose tolerance test (OGTT), newly diagnosed diabetes was found to be present in 22% of those with acute CAD, and in 14% of those with stable CAD [23].

Among subjects aged ≥80 years with acute myocardial infarction in the Glucose tolerance in Acute Myocardial Infarction (GAMI) study, the prevalence of type 2 diabetes at discharge was 34% [24]. Of these patients, 93% still had abnormalities of glucose tolerance after 12 months (64% with type 2 diabetes, 29% with IGT).

In a cohort of 3266 people (mean age ca. 65 years) scheduled for coronary angiography, the prevalence of diabetes was 32% (17% known diabetes, 15% undiagnosed diabetes) [25].

Diabetes is also common in patients with cerebrovascular disease. For example, when Matz and colleagues [26] examined the prevalence of glucose abnormalities in 238 people (mean age ca. 70 years) with acute stroke, they found 16% of the patients to have newly diagnosed type 2 diabetes, based on an OGTT. The prevalence of diabetes at discharge in 106 people (median age 71 years) with acute ischemic stroke and no history of known diabetes was 46%, also based on an OGTT [27]. On admission, however, a further 29% already had a diagnosis of diabetes.

2.10 Physical inactivity

There is a clear relationship between (a lack of) physical activity and the development of type 2 diabetes. A meta-analysis of 10 prospective cohort studies which included a total of 301 221 participants showed that, compared to being sedentary, the participation in moderate intensity physical activity had a relative risk (RR) of 0.69 for developing type 2 diabetes. In five of these cohort studies that specifically investigated the role of walking, the RR of type 2 diabetes was 0.70 for regular walking (usually ≥2.5 h per week brisk walking) compared with almost no walking [31].

Less information is available on the relationship between physical activity and undiagnosed diabetes. Baan and colleagues [32] assessed this relationship in 1016 people aged 55–75 years and without known diabetes, from the Rotterdam Study. The total time spent on physical activity per week was seen to decrease with increasing glucose intolerance, with adjusted odds ratios (ORs) for vigorous activities such as cycling (0.26 in men, 0.37 in women) and other sports (0.28 in men) showing an inverse association with the prevalence of newly diagnosed diabetes.

In an elderly French population (n = 2532, all aged ≥60 years), sporting activity showed a negative independent association with the prevalence of diagnosed and undiagnosed type 2 diabetes, with a significantly lower prevalence of type 2 diabetes in those who played for at least 30 min per day, compared to those who played for less than 30 min (OR 0.61 in men, 0.62 in women) [9].

2.11 Antipsychotic medication and Mental Illness

Certain mental illnesses and antipsychotic medications appear to be associated with an increase in type 2 diabetes, although study findings vary widely.

In a retrospective, chart-review in the US, the prevalence of type 2 diabetes was assessed in 243 psychiatric inpatients aged 50–74 years with a variety of mental illnesses [33]. The overall prevalence of type 2 diabetes was 25%, which was significantly greater than the rate expected for an age-, race- and gender-matched group in the general US population (14%). The rates of type 2 diabetes for each mental illness were: schizoaffective disorder (50%)⟩bipolar I disorder (26%)⟩major depression (18%) = dementia (18%)⟩schizophrenia (13%) (p <0.006), independent of the effects of age, race, gender, medication and body mass. Of these rates of type 2 diabetes, only those for schizoaffective disorder and bipolar I disorder were significantly higher than the national norms.

The data for antipsychotic medications were less clear. Here, a meta-analysis of 25 observational pharmaco-epidemiological studies found no significant difference in the risk of developing treatment-requiring type 2 diabetes using either second- or first-generation antipsychotics [34]. However, the data on two recent second-generation antipsychotics, aripiprazole and ziprasidone, were limited.

A systematic review of 17 pharmaco-epidemiologic studies examined the relationship between certain atypical antipsychotics and the risk of type 2 diabetes [35]. Treatment with olanzapine in people with major psychiatric illness, compared to no treatment, was associated with a significantly greater risk of new-onset diabetes. Risperidone was not associated with a greater RR of diabetes than conventional antipsychotics or no treatment. Of nine studies that compared the RR of diabetes with risperidone and olanzapine, six demonstrated a significantly greater risk with olanzapine, although the magnitude of the risk varied considerably across studies. Definitive conclusions could not be drawn for clozapine and quetiapine, due to insufficient evidence. Results from the review also showed that three out of four studies did not demonstrate any significant increase in risk for diabetes using atypical antipsychotics compared to conventional antipsychotics.

Bellantuono and colleagues [36] reviewed 21 studies (nine prospective, 11 retrospective) to evaluate the risk of type 2 diabetes in people treated with different antipsychotic drugs (conventional and second-generation). Subjects with schizophrenia treated with different antipsychotics had a higher risk of developing type 2 diabetes than the general population. It is not currently clear, however, whether the increased risk is due to the schizophrenia itself or to the antipsychotic treatment.

2.12　Sleep disorders

The association of sleep-disordered breathing and type 2 diabetes is increasingly recognized [37]. Among 2656 subjects (median age 68 years) from the Sleep Heart Health Study [38], the prevalence of diabetes was increased approximately twofold in people with an elevated respiratory disturbance index. Hence, those with this condition should be assessed routinely for undiagnosed diabetes.

2.13　Smoking

A meta-analysis of 25 prospective cohort studies involving 1.2 million participants found that active smoking is associated with an increased risk of type 2 diabetes [39]. The pooled adjusted RR of type 2 diabetes for active smoking compared to non-smoking was 1.44. Moreover, the risk of type 2 diabetes was greater for heavy smokers (≥ 20 cigarettes per day; RR = 1.61) than for lighter smokers (RR = 1.29), and lower for former smokers (RR = 1.23) compared to active smokers (RR = 1.44).

2.14　Conclusions

Diabetes-related risk factors are relevant and important in older people, and should be strongly considered when assessing the elderly for undiagnosed diabetes, and for the future risk of developing the condition. While undiagnosed diabetes carries significant morbidity in the elderly, diabetes prevention studies generally demonstrate equal or greater effectiveness when applied to older rather than to younger people.

References

1. Dunstan DW, Zimmet PZ, Welborn TA, De Courten MP, Cameron AJ, Sicree RA, Dwyer T, Colagiuri S, Jolley D, Knuiman M, Atkins R and Shaw JE. (2002) The rising prevalence of diabetes and impaired glucose tolerance: the Australian Diabetes, Obesity and Lifestyle Study. Diabetes Care, 25 (5), 829–34.
2. McBean AM, Li S, Gilbertson DT and Collins AJ. (2004) Differences in diabetes prevalence, incidence,

and mortality among the elderly of four racial/ethnic groups: whites, blacks, Hispanics, and Asians. Diabetes Care, 27 (10), 2317–24.

3. DECODE Study Group. (2003) Age- and sex-specific prevalences of diabetes and impaired glucose regulation in 13 European cohorts. Diabetes Care, 26 (1), 61–9.

4. Qiao Q, Hu G, Tuomilehto J, Nakagami T, Balkau B, Borch-Johnsen K, Ramachandran A, Mohan V, Iyer SR, Tominaga M, Kiyohara Y, Kato I, Okubo K, Nagai M, Shibazaki S, Yang Z, Tong Z, Fan Q, Wang B, Chew SK, Tan BY, Heng D, Emmanuel S, Tajima N, Iwamoto Y, Snehalatha C, Vijay V, Kapur A, Dong Y, Nan H, Gao W, Shi H and Fu F. (2003) Age- and sex-specific prevalence of diabetes and impaired glucose regulation in 11 Asian cohorts. Diabetes Care, 26 (6), 1770–80.

5. Harris MI, Flegal KM, Cowie CC, Eberhardt MS, Goldstein DE, Little RR, Wiedmeyer HM and Byrd-Holt DD. (1998) Prevalence of diabetes, impaired fasting glucose, and impaired glucose tolerance in U.S. adults. The Third National Health and Nutrition Examination Survey, 1988-1994. Diabetes Care, 21 (4), 518–24.

6. Magliano DJ, Barr EL, Zimmet PZ, Cameron AJ, Dunstan DW, Colagiuri S, Jolley D, Owen N, Phillips P, Tapp RJ, Welborn TA and Shaw JE. (2008) Glucose indices, health behaviors, and incidence of diabetes in Australia: the Australian Diabetes, Obesity and Lifestyle Study. Diabetes Care, 31 (2), 267–72.

7. Knowler WC, Barrett-Connor E, Fowler SE, Hamman RF, Lachin JM, Walker EA and Nathan DM. (2002) Reduction in the incidence of type 2 diabetes with lifestyle intervention or metformin. N Engl J Med, 346 (6), 393–403.

8. Tuomilehto J, Lindstrom J, Eriksson JG, Valle TT, Hamalainen H, Ilanne-Parikka P, Keinanen-Kiukaanniemi S, Laakso M, Louheranta A, Rastas M, Salminen V and Uusitupa M. (2001) Prevention of type 2 diabetes mellitus by changes in lifestyle among subjects with impaired glucose tolerance. N Engl J Med, 344 (18), 1343–50.

9. Defay R, Delcourt C, Ranvier M, Lacroux A and Papoz L. (2001) Relationships between physical activity, obesity and diabetes mellitus in a French elderly population: the POLA study. Pathologies Oculaires liees a l'Age. Int J Obes Relat Metab Disord, 25 (4), 512–18.

10. Huang KC, Lee MS, Lee SD, Chang YH, Lin YC, Tu SH and Pan WH. (2005) Obesity in the elderly and its relationship with cardiovascular risk factors in Taiwan. Obes Res, 13 (1), 170–8.

11. International Diabetes Federation. (2006) Diabetes Atlas, Third Edition.

12. Kim C, Newton KM and Knopp RH. (2002) Gestational diabetes and the incidence of type 2 diabetes: a systematic review. Diabetes Care, 25 (10), 1862–8.

13. Kobberling J and Tillil H. (1982) Empirical risk figures for first degree relatives of non-insulin dependent diabetics. In: The Genetics of Diabetes Mellitus. J. Kobberling and R. Tattershall (eds). Academic Press, London, New York, pp. 201–9.

14. Mooy JM, Grootenhuis PA, de Vires H, Valkenburg HA, Bouter LM, Kostense PJ and Heine RJ. (1995) Prevalence and determinants of glucose intolerance in a Dutch Caucasian population. The Hoorn study. Diabetes Care, 18, 1270–3.

15. Sugimori H, Miyakawa M, Yoshida K, Izuno T, Takahashi E, Tanaka C, Nakamura K and Hinohara S. (1998) Health risk assessment for diabetes mellitus based on longitudinal analysis of MHTS database. J Med Systems, 22, 27–32.

16. Costa A, Rios M, Casamitjana R, Gomis R and Conget I. (1998) High prevalence of abnormal glucose tolerance and metabolic disturbances in first degree relatives of NIDDM patients. A study in Catalonia, a Mediterranean community. Diabetes Res Clin Pract, 41, 191–6.

17. Saad MF, Knowler WC, Pettitt DJ, Nelson RG, Mott DM and Bennett PH. (1990) Insulin and hypertension. Relationship to obesity and glucose intolerance in Pima Indians. Diabetes, 39, 1430–5.

18. Chou P, Liao MJ and Tsai ST. (1994) Associated risk factors of diabetes in Kin-Hu, Kinmen. Diabetes Res Clin Pract, 26, 229–35.

19. Ruige JB, de Neeling JN, Kostense PJ, Bouter LM and Heine RJ. (1997) Performance of an NIDDM screening questionnaire based on symptoms and risk factors. Diabetes Care, 20, 491–6.

20. Welborn TA, Reid CM and Marriott G. (1997) Australian diabetes screening study: impaired glucose tolerance and non-insulin-dependent diabetes mellitus. Metabolism, 46 (Suppl. 1), 1–5.

21. Baan CA, Ruige JB, Stolk RP, Witteman JCM, Dekker JM, Heine RJ and Feskens EJM. (1999) Performance of a predictive model to identify undiagnosed diabetes in a health care setting. Diabetes Care, 22, 213–19.

22. Bog-Hansen E, Lindblad U, Bengtsson K, Ranstam J, Melander A and Rastam L. (1998) Risk factor clustering in patients with hypertension and non-insulin-dependent diabetes mellitus. The Skaraborg Hypertension Project. J Intern Med, 243, 223–32.

23. Bartnik M, Ryden L, Ferrari R, Malmberg K, Pyorala K, Simoons M, Standl E, Soler-Soler J and Ohrvik J. (2004) The prevalence of abnormal glucose regulation in patients with coronary artery disease across Europe.

The Euro Heart Survey on diabetes and the heart. Eur Heart J, 25 (21), 1880–90.

24. Wallander M, Malmberg K, Norhammar A, Ryden L and Tenerz A. (2008) Oral glucose tolerance test: a reliable tool for early detection of glucose abnormalities in patients with acute myocardial infarction in clinical practice: a report on repeated oral glucose tolerance tests from the GAMI study. Diabetes Care, 31 (1), 36–8.

25. Taubert G, Winkelmann BR, Schleiffer T, Marz W, Winkler R, Gok R, Klein B, Schneider S and Boehm BO. (2003) Prevalence, predictors, and consequences of unrecognized diabetes mellitus in 3266 patients scheduled for coronary angiography. Am Heart J, 145 (2), 285–91.

26. Matz K, Keresztes K, Tatschl C, Nowotny M, Dachenhausenm A, Brainin M and Tuomilehto J. (2006) Disorders of glucose metabolism in acute stroke patients: an under-recognized problem. Diabetes Care, 29 (4), 792–7.

27. Vancheri F, Curcio M, Burgio A, Salvaggio S, Gruttadauria G, Lunetta MC, Dovico R and Alletto M. (2005) Impaired glucose metabolism in patients with acute stroke and no previous diagnosis of diabetes mellitus. Q J Med, 98 (12), 871–8.

28. Ostchega Y, Paulose-Ram R, Dillon CF, Gu Q and Hughes JP. (2007) Prevalence of peripheral arterial disease and risk factors in persons aged 60 and older: data from the National Health and Nutrition Examination Survey 1999-2004. Journal of the American Geriatric Society, 55 (4), 583–9.

29. Regensteiner JG, Hiatt WR, Coll JR, Criqui MH, Treat-Jacobson D, McDermott MM and Hirsch AT. (2008) The impact of peripheral arterial disease on health-related quality of life in the Peripheral Arterial Disease Awareness, Risk, and Treatment: New Resources for Survival (PARTNERS) Program. Vasc Med, 132 (1), 15–24.

30. Gorter PM, Olijhoek JK, van der Graaf Y, Algra A, Rabelink TJ, Visseren FL and the SMART Study Group. (2004) Prevalence of the metabolic syndrome in patients with coronary heart disease, cerebrovascular disease, peripheral arterial disease or abdominal aortic aneurysm. Atherosclerosis, 173 (2), 363–9.

31. Jeon CY, Lokken RP, Hu FB and Van Dam RM. (2007) Physical activity of moderate intensity and risk of type 2 diabetes: A systematic review. Diabetes Care, 30 (3), 744–52.

32. Baan CA, Stolk RP, Grobbee DE, Witteman JC and Feskens EJ. (1999) Physical activity in elderly subjects with impaired glucose tolerance and newly diagnosed diabetes mellitus. American Journal of Epidemiology, 149 (3), 219–27.

33. Regenold WT, Thapar RK, Marano C, Gavirneni S and Kondapavuluru PV. (2002) Increased prevalence of type 2 diabetes mellitus among psychiatric inpatients with bipolar I affective and schizoaffective disorders independent of psychotropic drug use. Journal of Affective Disorders, 70 (1), 19–26.

34. Citrome LL, Holt RIG, Zachry WM, Clewell JD, Orth PA, Karagianis JL and Hoffmann VP. (2007) Risk of treatment-emergent diabetes mellitus in patients receiving antipsychotics. Annals of Pharmacotherapy, 41 (10), 1593–603.

35. Ramaswamy K, Masand PS and Nasrallah HA. (2006) Do certain atypical antipsychotics increase the risk of diabetes? A critical review of 17 pharmacoepidemiologic studies. Annals of Clinical Psychiatry, 18 (3), 183–94.

36. Bellantuono C, Tentoni L and Donda P. (2004) Antipsychotic drugs and risk of type 2 diabetes: An evidence-based approach. Human Psychopharmacology, 19 (8), 549–58.

37. Shaw JE, Punjabi NM, Wilding JP, Alberti KG and Zimmet PZ. (2008) Sleep-disordered breathing and type 2 diabetes: a report from the International Diabetes Federation Taskforce on Epidemiology and Prevention. Diabetes Res Clin Pract, 81 (1), 2–12.

38. Punjabi NM, Shahar E, Redline S, Gottlieb DJ, Givelber R and Resnick HE. (2004) Sleep-disordered breathing, glucose intolerance, and insulin resistance: the Sleep Heart Health Study. American Journal of Epidemiology, 160 (6), 521–30.

39. Willi C, Bodenmann P, Ghali WA, Faris PD and Cornuz J. (2007) Active smoking and the risk of type 2 diabetes: A systematic review and meta-analysis. Journal of the American Medical Association, 298 (22), 2654–64.

SECTION II
Screening and Diagnosis

3

Diabetes in the Elderly: Diagnosis, Testing and Screening

Simon Croxson

United Bristol Healthcare NHS Trust, Bristol General Hospital, Bristol, UK

Key messages

- Undiagnosed diabetes is common in the older population.
- Diagnosis is probably beneficial to the subjects.
- Elderly subjects with undiagnosed diabetes characteristically have isolated post-challenge hyperglycaemia.
- A non-diabetic fasting plasma glucose level does not exclude diabetes, and glucose tolerance tests are often required.

3.1 Introduction

In this chapter, attention is focused on the diagnosis, testing and screening of diabetes in the elderly, mainly in relation to type 2 diabetes (T2DM).

Although type 1 diabetes (T1DM) does occur in the elderly, and is not uncommon, it is often clinically apparent that the problem with diabetes is not its detection but rather the recognition of its type. Secondary diabetes is a disease of the elderly, often as a result of chronic pancreatitis and steroid therapy rather than being secondary to other endocrine conditions or pregnancy; this presents in similar fashion to T2DM, with problems being related to both the diagnosis and recognition of type.

Here, we will consider the diagnosis of diabetes in the elderly – why a diagnosis should be made, the tests to be made for such diagnosis, and the types of diabetes encountered. We will consider these points from the settings of older people at home in the community ('free range'), of those in residential care, and of those being admitted as hospital inpatients.

3.2 Definition of diabetes in the elderly

Although many different diagnostic criteria for diabetes have previously been defined, they were rationalized in 1979/1980 in reports from both the National Diabetes Data Group (NDDG) and the World Health Organization (WHO) [1, 2]. At that time, the 'gold standard' definition was to wait for 3 to 10 years without any formal diagnosis or treatment; then, if diabetes-specific complications (generally retinopathy) or overt diabetes symptoms were shown to be present, a diagnosis of diabetes was made [3–7]. These studies showed that a 2 h post-glucose challenge (generally 75 g anhydrous glucose) venous plasma glucose level of 11.1 mmol 1^{-1} or more predicted the presence of specific complications, and that 'normal' or elevated fasting plasma glucose levels (using the criteria of the time) did not predict the absence of specific complications [4, 6].

Diabetes in Old Age. Third Edition. Edited by Alan J. Sinclair
© 2009 John Wiley & Sons, Ltd

However, as these studies were conducted predominantly middle-aged populations, would the same criteria apply to elderly subjects?

If the prevalence of undiagnosed diabetes is $\geq 10\%$, then a histogram of the results of oral glucose tolerance tests (OGTTs) would show a bimodal distribution of normal and diabetic groups, with a plasma level of 11.1 mmol l^{-1} dividing the two [4, 8–11]. This has been shown not only in middle-aged populations, but also in elderly and old populations. It is believed, therefore, that the modern criteria apply in the elderly, although no long-term follow- up studies of specific complications to confirm have been conducted, for obvious reasons.

As will be noted later, the elderly diabetic person generally has an elevated post- challenge glucose level but a normal fasting level; this is termed 'isolated post-challenge hyperglycaemia'. Whether this is a real illness, and whether it matters, remains the subject of debate, with several population-based studies, as well as the DECODE review, having shown isolated post-challenge hyperglycaemia in elderly people to be associated with an adverse outcome (often death) when compared to normal glucose tolerance [12–15].

3.2.1 The oral glucose tolerance test (OGTT)

At present, the clinical gold standard for the diagnosis of diabetes is the OGTT, in which venous plasma glucose samples are measured. Although values for other types of sample have been described, they seem not to provide the same diagnoses [16].

Previously, it has been reported by many that the OGTT can be a 'variable' test [17]. For example, when Feskens *et al.* repeated OGTTs in 237 subjects, aged 64–87 years, annually between 1971 and 1975, the co-efficients of intra-individual variation for fasting and 30, 60 and 120 min glucose ranged from 12% to 18% [18]. Such variability was not associated with age, gender, drug use or disease prevalence, although the reliability coefficient was shown to depend on the prevalence of diabetes in the population, this being higher than was observed in younger populations. When classifying according to the WHO criteria, the variability was comparable to that of other cardiovascular risk factors, such as serum total cholesterol.

The variability of the OGTT has been shown similar to that of other biochemical measures. A degree of the variability might in fact be due to variability among the subjects; for example, should a prolonged time elapse between the OGTTs (as in Feskens' study), the subjects might adopt a more healthy lifestyle, or develop diabetes. Feskens *et al.* used a 50 g glucose load, and cited evidence that such a load would induce minimal variability. In contrast, others have shown higher glucose loads to be more consistent than smaller loads [19]. Nonetheless, care must be taken to perform the OGTT correctly, including an overnight fast of 9 h or more, no food or medication to be ingested on the morning of the test, and only water to be drunk. In addition, no exercise should be taken during the test, which should be performed in the morning (in general, a higher result is obtained during the afternoon). Several major, incorrectly conducted surveys have resulted in prevalences higher than reported in comparable surveys, as noted by Mykkanen and colleagues [20].

3.2.2 Other categories of glucose intolerance

There are two other categories of glucose intolerance, namely impaired glucose tolerance (IGT) and impaired fasting glucose (IFG):

- The concept of IGT was introduced in 1979/1980 [1, 2] as a statement of between what was regarded as 'normal' and 'diabetic', with subjects having a higher risk of progressing to diabetes over time, in proportion to the prevalence of diabetes among the population. IGT is also associated with large-vessel disease and an increased mortality rate [21] (Table 3.1). Among the population of Asturas, aged 30–75 years, progression from IGT to diabetes was ascertained by conducting repeat OGTTs at 6-year intervals; the independent risk factors for progression were fasting and 2 h plasma glucose levels, triglyceride levels and the body mass index (BMI) [22]. Age, gender, education level, physical activity, family history of diabetes, systolic and diastolic blood pressures, total cholesterol and HDL-cholesterol each also increased the risk of progression, and were dependent on the preceding variables.

- Impaired Fasting Glucose (IFG) was first introduced in the 1997 American Diabetes Association (ADA) diagnostic criteria [23] and, as its name implies, is a state with a fasting plasma glucose between 'normal' and diabetic. People with IFG should be subjected to an OGTT (despite the fasting level already having been checked) to accurately clarify their glucose tolerance status.

- Considerable interest has also been expressed in using the fasting plasma glucose (FPG) or glycosylated haemoglobin in lieu of the OGTT. Both, McCance *et al.* and others have shown that the use of various cut-offs for these values provides a good sensitivity for predicting future retinopathy, though not quite as effective as the 2 h post-challenge value [24]. This report was the subject of much constructive and critical correspondence [25–27], as it highlighted the 5-year incidence of retinopathy (17.0% by raised 2 h glucose; 11.3% by raised FPG; and 9.16% by raised glycosylated haemoglobin). It was noted, however, that the high performance of these tests in McCance's study was increased by performing the study in Pima Indians, a population with a naturally high prevalence of diabetes [28].

Because a single raised plasma glucose level does not serve as a diagnosis of diabetes (despite almost all epidemiological surveys using just one test), confirmatory evidence is required in clinical practice; this might be a further raised plasma glucose level at a different time, and/or include osmotic symptoms or specific complications (e.g., retinopathy).

The latest WHO and International Diabetes Federation (IDF) criteria [29] have simplified matters greatly by introducing 'intermediate hyperglycaemia' as locating somewhere between a normal glucose tolerance (venous FPG <6.1 mmol l^{-1} and 2 h post challenge <7.8 mmol l^{-1}) and diabetes (venous FPG ≥ 7.0 mmol l^{-1} and 2 h post challenge ≥ 11.1 mmol l^{-1}).

3.3 Why detect diabetes?

Although opinion varies as to whether diabetes should be actively detected, or simply allowed to be presented in the clinical situation, detection may be preferred for a variety of reasons:

- Diabetes is a common condition, with its prevalence varying depending on the age, ethnic origin, residence and country of the population [30–35]. Approximately 30–50% of diabetes cases are undiagnosed, such that between 3% and 15% of the elderly population may have undiagnosed diabetes.

- The identification of diabetes allows the aggressive management of vascular risk factors such as dyslipidaemia, hypertension and the use of antiplatelet agents, as diabetes represents Coronary Heart Disease equivalence [36, 37]. Having diabetes has an equivalent vascular morbidity and mortality to myocardial infarction, and both have a 7-year vascular death rate of 42% [36].

- There is some evidence that a delayed diagnosis leads to greater complications [38–40], but of course this may be due to other factors such as lead time bias. The behaviour of those patients who delay seeking medical help might also lead them to harm.

- The identification of diabetes allows hyperglycaemia to be controlled; this in turn would improve cognition and the quality of life [41]; it might also avoid microvascular complications [42].

- The identification of diabetes allows screening for eye disease.

- Identification should also reduce the risk of metabolic decompensation; in the Rhode Island study, hyperglycaemic coma was more likely to be fatal if the diabetes had not been previously diagnosed [43].

- The identification of diabetes enables secondary care providers to claim for more complex (expensive) inpatient episodes; early identification also allows an easy attainment of Quality and Outcomes Framework targets, increasing the UK GP's income.

- An accurate ascertainment of glucose tolerance status is important not only for diabetes-specific research, but also for other studies where diabetes is an important predictor variable.

Although I believe that the detection of diabetes in older people is unquestionably valuable, no formal controlled trials have been conducted to confirm this proposal. At this point, it is worth considering the different tests for diabetes in comparison to the OGTT using 'modern' criteria – that is, a 2 h post-challenge plasma glucose level of 11.1 mmol l^{-1} or more. Before the IGT concept was introduced in 1979/1980, approximately 17% of all subjects in Rochester Minnesota who had been diagnosed diabetic in fact had IGT rather than diabetes [44, 45]. One should examine whether a simple test such as glycosuria or a raised FPG could be used to identify subjects in whom an OGTT is worth performing, rather than a screening test to instantly identify diabetic subjects (although this may occur with some screening tests, such as a dramatically elevated FPG). In particularly, the settings of the test – whether in the community, in residential

Table 3.1 The 1999 WHO criteria for the diagnosis of diabetes. Values shown are glucose concentrations (mmol l^{-1}).

Diagnostic category	Plasma glucose		Whole-blood glucose	
	Venous	Capillary	Venous	Capillary
Diabetes				
Fasting or	≥7.0	≥7.0	≥6.1	≥6.1
2-h post load	≥11.1	≥12.2	≥10.0	≥11.1
IGT				
Fasting and	<7.0	<7.0	<6.1	<6.1
2-h post load	7.8–11.0 (incl.)	8.9–12.1 (incl.)	6.7–9.9 (incl.)	7.8–11.0 (incl.)
IFG				
Fasting and	6.1–6.9 (incl.)	6.1–6.9 (incl.)	5.6–6.0 (incl.)	5.6–6.0 (incl.)
2-h post load	<7.8	<8.9	<6.7	<7.8

Note: To convert mmol l^{-1} to mg dl^{-1}, the value should be divided by 0.0555.

care or in an acute medical admission – will be considered

It is also important to be aware that, as the prevalence of an illness increases, then the performance of any screening test will be improved. When studies are conducted in high-risk populations, such as Hispanics or Pima Indians of the USA, a screening test will perform better than in a low-prevalence population [28].

A variety of other problems have been identified with many of the studies; for example, while some use a screening test and concentrate on those patients who screen positive compared to just a handful of negative 'screenees', and elderly participants may be limited not only in numbers but also in age, often up to only 75 years.

3.4　The symptoms of diabetes

The classic osmotic diabetic symptoms of polyuria and polydipsia occur when the renal threshold for glycosuria has been exceeded. As the renal threshold of glucose rises with age [46], it would be anticipated that symptoms should occur quite late in disease progression. The questioning of newly presenting diabetic subjects of all ages at a diabetes centre revealed that only 39% of patients had noticed symptoms of their diabetes, yet 80% had symptoms when directly questioned [47]. When considering all age groups of the UK general population, the elderly were considered more likely to recognize the symptoms of diabetes than were the young [48].

Very few screening surveys have investigated the presence of symptoms, but of course if the subjects were shown to be symptomatic then it might be hoped that they would seek – and receive – appropriate medical attention.

In the Melton screening survey, among 24 elderly people aged 65–85 years found to have (previously undiagnosed) diabetes by OGTT, seven of them had thirst or polyuria on questioning. An absence of symptoms was more likely in those subjects aged over 79 years and none of the eight octogenarians had symptoms [49, 50]. Among 210 non-diabetic subjects, five had thirst or polyuria for no obvious reason (non-diabetic OGTT, no diuretic use, normal renal function, calcium and potassium levels). Interestingly, one of the symptomatic subjects had consulted his GP and been reassured that there was not a problem; another subject denied osmotic symptoms, but had a glass of water in every room because he liked water.

In the Tampere screening survey [51], none of 19 elderly (aged 80+ years) new diabetic subjects was found to have symptoms of diabetes.

Thus, in the 'free range' population, osmotic symptoms are specific but insensitive.

In the Birmingham Care Home Study [31], care home residents received an OGTT and were asked about their osmotic symptoms; among 44 found to have diabetes, 22 had polyuria, 22 had thirst and 22 felt tired; the corresponding figures for 227 non-diabetic residents were 116, 116 and 121. Thus, among care home residents, osmotic symptoms are insensitive and as non-specific as possible.

Overall, it is hoped that the public will come to recognize the significance of osmotic symptoms, and report to medical care and receive appropriate diagnostic testing.

3.5 Glycosuria

In the Bedford diabetes survey, approximately half pf the subjects with undiagnosed diabetes had postprandial glycosuria at all ages [52]; among undiagnosed diabetic subjects in the Islington diabetes survey, 33% had fasting glycosuria and 73% had postprandial glycosuria [53].

In the Melton diabetes survey in the elderly, glycosuria was present in 13 of 25 diabetic subjects, in three of 20 IGT subjects, and in 12 of 225 normal subjects. Ignoring those subjects with known diabetes and those who were not tested, and extrapolating to those who had OGTT but no urinalysis, provides a sensitivity 53%, a specificity of 94%, and predictive values of positive and negative tests of 23% and 98%, respectively [49, 50].

Very few other studies have been reported examining glycosuria as a means of diabetes detection [54] using post 1979/1980 criteria. Glycosuria was assessed in both Ipswich [55] and Ringkøbing, Denmark [56], where the population tested their urine and a small number of negative screenees were invited to take an OGTT. In both studies, the elderly tended to have a higher participation rate than the young, and this difference was significant in elderly Danish men.

In the Ringkøbing study, when 106 subjects without glycosuria were tested using a fasting capillary whole blood glucose, three were found to have diabetes [56]. Although, the prevalence of diabetes was shown to be 9-11% for Danes aged 60–70 years by other OGTT screening studies, the Ringkøbing screening study showed only 0-2% of the elderly subjects to have diabetes. Among all age groups, however, the sensitivity of urinalysis for glycosuria was calculated to be 20%.

In the Ipswich study, OGTTs were conducted in people with glycosuria and in 442 participants in the Isle of Ely OGTT screening project; the two groups were subsequently amalgamated and the data analyzed together [55]. This provided a sensitivity of 89% (albeit across subjects of all ages) and, by enriching the sample with positive urinalysis subjects, made the test results appear better than they in fact were. Friderichsen subsequently calculated that a sensitivity of 17% would be more realistic for the Ipswich data [56].

Thus, very few studies have been conducted to assess the value of urinalysis in elderly populations compared to an OGTT; where performed, the sensitivity was found to be low (e.g., 50%) but the test was relatively specific (e.g., 90%). Urinalysis has the advantage that it provides a cheap and simple means of selecting people for an OGTT, rather than simply testing the entire population with an OGTT; unfortunately, however, half of the subjects with undiagnosed diabetes will remain undiagnosed and be falsely reassured. An example of this can be deduced from the approximate costs of the Ipswich and Melton studies; if £900 (1988 prices) was available to spend, then screening with OGTTs would identify one diabetic person in the Melton survey, and miss none. In contrast, a pre-screening with urinalysis would identify 10 diabetics but would probably miss a similar number, despite screening a much larger population.

3.6 Fasting plasma glucose and the modified oral glucose tolerance test

Although, in the past the FPG has often been favoured because of its simplicity, it has long been realized that elderly subjects may have a clearly elevated 2 h post-challenge glucose level, despite non-diabetic FPG levels [57, 58]. Based on population-wide information, this was apparent from the NHANES 2 data, which showed the average FPG to vary very little with age, while the average post-challenge level tends to rise significantly with age [32].

There is a tendency to use the above data to support the premise that the FPG should be used for diagnostic purposes because, by using the post-challenge value, too many 'diabetic' subjects would be identified. However, the original OGTT data indicated that the incidence of specific complications was related to the post-challenge glucose levels, and that this occurred whether the FPG was raised, or not. This effect has recently been confirmed in a series of larger, multi-ethnic studies [59].

Data from Rancho Bernardo's elderly population, NHANES 2 and the DECODE group has indeed shown that isolated post-challenge hyperglycaemia is associated with adverse outcome (death) compared to normal glucose-tolerant individuals of similar age from the same populations [12–15, 60].

Other studies from the DECODE group have shown that the FPG tends to be raised in fatter, younger patients, but not in older, slimmer patients [61].

One further area of confusion is the difference between a diabetic FPG ($\geq$7.8 mmol l^{-1} from 1979,

≥ 7.0 mmol 1^{-1} from 1997) and a value above normal (6.0 mmol 1^{-1} from 1997 onwards); one of these is definitely a diabetic value (although confirmatory evidence of the diagnosis is required clinically) and the other is not normal.

Subjects with a FPG that is above normal, but not in the diabetic range, are labelled as having IFG; this is not regarded as an adequate diagnosis clinically, because in Bristol 30% of the subjects would have diabetes on the 2 h values [62], while in the Leicester Gujerati population 85% would have diabetes [63]. Thus, subjects with IFG require their glucose level to be monitored post challenge (the fasting level for the OGTT has already been done). Further evidence that subjects with non-diabetic FPGs can still not be normal comes from the Quebec Family Study, where subjects with non-diabetic OGTTs were divided into tertiles of FPG [64]. Those in the highest FPG tertile had more insulin resistance, less insulin secretion (corrected for their insulin resistance) and more lipid abnormalities than subjects in the lowest tertile. Also, within the 'normal range' with post-challenge hyperglycaemia excluded, a higher FPG is associated with an increased mortality [65].

In the Rancho Bernardo study of retirees aged 50–89 years, only 69 of 254 newly diagnosed diabetic people had a raised FPG of ≥ 7.8 mmol 1^{-1} [58]. More usefully by modern criteria, Modan and colleagues found that 49 of 134 newly diagnosed diabetic subjects from a community survey of subjects aged 40–70 years had a FPG below 6.4 mmol 1^{-1} [66]. In Pima Indians of all ages, the screening of those not known to have diabetes by OGTT showed that 8% of the subjects with previously undiagnosed diabetes had a FPG under 6.1 mmol 1^{-1} [67], with corresponding figures for Taiwanese of all ages of 27% [68] and for Australians of all ages of approximately 30% [69].

In elderly Koreans with previously undiagnosed diabetes, 50% of the men and 40% of the women had a FPG under 6.1 mmol 1^{-1} [70] and in elderly African Americans 30% had a FPG under 7.0 mmol 1^{-1} [71]. Thus, the FPG in free range individuals and elderly misses many people with undiagnosed diabetes.

The over-riding difference between the ADA criteria and the WHO criteria has been the ADA's preoccupation with using the FPG. Not surprisingly, the prevalence of diabetes in the elderly Korean is approximately twice that by WHO criteria than by ADA criteria [70], and similar findings occur in elderly African Americans [71]. However, this is not always the case,

and in testing people of different races aged 25 to 74 years in Newcastle, the prevalence of diabetes was higher in all three ethnic groups using the new fasting ADA criteria compared to the WHO post-challenge criteria: 7.1% versus 4.8% in Europeans; 6.2% versus 4.7% in Chinese; and 21.4% versus 20.1% in South Asians [72]. Unfortunately, these are younger subjects and are possibly overweight, thereby emphasizing the DECODE findings of different phenotypes with different abnormalities on OGTT in the young and old [61].

Ultimately, this is all of historical interest, since the 1999 WHO and 2003 ADA criteria for diabetes diagnosis are very similar, and the ADA now advocates the use of the OGTT [29].

Recently, the ADA has altered its definition of 'normal'; since the introduction of the 1979 National Diabetes Data Group and the 1980 WHO criteria, the USA and the rest of the world have used the same criteria, apart from minor differences converting mg per deciliter to millimoles per litre. However, in 2003, the ADA decreased the normal FPG to under 5.6 mmol 1^{-1} [73], while the WHO and International Diabetes Federation adhered to under 6.1 mmol 1^{-1} [29].

We recently examined the data from routine OGTTs with regards to different FPG cut-offs in middle-aged and elderly subjects [74], the term 'elderly' was taken as ≥ 60 years, following the WHO criteria [75]. Among 334 younger people tested, 121 had diabetes (FPG 7.0+ mmol 1^{-1} or post-challenge glucose 11.1+ mmol 1^{-1}); of these, one person (1%) had a FPG <5.6 mmol 1^{-1} and two people (2%) had a FPG of 5.6–6.0 mmol 1^{-1}. Among 265 older people tested, 151 had diabetes; of these, 10 (7%) had a FPG <5.6 mmol 1^{-1} and 11 (7%) had a FPG of 5.6–6.0 mmol 1^{-1}. In young people, changing the normal plasma glucose value has little effect, as only 2.5% (95% CI: 0.5–7.0%) with undiagnosed diabetes have a FPG <6.1 mmol 1^{-1}. On the other hand, again older people with undiagnosed diabetes often had a low FPG, with 10 (7%; 95% CI: 3–12%) having a value <5.6 mmol 1^{-1} and 21 (14%; 95% CI: 9–21%) a value <6.1 mmol 1^{-1}; that is, 7% (95% CI: 4–13%) of undiagnosed elderly diabetic subjects had a FPG of 5.6 to 6.0 mmol 1^{-1}, inclusive. Thus, in young people, the FPG is reasonable at excluding diabetes, whichever 'normal' FPG is used. However, in older people the lower ADA cut-off of <5.6 mmol 1^{-1} as 'normal' is needed to detect many of the diabetic subjects (although even this will still miss some subjects with undiagnosed diabetes). Unfortunately, among the 151 diabetic elderly subjects,

29 (6%: 95% CI: 13–25%) did not have a diabetic 2 h post-challenge value but rather had a diabetic FPG level. Consequently, it would seem that both fasting and post-challenge glucose values are required for a comprehensive assessment of glucose tolerance status in older people.

In the Birmingham Care Home Study, the fasting capillary plasma glucose data were acquired alongside the OGTT results [31, 76]. From this, it is possible to draw a receiver operator characteristics (ROC) curve (this may be drawn using statistical software) in which sensitivity is plotted against 1-specificity for all possible cut-offs (Figure 3.1). It is important to emphasize that the aim here is to identify the optimum FPG as a diabetes screen, and not to redefine the criterion for a diabetic FPG. Ideally, the ROC curve for the data would include a point with maximum sensitivity and specificity (i.e., at the top left-hand corner of the graph), which would also have the largest area under the ROC curve and may be a useful value to compare screening tests (again the statistics software performs the calculations). A clear example is in the Coventry Study, where the optimum cut-off for a random blood glucose to find diabetes was examined [77].

In the Birmingham Care Home Study, the optimum fasting capillary plasma glucose was ≥ 5.8 mmol l^{-1}, with sensitivity 42% and specificity 96%; the corresponding values for cut-offs for 5.0 mmol l^{-1} were 61% and 70%, and for 6.0 mmol l^{-1} were 35% and

97%. Thus, many care home residents with undiagnosed diabetes will have a low FPG; for example, 40% had a FPG <5.0 mmol l^{-1} and only 18% had a FPG ≥ 7.0 mmol l^{-1}. The converse is that the modified oral glucose tolerance test (MOGTT) using just the 2 h post-challenge value is extremely useful; among the Birmingham Residential Home subjects, 43 of the 46 new diabetic subjects had post-challenge hyperglycaemia, often with unremarkable fasting glucose levels. This has a sensitivity of 0.93, a specificity of 1.0, predictive value positive test of 1.0 and predictive value negative test of 0.99.

3.7 Random and postprandial plasma glucose

Postprandial glucose levels were comprehensively assessed by Engelgau *et al.* in Egypt [78], when a total of 828 subjects had a random capillary whole blood estimation timed relative to their last meal, followed by an OGTT. This was a very practical 'real world' study using a One Touch II meter, testing whenever possible (but often afternoon) and with a variable time after a variable meal. By using an ROC curve, the random blood glucose level was found to have an optimum sensitivity with shorter postprandial periods, while the cut-off level needed to decrease with longer postprandial periods yet to increase with advancing age. Thus, for subjects aged 75 years the optimal cut-off was

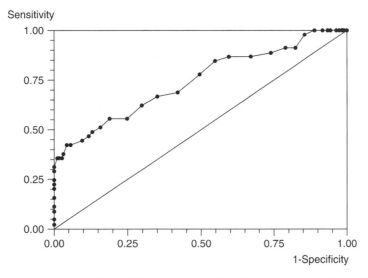

Figure 3.1 Receiver operator characteristics (ROC) curve from the Birmingham Care Home Study of fasting plasma glucose for diabetes diagnosis

7.8 mmol l^{-1} at 1 h postprandial, with a sensitivity of 81% and specificity of 80%. Again, the study results emphasized that different cut-offs were required in the young and old; for example, for 30-year-old subjects the optimal level was 1 h postprandial, with a glucose level of 6.55 mmol l^{-1}, and a sensitivity of 82% and specificity of 78%.

In the Coventry Study, the bi-ethnic population of Coventry was prescreened with a random glucose level, and then subjected to OGTT if screen-positive (capillary whole blood glucose ≥6.0 mmol l^{-1} within 2 h of meal, or ≥5.0 mmol l^{-1} at more than 2 h postprandially); a group of screen-negative subjects was also subjected to an OGTT [34, 77, 79]. Interestingly, there was a significant difference in sensitivity for a random capillary whole blood glucose cut-off of 8.0 mmol l^{-1} between elderly Europeans (sensitivity 36%) and elderly South Asian subjects (sensitivity 68%) (the sensitivity values for a 7.0 mmol l^{-1} cut-off were 50% and 75%, respectively), while the addition of testing within 2 h of a meal improved the sensitivity in South Asian, but not European, people. At all cut-offs, the sensitivity was greater in South Asian subjects than Europeans, presumably due to the much higher prevalence. However, very few elderly screen-negative subjects [43] were available, and the two subjects who had undiagnosed diabetes but were screen-negative were both elderly.

Again, there are other community-based studies using random plasma glucose (RPG) estimations, and Andersson's study is such an example [80]. Here, subjects aged up to age 79 years and with a positive urinalysis for glucose or random capillary whole blood glucose ≥8.0 mmol l^{-1} were followed up, with a fasting whole blood glucose (FBG) assessment; if the FBG was neither diabetic nor very low (FBG 5.5–6.6 mmol l^{-1}, inclusive), an OGTT was performed; as a consequence, 3268 people (85% of the target population) were tested over 3 years, and 66 were found to be diabetic. Urinalysis detected 20 diabetic subjects, while blood glucose testing detected 64; other similar studies confirmed the much higher sensitivity of blood testing over urine testing [81]. The drawbacks to this study were that it excluded subjects aged >79 years, there was no assessment of screen-negative subjects, and it was not possible to compare the final prevalence in the general practice population to that of a screened population. On the other hand, the results showed that a keen general practice can use a screening system to identify many (although not all) diabetic subjects. It is unknown how many would have surfaced naturally if left to their own devices.

The use of a random blood glucose measurement was investigated in the Birmingham Care Homes Study using BM-test 1–44 test strips and Reflolux S meter [Boehringer Mannheim (BM), Mannheim, Germany]. An ROC curve analysis gave an optimum BM test cut-off of 5.3 mmol l^{-1} [31, 76], with a sensitivity of 56% and a specificity of 82%. Given the findings in Egypt above and Bristol below, an ≥8.0 mmol l^{-1} cut-off was examined that showed a sensitivity of 4% and a specificity of 100% (it is standard finding that either sensitivity or specificity is gained at the expense of the other).

Previously, the use of a random venous plasma glucose for diabetes detection in elderly medical admissions to the hospital in Bristol, has been investigated. In this predominantly white, European population [82], the ultimate prevalence of diabetes was 1% if the admission plasma glucose (APG) was 7.0–7.9 mmol l^{-1}, 10% if it was 8.0–12.9 mmol l^{-1}, and 50% if ≥13.0 mmol l^{-1}. Other interesting findings were that, in patients found to have diabetes as an inpatient, 50% were non-diabetic on retesting at 6 weeks after discharge. The lowest APG found to be positive for diabetes was 7.0 mmol l^{-1}, while the highest APG to be negative for diabetes was >20 mmol l^{-1}. As a consequence, any patient admitted to the Bristol hospital with an APG ≥8.0 mmol l^{-1} will be screened; in this way one subject with undiagnosed diabetes will be missed every per 6 months. Unfortunately, these tests are not 100% accurate, and a diagnosis of diabetes made during a hospital admission should be reviewed at a later date.

Thus, while a RPG in a care home resident is generally unhelpful, within the free range population a 1 h postprandial plasma glucose ≥7.8 mmol l^{-1} or, in the acute hospital admission a RPG ≥8.0 mmol l^{-1}, represent useful tests to determine which patients should receive an OGTT to check for diabetes.

3.8   Blood glucose meters

Modern studies measuring venous plasma glucose use a glucose oxidase method which is specific for glucose. However, meters for self glucose monitoring measure whole blood glucose, and either report whole blood glucose or report a plasma glucose equivalent [83]. Occasionally, in fact, it is difficult to determine from the manufacturer exactly what is being reported by the meter. Typically, whole blood glucose is approximately 10–15% (1 mmol l^{-1}) lower than plasma glucose due to the presence of red blood cells; hence, anaemic subjects will record higher readings on whole blood glucose measurements, as are used in self blood glucose meters. The plasma/whole blood difference depends on the haematocrit; a 15% decrease in glucose level is evident when the haematocrit is 0.55, but only 8% when the haematocrit is 0.31 [83]. Thus, attention must be paid to the meters used in the studies, as well as remaining aware of other factors that might influence the results obtained with glucose meters.

It is also important to remember that fingerprick capillary glucose values may be falsely low in sick patients, and this may lead to an underestimation of their hyperglycaemia [84, 85].

3.9   Glycosylated haemoglobin

Glycosylated haemoglobin (GHb) assays have been developed and enhanced over the past three decades, and now measure the more specific HbA$_{1c}$ than the original HbA$_1$; there are, however, several different assay methods which can produce slightly different results. In addition, a variety of factors can influence GHb other than plasma glucose [86]. For example, a rapid turnover of red blood cells due to haemolysis, sickle cell disease or thalassemia will reduce GHb levels, whereas the persistence of fetal Hb will cause an increase in GHb. In particular, the effect of variant haemoglobins differs with different assays.

Interestingly, some subjects are higher 'glycators' than others; this is unrelated to glycaemic levels, and most likely due to a longer red cell survival in high glycators. It may lead to a GHb difference of 2% between high and low glycators with normal glucose tolerance [87].

It is often written that the GHb normal range increases with age. In the France Telecom project, workers were screened using OGTT and HbA$_{1c}$ measurements. Among 3240 subjects aged 18 to 80 years, very few had abnormal glucose tolerance (22 diabetic, 210 IGT subjects) and the HbA$_{1c}$ was seen to rise significantly with age, before falling in males [88]. Certainly, splitting the OGTT data into standard categories, rather than treating it as a continuous variable [89], would have lost some of the power of the data to detect whether age itself or an increase in glucose levels with age cause this rise in HbA1c. In a further

study, 232 subjects with FPG <6.4 mmol l^{-1} showed an increase in HbA$_{1c}$ with age [90], although it was not known how many of these subjects would have isolated post-challenge hyperglycaemia, which is more common with age. Others have shown that, in a group of 93 subjects, age was not associated with any change in FPG or GHb [91], although this size sample would have been highly prone to a type 2 error. Thus, there is still scope to determine whether older folk with normal glucose tolerance have a significantly higher HbA$_{1c}$ than do younger folk.

GHb has been assessed as a tool for diabetes diagnosis in many studies, and is indeed an almost standard investigation in such trials.

An analysis of data from a large database of the Meta-analysis Research Group (MRG) and the NHANES III data (subjects aged 40–74 years) showed that two-thirds of subjects with a 2 h post-challenge plasma glucose of 11.1–13.3 mmol l^{-1} had a normal HbA$_{1c}$ (up to 6.3%), while only one-third with an OGTT result >13.3 mmol l^{-1} had a raised HbA$_{1c}$ [92]. The data from the MRG study over-represented subjects with undiagnosed diabetes, which again makes screening tests perform better, although the sensitivities were low. The finding that an elevated HbA$_{1c}$ missed many diabetic subjects and only identified those with an elevated HbA$_{1c}$, was described as being advantageous, as it only finds those diabetic subjects with raised HbA$_{1c}$ in whom an intervention would be made to lower such levels (a rather self-recursive argument); this clearly misses the majority of diabetic subjects in whom aggressive intervention would be made for vascular protection.

A recent systematic review of HbA$_{1c}$ compared to formal OGTT was prepared by Bennett *et al.* [93]. Here, the most interesting point was that only nine studies met the inclusion criteria which were that the study had to be written in English, the majority of subjects had to have had OGTT by modern criteria, and the HbA$_{1c}$ result could be aligned to Diabetes Control and Complications Trial values. The results showed HbA$_{1c}$ to have a slightly lower sensitivity than FPG in detecting diabetes, but a slightly higher specificity. At an HbA$_{1c}$ cut-off of $\geq$6.1%, the sensitivity ranged from 78 to 81%, and specificity from 79 to 84%. For FPG at a cut-off point of $\geq$6.1 mmol l^{-1}, the sensitivity ranged from 48 to 64% and specificity from 94 to 98%. Both, HbA$_{1c}$ and FPG have a low sensitivity for the detection of IGT (ca. 50%).

In the Melton diabetes survey the HbA_1 levels were measured, using a Corning Gel electrophoresis method, in subjects with diabetes and in a random selection of other subjects with normal and impaired glucose tolerance, with an upper limit normal range of 8.5% [50]. Fifteen of 25 new diabetic subjects had an elevated HbA_1, while only one of 26 normal glucose-tolerant subjects had a raised HbA_1. The extrapolation of these data to the whole population, including IGT subjects, provided a sensitivity of 63% but a specificity of 91%

In the Birmingham Care Home Study, HbA_{1c} was measured using a latex-enhanced competitive turbidimetric immunoassay (Unimate 5 HbA_{1c}; Roche Diagnostics Division, F. Hoffmann-La Roche Ltd, Basel, Switzerland) with a reference range of 3.5–6.5% [31, 76]. When considering an HbA_{1c} elevated above the normal range (>6.5%), 10 of 38 diabetic subjects and 12 of 189 non-diabetic subjects had elevated HbA_{1c} levels (sensitivity 26%, specificity 94%, predictive value positive test = 0.45, predictive value negative test = 0.86). The ROC curve analysis gave an optimum cut-off of 6.2%, with elevated HbA_{1c} in 19 diabetic and 32 non-diabetic residents (sensitivity 0.5, specificity 0.83, predictive value of positive test = 0.37, predictive values of negative test = 0.89).

The use of HbA_{1c} (DCCT aligned) has been studied in acutely admitted stroke patients; this included all subjects who had an admission plasma glucose level ≥ 6.1 mmol l^{-1} who were later subjected to an OGTT at 12 weeks [94]. Here, a HbA_{1c} level of $\geq 6.2\%$ had a sensitivity of 86% and a specificity of 94%. It would be expected that few subjects with undiagnosed diabetes would have an admission plasma glucose <6.1 mmol l^{-1}. Hence, in this study the HbA_{1c} test performed well, possibly due to the high underlying prevalence of diabetes (21%) in this group.

Although, in older people HbA_{1c} is poorly sensitive, it is specific for undiagnosed diabetes. Yet, this may prove beneficial in the clinical situation, when an ill patient has hyperglycaemia: if their HbA_{1c} level is raised, they are highly likely to have diabetes; however, if it is not raised they might still be diabetic.

3.10 Fructosamine

Fructosamine is misleadingly named as it consists of glycosylated plasma proteins (mainly albumin), and does not involve fructose at all. Current clinical experience with fructosamine is far inferior to that with GHb, and the measurement is less well standardized.

The attraction of fructosamine is that its assay is easily automated, which makes it less costly. However, fructosamine levels are affected not only by the glucose level and the assay method, but also by albumin and lipid levels, and the time of day when the sample is taken [95].

In the Melton study, fructosamine levels were measured in 264 normal glucose-tolerant subjects using a standard method with the Cobas biocentrifugal analyzer, standardized against a human albumin solution [50, 96]. The upper limit of the normal range was taken as the 95th centile (1.92 mmol l^{-1}), which gave a sensitivity of 74%, and specificity and specificity of 95%. However, the authors noted that the upper limit of the 'normal' range varied widely, from 1.18 to 3.12 mmol l^{-1} in different populations reported elsewhere.

In recent years the fructosamine assay has been improved by removing other substances that interact with the assay, and by using improved standardization [97].

Among 157 free range elderly subjects (aged 65–88 years), serum fructosamine levels (first- and second-generation assays) were monitored and OGTTs performed [98]. As a consequence, 16 undiagnosed asymptomatic diabetic subjects were identified. ROC curves were used to provide the optimum cut-offs. When using a cut-off ≥ 2.3 mmol l^{-1} for the first-generation assay, the sensitivity to detect diabetes was 75%, specificity 83%, and positive predictive value 35%. With a cut-off of 250 μmol l^{-1} for the second-generation assay, the sensitivity to detect diabetes was 81%, specificity 87%, and positive predictive value 43%. Consequently, while the two fructosamine assays performed similarly in the elderly, the enhancement of the assay contributed little, as did adjustments for serum albumin or protein levels in other studies.

It may be useful to combine several blood tests. For instance, in a Hong Kong population, the paired values of an FPG of 5.6 mmol l^{-1} and a HbA_{1c} of 5.5% gave a sensitivity of 83.8% and specificity of 83.6% to predict a 2 h plasma glucose of ≥ 11.1 mmol l^{-1}, while the paired values of an FPG of 5.4 mmol l^{-1} and a fructosamine level of 235 μmol l^{-1} gave an optimal sensitivity of 81.5% and specificity of 83.2% [99]. Although these figures were impressive, again the population was selected to be at high risk of glucose intolerance, which improves the performance of the diagnostic tests; nonetheless, the result proved to be excellent in these subjects. However, these findings should be counterbalanced by Modan's study in an

Israeli general population, the results of which showed that the addition of HbA_1 to the FPG contributed zero [57].

3.11 Diabetes prediction calculators

In recent years there has been a growing interest in using patient information to select subjects at high risk of diabetes and in their screening, rather than to pre-screen with a blood or urine test. Examples include the Finnrisk calculator [100] and the USA Diabetes Prevention Program calculator [101], both of which were developed for populations with a high risk of diabetes. It has been shown, however, that calculators that function well in one population often do not do so in a different population.

The San Antonio clinical model formula used age, gender, ethnicity, fasting glucose level, systolic blood pressure, HDL-cholesterol level, BMI and parental or sibling history of diabetes [102]. In this predominantly middle-aged Hispanic population the model predicted the development of diabetes over the next 7.5 years, and probably worked well because the population was at very high risk of developing diabetes. When the San Antonio formula was applied to Japanese Americans of all ages, the model was good at predicting diabetes development in subjects under the age of 55 over a 5-year period, but was not helpful in subjects aged over 55 years [103].

Four screening tests – the Rotterdam Diabetes Study, the Cambridge Risk Score, the San Antonio Heart Study and the Finnish Diabetes Risk Score – were performed in 1353 participants (aged 55–74 years) without known diabetes in the Cooperative Health Research in the Region of Augsburg (KORA) Survey, and compared to OGTT results [104]. The sensitivity, specificity and the area under the ROC curve (termed the AUC) for undiagnosed diabetes were calculated. The AUCs were 61% (95% CI: 56–66%) for the Rotterdam Diabetes Study, 65% (95% CI: 60–69%) for the Finnish Diabetes Risk Score ($P = 0.10$ versus Rotterdam), and 67% (95% CI: 62–72%) for the Cambridge Risk Score ($P < 0.001$ versus Rotterdam). The San Antonio Heart Study model, which includes the fasting glucose level, yielded an AUC of 90% ($P < 0.01$ versus all three questionnaires); however, this was not significantly different from fasting glucose level alone (AUC, 89%; $P = 0.46$). The sensitivities, specificities and predictive values of questionnaires were substantially lower than originally described, which was mainly due to population variation of risk factors compared to the KORA sample (age, BMI, antihypertensive medication and smoking).

The Atherosclerosis Risk in Communities cohort study examined 7915 participants aged 45–64 years who were free of diabetes at baseline, and ascertained 1292 incident cases of diabetes by clinical diagnosis or OGTT [105]. A risk function based on waist, height, hypertension, blood pressure, family history of diabetes, ethnicity and age performed similarly to the fasting glucose level (AUC 0.71 and 0.74, respectively; $P = 0.2$). The addition of fasting glucose to the clinical model improved the AUC marginally (to 0.78), and including triglycerides and HDL-cholesterol provided an even better performance (AUC 0.80; $P < 0.001$). These models achieved sensitivities of 40–87% and specificities of 50–86% – similar to when using a diagnosis of metabolic syndrome.

In the NHANES 3 study, which was conducted in the USA in subjects aged up to 75 years, a Diabetes Risk Calculator that included questions on age, waist circumference, gestational diabetes, height, race/ethnicity, hypertension, family history and exercise, was developed [106]. This had sensitivity, specificity, positive and negative predictive values, and ROC for detecting undiagnosed diabetes of 88%, 75%, 14%, 99.3% and 0.85, respectively.

The Rancho Bernardo population was used to derive a prediction tool for abnormal glucose tolerance based on age, gender, FPG and triglyceride levels, where a cut-off of 4 points on the equation had a sensitivity of 46% and a specificity of 83% [107]. This was derived in a retired white population, but similar values were found in white and black populations aged 70–79 years.

Thus, while many prediction formulae may become available for the prediction of diabetes or abnormal glucose tolerance, they are highly dependent on the individual population being studied. Their performances are clearly altered by the age and ethnicity of the subjects such that, in some cases, it is no better than FPG. In fact, some other models actually include the FPG within the formula.

3.12 Known diabetes

It must be appreciated that the diagnosis of diabetes is not always correct; in the Melton diabetes survey, for example, 48 subjects were diagnosed as diabetic and had confirmatory blood tests in their medical records.

However, a further three subjects had a diagnosis of diabetes which was incorrect on diabetes testing; among these three, one subject had impaired glucose tolerance, one had a low renal threshold for glycosuria, and one simply had a name similar to another person who *did* have diabetes [30, 50].

In the Bristol admission plasma glucose study [82], 70 subjects were 'known' to have diabetes, but on testing this was refuted in five cases.

In the NHANES II study, a selected subgroup of 'known diabetic' subjects was tested, and 19% were shown *not* to have diabetes [32].

As well as the causes given above, other causes include stress-induced hyperglycaemia, drug-induced hyperglycaemia and incorrect application of the diagnostic criteria.

So, in a subject with 'known diabetes', the diagnosis should be questioned, although continuing with the incorrect diagnosis does help to achieve glycaemic targets.

3.13   Types of diabetes

It is clear that the majority of diabetes in the elderly is T2DM. For example, in the Oxford study 95% of subjects known to have diabetes had T2DM, as did 75% of the insulin-treated patients [108]. Nonetheless, T1DM does occur in the elderly, with studies conducted in Denmark and Rochester, USA, having shown that the incidence is similar at ages 30 to 80 years [44, 109].

The standard clinical criteria for classification as T1DM are either spontaneous significant ketosis, or any two of personal history of autoimmune disease, T1DM in a first-degree relative, significant osmotic symptoms, or significant weight loss (even if overweight at onset and still overweight) [110].

In some subjects, autoimmune diabetes can have an insidious onset, and is known as 'latent autoimmune diabetes of the adult' (LADA); the criteria include age ≥ 35 years, a 6–12 months period of diabetes prior to insulin initiation and the presence of glutamic acid decarboxylase (GAD) antibodies [111]. These subjects have an HLA genotype between T1DM and T2DM, their β-cell function deteriorates faster than in T2DM but slower than in T1DM, and they tend not to have the features of the metabolic syndrome. Although some question the rationale for the designation of LADA [112], it is important to realize that an elderly person presenting with diabetes that has the appearance of

T2DM, may rapidly fail if prescribed oral agents, and the need for insulin must not be overlooked.

As well as T1DM having an insidious onset in the elderly, T2DM can – at all ages – present with ketosis resembling T1DM, particularly in non-white ethnic groups; this is known by many names, of which 'ketosis-prone T2DM' seems most appropriate. Umpierrez and colleagues recently published an extremely succinct, yet comprehensive, review of the subject [113]. Features suggestive of ketosis-prone T2DM include non-white ethnic origin, newly diagnosed diabetes, obesity, family history of T2DM, negative autoantibodies (e.g., GAD or islet cells), fasting C-peptide levels of ≥ 0.33 nmol l^{-1} within one week after resolution of diabetic ketoacidosis (DKA), or ≥ 0.5 nmol l^{-1} after 6–8 weeks, and a glucagon-stimulated C-peptide level of 0.5 nmol l^{-1} at presentation and 0.75 nmol l^{-1} during follow-up.

Some subjects with T2DM are relatively slim, and are diagnosed with T2DM by virtue of a lack of autoantibodies; however, on testing their main defect is β-cell dysfunction and not insulin resistance [114]. T2DM with predominantly impaired β-cell function is particularly common among Oriental people.

Secondary diabetes is a disease of the elderly in which the incidence increases dramatically with age [44]; although this may be due to altered endocrine conditions, in practice it is due to chronic pancreatitis, and also to diabetogenic drugs such as glucocorticosteroids, thiazides, beta-receptor agonists (e.g., salbutamol tablets), β-blockers and the atypical antipsychotics [1, 115].

Although, it may be difficult to decide at the time of presentation of DKA, which type of diabetes a patient has, the recent Aβ classification [116] can be extremely helpful, by using immunologic and β-cell function measures (Table 3.2). This examines the autoantibodies and whether the β-cell function is preserved by virtue of a fasting serum C-peptide level ≥ 1 ng ml^{-1} or maximum glucagon-stimulated C-peptide ≥ 1.5 ng ml^{-1}, measured both at the time of DKA and at 6–12 months later; usefully, the 6–12 month results are often equivalent to the acute result, while the fasting result is often equivalent to the stimulated value. The significance of GAD positivity is still uncertain, however, since in a small group of elderly diabetic subjects GAD-positive individuals showed a greater insulin response than did GAD-negative individuals [117].

Table 3.2 Diagnostic outcomes of Aβ classification in USA subjects with DKA [116].

	β-Cell reserve present	β-Cell reserve absent
Antibodies −ve	Ketosis-prone T2DM: 55% of population	Insulin-requiring DM: 21% of population
Antibodies +ve	$1/2$ T1DM $1/2$ T2DM: 5% of population	T1DM: 19% of population

Adapted from Balasubramanyam *et al.* Diabetes Care. 2006; 29(12): 2575–9.

3.14 Metabolic syndrome

This condition is the clustering of obesity, insulin resistance, dyslipidaemia and hypertension; previously, this has also been referred to as Reaven's syndrome, syndrome X and the 'deadly quartet'. Its significance is that it predicts a doubling of the risk of vascular events and also multiplies the risk of developing diabetes in non-diabetic subjects fivefold [118]. Some studies have suggested that the increasing risk of vascular events with increasing number of components of metabolic syndrome is additive, whilst others have suggested that the effect is greater [118].

The criteria for the diagnosis of metabolic syndrome from bodies such as the WHO and National Cholesterol Education Program – Third Adult Treatment Panel, have been evolving and converging over recent years, and have culminated in the recent International Diabetes Federation (IDF) consensus guidelines [118].

The key component of metabolic syndrome is central obesity, assessed by waist measurement (with IDF cut-offs of ≥ 94 cm for Europid men and ≥ 80 cm for Europid women); the IDF cite waist cut-offs for different ethnic groups and gender, which should be applied to subjects wherever they live. The IDF committee make the point that the waist cut-offs are pragmatic, from various sources, and should be refined with time; there is no consideration of change in waist measurement with age.

The IDF definition of the metabolic syndrome [118] consists of central obesity (a waist circumference greater than ethnic-specific cut-offs, or BMI > 30), plus any two of: raised triglycerides (> 1.7 mmol l^{-1}); low HDL-cholesterol (< 1.03 mmol l^{-1} in males, 1.29 mmol l^{-1} in females); raised blood pressure (> 129 mmHg systolic or 84 mmHg diastolic, or treated hypertension); or a raised fasting plasma glucose (> 5.5 mmol l^{-1} or diabetes diagnosed).

The management of metabolic syndrome is via lifestyle modulation and the administration of drugs to avoid the development of diabetes and adverse vascular events

3.15 Future research

Although, for future investigations, the use of HbA$_{1c}$ as a screening tool might not be worthwhile, it would be intriguing to determine whether this parameter is affected by patient age. Likewise, while second-generation fructosamine assays may be of interest as a screening tool, in large studies they would most likely perform in similar fashion to the HbA$_{1c}$ assay.

It might also be important to ascertain whether diabetes detection in frail care home residents would lead to interventions that were beneficial, and this could perhaps be achieved via an audit.

Patient characteristics might also be used, either to provide a score suggesting that an OGTT should be performed in the short term, or which other test(s) to perform. For example, whereas very thin people require the post-challenge glucose level to be measured, the FPG may suffice in an obese patient. Other important variables to consider in this model would be the type of patient (e.g., care home resident, free range or acute hospital admission) and the BMI.

It is clear that paying more attention to postprandial glucose levels would be valuable, as might the combination of variables such as FPG and HbA$_{1c}$ or fructosamine.

Finally, further studies of the Aβ classification in other population groups to ensure the most appropriate treatment for subjects presenting with DKA would not only be of interest but also of great therapeutic value.

3.16 Conclusions

The detection of diabetes in elderly people is clearly worthwhile, not only because the undiagnosed disease is common but also that treatment can benefit these patients in several ways. However, no controlled trials have been conducted to justify this view.

A full ascertainment of glucose tolerance status requires a two-point OGTT to be performed, but in routine clinical practice it is impractical to test every potential patient. Thus an initial test is required to screen for those subjects at high risk of diabetes and, if identified, subsequently to perform the OGTT. While some subjects will be found to have glycosuria on urinalysis, a few will show osmotic symptoms. Although these features are less common with advancing age, public education and opportunistic urine testing might allow the identification of those people likely to have diabetes and in whom further testing is required. However, the evidence acquired from residential home settings suggests that osmotic symptoms are meaningless, although it would still be necessary to conduct a blood glucose test in the presence of any relevant symptoms (i.e., in half of all residents). At present, random blood/plasma glucose measurements (notably 1 h postprandial) offer the best sensitivity and specificity in both free range and acute hospital admission settings, but perform poorly in the residential care setting, where the modified OGTT shows superior sensitivity and specificity but it is complicated to carry out.

It is important to appreciate that the above details apply to the different populations studied; with different ages, diabetes prevalences and/or BMIs, these screening tests are likely to perform differently. The findings of any pre-screening test will vary depending on the population characteristics (notably age, residence, BMI), the technical details of the test used, and the prevalence of diabetes in the population, with screening tests performing better in high-prevalence populations.

When considering a screening program, it is also necessary to consider not only the scientific aspects – whether a specific population is being tested – but also the practical aspects. For example, although a simple screening test might only show 50% sensitivity, it would be much more easy to perform in all patients than would a two-point OGTT.

Whichever screening test is carried out, the most important point to appreciate is that all may provide false-negative results (some more than others). Consequently, a deteriorating patient will, at the bare minimum, require a glucose estimation to be made in a fingerprick capillary blood sample.

References

1. National Diabetes Data Group. Classification and diagnosis of diabetes mellitus and other categories of glucose intolerance. Diabetes 1979; 28: 1039–57.

2. WHO Study Group. (1980) Technical Report Series 646: Diabetes Mellitus. World Health Organization, Geneva.

3. Sayegh H and Jarrett R. Oral glucose-tolerance tests and the diagnosis of diabetes: results of a prospective study based on the Whitehall survey. Lancet 1979, 2 (8140), 431–3.

4. Dorf A, Ballintine E, Bennett P and Miller M. Retinopathy in Pima Indians. Relationships to glucose level, duration of diabetes, age at diagnosis of diabetes, and age at examination in a population with a high prevalence of diabetes mellitus. Diabetes 1976, 25(7), 554–60.

5. Jarrett R and Keen H. Hyperglycaemia and diabetes mellitus. Lancet 1976, 2 (7993), 1009–12.

6. Saad M, Knowler W, Pettitt D, Nelson R, Mott D and Bennett P. The natural history of impaired glucose tolerance in the Pima Indians. N Engl J Med 1988, 319 (23), 1500–6.

7. Pettitt D, Knowler W, Lisse J and Bennett P. Development of retinopathy and proteinuria in relation to plasma-glucose concentrations in Pima Indians. Lancet 1980, 2 (8203), 1050–2.

8. Rushforth N, Bennett P, Steinberg A, Burch T and Miller M. Diabetes in the Pima Indians. Evidence of bimodality in glucose tolerance distributions. Diabetes 1971, 20 (11), 756–65.

9. Zimmet P and Whitehouse S. The effect of age on glucose tolerance. Studies in a Micronesian population with a high prevalence of diabetes. Diabetes 1979, 28 (7), 617–23.

10. Lim T, Bakri R, Morad Z and Hamid M. Bimodality in blood glucose distribution: is it universal? Diabetes Care 2002, 25 (12), 2212–17.

11. Fan J, May S, Zhou Y and Barrett-Connor E. Bimodality of 2-h plasma glucose distributions in whites: the Rancho Bernardo study. Diabetes Care 2005, 28 (6), 1451–6.

12. Barrett-Connor E and Ferrara A. Isolated postchallenge hyperglycemia and the risk of fatal cardiovascular disease in older women and men. The Rancho Bernardo Study. Diabetes Care 1998, 21 (8), 1236–9.

13. Saydah S, Miret M, Sung J, Varas C, Gause D and Brancati F. Postchallenge hyperglycemia and mortality in a national sample of U.S. adults. Diabetes Care 2001, 24 (8), 1397–402.

14. THE DECODE study group on behalf of the European Diabetes Epidemiology Group. Glucose tolerance and cardiovascular mortality. Comparison of fasting and 2-h diagnostic criteria. Arch Intern Med 2001, 161, 397–404.

15. Shaw J, Hodge A, de Courten M, Chitson P and Zimmet P. Isolated post-challenge hyperglycemia confirmed as a risk factor for mortality. Diabetologia 1999, 42, 1050–4.

16. Neely R, Kiwanuka J and Hadden D. Influence of sample type on the interpretation of the oral glucose tolerance test for gestational diabetes mellitus. Diabetic Medicine 1991, 8, 129–34.

17. Home P. The OGTT: gold that does not shine. Diabetic Medicine 1988, 5 (4), 313–14.

18. Feskens E, Bowles C and Kromhout D. Intra- and interindividual variability of glucose tolerance in an elderly population. J Clin Epidemiol 1991, 44 (9), 947–53.

19. Toeller M and Knussmann R. Reproducibility of oral glucose tolerance tests with three different loads. Diabetologia 1973, 9 (2), 102–7.

20. Mykkänen L, Laakso M, Uusitupa M and Pyorala K. Prevalence of diabetes and impaired glucose tolerance in elderly subjects and their association with obesity and family history of diabetes. Diabetes Care 1990, 13 (11), 1099–105.

21. Croxson SCM, Price DE, Burden M, Jagger C and Burden AC. The mortality of elderly people with diabetes. Diabetic Medicine 1994, 11 (3), 250–2.

22. Valdés S, Botas P, Delgado E, Alvarez F, Cadórniga FD. Population-based incidence of type 2 diabetes in northern Spain: the Asturias Study. Diabetes Care 2007, 30 (9), 2258–63.

23. The Expert Committee on the Diagnosis and Classification of Diabetes Mellitus. Report of the Expert Committee on the Diagnosis and Classification of Diabetes Mellitus. Diabetes Care 1997, 20, 1183–97.

24. McCance D, Hanson R, Charles M, Jacobsson L, Pettitt D, Bennett P, et al. Comparison of tests for glycated haemoglobin and fasting and two hour plasma glucose concentrations as diagnostic methods for diabetes. British Medical Journal 1994, 308 (6840), 1323–8.

25. McHugh D. Letters: Tests for diagnosing diabetes mellitus. Glucose tolerance test is most sensitive. British Medical Journal 1994, 309, 537–8.

26. Simon K. Letters: Tests for diagnosing diabetes mellitus. Glucose tolerance test is most sensitive. British Medical Journal 1994, 309, 537–8.

27. Sinclair A. Letters: Tests for diagnosing diabetes mellitus. Glucose tolerance test is most sensitive. British Medical Journal 1994, 309, 537–8.

28. Brenner H and Gefeller O. Variation of sensitivity, specificity, likelihood ratios and predictive values with disease prevalence. Statistics in Medicine 1997, 16 (9), 981–91.

29. World Health Organization and International Diabetes Federation. Definition and diagnosis of diabetes mellitus and intermediate hyperglycemia: Report of a WHO/IDF Consultation. World Health Organization, Geneva, 2006.

30. Croxson SCM, Burden AC, Bodington M and Botha JL. The prevalence of diabetes in elderly people. Diabetic Medicine 1991, 8 (1), 28–31.

31. Sinclair AJ, Gadsby R, Penfold S, Croxson SC and Bayer AJ. Prevalence of diabetes in care home residents. Diabetes Care 2001, 24 (6), 1066–8.

32. Harris MI, Hadden WC, Knowler WC and Bennett PH. Prevalence of diabetes and impaired glucose tolerance and plasma glucose levels in U.S. population aged 20-74 yr. Diabetes 1987, 36 (4), 523–34.

33. Harris MI, Flegal KM, Cowie CC, Eberhardt MS, Goldstein DE, Little RR, et al. Prevalence of diabetes, impaired fasting glucose, and impaired glucose tolerance in U.S. adults. The Third National Health and Nutrition Examination Survey, 1988-1994. Diabetes Care 1998, 21 (4), 518–24.

34. Simmons D and Williams D. Diabetes in the elderly: an underdiagnosed condition. Diabetic Medicine 1993, 10 (3), 264–6.

35. Wang S-L, Pan W-H, Hwu C-M, Ho L-T, Lo C-H, Lin S-L, et al. Incidence of NIDDM and the effects of gender, obesity and hyperinsulinaemia in Taiwan. Diabetologia 1997, 40, 1431–8.

36. Haffner S, Lehto S, Rönnemaa T, Pyörälä K and Laakso M. Mortality from coronary heart disease in subjects with type 2 diabetes and in nondiabetic subjects with and without prior myocardial infarction. N Engl J Med 1998, 339 (4), 229–34.

37. British Cardiac Society, British Hypertension Society, Diabetes UK, HEART UK, Primary Care Cardiovascular Society, Stroke Association. JBS 2: Joint British Societies' guidelines on prevention of cardiovascular disease in clinical practice. Heart 2005; 91 (Suppl. 5), v1–v52.

38. Howard-Williams J, Hillson R, Bron A, Awdry P, Mann J and Hockaday T. Retinopathy is associated with higher glycaemia in maturity-onset type diabetes. Diabetologia 1984, 27 (2), 198–202.

39. Hillson R, Hockaday T, Newton D and Pim B. Delayed diagnosis of non-insulin-dependent diabetes is associated with greater metabolic and clinical abnormality. Diabetic Medicine 1985, 2 (5), 383–6.

40. Colagiuri S, Cull C, Holman R and the UKPDS Group. Are lower fasting plasma glucose levels at diagnosis of type 2 diabetes associated with improved outcomes?: UK prospective diabetes study 61. Diabetes Care 2002, 25 (8), 1410–17.

41. Testa MA and Simonson DC. Health economic benefits and quality of life during improved glycemic

control in patients with type 2 diabetes mellitus: a randomized, controlled, double-blind trial. JAMA 1998, 280 (17), 1490–6.

42. Stratton IM, Adler AI, Neil HA, Matthews DR, Manley SE, Cull CA, *et al.* Association of glycaemia with macrovascular and microvascular complications of type 2 diabetes (UKPDS 35): prospective observational study. British Medical Journal 2000, 321 (7258), 405–12.

43. Wachtel TJ, Tetu-Mouradjian LM, Goldman DL, Ellis SE and O'Sullivan PS. Hyperosmolarity and acidosis in diabetes mellitus: a three-year experience in Rhode Island. J Gen Intern Med 1991, 6 (6), 495–502.

44. Melton LJ, 3rd, Palumbo PJ, Chu CP. Incidence of diabetes mellitus by clinical type. Diabetes Care. 1983; 6(1): 75–86.

45. Melton LJ, III, Palumbo PJ, Dwyer MS and Chu CP. Impact of recent changes in diagnostic criteria on the apparent natural history of diabetes mellitus. Am J Epidemiol 1983, 117 (5), 559–65.

46. Butterfield WJ, Keen H and Whichelow MJ. Renal glucose threshold variations with age. British Medical Journal 1967, 4 (5578), 505–7.

47. Singh BM, Jackson DM, Wills R, Davies J and Wise PH. Delayed diagnosis in non-insulin dependent diabetes mellitus. British Medical Journal 1992, 304 (6835), 1154–5.

48. Jackson DM, Wills R, Davies J, Meadows K, Singh BM and Wise PH. Public awareness of the symptoms of diabetes mellitus. Diabetic Medicine 1991, 8 (10), 971–2.

49. Croxson SCM and Burden AC. Polyuria and polydipsia in an elderly population: Its relationship to previously undiagnosed diabetes. Practical Diabetes International 1998, 15 (6), 170–2.

50. Croxson S. Diabetes in the elderly. PhD thesis, University of Leicester, Leicester, 1995.

51. Haavisto M, Mattila K and Rajala S. Blood glucose and diabetes mellitus in subjects aged 85 years or more. Acta Med Scand 1983, 214 (3), 239–44.

52. Sharp CL, Butterfield WJ and Keen H. Diabetes Survey in Bedford 1962. Proceedings of the Royal Society of Medicine 1964, 57, 193–202.

53. Forrest R, Jackson C and Yudkin J. Glucose intolerance and hypertension in north London: the Islington Diabetes Survey. Diabetic Medicine 1986, 3 (4), 338–42.

54. Wei O and Teece S. Best evidence topic report. Urine dipsticks in screening for diabetes mellitus. Emerg Med J 2006, 23 (2), 138.

55. Davies MJ, Williams DR, Metcalfe J and Day JL. Community screening for non-insulin-dependent diabetes mellitus: self-testing for post-prandial glycosuria. Q J Med 1993, 86 (10), 677–84.

56. Friderichsen B and Maunsbach M. Glycosuric tests should not be employed in population screenings for NIDDM. J Public Health Med 1997, 19, 55–60.

57. Modan M, Halkin H, Karasik A and Lusky A. Effectiveness of glycosylated hemoglobin, fasting plasma glucose, and a single post load plasma glucose level in population screening for glucose intolerance. Am J Epidemiol 1984, 119 (3), 4431–44.

58. Wingard DL, Sinsheimer P, Barrett Connor EL and McPhillips JB. Community-based study of prevalence of NIDDM in older adults. Diabetes Care 1990, 13 (Suppl. 2), 3–8.

59. Wong T, Liew G, Tapp R, Schmidt M, Wang J, Mitchell P, *et al.* Relation between fasting glucose and retinopathy for diagnosis of diabetes: three population-based cross-sectional studies. Lancet 2008, 371, 736–43.

60. The DECODE study group on behalf of the European Diabetes Epidemiology Group. Glucose tolerance and mortality: comparison of WHO and American Diabetes Association diagnostic criteria. Lancet 1999, 354, 617–21.

61. The DECODE Study Group. Will new diagnostic criteria for diabetes mellitus change phenotype of patients with diabetes? Reanalysis of European epidemiological data. British Medical Journal 1998, 317, 371–5.

62. Croxson SCM and Thomas PH. Glucose tolerance test results reappraised using recent ADA criteria. Practical Diabetes International 1998, 15 (6), 178–80.

63. Davies MJ, Ammari F, Sherriff C, Burden ML, Gujral J and Burden AC. Screening for Type 2 diabetes mellitus in the UK Indo-Asian population. Diabetic Medicine 1999, 16 (2), 131–7.

64. Piché M, Arcand-Bossé J, Després J, Pérusse L, Lemieux S and Weisnagel S. What is a normal glucose value? Differences in indexes of plasma glucose homeostasis in subjects with normal fasting glucose. Diabetes Care 2004, 27 (10), 2470–7.

65. Balkau B, Shipley M, Jarrett R, Pyörälä K, Pyörälä M, Forhan A, *et al.* High blood glucose concentration is a risk factor for mortality in middle-aged nondiabetic men. 20-year follow-up in the Whitehall Study, the Paris Prospective Study, and the Helsinki Policemen Study. Diabetes Care 1998, 21 (3), 360–7.

66. Modan M, Halkin H, Karasik A and Lusky A. Effectiveness of glycosylated hemoglobin, fasting plasma glucose, and a single post load plasma glucose level in population screening for glucose intolerance. Am J Epidemiol 1984, 119 (3), 431–44.

67. Gabir M, Hanson R, Dabelea D, Imperatore G, Roumain J, Bennett P, *et al.* The 1997 American Diabetes Association and 1999 World Health Organization criteria for hyperglycemia in the diagnosis

and prediction of diabetes. Diabetes Care 2000, 23 (8), 1108–12.

68. Chang C, Wu J, Lu F, Lee H, Yang Y and Wen M. Fasting plasma glucose in screening for diabetes in the Taiwanese population. Diabetes Care 1998, 21 (11), 1856–60.

69. Dunstan DW Zimmet PZ, Welborn TA, De Courten MP, Cameron AJ, Sicree RA, Dwyer T, Colagiuri S, Jolley D, Knuiman M, Atkins R and Shaw JE. The rising prevalence of diabetes and impaired glucose tolerance: the Australian Diabetes, Obesity and Lifestyle Study. Diabetes Care 2002, 25 (5), 829–34.

70. Choi K, Lee J, Kim D, Kim S, Shin D, Kim N, et al. Comparison of ADA and WHO criteria for the diagnosis of diabetes in elderly Koreans. Diabetic Medicine 2002, 19 (10), 853–7.

71. Wahl P, Savage P, Psaty B, Orchard T, Robbins J and Tracy R. Diabetes in older adults: comparison of 1997 American Diabetes Association classification of diabetes mellitus with 1985 WHO classification. Lancet 1998, 352, 1012–15.

72. Unwin N, Alberti K, Bhopal R, Harland J, Watson W and White M. Comparison of the current WHO and new ADA criteria for the diagnosis of diabetes mellitus in three ethnic groups in the UK. Diabetic Medicine 1998, 15 (7), 554–7.

73. The Expert Committee on the Diagnosis and Classification of Diabetes Mellitus. Report of the Expert Committee on the Diagnosis and Classification of Diabetes Mellitus. Diabetes Care 2003, 26 (Suppl. 1), S5–S20.

74. Croxson S and Mostafa S. What is normal Fasting Plasma Glucose? Practical Diabetes International 2008, 25 (5), 209.

75. WHO Expert Committee. Health of the Elderly. World Health Organization, Geneva, 1989.

76. Croxson S, Bayer A and Sinclair A. Screening for diabetes in care homes. Diabetic Medicine 2005, 22(Suppl. 2), 100 (P928).

77. Simmons D and Williams D. Random blood glucose as a screening test for diabetes in a bi-ethnic population. Diabetic Medicine 1994, 11 (9), 830–5.

78. Engelgau M, Thompson T, Smith P, Herman W, Aubert R, Gunter E, et al. Screening for diabetes mellitus in adults. The utility of random capillary blood glucose measurements. Diabetes Care 1995, 18 (4), 463–6.

79. Simmons D, Williams D and Powell M. Prevalence of diabetes in a predominantly Asian population; preliminary findings of the Coventry diabetes study. British Medical Journal 1989, 298, 18–21.

80. Andersson D, Lundblad E and Svärdsudd K. A model for early diagnosis of type 2 diabetes mellitus in

primary health care. Diabetic Medicine 1993, 10 (2), 167–73.

81. Bitzén P and Scherstén B. Assessment of laboratory methods for detection of unsuspected diabetes in primary health care. Scand J Prim Health Care 1986, 4 (2), 85–95.

82. Croxson SCM, Keir SL and Ibbs L. Admission plasma glucose and diabetes mellitus in elderly admissions to hospital. Diabetic Medicine 1997, 14 (5), 381–5.

83. US Food and Drug Administration. Glucose Meters and Diabetes Management. 2008 [updated 2008; cited 05/03/2008]. Available from: http://www.fda.gov/diabetes/glucose.html#8 (accessed 1 August 2008).

84. Atkin S, Dasmahapatra A, Jaker M, Chorost M and Reddy S. Fingerstick glucose determination in shock. Ann Intern Med 1991, 114 (12), 1020–4.

85. Desachy A, Vuagnat A, Ghazali A, Baudin O, Longuet O, Calvat S, et al. Accuracy of bedside glucometry in critically ill patients: Influence of clinical characteristics and perfusion index. Mayo Clin Proc 2008, 83, 400–5.

86. Kilpatrick E. Problems in the assessment of glycaemic control in diabetes mellitus. Diabetic Medicine 1997, 14, 819–31.

87. Jiao Y, Okumiya T, Saibara T, Park K and Sasaki M. Abnormally decreased HbA1c can be assessed with erythrocyte creatine in patients with a shortened erythrocyte age. Diabetes Care 1998, 21 (10), 1732–5.

88. Simon D, Senan C, Garnier P, Saint-Paul M and Papoz L. Epidemiological features of glycated haemoglobin A1c-distribution in a healthy population. The Telecom Study. Diabetologia 1989, 32 (12), 864–9.

89. Altman D and Royston P. The cost of dichotomising continuous variables. British Medical Journal 2006, 332, 1080.

90. Kilpatrick ES, Dominiczak MH and Small M. The effects of ageing on glycation and the interpretation of glycaemic control in Type 2 diabetes. Q J Med 1996, 89 (4), 307–12.

91. Kabadi U. Glycosylation of proteins. Lack of influence of aging. Diabetes Care 1988, 11 (5), 429–32.

92. Davidson M, Schriger D, Peters A and Lorber B. Revisiting the oral glucose tolerance test criterion for the diagnosis of diabetes. J Gen Intern Med 2000, 15 (8), 551–5.

93. Bennett C, Guo M and Dharmage S. HbA1c as a screening tool for detection of Type 2 diabetes: a systematic review. Diabetic Medicine 2007, 24 (4), 333–43.

94. Gray CS, Scott JF, French JM, Alberti KGMM and O'Connell JE. Prevalence and prediction of unrecognised diabetes mellitus and impaired glucose tolerance

following acute stroke. Age Ageing 2004, 33 (1), 71–7.

95. Flückiger R, Woodtli T and Berger W. Evaluation of the fructosamine test for the measurement of plasma protein glycation. Diabetologia 1987, 30 (8), 648–52.

96. Croxson SCM, Absalom S and Burden AC. Fructosamine in diabetes screening of the elderly. Annals of Clinical Biochemistry 1991, 28 (3), 279–82.

97. Cefalu W, Bell-Farrow A, Petty M, Izlar C and Smith J. Clinical validation of a second-generation fructosamine assay. Clin Chem Lab Med 1991, 37 (7), 1252–6.

98. Cefalu WT, Ettinger WH, Bell-Farrow AD and Rushing JT. Serum fructosamine as a screening test for diabetes in the elderly: a pilot study. Journal of the American Geriatrics Society 1993, 41 (10), 1090–4.

99. Ko G, Chan J, Yeung V, Chow C, Tsang L, Li J, et al. Combined use of a fasting plasma glucose concentration and HbA1c or fructosamine predicts the likelihood of having diabetes in high-risk subjects. Diabetes Care 1998, 21 (8), 1221–5.

100. Lindström J and Tuomilehto J. The diabetes risk score: a practical tool to predict type 2 diabetes risk. Diabetes Care 2003, 26 (3), 725–31.

101. Diabetes Prevention Program Research Group. Strategies to identify adults at high risk for type 2 diabetes: the Diabetes Prevention Program. Diabetes Care 2005, 28 (1), 138–44.

102. Stern M, Williams K and Haffner S. Identification of persons at high risk for type 2 diabetes mellitus: do we need the oral glucose tolerance test? Ann Intern Med 2002, 136 (8), 575–81.

103. McNeely M, Boyko E, Leonetti D, Kahn S and Fujimoto W. Comparison of a clinical model, the oral glucose tolerance test, and fasting glucose for prediction of type 2 diabetes risk in Japanese Americans. Diabetes Care 2003, 26 (3), 758–63.

104. Rathmann W, Martin S, Haastert B, Icks A, Holle R, Löwel H, et al. Performance of screening questionnaires and risk scores for undiagnosed diabetes; The KORA Survey 2000. Arch Intern Med 2005, 165 (436-441), 436.

105. Schmidt M, Duncan B, Bang H, Pankow J, Ballantyne C, Golden S, et al. Identifying individuals at high risk for diabetes: The Atherosclerosis Risk in Communities study. Diabetes Care 2005, 28 (8), 2013–18.

106. Heikes KE, Eddy DM, Arondekar B and Schlessinger L. Diabetes Risk Calculator: a simple tool for detecting undiagnosed diabetes and pre-diabetes. Diabetes Care 2008, 31(5), 1040–5.

107. Kanaya A, Wassel Fyr C, de Rekeneire N, Shorr R, Schwartz A, Goodpaster B, et al. Predicting the development of diabetes in older adults: the derivation and validation of a prediction rule. Diabetes Care 2005, 28 (2), 404–8.

108. Neil H, Thompson A, Thorogood M, Fowler G and Mann J. Diabetes in the elderly: the Oxford Community Diabetes Study. Diabetic Medicine 1989, 6 (7), 608–13.

109. Molbak AG, Christau B, Marner B, Borch-Johnsen K and Nerup J. Incidence of insulin-dependent diabetes mellitus in age groups over 30 years in Denmark. Diabetic Medicine 1994, 11 (7), 650–5.

110. Gale E and Tattersall R. (1990) The new patient: assessment & management. In: R. Tattersall and E. Gale (eds), Diabetes: Clinical Management. Churchill Livingstone, Edinburgh, pp. 3–16.

111. Groop L, Tuomi T, Rowley M, Zimmet P and Mackay I. Latent autoimmune diabetes in adults (LADA) – more than a name. Diabetologia 2006, 49 (9), 1996–8.

112. Gale E. Latent autoimmune diabetes in adults: a guide for the perplexed.. Diabetologia 2005, 48 (11), 2195–9.

113. Umpierrez G, Smiley D and Kitabchi A. Narrative review: ketosis-prone type 2 diabetes mellitus. Ann Intern Med 2006, 144 (5), 350–7.

114. Meneilly G and Elahi D. Metabolic alterations in middle-aged and elderly lean patients with type 2 diabetes. Diabetes Care 2005, 28 (6), 1498–9.

115. Livingstone C and Rampes H. Atypical antipsychotic drugs and diabetes. Practical Diabetes International 2003, 20 (9), 327–31.

116. Balasubramanyam A, Garza G, Rodriguez L, Hampe C, Gaur L, Lernmark A, et al. Accuracy and predictive value of classification schemes for ketosis-prone diabetes. Diabetes Care 2006, 29 (12), 2575–9.

117. Meneilly G, Tildesley H, Elliott T, Palmer J and Juneja R. Significance of GAD positivity in elderly patients with diabetes. Diabetic Medicine 2000, 17 (3), 247–51.

118. Alberti G, Zimmet P, Shaw J and Grundy SM, for the International Diabetes Federation Task Force on Epidemiology and Prevention. The IDF consensus worldwide definition of the METABOLIC SYNDROME, Brussels, International Diabetes Federation, 2006 (http://www.idf.org/webdata/docs/IDF_Meta_def_final.pdf).

SECTION III
Vascular Complications

4

Peripheral Arterial Disease in Old People with Diabetes

Leocadio Rodríguez Mañas, Cristina Alonso Bouzon and Marta Castro Rodríguez

Servicio de Geriatría, Hospital Universitario de Getafe, Madrid, Spain

Key messages

- Peripheral arterial disease (PAD) is a very prevalent disease in the elderly. Often, the clinical presentation is atypical, and on many occasions the only manifestation is a functional impairment.
- PAD is a cardiovascular risk factor and a marker of mortality.
- The treatment of PAD can improve the patient's quality of life. Hence, an early diagnosis must be actively sought in the elderly patient with diabetes.

4.1   Introduction

Peripheral arterial disease (PAD) is a condition that is often ignored, underdiagnosed and poorly treated in everyday medical practice. This reality is even greater among the elderly, in whom the typical symptoms of PAD (e.g., pain, claudication) appear in less than 50% of cases. Unfortunately, these symptoms may also be mistaken for others that are attributable to conditions that are very prevalent in the elderly, such as osteoarthritis or neuropathy.

Very often – and typically in older patients – the only manifestation of PAD is a loss of function, which translates into a progressive loss of autonomy to perform daily activities. At present, the actual prevalence of PAD in the elderly population is unknown, which makes it even more difficult to identify those cases with gait disorders and/or falls where the underlying (or adjuvant) cause is PAD. Accordingly, a high index of suspicion has been accorded to PAD when it is identified as a cause of functional impairment and falls in old patients.

Another reason which leads us to 'ignore' this disease is its relatively 'benign' evolution. By not compromising key organs, such as the heart or brain, PAD has traditionally been regarded as less important than coronary disease or brain vascular disease. This, in turn, has led us to ignore the serious consequences of the evolution of PAD, including amputation, and the serious prognostic implications of the presence of atherosclerotic lesions in the legs. The mortality rate for PAD at 5 years, of approximately 30%, is higher than that of many cancers. The majority of these patients will die from vascular complications that do not occur in the lower limbs, but occur rather in coronary and cerebral territories. The results of recent studies have suggested that the risk of a vascular event of any territory is approximately twice in patients with PAD as in those with coronary or cerebral vascular involvement.

For this reason, PAD has in recent years become an important marker of cardiovascular risk, allowing the identification of subjects who are at very high cardiovascular risk and who require an intensive treatment

Diabetes in Old Age. Third Edition. Edited by Alan J. Sinclair
© 2009 John Wiley & Sons, Ltd

of risk factors in order to delay the risk of functional impairment.

4.2 Epidemiology of peripheral arterial disease

From an epidemiological standpoint, atherothrombosis accounts – either directly or indirectly – for 70% of all deaths in people aged over 70 years. The factors that lead to atherosclerotic disease are multiple, and include genetic aspects, metabolic diseases, inflammatory diseases, lifestyle and local and systemic conditions of the vascular system. Among these conditions and diseases are included the major risk factors, namely older age, smoking, hypertension, dyslipidaemia, type 2 diabetes mellitus, physical inactivity and abdominal obesity. Indeed, the INTERHEART study showed that while nine of these factors were responsible for 90% of cardiovascular diseases, older age was the only *unmodifiable* risk factor.

While older age is also the main risk factor for PAD, other risk factors include smoking, diabetes, hypertension, dyslipidaemia and hyperhomocysteinaemia.

- *Smoking* not only predisposes to develop PAD but also increases its severity. Smoking may also affect the prognosis of revascularization interventions.

- *Diabetes mellitus* as a risk factor is both qualitative and quantitative. In fact, glycemic control represents one of the most powerful risk factors for illness and for the main consequence of this disease, amputation. In this regard, amputation is 10-fold more frequent in diabetic than in non-diabetic patients.

- Although, as a risk factor, *hypertension* contributes to a lesser extent than either smoking or diabetes mellitus to the development of PAD, it must also be controlled.

- With regards to *dyslipidaemia*, a high total cholesterol:HDL-cholesterol ratio seems to be the best predictor of PAD, and its lowering has been shown to reduce progression of the disease and in turn the risk of developing critical ischemia.

- An alteration in the metabolism of *homocysteine* is an important risk factor for atherosclerosis; however, its role is most likely age-dependent, as it is more relevant in young people.

While the prevalence of PAD in the elderly (considered as aged >70 years) is generally 15–20%, this figure would be even higher if the proportion of apparently healthy elderly people investigated for its detection were to be increased. The most widely used diagnostic test to detect PAD is the ankle–brachial index, for which a value <0.9, with a sensitivity >95% and specificity close to 100%, is effective in the diagnosis of PAD (see Figure 4.1). In the recently conducted MERITO I study, the prevalence of a low ankle–brachial index (ABI) was evaluated in older patients with metabolic syndrome and the risk factors associated with its development. The study showed that in those patients with metabolic syndrome, factors associated with a low ABI (<0.9) were age, higher serum creatinine levels and the presence of proteinuria. After multivariate adjustment, only age and active smoking continued to be significantly associated with a low ABI [1].

Typically, patients with PAD have a cardiovascular mortality of 2.5%, compared to only 0.5% for healthy controls. In patients with coronary artery disease, if PAD is present then the cardiovascular mortality is 25%. In conjunction with PAD serving as an overall predictor for cardiovascular risk, the ABI may also be used as a marker of subclinical functional decline.

4.3 Pathophysiology

Atherosclerosis is a process of thickening and stiffening of the arteries, the basic lesion being the *atherosclerotic plaque*. Until recently, the classic concept of atherosclerosis was the mechanical accumulation of lipids and a fibrodegenerative response of the arterial wall by changes in its structure, which in turn caused a progressive failure of tissue perfusion.

Today, these previous ideas have been added to the concept of inflammation, such that atherosclerotic disease is regarded as a true multifactorial disease in which metabolic, inflammatory, hemodynamic and haemostatic factors are involved, with both local and systemic roles. There is no correlation between the histological phases of the atheroma lesion and clinical symptoms in the elderly patients. Frequently, the first sign appears when the local lesion is advanced; consequently, the early active diagnosis of atherosclerosis is very important (see Figure 4.2).

It is important, therefore, that the presence of atherosclerosis is detected at an early stage. To that end, it is essential to identify any physiological disorders associated with endothelial dysfunction and its progression toward atherothrombosis, long before these become visible obstructive lesions. This highlights the

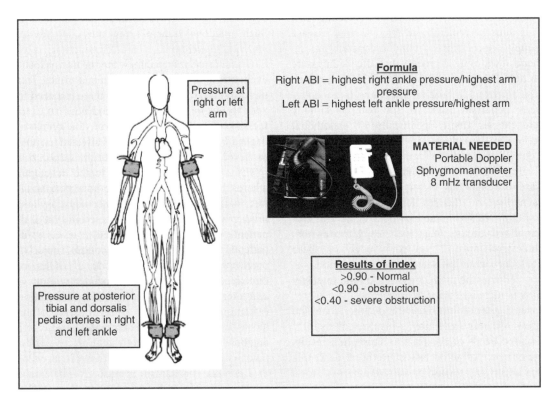

Figure 4.1 The ankle–brachial index.

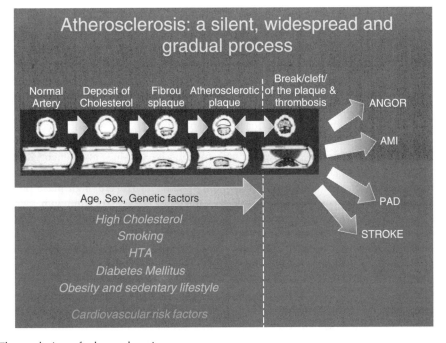

Figure 4.2 The evolution of atherosclerosis.

importance of the early treatment of vascular risk factors. It must be remembered that vascular disease is not simply a local process within a concrete plaque, but rather is a widespread process that affects the entire vascular tree. This concept has therapeutic implications because it forces us to raise an integrated treatment.

Another important aspect of the pathophysiology of atherosclerosis (more specifically of endothelial dysfunction) in the elderly is which of the processes that occur at the endothelium can be attributed to physiological aging, and which to the presence of other cardiovascular risk factors. Some of the mechanisms involved in the development of endothelial dysfunction are in fact shared by both aging and cardiovascular risk factors (e.g., diabetes, hypertension, hypercholesterolemia) [2]. A knowledge of these issues has deep practical therapeutic implications, as they may serve as the main constraint on the intensity of cardiovascular risk factor treatment.

Peripheral arterial insufficiency occurs when the blood flow reaching the limbs is insufficient to fulfil the metabolic needs of the tissues. This often results from the presence of an occlusive arterial disease, this being the underlying disease process of atherosclerosis and affecting primarily – though not exclusively – the vascularization of the lower limbs.

Although atherosclerosis – and in particular the formation of atherosclerotic plaque – is an universal process, it does show certain pathophysiological differences, depending on the anatomic location in question. Atherosclerotic plaques located in high-risk lower limbs are very fibrous and strictures and, when associated with a hypercoagulable state, this gives rise to an acute event. By contrast, at level of the coronary arteries, the atherosclerotic plaque consists of a large extracellular lipid core and a large number of foam cells, coated with a thin cover that is susceptible to breakage; such breakage is the ultimate cause of any acute event that might happen. In any event, common to all these injuries there is a consequence of an imbalance between the needs of the tissues and blood flux. If this mismatch occurs suddenly, as in a thrombotic event, then it will lead to acute ischemia. However, if the establishment of a stenosis is gradual, allowing the development of a collateral circulation, and/or a metabolic adaptation of the muscle mass involved and the use of non-ischemic muscle groups, then ischemia may persist as a chronic state (see Figure 4.2).

From the pathophysiological point of view, it is possible to refer to *functional ischemia* when the blood flow is insufficient for any demand that involves

exercise, but is sufficient when the patient is resting. Such functional ischemia translates clinically as *intermittent claudication*.

Critical ischemia occurs when the flow is insufficient even at rest, and appears as pain and trophic lesions in the extremities. In this situation there is a need to intervene to restore an adequate blood flow, so as to avoid the risk of amputation. However, the symptoms will depend largely on the number of affected territories and the level of physical activity that the subject demands.

Glyco-oxidation contributes to the development of atherosclerosis in the below-the-knee peripheral artery tree in type 2 diabetes. Advanced glycosylation end product (AGE) levels are increased in type 2 diabetic patients with PAD, as compared to levels in diabetic patients without PAD and in control subjects. More precisely, among the components of AGEs, pentosidine appears to be strongly associated with the peripheral artery status of diabetic patients. In addition, lipid oxidation, as estimated by the serum levels of malondialdehyde (MDA), is associated with diabetic peripheral angiopathy. In contrast, both total reactive antioxidant potentials (TRAP) and vitamin E levels, as expressions of a defence mechanism against glycolipid oxidation, are lower in type 2 diabetic patients with PAD than in those without PAD and in healthy subjects [3].

However, the presence of several cardiovascular risk factors, which act in synergistic manner, is an important factor in progression of the disease and amputation. However, not all cardiovascular risk factors contribute equally: for example, diabetes mellitus increases the risk of critical ischemia fourfold and smoking threefold, while an ABI <0.5 increases such risk 2.5-fold. In addition to these factors, in the case of amputation, there are other independent risk factors for amputation, notably sensory neuropathy, PAD, previous minor amputations and the use of insulin [4].

In the Wisconsin study, which followed a cohort that included elderly patients for 14 years, male gender, high levels of HbA1c, high pulse pressure and severe retinopathy were associated with a greater power to a need for amputation, while regular aspirin consumption was protective [5].

In addition, other factors that are very prevalent in the elderly (e.g., physical disability, loss of vision or a shortage of social resources) act as facilitators of the amputation. However, in the pathogenesis of diabetic amputations in the elderly, coexisting involvement of the peripheral nervous system, microvascular damage and infection are the most important concurrent factors. Peripheral neuropathy diminishes pain perception, placing the skin at risk for suffering from continuous damage and muscle atrophy. As a consequence, changes in the points of support occur, downloading the pressure on areas not prepared for such change. As a result the metatarsal heads may suffer ischemic necrosis which, in the presence of ulcers, might facilitate the development of osteomyelitis. Sensory neuropathy hinders the perception of pain as a symptom of alarm, thereby facilitating the emergence of pressure ulcers. The autonomic neuropathy facilitates the opening of artery–vein shunts and causes skin hydration to become difficult.

The involvement of the *microcirculation* has been widely discussed. Although the basement membrane is seen to become thickened, this does not seem to be clinically significant in the absence of peripheral and autonomic neuropathy. Other factors, which are related both directly and indirectly to vascular injury, cooperate in the development of clinically apparent damage: the ischemia causes pain, especially in patients with high blood glucose levels, and difficulty may be encountered in the healing of existing injuries while the sterilization of infected lesions may be delayed. Other mechanisms that can hinder healing include AGEs or a zinc shortfall in relation to its increased renal elimination in patients with poor glycemic control. It is quite possible that this mechanism should be enhanced in the elderly. The ischemia that occurs due to a poor circulation also prevents the antibiotic from targeting the infected ulcers.

Finally, other mechanisms associated with hyperglycemia may participate in the pathogenesis of the diabetic foot, but this is more controversial. It is especially the case for the decline in chemotaxis, phagocytosis and bacterial lysis secondary to hyperglycemia [6].

Among elderly patients, while amputation remains the most dramatic complication, as it creates not only disability but also psychological damage, it must not be forgotten that on many occasions the cause of functional decline – notably in those with sarcopenia – is that of PAD.

4.4 Clinical presentation

4.4.1 Asymptomatic

Although intermittent claudication (see Section 4.4.2) is the most common symptom in patients with PAD, the majority of individuals with this pathology do not experience this typical limb ischemic symptom. Rather, some studies [7, 8] have demonstrated how intermittent claudication may underestimate the prevalence of PAD. The reasons for such asymptomatic presentation might be the development of collateral arteries, a muscular adjustment to the ischemia, and the employment of muscular groups least affected. Added to this, the presence of comorbidity and functional impairment in some elderly patients do not allow them to perform a sufficiently active life to provoke intermittent claudication. On the other hand, chronic ischemia can modify the muscle function. In a sub-study from the Women's Health and Aging Study [9], those patients with a low ABI but without claudication were characterized by a slow walking, a longer time to arise from a seated position than normal, a poor standing balance score, and a shorter weekly walking distance, even after making adjustments for age, gender, race, cigarette smoking and comorbidities. Similar results were found elsewhere [10, 11], highlighting the importance of functional impairment as a frequent means of clinical presentation of PAD in older people. Furthermore, those patients with a low ABI but no claudication do not enjoy a benign functional [9, 12] and cardiovascular [13, 14] prognosis. In fact, it is important to note that there is no relationship between the injury severity and the clinical presentation of the disease, with the severity of the vascular injuries being the most important prognostic factor.

4.4.2 Claudication

Claudication is defined as fatigue, discomfort or pain that occurs in specific limb muscle groups during effort, as a result of exercise-induced ischemia [15]. These symptoms are absent at rest. It is important to determine a differential diagnosis from other causes of ischemia (e.g., emboli, Berger's disease, other arteritides), and in particular claudication must be distinguished from other illnesses that cause exertional leg pain – so-called 'pseudoclaudication' – as a result perhaps of lumbar disease and spinal stenosis, osteoarthritis, severe venous obstructive disease and peripheral neuropathy.

The anatomic site of an arterial stenosis has been associated frequently with specific leg symptoms. For example, obstructions in the femoral and popliteal arteries are associated with calf pain, while affectation in the tibial arteries may produce calf pain, foot pain or numbness. Occlusive disease in the iliac arteries could produce hip, buttock, thigh pain and calf pain.

Table 4.1 Fontaine's stages of the severity of clinical symptoms of patients with PAD. Values in parentheses indicate walking distances.

Fontaine stage	Clinical finding
I	Asymptomatic
IIa	Mild claudication (>150 m)
IIb	Moderate-severe claudication (<150 m)
III	Ischemic rest pain
IV	Ulceration or gangrene

The severity of the clinical symptoms allows patients with PAD to be categorized (see Table 4.1). This is not only especially useful for facilitating communication between different specialists, but also has important therapeutic value. Although intermittent claudication is often poorly correlated with the actual stenosis, the symptoms, their repercussions on the quality of life and the potential benefits with different treatment strategies, are each keys to decide between revascularization and conservative treatment.

4.4.3 Critical limb ischemia

Critical limb ischemia is defined as limb pain which occurs at rest, or as the immediate limb loss caused by a severe compromise of blood flow to the affected extremity [15]. This pain, which may be sharp in nature, occurs typically at rest, especially when the patient is supine or when the leg is held in an elevated position. Occasionally, narcotics may be needed to control the pain, but these may often cause severe side effects in the elderly. Consequently, such drugs should be avoided whenever possible, but if unavoidable they should be used with extreme caution. These patients may also suffer trophic skin changes or tissue loss, ulcers or gangrene. Ischemic ulcers are very painful (unless they are associated with neuropathy), and have irregular margins, no pulses, are dry, and occur frequently on the toes with a cold, pale or cyanotic foot. These ulcers are usually associated with infection in the surrounding tissues.

Critical limb ischemia may represent the initial presentation of a lower-extremity PAD, and occur more frequently among elderly diabetic patients. This situation arises because the arterial disease develops especially on small arteries [16]; there is also often an important comorbidity such that the intermittent claudication is suppressed.

Although generally the progression of PAD from asymptomatic and intermittent claudication to critical limb ischemia will occur gradually, occasionally a rapid or sudden decrease in limb perfusion will threaten tissue viability. Pain, paralysis, paresthesias, pulselessness and pallor are the five 'P's that suggest this syndrome. In this case it is imperative that the patient is evaluated by a vascular surgeon as an emergency case.

4.5 Diagnostic methods

4.5.1 Anamnesis and physical assessment

The diagnosis of PAD is based mainly on a clinical evaluation, and the medical history. Very often, a patient will minimize the symptoms, attributing them to normal aging; consequently, an active search for intermittent claudication or any atypical presentation of PAD must be carried out, thereby distinguishing any symptoms from those of a non-vascular cause (pseudoclaudication) [15, 17]. A careful history, including a comprehensive geriatric assessment, may allow the discovery of functional impairment at clinical presentation.

A physical assessment should include an examination with the patient's shoes and socks removed, paying special attention to pulses (femoral, popliteal, posterior tibial and pedal), bruits, hair loss, skin colour, temperature, ulcers and trophic skin changes [18].

The clinical guidelines for type 2 diabetes mellitus (European Diabetes Working Party for Older People 2004) [19] suggest that a comprehensive geriatric assessment should be routine in older people with type 2 diabetes, both at the initial diagnosis and thereafter at regular intervals. Further recommendations include (at minimum) an annual inspection of the feet by a health care professional, including vascular and neurological examinations, even in the absence of any symptoms.

Other physical measures, such as a slow walking speed, a longer time to rise from a seated position, or a poor standing balance score, have been related to the presence of subclinical disease [9]. At present, no evidence is available of the sensitivity and prognostic values of these latter symptoms/signs within the usual clinical setting.

4.5.2 Vascular diagnostic techniques

These tests allow the objective establishment of a diagnosis of PAD, for the severity of the disease to be quantified, the stenosis to be localized, a plan of treatment to be organized, and the progression of disease or its response to treatment to be determined.

The ABI is a quick and cost-effective method for providing sufficient information for the screening, diagnosis and follow-up. In order to calculate the ABI, the systolic blood pressures are determined in both arms and both ankles, using a hand-held Doppler instrument (see Figure 4.1). Although the ABI has been validated against the 'gold standard' of lower-extremity contrast angiography [20, 21], in patients with non-comprehensible arteries, such as long-term diabetics and very old patients, it may not be sufficiently accurate, raising the probability of obtaining false-negative results. In these cases, other alternative non-invasive diagnostic tests (e.g., the toe–brachial index, exercise ABI test, pulse volume recording) should be performed [15].

An altered ABI has been associated with systemic atherosclerotic disease, total and cardiovascular mortality [22, 23] and functional impairment [9]. Today, the American Diabetes Association (ADA) suggests that the ABI must be performed by the general practitioner for all patients with diabetes who are aged ≥50 years (i.e., in every old patient), in diabetic individuals aged <50 years who have other atherosclerosis risk factors, and in those patients who have been diabetic for at least 10 years [24].

Other possible diagnostic techniques include magnetic resonance angiography and computed tomographic angiography, both of which can be used to identify the anatomic location and degree of a stenosis. These methods are valuable when selecting patients, notably those for endovascular treatment. The diagnostic performance of both imaging procedures is quite similar, but computed tomographic angiography is preferred when magnetic resonance is contraindicated. Today, contrast angiography is regarded as the 'gold standard', and is the definitive method before revascularization procedures. However, it may be associated with a higher risk of medical complications (e.g., bleeding, infection, contrast allergy) than non-invasive techniques and should be performed only in selected (surgical) patients [15].

4.6 Treatment

4.6.1 Foot care

The use of appropriate footwear to avoid pressure injuries, the use of moisturizing cream to prevent dryness and fissuring, as well as daily inspections and cleansing by the patient and chiropodist, are necessary measures to reduce the risk of skin ulceration, necrosis and amputation. These measures are recommended based on the results of studies in which their effects in diabetic patients have been analyzed [25, 26]; however, no investigations appear to have been carried out analyzing the impact of such measures in elderly diabetic patients with PAD.

4.6.2 Cardiovascular risk reduction

The treatment of patients with PAD requires that each modifiable risk factor associated with the development and evolution of the condition be addressed, including cigarette smoking, diabetes mellitus, sedentary lifestyle, dyslipidaemia, hyperhomocystinaemia and hypertension. To date, no conclusive evidence has been reported regarding the relationship between the control of risk factors and the prognosis of PAD. Nevertheless, the need to control cardiovascular risk factors in the manifestation of atherosclerosis has been well established, as has the association between PAD and systemic atherosclerosis. Consequently, the screening and treatment of cardiovascular risk factors should be regarded as a priority in all patients with PAD, independent of their clinical manifestations.

No evidence has yet been provided to suggest the preferred control level of cardiovascular risk factors in elderly diabetic patients with PAD. Hence, the treatment goals are similar to those for diabetic elderly patients [15].

Antiplatelet therapy with aspirin, using daily doses of 75 to 325 mg, reduces the risk of vascular death, myocardial infarction and stroke in patients with PAD [27]. Although clopidogrel appears to be more effective than aspirin in preventing ischemic events in individuals with symptomatic PAD [28], the size effect does not allow any broad recommendation to be made regarding its use instead of aspirin. Thus, the more expensive thienopyridines (ticlopidine and clopidogrel) may be considered as alternatives to aspirin when patients are unable to tolerate the latter. Currently available data have not indicated any advantage of dual antiplatelet therapy over single-agent therapy.

4.6.3 Intermittent claudication

In addition to the previously described approaches to treat intermittent claudication, it is important also to consider exercise and rehabilitation, as well as pharmacological and endovascular treatments focused on specific manifestations of the condition [15]. There is strong evidence supporting the beneficial effects of exercise [29, 30], with regular walking, within a supervised claudication exercise program, having been shown to improve walking time free of pain by an average of 150% (range: 74 to 230%). Such a program was based on certain specifications, with the patient walking at close to the maximum tolerable pain, for more than 30 min per session, three times each week for more than six months.

Cilostazol is a phosphodiesterase type 3 inhibitor with vasodilatory and antiplatelet properties. Following cilostazol treatment (100 mg, twice daily), the walking distance was increased by approximately 50% compared to placebo, after 3–6 months of therapy [31]. Unfortunately, cilostazol is contraindicated in patients with heart failure, which limits its use in old people with diabetes, where heart failure is very common. Pentoxifylline has been considered a second-line therapy to improve walking distances, but its efficacy is not well established; indeed, this is also the case for other pharmacological agents, including oral vasodilator prostaglandins, vitamin E and ginkgo biloba.

Endovascular or surgical revascularization therapy is reserved for those patients in whom the functional capacity is compromised only by claudication (not for other comorbidities), for those who have not responded to exercise and pharmacotherapy, and for those in whom the risk–benefit ratio with revascularization is favourable [15]. These patients, and those with critical and acute limb ischemia, should be referred to a vascular surgeon.

Recently, the role of stem or progenitor cells in vascular disease, including atherosclerosis and post-angioplasty restenosis, has been demonstrated [32–35]. Although such studies utilized animal models, this line of investigation clearly constitutes a new approach in the treatment of PAD.

References

1. Suarez C, Manzano L, Mostaza J, Cairols M and Palma JC. Prevalence of peripheral artery disease evaluated by ankle brachial index in patients with metabolic syndrome. MERITO I study. *Rev Clin Esp*. 2007; 207: 228–33.

2. Serrano Hernando FJ and Martín Conejero A. Peripheral artery disease: pathophysiology, diagnosis and treatment. *Rev Esp Cardiol* 2007; 60: 969–82.

3. Lapolla A, Piarulli F, Sartore G, Ceriello A and Ragazzi E. Advanced glycation end products and antioxidant status in type 2 diabetic patients with and without peripheral artery disease. *Diabetes Care* 2007; 30: 670–6.

4. Adler AJ, Boyko EJ, Ahroni JH and Smith DG. Lower extremity amputation in diabetes. The independent effects of peripheral vascular disease, sensory neuropathy and foot ulcers. *Diabetes Care* 1999; 22: 1029–35.

5. Moss SE, Klein R and Klein BEK. The 14-year incidence of lower-extremity amputations in a diabetic population. *Diabetes Care* 1999; 22: 951–9.

6. Rodríguez-Mañas L and Monereo Megías S. (2002) *El anciano con diabetes*. Sociedad Española de Medicina Geriátrica (Spanish Society of Geriatric Medicine)/Sociedad Española de Endocrinología y Nutrición. Villanueva, Madrid.

7. Meijer WT, Hoes AW, Rutgers D, Bots ML, Hofman A and Grobbee DE. Peripheral arterial disease in the elderly: the Rotterdam Study. *Arterioscler Thromb Vasc Biol* 1998, 18: 185–92.

8. Criqui MH, Fronek A, Barret-Connor E, Klauber MR, Gabriel S and Goodman D. The prevalence of peripheral arterial disease in a defined population. *Circulation* 1985, 71: 510–15.

9. McDermott MM, Ferrucci L, Simonsick EM, Balfour J, Fried L, Ling S, Gibson D and Guralnik JM. The ankle brachial index and change in lower extremity functioning over time: the Women's Health and Aging Study. *J Am Geriatr Soc* 2002; 50: 238–46.

10. McDermott MM, Greenland P, Liu K, Guralnik JM, Criqui MH, Dolan NC, Chan C, Celic L, Pearce WH, Schneider JR, Sharma L, Clark E, Gibson D and Martin GJ. Leg symptoms in peripheral arterial disease: associated clinical characteristics and functional impairment. *JAMA* 2001, 286: 1599–606.

11. Doland NC, Liu K, Criqui MH, Greenland P, Guralnik JM, Chan C, Schneider JR, Mandapat AL, Martin G and McDermott MM. Peripheral artery disease, diabetes, and reduced lower extremity functioning. *Diabetes Care* 2002, 25: 113–20.

12. McDermott MM, Liu K, Greenland P, Guralnik JM, Criqui MH, Chan C, Pearce WH, Schneider JR, Ferrucci L, Celic L, Taylor LM, Vonesh E, Martin GJ and Clark E. Functional decline in peripheral arterial disease: associations with the ankle brachial index and leg symptoms. *JAMA* 2004, 292: 453–61.

13. Long TH, Criqui MH, Vasilevskis EE, Denenberg JO, Klauber MR and Fronek A. The correlation between the severity of peripheral arterial disease and carotid occlusive disease. *Vasc Med* 1999; 4: 135–42.

14. Criqui MH and Denenberg JO. The generalized nature of atherosclerosis: how peripheral arterial disease may predict adverse events from coronary artery disease. *Vasc Med* 1998, 3: 241–5.

15. Hirsch AT, Haskal ZJ, Hertzer NR, *et al.* ACC/AHA 2005 Practice Guidelines for the management of patients with peripheral arterial disease (lower extremity, renal, mesenteric, and abdominal aortic): a collaborative report from the American Association for Vascular Surgery/Society for Vascular Surgery. *Circulation* 2006, 113: e463–e654.

16. Aboyans V, Criqui MH, Denenberg JO, Knoke JD, Ridker PM and Fronek A. Risk factors for progression of peripheral arterial disease in large and small vessels. *Circulation* 2006, 113: 2623–9.

17. Schmieder FA and Comerota AJ. Intermittent claudication: magnitude of the problem, patient evaluation, and therapeutic strategies. *Am J Cardiol* 2001, 87: 3D–13D.

18. White, C. Intermittent claudication. *N Engl J Med* 2007; 356: 1241–50.

19. European Diabetes Working Party for Older People. (2004) Clinical guidelines for Type 2 Diabetes Mellitus. www.eugms.org/index.php?pid=30 (accessed 6 December 2008).

20. Lijmer JG, Hunink MG, van den Dungen JJ, Loonstra J and Smit AJ. ROC analysis of noninvasive tests for peripheral arterial disease. *Ultrasound Med Biol* 1996, 22: 391–8.

21. Feigelson HS, Criqui MH, Fronek A, Langer RD and Molgaard CA. Screening for peripheral arterial disease: the sensitivity, specificity and predictive value of noninvasive tests in a defined population. *Am J Epidemiol* 1994, 140: 526–34.

22. Newman AB, Siscovick DS, Manolio TA, Polak J, Fried LP, Borhani NO and Wolfson SK. Ankle-arm index as a marker of atherosclerosis in the Cardiovascular Health Study (CHS) Collaborative Research Group. *Circulation* 1993, 88: 837–45.

23. Newman AB, Sutton-Tyrrel K, Vogt MT and Kuller LH. Morbidity and mortality in hypertensive adults with a low ankle/arm blood pressure index. *JAMA* 1993, 270: 487–9.

24. American Diabetes Association. Peripheral arterial disease in people with diabetes. *Diabetes Care* 2003, 26: 3333–41.

25. Plank J, Haas W, Rakovac I, Görzer E, Sommer R, Siebenhofer A and Pieber TR. Evaluation of the impact of chiropodist care in the secondary prevention of foot ulcerations in diabetic subjects. *Diabetes Care* 2003, 26: 1691–5.

26. Reiber GE, Smith DG, Wallace C, Sullivan K, Hayes S, Vath C, Maciejewski ML, Yu O, Heagerty PJ and LeMaster J. Effect of therapeutic footwear on foot reulceration in patients with diabetes: a randomized controlled trial. *JAMA* 2002, 287: 2552–8.

27. Antithrombotic Trialists' Collaboration. Collaborative metaanalysis of randomised trials of antiplatelet therapy for prevention of death, myocardial infarction and stroke in high risk patients. *Br Med J* 2002, 324: 71–86.

28. CAPRIE Steering Committee. A randomised, blinded, trial of clopidogrel versus aspirin in patients at risk of ischaemic events (CAPRIE). *Lancet* 1996, 348: 1329–39.

29. Leng GC, Fowler B and Ernst E. Exercise for intermittent claudication. *Cochrane Database Syst Rev*, 2000: CD000990

30. Bendermacher BL, Willigendael EM, Teijink JA and Prins MH. Supervised exercise therapy versus non-supervised exercise therapy for intermittent claudication. *Cochrane Database Syst Rev*, 2006: CD005263.

31. Strandness DE, Jr, Dalman RL, Panian S, Rendell MS, Comp PC, Zhang P and Forbes WP. Effect of cilostazol in patients with intermittent claudication: a randomized, double-blind, placebo-controlled study. *Vasc Endovascular Surg* 2002, 36: 83–91.

32. Nevskaya T, Ananieva L, Bykovskaia S, Eremin I, Karandashov E, Khrennikov J, Mach E, Zaprjagaeva M, Guseva N and Nassonov E. Autologous progenitor cell implantation as a novel therapeutic intervention for ischaemic digits in systemic sclerosis. *Rheumatology* 2009; 48 (1): 61–4.

33. Werner N and Nickenig G. Clinical and therapeutical implications of EPC biology in atherosclerosis. *J Cell Mol Med.* 2006; 10 (2): 318–32.

34. Versari D, Lerman LO and Lerman A. The importance of reendothelialization after arterial injury. *Curr Pharm Des.* 2007; 13 (17): 1811–24.

35. Kiernan TJ, Yan BP, Cruz-Gonzalez I, Cubeddu RJ, Caldera A, Kiernan GD and Gupta V. Pharmacological and cellular therapies to prevent restenosis after percutaneous transluminal angioplasty and stenting. *Cardiovasc Hematol Agents Med Chem.* 2008; 6 (2): 116–24.

5

Coronary Heart Disease

Ahmed H. Abdelhafiz

Department of Elderly Medicine, Rotherham General Hospital, Rotherham, UK

Key messages

- Cardiovascular disease is the single most important cause of death in patients aged 70 years and over, and diabetes is an independent risk factor for cardiovascular disease.
- In older people with diabetes, significant evidence of coronary heart disease may be present, with few or no symptoms.
- Optimizing cardiovascular care requires a multifaceted approach that targets risk factor identification, hypertension, dyslipidaemia, the hypercoagulable state, as well as glucose control.

5.1 Introduction

Diabetes mellitus has been recognized as an independent major cardiovascular risk factor since the publication of the Framingham study in 1979 [1]. In spite of various known metabolic and microvascular complications of diabetes, cardiovascular disease (CVD) remains the most common cause of death in all age groups. Diabetes itself, in the absence of associated CVD, constitutes a risk similar to those of non-diabetic individuals with previous history of myocardial infarction (MI) [2]. In that sense, diabetes is considered as a 'coronary risk equivalent', and any prevention in this population should be considered as a secondary prevention. In fact, it may be appropriate to say that diabetes is a CVD. On top of that, when diabetics

develop coronary heart disease (CHD) they have at least twice excess risk of morbidity and worse cardiovascular outcomes compared to non-diabetics. Moreover, myocardial ischemia due to coronary atherosclerosis is commonly silent in diabetics. As a result, CHD is often present before ischemic symptoms occur. Hyperglycemia, insulin resistance, hyperinsulinaemia and visceral obesity, in addition to 'traditional' risk factors, are the major contributors to CVD in diabetics. In this chapter we review the major risk factors for CHD, MI and heart failure (HF) in diabetes, with particular emphasis on evidence relevant to older people (as much as available). Because type 2 diabetes affects the vast majority of older people diagnosed with diabetes, it will be the primary focus of the chapter.

5.2 Effect of ageing and diabetes on the cardiovascular system

Both, ageing and diabetes have profound effects on the cardiovascular system structure and function. Indeed, such related changes to the cardiovascular system are themselves increasingly recognized as risk factors for CVD.

5.2.1 The effect of ageing

Vascular ageing contributes to the age-dependent rise in hypertension and atherosclerotic disease. With increasing age, the intima of the arterial wall becomes less smooth, with an increased deposition of lipid, cal-

Diabetes in Old Age. Third Edition. Edited by Alan J. Sinclair
© 2009 John Wiley & Sons, Ltd

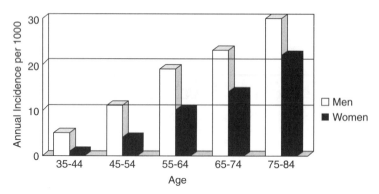

Figure 5.1 Incidence of coronary heart disease by age in men (light bars) and women (dark bars). Reproduced with permission from Ref. [12].

cium and connective tissue. In the media, there is an increased deposition of elastic fibres and smooth muscle cells, which in turn leads to a stiffening of the vascular wall and a loss of compliance of the aorta and major arteries [3]. This loss of compliance plays a central pathophysiological role in systolic hypertension in older people. Isolated systolic hypertension and a wide pulse pressure are a result of reduced compliance, and are a powerful determinant of cardiovascular risk [4]. The elastic recoil of the central arteries in diastole is important for coronary perfusion, as a loss of such elasticity impairs the coronary blood flow and may also contribute to the development of CHD. Both, arterial function and vascular ageing, could be programmed during fetal life or influenced by adverse growth patterns in early postnatal life [5]. However, interindividual variations in the risk of occurrence of ageing changes, and the development of CVD may be genetic in origin [6, 7]. The responsiveness of arterioles to the catecholamine alpha-adrenergic receptor also decreases with ageing, and this prevents an adequate increase in systemic vascular resistance from occurring in older individuals during orthostasis [8], making them prone to drug-induced orthostatic hypotension [9].

At the level of the myocardium, a prolonged exposure to a high systolic pressure leads to an increased myocyte turnover, with subsequent hypertrophy and interstitial fibrosis. This results in a stiff, non-compliant myocardium, which in turn leads to diastolic dysfunction and an impaired early diastolic filling of the ventricles [10]. Left ventricular hypertrophy has been shown to be associated with an increased risk of CVD [11]. The increased large artery thickening, stiffness

and endothelial dysfunction in apparently healthy older people lead to increases in the systolic and pulse pressures that were formerly thought to be part of normal ageing. This vascular ageing precedes and predicts a higher risk for the development of clinical disease; indeed, what is now referred to as vascular disease could be regarded as the vascular ageing–vascular disease interaction [12]. This results in a steep increase in the prevalence and incidence of CHD by increasing age (Figure 5.1) [12].

5.2.2 The effect of diabetes

Arterial endothelium normally produces vasoactive substances such as nitric oxide (vasodilator) and endothelin (vasoconstrictor and procoagulant). In diabetes, when endothelin production increases and nitric oxide production decreases; this favours a procoagulant state and promotes vascular smooth muscle growth, causing in turn an increased risk of cardiovascular events [13]. The formation of advanced glycosylation end products also increases in diabetes, and this leads to structural wall changes and endothelial dysfunction [14, 15]. The increased risk of CVD in diabetes is not fully explained by the traditional risk factors, and there is some evidence to suggest that abnormalities of insulin-like growth factor-1 and one of its binding proteins, insulin-like growth factor binding protein-1, occur in insulin-resistant states and may be significant factors in the pathophysiology of CVD [16].

At the level of the myocardium, diabetes is associated with an abnormal left ventricular structure and function in older people; typically, the left ventricular mass increases in diabetes. In the Cardiovascular

Health Study, among a cohort of 5201 men and women aged ≥ 65 years, the echocardiographically measured ventricular septal and left posterior wall thicknesses were greater in diabetic than in non-diabetic subjects, showing a significant linear trend with increased duration of diabetes ($p = 0.025$ for ventricular septal thickness; $p = 0.002$ for posterior wall thickness). An increased wall thickness of the ventricular septum or the left posterior wall was not associated with prevalent CHD in the cohort. After adjusting for body weight, blood pressure, heart rate and prevalent coronary or cerebrovascular disease, diabetes remained an independent predictor of increased left ventricular mass among men and women (174.2 g in diabetic men versus 169.8 g in normal men; 138.2 g versus 134.0 g, respectively, for women; $p = 0.043$ for both genders combined). This association between diabetes and left ventricular mass appeared to be both duration- and severity-dependent [17]. Diabetes also impairs cardiac diastolic function, leading to a myopathic state known as *diabetic cardiomyopathy*. This involves a prolongation of contraction and relaxation, as well as a slowing in relaxation velocity [18]. Potential abnormalities underlying this cardiomyopathy include hyperglycemia, hyperinsulinaemia and alterations in cell membrane electrolyte channels functions [19]. An impaired left ventricular function occurs before clinical diabetes, and affects individuals with an impaired glucose tolerance [20]. As a result, diabetics may be more prone to HF and other cardiovascular events, independently of traditional cardiovascular risk factors.

To summarize:

- The effects of ageing include:
  - Increased arterial wall thickness and stiffness
  - Predisposition to systolic hypertension and wide pulse pressure
  - Loss of elastic recoil of aorta and impaired coronary filling
  - Predisposition to orthostatic hypotension
  - Hypertrophy and diminished compliance of the ventricles

- The effects of diabetes include:
  - Structural arterial wall changes and endothelial dysfunction
  - Predisposition to a procoagulant state
  - Diastolic dysfunction and diabetic cardiomyopathy
  - Increased ventricular mass

5.3 Epidemiology

Today, as the prevalence of type 2 diabetes continues to increase rapidly in the developed world, due to the ageing of the population and an increased frequency of obesity, the prevalence of associated CVD is also increasing [21]. This is likely to lead to an epidemic of CHD over the next decades. Currently, CVD is the most common cause of death in diabetic patients, affecting between 65% and 80%, compared to only one-third of all deaths in the general population [22]. The prevalence of CHD is approximately 80% of elderly Americans with type 2 diabetes [23]. Silent or asymptomatic CHD is also highly prevalent among diabetics, with autopsy studies having reported a prevalence of CHD in diabetics but without ante-mortem evidence of clinical CHD, ranging from 50% to 75% [24, 25]. Screening for CHD in diabetic patients will not alter risk factor management, because these patients are considered at high risk on the basis of diabetes alone [26]. However, screening may be useful in high-risk patients in whom revascularization therapy will be indicated. This is particularly important as CHD in diabetic patients may be asymptomatic or present atypically (shortness of breath instead of chest pain) than in non-diabetic patients [27]. The incidence of CHD is also higher in the diabetic population more than in non-diabetics. In a prospective study of a diabetic cohort aged >65 years and followed up for six years after first diagnosed as having diabetes, approximately 40% were shown to have HF compared to 20% for controls. Similarly, the rate of MI among the diabetic cohort was almost twice that for controls [28].

5.4 Cardiovascular risks

The National Cholesterol Education Program (NCEP) recommends that diabetic patients do not need specific CHD risk assessment, but instead that they be managed as if they had CHD [29]. Consequently, by definition:

- *Relative risk* is a measure of the likelihood of occurrence of the target event (death or disease) in those exposed in comparison to those not exposed to the agent of interest.

- *Absolute risk* is the likelihood or probability of occurrence of an event (death or disease) after exposure to an agent (risk factor) of interest.

- *Intervention* is the application of a modifying agent (e.g., drug or procedure) of the baseline risk of individual or population.

- *Relative risk reduction* is the percentage reduction in occurrence of an event in the population exposed to intervention, compared to that in the population not exposed to intervention (control).

- *Absolute risk reduction* is the percentage reduction in occurrence of the event in the population exposed to intervention from their baseline risk.

- *Number needed to treat (NNT)* is the number of patients needed to treat to prevent the occurrence of one event over a certain period of time.

Although the relative risk reduction might be similar in both diabetics and non-diabetics, the absolute risk reduction is likely to be more significantly beneficial in diabetics due to their higher baseline risk, while the number needed to treat would be expected to be lower. As a result, the aggressive control of all risk factors is especially important in diabetics, and includes both lifestyle modification and pharmacological intervention. This aggressive treatment is appropriate for elderly diabetics with a life expectancy of at least 10 years, but for those with a limited life expectancy, or multiple comorbidities, the objectives should be more conservative [30]. Between 50% and 75% of all deaths among patients with diabetes mellitus are cardiovascular-related, and type 2 diabetes increases the risk of death from CHD by between twofold and fourfold [31]. In The Cardiovascular Health Study, diabetes and increasing age were each seen to be independent predictors of CHD fatality [Odds ratio (OR) 1.66, 95% CI: 1.10 to 2.31 and 1.21 per 5 years; 95% CI: 1.07 to 1.37, respectively] among 5888 adults aged >65 years and followed up for a median of 8.2 years. Of the traditional CHD risk factors (hypertension, cholesterol, obesity), only diabetes was found to be an independent predictor for case fatality in this population [32].

The major cardiovascular risks include traditional risk factors of smoking, hypertension, dyslipidaemia in addition to hyperglycemia, visceral obesity, insulin resistance and hyperinsulinaemia. The identification of these risk factors is vitally important in the initial evaluation of diabetic patients. Hyperglycemia should not be treated in isolation, but the holistic view of the collective cardiovascular risk should constitute a comprehensive plan of intervention and risk

reduction in these patients. In a small randomized controlled trial of patients with type 2 diabetes, when a structured multifactorial intervention management (including behaviour modification and tight targets for blood glucose, blood pressure and lipids) in a specialist setting was compared with a conventionally managed group receiving the usual care in a primary care setting, the risks of CVD were reduced by 0.47 (95% CI: 0.24 to 0.73) in the multifactorial intervention group after eight years of follow up [33]. This comprehensive approach is currently suboptimal. In a recent study to assess whether elderly patients with type 2 diabetes (n = 48 505; aged >66 years) could use a comprehensive cardioprotective regimen (CCR) of anti-hypertensive, lipid-lowering and anti-platelet drugs in the year following oral anti-diabetic drug initiation, only 9912 (20.4%) used a CCR during the year following the first anti-diabetic medication [34].

5.4.1 Behaviour modification

Behaviour modifications include changes in diet, exercise, weight reduction and smoking cessation. Smoking cessation may be the single most effective means of reducing mortality in high-risk populations [35], as smoking is known to induce vasoconstrictive and toxic effects on the endothelium. After only one year of smoking cessation, the excess risk associated with current smoking was reduced by over 50%. However, many years of abstinence are required to reduce the risk of an ex-smoker to the level of a non-smoker. A diet that is high in fibre and potassium, and lower in saturated fats and refined carbohydrates and salt, will improve the lipid profile and significantly lower the blood pressure [36]. The achievement of an ideal body weight through diet changes and exercise will reduce the overall cardiovascular risk and have a favourable effect on the metabolic profile of lipids, glycaemia and blood pressure.

5.4.2 Metabolic syndrome

Cardiovascular risk factors rarely occur in isolation but rather tend to cluster in what is known as the *metabolic syndrome*. This is characterized by a group of risk factors including visceral obesity, dyslipidaemia [low high-density lipoprotein (HDL) cholesterol, high triglycerides], hypertension, impaired glucose/insulin homeostasis (insulin resistance, hyperinsulinaemia, glucose intolerance), increased cardiovascular oxidative stress, impaired endothelial

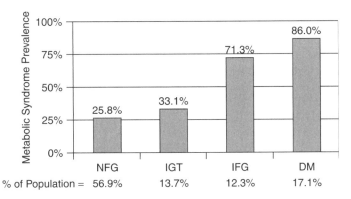

Figure 5.2 Age-adjusted prevalence of metabolic syndrome in the U.S. population over 50 years of age, categorized by glucose intolerance (NFG = normal fasting glucose; IGT = impaired glucose tolerance without impaired fasting glucose; IFG = impaired fasting glucose with or without impaired glucose tolerance; DM = diabetes mellitus). Reproduced with permission from Ref. [47].

function and abnormal coagulation and fibrinolytic profiles. Depending on various combinations of these risk factors, five definitions of metabolic syndrome exist [37–41]. The World Health Organization definition includes microalbuminuria (30–300 mg per 24 h) as a final component [37]. Microalbuminuria is a significant marker of CVD, and is highly associated with hypertension and diabetes [42]. The prevalence of metabolic syndrome increases with age; in a cohort of 2175 older people (>65 years) from the Cardiovascular Health Study, the prevalence was 21–28% (depending on the definition used) [43]. In the Three City Study, which included 5585 French, non-institutionalized, non-diabetic elderly subjects aged 65–85 years, the prevalence of metabolic syndrome was 12.1% [44]. In a Norwegian study, the prevalence of metabolic syndrome was increased from 11.0% in the 20–29 year-old group to 47.2% in the 80–89 year-old group in men, and from 9.2% to 64.4% in the corresponding age groups in women [45]. However, the magnitude of metabolic syndrome in elderly diabetic individuals is higher. For example, in a population-based study of 5632 Caucasians (aged 65–84 years), prevalences of 64.9% and 87.1% were found in diabetic men and women, respectively, compared to 25.9% and 55.2% in non-diabetics [46]. The prevalence of metabolic syndrome also increases with increasing glucose intolerance. In the Third National Health and Nutrition Examination survey (NHANES III) of the United States (US) population aged ≥50 years, there was a stepwise increase in the prevalence of metabolic syndrome with worsening glucose tolerance, from almost 26% in those with normal fasting glucose rising to 86% in those with diabetes [47] (Figure 5.2).

The metabolic syndrome is increasingly recognized as a risk factor for CVD [48], and was associated with ischemic electrocardiographic changes in 2274 elderly subjects enrolled in the Rancho Bernardo cross-sectional study [49]. The syndrome may also have adverse effects on the structural and functional properties of the arteries, such as increasing arterial wall stiffness and thickness, through a synergistic effect of the clustering of its components [50]. In a prospective study of 888 subjects aged 40–79 years, metabolic syndrome conferred a significantly increased risk for developing new carotid plaques [hazard ratio (HR) 1.5], new carotid stenosis (HR 2.5) and new coronary events (HR 2.3) [51]. In the Three City Study, subjects with metabolic syndrome had higher frequency of carotid plaques (OR 1.30, 95% CI: 1.09 to 1.55) and higher intima-media thickness of the common carotid artery (OR 1.81, 95% CI: 1.37 to 2.41) [44]. However, in a recent prospective study of 1025 elderly subjects aged between 65 and 74 years, metabolic syndrome was shown to be a marker of CVD, but not above and beyond the risk associated with its individual components [52]. In a more recent analysis of the outcome of two prospective studies in an elderly population aged >60 years, metabolic syndrome and its components were associated with type 2 diabetes but showed only a modest association with vascular risk in elderly populations. Therefore, metabolic syndrome in the elderly may not enhance risk prediction, and the criteria of metabolic syndrome may not offer more than the sum of its components [53].

5.4.3 Dyslipidaemia

Cholesterol levels tend to fall normally with increasing age, and low cholesterol levels are often associated with increased non-cardiovascular mortality, particularly cancer [54]. Low cholesterol levels appears to be associated with a lower body weight, disability, infections and other markers of general ill health, such as low serum albumin and iron [55]. This may be related to reduced hepatic cholesterol synthesis, poor appetite and low food intake in frail, older people [56]. Low cholesterol and low albumin levels could also be taken as markers of poor general health. In other words, a low plasma cholesterol in an elderly subject does not necessarily cause premature death, but instead may reflect the presence of subclinical disease. In contrast, a high cholesterol level is associated with increased cardiovascular events and mortality in all age groups. Indeed, there is a positive relationship between serum cholesterol level and cardiovascular risk. Statins are effective in lowering cholesterol, and reducing the risk of cardiovascular events, their efficacy having been demonstrated in numerous clinical trials with high-risk individuals having both high and normal cholesterol levels. The benefit of cholesterol-lowering therapy continues to lower levels than the normal range. In fact, there is no evidence of any threshold below which lower cholesterol levels are not associated with a lower risk, which suggests that cholesterol reduction would be useful for all those individuals at high cardiovascular risk, regardless of their baseline cholesterol level.

While the evidence for cholesterol lowering is clear for individuals aged up to 80 years, for older patients there is also some evidence of benefit from observational studies [57–59]. Whereas no mortality benefit was identified in patients aged >80 years and treated with a statin, those aged 65–79 years showed a significant (11%) reduction in mortality. There was evidence, however, of a greater trend towards benefit in those aged 80–85 years versus those aged >85 years [59]. The positive association between total and LDL-cholesterol and cardiovascular risk becomes attenuated with advancing age (and more so in men than in women [60]). However, in the Cholesterol Treatment Trialists Collaborators (CTTC) systematic prospective meta-analysis, which reported data from 14 randomized trials, those patients aged >65 years (n = 6446) had 19% reduction in the risk of major cardiovascular events, a benefit similar to the 22% reduction in risk experienced by those aged <65 years (n = 7902) [61].

Although statins are known to reduce the proportional risk to equal effect in older and younger patients, only limited data are available for elderly patients with type 2 diabetes. In the CTTC meta-analysis, which included 18 686 patients with diabetes out of a total of 90 056 participants, there was a 21% reduction (95% CI: 19–23) in major vascular events per 1 mmol l^{-1} reduction in LDL-cholesterol, and no difference in treatment effect between patients with and without diabetes [61]. The heart protection study included a total of 20 536 patients between the ages of 40–80 years, among which the older patients (>70 years) numbered 5806 (28%), and total diabetics 5963 (29%). The reduction in cardiovascular events following simvastatin therapy (40 mg daily) was 25% after five years of follow up in all subgroups, irrespective of the cholesterol level at the start of treatment. Although the relative risk reduction was similar in all subgroups, the absolute benefit was seen to depend on the individual's baseline risk, which is higher in diabetics [62, 63]. In a meta-analysis of 12 studies, conducted to evaluate the clinical benefit of lipid-lowering in patients with and without diabetes mellitus, the risk reduction for major coronary events was 21% (95% CI: 11–30%, P < 0.0001) in diabetic patients and 23% (95% CI: 12–33%; P = 0.0003) in non-diabetic patients for primary prevention. In secondary prevention, the corresponding risk reductions were 21% (95% CI: 10–31%; P = 0.0005) and 23% (95% CI: 19–26%, P ≤ 0.00001). However, the absolute risk difference was threefold higher in the secondary prevention. When results were adjusted for baseline risk, however, the benefit was greater in diabetic patients, and blood lipids were reduced to a similar degree in both groups [64]. The *post hoc* analysis of the Collaborative Atorvastatin Diabetes Study (CARDS) compared the efficacy and safety of atorvastatin among 1129 patients aged 65–75 years at randomization with 1709 younger patients without elevated LDL-cholesterol levels. Treatment with atorvastatin at 10 mg per day resulted in a 38% reduction in relative risk (95% CI: –58 to –8, P = 0.017) of the first major cardiovascular event in older patients, and a 37% reduction (95% CI: –57 to –7, P = 0.019) in younger patients. The corresponding absolute risk reductions were 3.9 and 2.7%, respectively (difference 1.2%, 95% CI: –2.8 to 5.3; P = 0.546), while the numbers needed to treat (NNT) for four years to avoid one event were 21 and 33, respectively. The higher absolute risk reduction and lower NNT in the elderly reflect their higher baseline risk. All-cause mortality was reduced non-significantly, by 22% (95% CI:

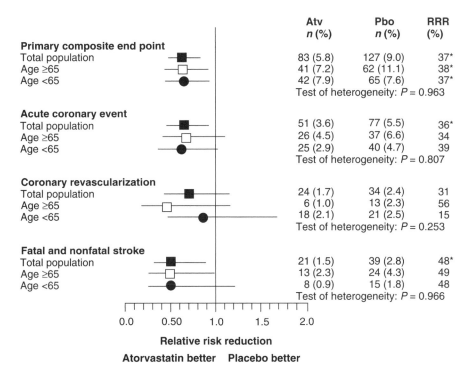

	Atv n (%)	Pbo n (%)	RRR (%)
Primary composite end point			
Total population	83 (5.8)	127 (9.0)	37*
Age ≥65	41 (7.2)	62 (11.1)	38*
Age <65	42 (7.9)	65 (7.6)	37*
	Test of heterogeneity: P = 0.963		
Acute coronary event			
Total population	51 (3.6)	77 (5.5)	36*
Age ≥65	26 (4.5)	37 (6.6)	34
Age <65	25 (2.9)	40 (4.7)	39
	Test of heterogeneity: P = 0.807		
Coronary revascularization			
Total population	24 (1.7)	34 (2.4)	31
Age ≥65	6 (1.0)	13 (2.3)	56
Age <65	18 (2.1)	21 (2.5)	15
	Test of heterogeneity: P = 0.253		
Fatal and nonfatal stroke			
Total population	21 (1.5)	39 (2.8)	48*
Age ≥65	13 (2.3)	24 (4.3)	49
Age <65	8 (0.9)	15 (1.8)	48
	Test of heterogeneity: P = 0.966		

Relative risk reduction

Atorvastatin better   Placebo better

*p <0.05 for atorvastatin vs. placebo.

Figure 5.3 Composite primary end point and components. The total number of acute coronary events, coronary revascularizations and strokes (separately) do not equal the total number of primary events shown above, because only the first of these events is included in the primary end point. Atv = atorvastatin; Pbo = placebo; RRR = relative risk reduction. Reproduced with permission from Ref. [65].

−49 to 18, P = 0.245) and 37% (95% CI: −64 to 9, P = 0.98), respectively. The reduction in total cholesterol, LDL-cholesterol and triglyceride was similar in both age groups, as was the overall safety profile of atorvastatin. The authors concluded that the absolute and relative benefits of statin therapy in older patients with type 2 diabetes were substantial, and that all older patients warranted treatment, unless specifically contraindicated [65] (Figure 5.3).

It appears from the above that statins should be prescribed for all older people with diabetes who have a reasonable life expectancy. Chronological age, in and of itself, should not exclude patients from receiving therapy, while the functional or biological age of the patient, and the impact of long-term drug therapy on safety and quality of life, should be considered. Given the larger reduction in event rates among older patients, treatment would also be expected to be more cost-effective in older than in younger patients [66]. Moderate-dose statins appear to be well tolerated in elderly persons participating in clinical trials, although

the risk of serious muscle adverse effects may be slightly higher. Higher doses of statins should be used with caution in frail elderly patients, who may be more susceptible to drug-related myopathy and other side effects, as statin toxicity has been shown to be dose-related.

5.4.4 Hypertension

The prevalence of hypertension in diabetics is up to threefold that in non-diabetics [67]. Hypertension affects up to 60% of patients with type 2 diabetes [68], with increasing age, obesity and the onset of renal disease being the contributory factors to increasing its prevalence among these patients. The development of type 2 diabetes is also about twice as likely in persons with hypertension than in normotensive people, which suggests a frequent coexistence of these two common chronic diseases [69]. Hypertension markedly increases the risk of CVD in patients with type 2 diabetes compared to those without diabetes [67].

Hypertension should be managed aggressively in diabetic patients. A tight blood pressure control below the recommended levels of 140/90 mmHg [70] markedly reduced not only CVD but also the development of end-stage renal disease in persons with type 2 diabetes mellitus. This risk reduction was even more impressive than the tight blood glucose control in the United Kingdom Prospective Diabetes Study (UKPDS), where the benefits of a diastolic blood pressure reduction to 82 mmHg in the tight control group compared to 87 mmHg in the usual care group, dramatically outweighed those of intensive glucose control of mean hemoglobin A_{1c} (HbA_{1c}) reduction to 7.0% versus 7.9% in both groups, respectively [71]. The reduction of diastolic blood pressure to <80 mmHg reduced CVD events by 51% in comparison to a diastolic blood pressure of 90 mmHg in the diabetic subgroup of the Hypertension Optimal Treatment (HOT) study [72]. In contrast, those HOT study participants without diabetes received no benefit from this further diastolic blood pressure reduction. The reduction of systolic pressure, from 175 to 153 mmHg, led to a significant reduction in CVD-related events in the Systolic Hypertension in Europe (Syst-Eur) trial [73]. Here, diabetic patients showed more benefit from an aggressive blood pressure lowering than did non-diabetics. In that trial, despite the systolic pressure being reduced by a comparable amount in each group (22.0 ± 16 mmHg in non-diabetics versus 22.1 ± 14 mmHg in diabetics), the risk reduction in mortality from CVD was 13% in non-diabetic patients compared to 76% for diabetics. The same effect was apparent in the Systolic Hypertension in the Elderly Program (SHEP) study, where elderly persons with type 2 diabetes derived more benefit from an aggressive systolic blood pressure lowering in reduction of CVD than did those without diabetes [74]. Based on the above findings, it appears that the benefit per mmHg blood pressure reduction is greater in diabetic patients than in those who are hypertensive but have no concomitant diabetes mellitus, and this confirms the need for an aggressive reduction of arterial pressure in diabetic patients. In order to achieve these goals, most older diabetic people will require a combination of at least two or three antihypertensive medications [75].

Angiotensin-converting enzyme (ACE) inhibitors may have a role in reducing cardiovascular risk in older diabetics. The elderly Heart Outcomes Prevention Evaluation (HOPE) trial included 2755 older patients who were aged ≥70 years with vascular disease or diabetes, had at least one additional cardiovascular risk factor, and were without HF or a low ejection fraction. Patients were randomized to ramipril (10 mg/day) or placebo for four-and-a-half-years of follow up. Those assigned to ramipril had fewer major vascular events compared to those receiving to placebo (18.6 versus 24.0%, HR = 0.75, P = 0.0006), cardiovascular deaths (9.3 versus. 13.0%, HR = 0.71, P = 0.003), MI (12.0 versus 15.6%, HR = 0.75, P = 0.006) and strokes (5.4 versus 7.7%, HR = 0.69, P = 0.013). These were of similar magnitude to the proportional reductions in risk observed in patients aged <70 years. Ramipril was generally safe, and equally well tolerated in patients aged ≥70 years and <70 years. Importantly, due to the high risk of cardiovascular events in elderly patients, the absolute risk reductions attained with ramipril were higher in patients aged ≥70 years than in those aged <70 years, for most endpoints. As an example, the absolute risk reduction for the primary endpoint was 5.4% in patients aged ≥70 years and 3% for those aged <70 years; consequently, for elderly patients the NNT to prevent one major cardiovascular event over four-and-a-half years was 18, compared to 33 for younger patients [76]. These cardiovascular and renoprotective beneficial effects of ACE inhibitors in patients with type 2 diabetes were independent of any blood pressure lowering, and may occur whether albuminuria is present, or not [77, 78].

Beta-blockers are associated with an increased risk for new-onset diabetes mellitus, with no benefit for the end point of death or MI, and with a 15% increased risk for stroke compared to other agents. A meta-analysis of 12 studies evaluating 94 492 patients taking beta-blockers as first-line therapy for hypertension with data on new-onset diabetes and a follow up for more than one year showed beta-blocker therapy to result in a 22% increased risk for new-onset diabetes (relative risk 1.22, 95% CI: 1.12 to 1.33) compared to non-diuretic antihypertensive agents. A higher baseline fasting glucose level was a significant predictor of new-onset diabetes (OR 1.01, 95% CI: 1.00 to 1.02, p = 0.004). The risk for diabetes was greater with atenolol in the elderly and in studies in which beta-blockers were less efficacious antihypertensive agents, and increased exponentially with an increased duration of beta-blocker therapy. On the other hand, calcium channel blockers (CCBs) and ACE inhibitors or angiotensin II receptor blockers (ARBs) resulted in 21% and 23% reductions, respectively, in the risk for new-onset diabetes compared to beta-blockers [79]. Also, in comparison with other agents, the antihypertensive efficacy of beta-blockers was inferior.

In this analysis, however, diuretics resulted in an increased risk for new-onset diabetes compared to beta-blockers, although their blood pressure-lowering efficacy was superior. In the UKPDS, although atenolol efficacy was similar to that of the ACE inhibitor, captopril, those patients receiving atenolol gained more weight and required a more frequent addition of new glucose-lowering agents than those taking captopril [71]. A recent meta-analysis showed that the association of antihypertensive drug class on incident diabetes was lowest for ARBs, ACE inhibitors followed by CCBs, beta-blockers and diuretics, in rank order [80]. Beta-blockers worsen glycemic control by inhibiting pancreatic insulin secretion, increasing both insulin resistance and glycogenolysis [81]. However, the newer, non-cardioselective beta-blockers with vasodilating properties (e.g., carvedilol) have minimal effects on glycemic control [82].

The Antihypertensive and Lipid-Lowering treatment to prevent Heart Attack Trial (ALLHAT) compared ACE inhibitors, CCBs and thiazide diuretics. In a subgroup analysis of 12 063 patients with type 2 diabetes, no significant differences were seen between different groups in the primary outcomes of non-fatal MI plus CHD death or all-cause mortality. However, the risk for HF was lowest in the diuretic group [83].

The ARBs reduce not only renal end points but also cardiovascular events [84–86]. In the Losartan Intervention for Endpoint Reduction (LIFE) study, patients with hypertension and signs of left ventricular hypertrophy on electrocardiography were assigned randomly to an ARB (losartan) or a beta-blocker (atenolol). In a subgroup analysis of 1195 patients with diabetes, the losartan group had a substantially lower risk for cardiovascular end-points and total mortality [87]. A recent meta-analysis to compare the benefits and adverse effects of ACE inhibitors versus ARBs for treating essential hypertension showed that both agents had similar effects on blood pressure control, but ACE inhibitors caused higher rates of cough than did ARBs. The data regarding other outcomes were limited [88].

The above evidence applies to older people (up to the age of 80 years), as clinical trials have either excluded this group of the population, or included only very few. The recently published Hypertension in the Very Elderly Trial (HYVET) has provided evidence that antihypertensive treatment with the diuretic indapamide (sustained release), with or without the ACE inhibitor perindopril, in persons aged ≥80 years, is beneficial and associated with reduced risks of HF,

death from stroke or from any cause, although only approximately 7% of the subjects were diabetics [89].

In summary, risk reduction via hypertension control in patients with diabetes is substantially greater than that in non-diabetic persons, who have similar blood pressure levels [72]. Blood pressure in diabetics should be treated aggressively, and indeed the control of this parameter may be the most important factor in preventing adverse outcomes. Most patients will need to be administered more than one antihypertensive agent, and in this respect thiazide diuretics, ARBs, ACE inhibitors and CCBs seem to be reasonable first-choice agents, although higher doses of diuretics may worsen blood glucose and lipid levels [90]. The addition of other agents may be necessary in order to achieve blood pressure targets.

5.4.5 Hyperglycemia

While diabetes has long been recognized as a risk factor for CHD, it is not clear whether hyperglycemia itself is a risk for CVD. Hyperglycemia leads to an increase in oxidative stress, an enhanced leukocyte–endothelial interaction and the glycosylation of proteins in the body, including lipoproteins, apolipoproteins and clotting factors [91]. This may have a role in increasing cardiovascular risk. In combination with other risk factors, hyperglycemia may cause an accelerated progression of atherosclerosis in people with diabetes, although few data are available to assess whether lowering the blood glucose level will predict CVD outcome. Prospective studies have demonstrated that glucose is a continuous CHD risk factor in diabetics [92, 93], the results having suggested that the risk of CHD rises by 10–30% for each 1% increase in HbA_{1c} level. In the UKPDS, intensive treatment with metformin in a subgroup of patients with type 2 diabetes resulted in a decreased risk for MI and stroke compared to the conventional treatment group, while intensive treatment with sulfonylurea or insulin improved the long-term outcomes of diabetes (microvascular and macrovascular complications); however, the improvement in cardiovascular risk did not reach statistical significance [94]. In the same study, the data also indicated that with each 1% rise in HbA_{1c} the incidence of MI rose by about 14%. Moreover, the relationship between glycaemia and cardiovascular risk was seen to start within the normal blood sugar range, with a linear relationship, and showed no indication of any threshold effect. This suggested that CHD started before the onset of clinical diabetes [95, 96]. A meta-analysis of three studies involving persons with type 1 diabetes (n = 1688), and 10 studies involving persons with type 2 diabetes (n = 7435), showed a positive effect of blood glucose lowering on the risk of cardiovascular events, and the effect seemed to be greater in type 2 diabetics than in type 1. For each 1% increase in HbA_{1c} the relative risk of CVD was 1.18 (95% CI: 1.10 to 1.26) for type 2 diabetes and 1.15 (95% CI: 0.92 to 1.43) for type 1 diabetes [97]. The relationship of postprandial glycaemia, fasting blood glucose and cardiovascular risk in individuals with diabetes was less clear, although most reports have indicated a greater pathogenic potential of postprandial hyperglycemia rather than fasting hyperglycemia [98]. A meta-analysis of randomized trials targeting postprandial hyperglycemia showed cardiovascular benefit in type 2 diabetes. The treatment of postprandial hyperglycemia was associated with a reduction in the development of any CVD by 35% [99]. These observations support the hypothesis that the lowering of blood glucose to levels within the normal range may either prevent or postpone the development of CHD. However, as there are at present no data available specifically for older diabetics, evidence must be extrapolated to the older age groups.

5.4.6 Hypercoagulability

A procoagulant state has been demonstrated in individuals with diabetes [100]. Both, platelet aggregation and adhesion are increased in diabetics [101]. Diabetes increases intrinsic platelet activation and decreasing the endogenous inhibitors of platelet activity [102]. These changes are likely due to a chronic inflammatory state induced by diabetes. Consequently, older diabetics should be prescribed antiplatelet treatment as part of a multifactorial treatment to reduce their cardiovascular risk, regardless of whether they have a history of CHD, or not.

5.4.7 Race and ethnicity

Most present-day knowledge regarding cardiovascular risk is derived from the Framingham population, the majority of which was white people of European origin. It is uncertain whether baseline absolute risk is similar to that in other populations, but race and ethnicity will have a significant influence on the risk of CVD. Although, the most important risk factors associated with diabetes are largely similar in all countries, their expression and intensities may vary between races and ethnic groups. In southern Asia, for example, in recent years there has been a progressive increase in the prevalence of diabetes mellitus and CHD due to lifestyle changes, modernization and increasing urbanization and industrialization, all of which have led to physical inactivity and obesity [103]. Yet, the prevalence of diabetes has also increased in southern Asians who have migrated to western countries, with southern Asians living in the UK having a fourfold higher prevalence of diabetes than their British counterparts [104]. Southern Asians are also genetically prone to develop both diabetes and CHD, and this tends to occur about a decade earlier than in western countries [105]. In addition to the 'traditional' risk factors, southern Asians may have a higher prevalence of emerging and new atherogenic risk factors, such as lipoprotein abnormalities and hyperhomocysteinaemia, that make them more prone to develop CVD [106]. This higher risk should be considered when southern Asians living in the 'developed' world are evaluated.

Black race is associated with increased mortality from ischemic heart disease compared to whites, and risk factors such as diabetes and hypertension tend to be less well controlled in blacks than in whites [107, 108]. Although this might lead to an increased cardiovascular risk in black diabetics, the evidence is conflicting. While one American study [109] reported a greater CVD prevalence among black geriatric patients with diabetes, others have not found this to be the case [110-112]. Black diabetics of Afro-Caribbean descent who are resident in the UK have also been found to be at a lower risk of CVD than white Europeans with diabetes [113]. In a recent study, there was no significant difference in the incidence of CVD among diabetic elderly black (23.9%) and white (29.2%) Americans. However, the risk of CVD was lower among southern black men (HR 0.87, 95% CI: 0.82–0.92) and women (HR 0.95, 95% CI: 0.91–0.99) than their southern white counterparts. In the three other US regions combined (northeast, midwest and west), black men had a similar risk for CVD (HR 1.01, 95% CI: 0.95–1.07), while black women had a greater risk (HR 1.10, 95% CI: 1.05–1.16) than non-southern white men and women, respectively. The greater risk for CVD of black women with diabetes not residing in the south (versus white women with diabetes) argues against any genetic explanation, and suggests that regional differences in lifestyle, environment or quality of care may play some role [114].

To summarize:

- Absolute risk reduction is higher and more cost effective in diabetics than in non-diabetics.

- Metabolic syndrome in the elderly may not enhance the prediction of risks above its components.

- Statin therapy is equally beneficial in older and younger diabetics.

- Blood pressure control has a greater impression on risk reduction than does blood glucose control.

- The diabetic elderly benefit more than non-diabetics from tight blood pressure control.

- The benefits of blood pressure reduction are similar for patients of all age groups.

- All classes of antihypertensive medication are effective in both elderly and younger people.

- Southern Asians demonstrate a higher risk, at a younger age, than do whites.

- Hyperglycemia should not be treated in isolation, but as part of multifactorial intervention.

5.5 Myocardial infarction

The prevalence of CHD may be as high as 55% among adults with diabetes compared to only about 4% among those without diabetes [115]. The risk of MI in patients with diabetes mellitus without a history of MI is as high as that in patients without diabetes mellitus who have had an MI [2]. Following the development of CHD in diabetics, the prognosis is worse and mortality after the first MI higher than in non-diabetics [116]. Age is the most powerful predictor of CHD risk; by the age of 65 years, most men have a 20% risk of a CHD event occurring within the next 10 years, with diabetes conferring a risk equivalent to ageing 15 years. In men, the transition from intermediate to high-risk status occurs at an average age of 47.9 years, whereas in women the transition is about seven years later, at the age of 54.3 years [117]. Screening for CHD is based on symptoms of angina, with a low threshold for investigation. Asymptomatic MI or myocardial ischemia is more common in diabetic patients, especially the elderly [118]. Patients with diabetes may also present with atypical symptoms of myocardial ischemia, such as an unexplained shortness of breath on exertion, which may be an angina equivalent and

warrant early investigation. However, exercise tolerance test or stress echocardiography are not routinely recommended. A 12-lead resting electrocardiogram has low sensitivity and specificity, but is a useful baseline [119]. The current recommendation is that patients with diabetes and two additional risk factors should undergo stress myocardial perfusion scans, although most elderly diabetics will have multiple risk factors for CHD and the burden of such screening would not be practical [120]. Although cardiovascular risk factors should be treated in older diabetics on the basis of the diabetes alone, screening may be indicated in higher risk patients in whom revascularization therapy is thought to be indicated.

The increased risk for CHD by diabetes appears to be greater in women. In a meta-analysis to estimate the relative risk for fatal CHD associated with diabetes in 37 studies, which included a total of 447 064 patients (some studies included people aged >65 years), the rate of fatal CHD was higher in diabetic than in non-diabetic patients (5.4% versus 1.6%). The overall summary relative risk for fatal CHD in patients with diabetes compared with no diabetes was significantly greater among women than it was among men (3.50, 95% CI: 2.70–4.53 versus 2.06, 95% CI: 1.81–2.34). Following exclusion of the eight studies that had adjusted only for age, the difference in risk between the genders was substantially reduced, but still highly significant. The pooled ratio of the relative risks (female: male) from the 29 studies with multiple adjusted estimates was 1.46 (95% CI: 1.14–1.88). The gender difference in CHD risk might be a consequence of diabetes inducing a more adverse cardiovascular risk profile in women, combined with a reduced likelihood of women receiving recommended levels of cardioprotective treatment [121]. The Hoorn study also emphasized the increased hazard in women with diabetes in a population of patients aged 62 ± 7 years [122]. Diabetes also increases CHD mortality for older people; in a cohort study of older patients (average age 72 years), diabetes conferred a CHD mortality risk that was 2.5- to 2.75-fold greater than for patients without diabetes [123]. The duration of diabetes represents a risk for the development of CHD. For example, in the Framingham study, the risk of CHD events and CHD death were shown to be 1.38 (95% CI: 0.99–1.92) and 1.86 (95% CI: 1.17–2.93) times greater for each 10 years increase in the duration of diabetes, respectively [124]. However, there is an increased risk for CHD even before the clinical diagnosis of diabetes [125].

Beta-blockers are associated with a lower one-year mortality rate for elderly diabetic patients, similar to that in non-diabetics. In a retrospective cohort study of 45 308 patients admitted to hospital with acute MI, and after adjusting for potential confounders, beta-blockers were associated with a lower one-year mortality for insulin-treated diabetics (HR = 0.87, 95% CI: 0.72–1.07), non-insulin-treated diabetics (HR = 0.77, 95% CI: 0.67–0.88) and non-diabetics (HR = 0.87, 95% CI: 0.80–0.94). Although some concern was expressed regarding the use of beta-blockers in diabetic patients, such therapy was not significantly associated with any increase in the six-month readmission rates for diabetic complications among diabetics [126].

The outcome after MI is poor in older diabetics. For example, the outcome data of 1698 elderly (aged $\geq$65 years) diabetics after one year of hospitalization for MI showed a high risk of HF, recurrent MI and mortality. Comorbid conditions related to diabetes mellitus (previous HF, MI, chronic renal impairment, peripheral vascular disease, stroke) at the time of the index MI were important contributors to poorer outcomes in elderly patients with diabetes mellitus [127]. A higher blood glucose level ($>6.1 \, \text{mol} \, \text{l}^{-1}$) was also associated with an increased mortality risk in elderly acute MI patients, particularly those without recognized diabetes [128].

In addition to a poor outcome, older diabetics have more comorbidities and a greater resource use than non-diabetics. In another study of older people hospitalized for acute MI, older diabetics constituted 33% of the total admissions in one year. Comorbid conditions, including hypertension, prior acute MI, prior stroke and/or prior revascularization, were more frequent in diabetic than in non-diabetic patients. Congestive heart failure (CHF) also occurred more frequently in diabetic patients. The length of hospital stay (7.9 versus 7.0 days, P < 0.001), in-hospital mortality rates (16% versus 13%, P < 0.001) and rates for mortality within 30 days (21% versus 17%, P < 0.001) were each higher in diabetic patients [129]. The long-term survival after acute MI was also significantly decreased in diabetic patients compared to non-diabetics. Over a 12-year period, the relative risk of dying was 1.56-fold higher among diabetic men than among non-diabetic men (95% CI: 1.43–1.68), whereas diabetic women were 1.57-fold more likely to die than non-diabetic women (95% CI: 1.45–1.73) [130]. Diabetics with acute MI

also tended to have more severe diffuse three-vessel or left main stem disease than those without diabetes. Typically, such patients showed about 30% mortality before receiving thrombolytic therapy, while among patients receiving thrombolysis the mortality was about twice that of non-diabetics [131].

Details of the effect of glucose, insulin and potassium (GIK) therapy on the mortality of acute MI are conflicting. The Diabetes Insulin–Glucose in Acute Myocardial Infarction (DIGAMI) study, which was reported in 1995, concluded that in diabetic patients an insulin–glucose infusion followed by a multidose insulin regimen for 3 months after discharge improved long-term survival after an acute MI. At one year, mortality in the infusion group was 18.6% compared to 26.1% in the control group (P < 0.0273), with a relative reduction in mortality of 30% [132]. The positive results of DIGAMI continued for a mean of 3.4 years of follow up, with a 33% mortality occurring in the insulin–glucose infusion group compared to 44% in the control group (P = 0.011) [133]. However, the DIGAMI II study, the details of which were reported in 2005, did not support the concept that both short- and long-term insulin therapy would improve survival in patients with type 2 diabetes mellitus with acute MI compared to conventional therapy [134]. The evidence of GIK in trials which included non-diabetic patients was also conflicting. For example, in 1997 a meta-analysis of GIK therapy for acute MI showed a mortality of 21% in the placebo group and 16.1% in the GIK group. The risk reduction in mortality was 28% (OR 0.72, 95% CI: 0.57–0.90, P < 0.004). However, the studies included in the meta-analysis were conducted before the reperfusion therapy era [135]. After 1997, most of the clinical trials did not show any benefit of GIK therapy on mortality [136].

To summarize:

- The risk of MI in diabetics is at least twice that in non-diabetics

- Presentation may be atypical in older people

- The outcome of MI is worse in diabetics than in non-diabetics

- The medications used in MI treatment have similar efficacies in diabetics and non-diabetics

- The role of glucose, insulin and potassium infusion therapy remains controversial

5.6 Heart failure

Type 2 diabetes is associated with a greater risk of HF and, indeed, both conditions frequently coexist. The mechanisms underlying this association remain controversial, but may include diabetes-associated co-morbidities such as hypertension and obesity, diabetes-associated complications such as small and large vessel disease, and diabetic cardiomyopathy. Independent risk factors for the development of HF in diabetes include a higher HbA_{1c} level [137] and an increased body mass index (BMI) [137, 138]; increasing the BMI by 2.5 units increases the risk of HF by 12% [137]. In the UKPDS, for every 1% reduction in HbA_{1c} the risk of HF fell by 16% [139]. Other factors included increasing age [137], CHD [137, 138], the use of insulin [137], end-stage renal disease [137], microalbuminuria [138], retinopathy [140] and the duration of diabetes [137]. Diabetes also is a risk factor for the development of HF with a normal ejection fraction (HFNEF); this condition is commonly referred to as 'diastolic HF', although most such patients also have associated systolic dysfunction. An overlap occurs between diabetes, hypertension and ischemic heart disease in the development of HFNEF [141]. The prevalence, incidence and mortality of HF in older patients with diabetes is very high. In a population-based cohort study of 151 738 patients with diabetes, all of whom were aged >65 years, HF prevalence was 22.3% and the incidence rate 12.6% (95% CI: 12.5–12.7%). Increasing age, ischemic heart disease, nephropathy and peripheral vascular disease were strong predictors for the development of HF. Over a 60-month follow-up period, however, mortality among HF patients was almost 10-fold that in diabetic patients who remained HF free (32.7% versus 3.7%) [142]. In a recent study, the cumulative incidence of HF in older diabetics was 47.5% after six years of diagnosis of diabetes compared to 20% in a non-diabetic control group [28]. Higher rates of HF with a greater number of complications were related to poor glycemic and blood pressure control. This was consistent with the limited clinical trials data, which suggested that blood pressure control, treatment with ACE inhibitors and glycemic control might reduce the risk of HF [141, 143]. Ischemic heart disease and renal impairment, as predictors of HF, have been demonstrated previously [144, 145]. In nursing homes, the incidence of HF in residents with diabetes was seen to be almost twice that of those without diabetes (12.1% versus 6.2%) [146].

Few data are available about reducing the risk of developing HF in diabetics, specifically in older people. It is unclear whether an improvement in glycemic control would reduce the incidence of HF. While a high HbA_{1c} level has been shown to increase the risk of HF [139], intensive glycemic control did not significantly reduce the incidence of HF in the UKPDS [147], although in the same study a tight control of the blood pressure led to a reduction in the risk of developing HF (HR 0.44, 95% CI: 0.2–0.94, P = 0.0043) [71]. Some evidence has been produced for the use of ACE inhibitors, ARBs and statins in reducing the risk of HF, with the ACE inhibitor ramipril producing a 20% risk reduction (95% CI: 4–34, P = 0.019) in the MICROHOPE trial [148]. In the IDNT, the ARB irbesartan reduced the incidence of HF compared to placebo (HR 0.72, 95% CI: 0.52–1.00, P = 0.048) [86], while high-dose atorvastatin (80 mg/day) reduced the hospitalization time for HF in the Treating to New Targets study [149]. It appears, however, that no specific drug therapy, alternative glycemic control or different blood pressure target is available either to prevent or to treat HF in diabetic patients. Subgroup analyses of HF clinical trials have suggested similar treatment benefits from ACE inhibitors and beta-blockers, regardless of the patients' diabetes status [150].

In diabetics, the possibility of HF should be considered in the presence of risk factors such as CHD, hypertension, proteinuria [151] and retinopathy [140]. B-type natriuretic peptide may also represent a useful screening approach [152], although is no particular investigation is available for HF in diabetes which differs from those in non-diabetics. Neither is there any specific difference in the clinical presentation of HF in diabetics. The typical diabetic patient with HFNEF is an elderly woman with a history of hypertension, in whom the HF is episodic and often precipitated by an episode of atrial fibrillation, ischemia or infection [153].

Beta-blockers offer similar benefit for diabetics and non-diabetics in HF, with relative risk reductions in mortality of 0.84 (95% CI: 0.73–0.96, P = 0.011) having been shown in diabetics compared to 0.72 (95% CI: 0.65–0.79, P < 0.001) in non-diabetics [154]. The benefits in morbidity were also similar [155]. Diabetics are less likely than non-diabetics with HF to be discharged from hospital while receiving beta-blocker therapy (OR 0.72, 95% CI: 0.55–0.94) [156]. Beta-blockers are cautiously prescribed for older HF diabetics because of their perceived unfavourable effects on glucose metabolism and a paucity of available clinical data. However, the results of a recent study showed that diabetes does not negatively influence the safety, tolerability and efficacy of carvedilol in older diabetic patients (aged >70 years) with systolic HF. At a one year follow up, the tolerability (93.7% versus 92.2%) and mean daily dose (24 ± 17 versus 23 ± 14 mg) of carvedilol were similar in diabetics and non-diabetics. Neither was any worsening of fasting blood glucose level, HbA_{1c} and creatinine levels, nor of the incidence of death and hospitalization, observed in diabetics treated with carvedilol. Similar improvements in New York Heart Association class and mitral regurgitation severity were observed in diabetic and non-diabetic patients receiving carvedilol. Although beta-blockers have previously been well tolerated in older diabetic patients with HF, diabetes remains a strong prognostic factor that limits the reversibility of left ventricular systolic dysfunction and the effect of treatment on subsequent outcome [157]. Other medications used in HF have similar effects in diabetics and non-diabetics. The relative risk of mortality among ACE inhibitor-treated, compared to placebo-treated, patients was 0.85 (95% CI: 0.78–0.92) in non-diabetics and 0.84 (95% CI: 0.70–1.00) in diabetics [158]. A similar pattern was shown with ARBs therapy [159, 160]. Spironolactone has similar mortality benefits in diabetics (HR 0.70, 95% CI: 0.52–0.94, P = 0.019) and non-diabetics (HR 0.70, 95% CI: 0.60–0.82, P < 0.001) with severe HF [161]. No data are presently available to suggest that other medications used in HF treatment (e.g., diuretics, digoxin, nitrates, hydralazine) will have any different effects in diabetes. Diabetes worsens the outcome of both systolic and diastolic HF in older people, especially in women [162]. In the Digitalis Investigation Group trial, diabetes-associated increases in hospitalization and mortality in chronic HF were more pronounced in women, and these gender-related differences in outcome were primarily observed in elderly patients (aged ≥ 65 years). The absolute increase in all-cause hospitalizations due to HF in women was 74% and 61%, respectively, for patients with and without diabetes (p < 0.001), while the absolute increase in mortality in women was 39% and 25%, respectively, for patients with and without diabetes (p < 0.001). These findings suggest that diabetes has a significant negative impact on the natural history of HF, and an early diagnosis and a more tight control of diabetes is necessary to improve outcomes in HF, especially in elderly women [163].

To summarize:

- Heart failure and diabetes commonly coexist

- Diabetes is associated with both reduced and normal ejection fractions in HF

- The presence of CHD, hypertension, proteinuria and retinopathy should lead to a suspicion of HF in diabetics

- Diabetes worsens the outcome of HF, especially in older women

- All HF medications have similar efficacies in both diabetics and non-diabetics

5.7 Anti-diabetic medications and CHD

An early clinical trial suggested that sulphonylureas are cardiotoxic and may exacerbate diabetic cardiomyopathy [164], although this was not confirmed in the UKPDS [152]. In a retrospective cohort study, patients commenced on insulin had a higher incidence of HF hospitalization than those commenced on sulphonylureas (HR 1.56, 95% CI: 1.00–2.45, P = 0.05) [165]. In another retrospective cohort study, there was no effect of sulphonylureas on mortality (HR 0.99, 95% CI: 0.91–1.08) [166]. Although insulin therapy has been shown to predict the development of HF and mortality in diabetes [167, 168], this was not shown in the UKPDS. However, insulin use is likely to be started at a late stage in type 2 diabetes, when macrovascular disease could have been already established.

Cardiovascular outcome seems to be better among patients receiving metformin therapy. In the UKPDS, in a subgroup of overweight subjects with type 2 diabetes mellitus, metformin treatment caused a decrease in all-cause mortality, notably that due to MI [169]. In patients with newly diagnosed HF, metformin monotherapy was associated with a reduced one-year mortality when compared to sulfonylurea treatment (HR 0.66, 95% CI: 0.44–0.97) [170]. The one-year mortality was also lower in patients receiving a metformin/sulfonylurea combination therapy than in those with sulfonylurea monotherapy (HR 0.54, 95% CI: 0.42–0.70). Metformin use was also associated with a lower one-year mortality compared to insulin or sulphonylureas treatment in patients admitted to hospital with HF (24.7 versus 36%, P < 0.0001) [166]. It has been suggested that metformin be used with caution in HF patients due to a risk of lactic acidosis, although such risk does not appear to be high. Indeed, in a retrospective cohort study the rate of lactic acidosis was 2.3% in metformin-treated patients compared to 2.6% in those not treated (P = 0.40) [166]. A similar retrospective study reported no cases of lactic acidosis with metformin in diabetics with HF [170].

The thiazolidinediones (TZDs), rosiglitazone and pioglitazone, have been shown to improve glycemic control and to slow the progression of beta-cell failure [171]. These drugs have multiple therapeutic effects through their action on peroxisome proliferator activated receptor gamma, which is expressed diffusely in human tissues. Their beneficial effects include reductions in insulin resistance and hyperglycemia, anti-inflammatory effects and improvement of hypertension, microalbuminuria and hepatic steatosis. These TZDs effects may be independent of their effects on blood glucose. While improved glycemic control has been linked to better clinical outcomes [172] and TZDs have been suggested as having potential cardiovascular benefits [173], this group of drugs has recently been scrutinised for increased cardiovascular risk. TZDs are associated with weight gain, oedema [174] and an increased risk of CHF [173]. The frequency of oedema is approximately 5% when TZDs are used either in monotherapy or as combination oral therapy, and approximately 15% when used with insulin [175]. The mechanism of fluid retention is not clear, and is largely peripheral, but may result from changes in hemodynamics, with some contribution from molecules that regulate cell and tissue permeability. There may also be a direct effect of TZDs on sodium reabsorption via the renal medullary collecting ducts [175]. The results of two meta-analyses have also suggested that rosiglitazone might be associated with an increased risk of acute MI and death, although the majority of clinical trials with TZDs were limited to subjects aged <65 years [173, 176–178]. A recent study examined the association between TZD therapy and CHF, acute MI and mortality in older diabetics (aged ≥66 years) compared to treatment with other oral hypoglycaemic agents. In this population-based study of older patients with diabetes, TZD treatment – primarily with rosiglitazone – was associated with an increased risk of CHF, acute MI and mortality when compared with other combination oral hypoglycaemic agents. During a median follow up of 3.8 years, treatment with TZD monotherapy was associated with a significantly increased risk of CHF (RR 1.60, 95% CI: 1.21–2.10,

P < 0.001), acute MI (RR 1.40, 95% CI: 1.05–1.86, P = 0.02) and death (RR 1.29, 95% CI: 1.02–1.62, P = 0.03) The increased risks associated with TZDs were independent of baseline cardiovascular risk or diabetes duration. The increased risk of CHF, acute MI and mortality associated with TZDs use appeared limited to rosiglitazone [179]. A recent meta-analysis of 42 trials comparing rosiglitazone with placebo or active comparators in more than 27 000 patients with diabetes suggested that treatment with rosiglitazone was associated with an increased risk of MI and cardiovascular death [176]. Another meta-analysis to evaluate the effect of pioglitazone on ischemic cardiovascular events included a total of 19 trials enrolling 16 390 patients. Death, MI or stroke occurred in 4.4% of patients receiving pioglitazone and in 5.7% of patients receiving control therapy (HR 0.82, 95% CI: 0.72–0.94, P = 0.005). The individual components of the primary end point were each reduced by a similar magnitude with pioglitazone treatment, with HRs ranging from 0.80 to 0.92. However, serious HF was reported in 2.3% of the pioglitazone-treated patients and in 1.8% of the control patients (HR 1.41, 95% CI: 1.14–1.76, P = 0.002) (Table 5.1).

It appeared that pioglitazone was associated with a significantly lower risk of death, MI or stroke among a diverse population of patients with diabetes. However, serious HF was increased by pioglitazone, though without any associated increase in mortality [173]. The reason why these two TZDs have different effects on cardiovascular outcome is unclear, but it may be related to the fact that pioglitazone produces greater reductions in serum triglycerides and increases in HDL-cholesterol levels [180]. Although the cardiovascular outcome data for pioglitazone are reassuring, there is a need for randomized clinical trials to be conducted in order to define the appropriate role of TZDs for the treatment of type 2 diabetes, particularly in older people who are at increased risk of CVD.

To summarize:

- There is no clear evidence to suggest that insulin or sulphonylureas are cardiotoxic

- Metformin therapy seems to be cardioprotective

- The risk of metformin-induced lactic acidosis in HF does not appear to be high

- Rosiglitazone is associated with an increased risk of MI, HF and mortality in older diabetics

Table 5.1 Cardiovascular event rates for combined trials.

	Number (%)			
	Pioglitazone (n = 8554)	Control (n = 7836)	Hazard ratio (95% CI)	P-value
Death/myocardial infarction/stroke	375 (4.38)	450 (5.74)	0.82 (0.72–0.94)	0.005
Death	209 (2.44)	224 (2.86)	0.92 (0.76–1.11)	0.38
Myocardial infarction	131 (1.53)	159 (2.03)	0.81 (0.64–1.02)	0.08
Death/myocardial infarction	309 (3.61)	357 (4.56)	0.85 (0.73–0.99)	0.04
Stroke	104 (1.22)	131 (1.67)	0.80 (0.62–1.04)	0.09
Serious heart failure	200 (2.34)	139 (1.77)	1.41 (1.14–1.76)	0.002
Death/serious heart failure	361 (4.22)	321 (4.10)	1.11 (0.96–1.29)	0.17
Death/myocardial infarction/stroke/serious heart failure	508 (5.94)	523 (6.67)	0.96 (0.85–1.09)	0.54

Reproduced with permission from Lincoff A M, Wolski K, Nicholls S J, et al., JAMA 2007; 298: 1180–8.

- Pioglitazone reduces the risks of MI and mortality, but increases the risk of HF

- There is a need for additional clinical trials to define the role of thiazolidinediones in older diabetics

5.8 Conclusions

Both, ageing and diabetes have a significant impact on the cardiovascular system, increasing the risk for developing CHD and HF in older people with diabetes. Moreover, the size of the problem is likely to expand as the ageing population and incidence of diabetes continue to increase. The baseline risks for CVD are increased in diabetics and the elderly in comparison to non-diabetics and younger people, respectively. As the combination of diabetes and old age places older diabetics at the highest baseline risk for CVD, elderly diabetics stand to gain the most benefit from cardiovascular risk reduction. Medications for such reduction and the treatment of CHD and HF have similar efficacies in diabetics and non-diabetics. Older diabetics are likely to have multiple risk factors at their first presentation with diabetes, and consequently a multifactorial and comprehensive approach is vital to their management. Although most clinical trials have either excluded or included few older people, there is now sufficient evidence available to suggest that the aggressive treatment of risk factors in this age group is both beneficial and cost effective. Although many older diabetics may not achieve the recommended targets for risk factor reduction, for a variety of reasons (e.g., multiple comorbidities, polypharmacy and intolerance of higher doses or multiple medications), any reduction in the risk factors will be beneficial. Today, the patient's quality of life is seen as the primary target

when caring for older diabetics and, as not all will be suited to an aggressive risk reduction, treatment must be considered on an individual basis. Any subsequent individual care plan must involve not only the patients but also their families and carers. In particular, will be necessary to recognize a patient's diversity of beliefs and their attitude towards health care.

References

1. Kannel WB, McGee DL. Diabetes and cardiovascular disease: the Framingham study. JAMA 1979; 241: 2035–8.
2. Haffner SM, Lehto S, Rönnemaa T, et al. Mortality from coronary heart disease in subjects with type 2 diabetes and in nondiabetic subjects with and without prior myocardial infarction. N Engl J Med. 1998; 339: 229–34.
3. Franklin SS, Gustin W, IV, Wong ND, et al. Hemodynamic patterns of age related changes in blood pressure. The Framingham Heart Study. Circulation 1997; 96: 308–15.
4. Blacher J, Asmar R, Djane S, et al. Aortic pulse wave velocity as a marker of cardiovascular risk in hypertensive patients. Hypertension 1999; 33: 1111–17.
5. Nilsson PM, Lurbe E, Laurent S. The early life origins of vascular ageing and cardiovascular risk: the EVA syndrome J Hypertens 2008; 26: 1049–57.
6. Samani NJ, Harst P. Biological ageing and cardiovascular disease. Heart 2008; 94: 537–9.
7. Capell BC, Collins FS, Nabel EG. Mechanisms of cardiovascular disease in accelerated ageing syndromes. Circ Res. 2007; 101: 13–26.
8. Lyons D, Roy S, Patel M, et al. Impaired nitric oxide-mediated vasodilatation and total body nitric oxide production in healthy old age. Clin Sci 1997; 93: 519–22.

9. Wynne H A, Schofield S. (1996) Drug induced orthostatic hypotension, in: R. A. Kenny (ed.), Syncope in the older patient: causes, investigations and consequences of syncope and falls. Chapman & Hall, London, pp. 137–54.

10. Lakatta EG. Changes in cardiovascular function with ageing. Eur Heart J 1990; 11 (Suppl. C): 22–9.

11. Haider AW, Larson MG, Benjamin EJ, *et al*. Increased left ventricular mass and hypertrophy are associated with increased risk for sudden death. J Am Coll Cardiol. 1998; 32: 1454–9.

12. Lakatta EG, Levy D. Arterial and cardiac ageing: major shareholders in cardiovascular disease enterprises: Part I: Ageing arteries: a "set up" for vascular disease. Circulation 2003; 107: 139–46.

13. McVeigh GE, Alen PB, Morgan DR, *et al*. Nitric oxide modulation of blood vessel tone identified by arterial wave form analysis. Clin Sci 2001; 100: 387–93.

14. Cameron JD, Pinto E, Bulpitt CJ, *et al*. The ageing of elastic and muscular arteries: a comparison of diabetic and non-diabetic subjects. Diabetes Care 2003; 26: 2127–32.

15. Pinto E, Mensah R, Meeran K, *et al*. Peripheral arterial compliance differs between races-comparison among Asian, Afro-Caribbeans, and white Caucasians with type 2 diabetes. Diabetes Care 2005; 28: 496.

16. Ezzat VA, Duncan ER, Wheatcroft SB, *et al*. The role of IGF-I and its binding proteins in the development of type 2 diabetes and cardiovascular disease. Diabetes, Obesity and Metabolism 2008; 10: 198–211.

17. Lee M, Gardin JM, Lynch JC, *et al*. Diabetes mellitus and echocardiographic left ventricular function in free-living elderly men and women: The Cardiovascular Health Study Am Heart J 1997; 133: 36–43.

18. Ren J, Sowers JR, Walsh MF and Brown RA. Reduced contractile response to insulin and IGF-1 in ventricular myocytes from genetically obese Zucker rats. Am J Physiol. 2000; 279: H1708–H14.

19. Casis O, Gallego M, Iriarte M, *et al*. Effects of diabetic cardiomyopathy on regional electrophysiologic characteristics of rat ventricle. Diabetologia 2000; 43: 101–9.

20. Henry, R. M. A., Paulus, W. J., Kamp, O., *et al*. Deteriorating glucose tolerance status is associated with left ventricular dysfunction - The Hoorn study. Netherlands Journal of Medicine 2008; 66: 110–17.

21. Zimmet P, Alberti KG and Shaw J. Global and societal implications of the diabetes epidemic. Nature 2001; 414: 782–7.

22. Grundy SM, Benjamin IJ, Burke GL, *et al*. Diabetes and cardiovascular disease: a statement for healthcare professionals from the American Heart Association. Circulation 1999; 100: 1134–46.

23. Varas-Lorenzo C, Rueda de Castro A, Maguire A, *et al*. Prevalence of glucose metabolism abnormalities and cardiovascular co-morbidity in the US elderly adult population. Pharmacoepidemiol Drug Saf 2006; 15: 317–26.

24. Burchfiel CM, Reed DM, Marcus EB, *et al*. Association of diabetes mellitus with coronary atherosclerosis and myocardial lesions. An autopsy study from the Honolulu Heart Program. Am J Epidemiol 1993; 137: 1328–40.

25. Goraya TY, Leibson CL, Palumbo PJ, *et al*. Coronary atherosclerosis in diabetes mellitus. A population-based autopsy study. J Am Coll Cardiol 2002; 40: 946–53.

26. Grundy SM, Howard BV, Smith SC, Jr, *et al*. Prevention Conference VI: Diabetes and cardiovascular disease. Executive summary. Conference proceeding for healthcare professionals from a special writing group of the American Heart Association. Circulation 2002; 105: 2231–9.

27. Nesto RW. Screening for asymptomatic coronary artery disease in diabetes. Diabetes Care 1999; 22: 1393–5.

28. Sloan FA, Bethel MA, Ruiz D, Jr, *et al*. The growing burden of diabetes mellitus in the US elderly population. Arch Intern Med 2008; 168: 192–9.

29. Expert Panel on Detection, Evaluation, and Treatment of High Blood Cholesterol in Adults: Executive Summary of The Third Report of The National Cholesterol Education Program (NCEP) Expert Panel on Detection, Evaluation, and Treatment of High Blood Cholesterol in Adults (Adult Treatment Panel III). JAMA 2001; 285: 2486–97.

30. Canadian Diabetes Association. Clinical Practice Guidelines for the Prevention and Management of Diabetes in Canada. Can J Diabetes 2003; 27(Suppl. 2): S1–S152.

31. Colagiuri S and Best J. Lipid-lowering therapy in people with type 2 diabetes. Curr Opin Lipidol. 2002; 13: 617–23.

32. Pearte CA, Furberg CD, O'Meara ES, *et al*. Characteristics and baseline clinical predictors of future fatal versus nonfatal coronary heart disease events in older adults. The Cardiovascular Health Study. Circulation 2006; 113: 2177–85.

33. Gaede P, Vedel P, Larsen N, *et al*. Multifactorial intervention and cardiovascular disease in patients with type 2 diabetes. N Engl J Med 2003; 348: 383–93.

34. Sirois C, Moisan J, Poirier P, *et al*. Underuse of cardioprotective treatment by the elderly with type 2 diabetes. Diabetes and Metabolism 2008; 34: 169–76.

35. Rea TD, Heckbert SR, Kaplan, RC, *et al*. Smoking status and risk for recurrent coronary events after

myocardial infarction. Ann Intern Med. 2002; 137: 494–8.

36. Stewart KJ. Exercise training and the cardiovascular consequences of type 2 diabetes and hypertension: plausible mechanisms for improving cardiovascular health. JAMA 2002; 288: 1622–31.

37. World Health Organization. (1999) Definition, Diagnosis and Classification of Diabetes Mellitus and its Complications Report of a WHO Consultation. Part 1: Diagnosis and Classification of Diabetes and Mellitus. World Health Organization, Geneva.

38. Balkau B and Charles MA. Comment on the provisional report from the WHO consultation. European Group for the Study of Insulin Resistance (EGIR). Diabet Med 1999; 16: 442–3.

39. Grundy SM, Cleeman JI, Daniels SR, et al. Diagnosis and management of the metabolic syndrome: an American Heart Association/National Heart, Lung, and Blood Institute Scientific Statement. Circulation 2005; 112: 2735–52.

40. Einhorn D, Reaven GM, Cobin RH, et al. American College of Endocrinology position statement on the insulin resistance syndrome. Endocr Pract 2003; 9: 237–52.

41. Alberti KG, Zimmet P and Shaw J. The metabolic syndrome – a new worldwide definition. Lancet 2005; 366: 1059–62.

42. Ravera M, Ratto E, Vettoretti S, et al. Microalbuminuria and subclinical cerebrovascular damage in essential hypertension. J Nephrol 2002; 15: 519–24.

43. Scuteri A, Najjar SS, Morrell CH, et al. The metabolic syndrome in older individuals: prevalence and prediction of cardiovascular events. Diabetes Care 2005; 28: 882–7.

44. Empana JP, Zureik M, Gariepy J, et al. The metabolic syndrome and the carotid artery structure in noninstitutionalized elderly subjects. The Three-City Study. Stroke 2007; 38: 893–9.

45. Hildrum B, Mykletun A, Hole T, et al. Age-specific prevalence of the metabolic syndrome defined by the International Diabetes Federation and the National Cholesterol Education Program: the Norwegian HUNT 2 study. BMC Public Health 2007, 7: 220.

46. Maggi S, Noale M, Gallina P, et al. Metabolic syndrome, diabetes, and cardiovascular disease in an elderly Caucasian cohort: the Italian longitudinal study on ageing. J Gerontol 2006; 61: 505–10.

47. Alexander CM, Landsman PB, Teutsch SM, et al. NCEP-defined metabolic syndrome, diabetes, and prevalence of coronary heart disease among NHANES III participants age 50 years and older. Diabetes 2003; 52: 1210–14.

48. Isommaa B, Almgren P, Tuomi T, et al. Cardiovascular morbidity and mortality associated with the metabolic syndrome. Diabetes Care 2001; 24: 683–9.

49. Lindblad U, Langer RD, Wingard DL, et al. Metabolic syndrome and ischaemic heart disease in elderly men and women. Am J Epidemiol 2001; 153: 481–9.

50. Scuteri A, Najjar SS, Muller DC, et al. Metabolic syndrome amplifies the age associated increases in vascular thickness and stiffness. J Am Coll Cardiol 2004; 43: 1388–95.

51. Bonora E, Kiechl S, Willeit J, et al. Carotid atherosclerosis and coronary heart disease in the metabolic syndrome: prospective data from the Bruneck Study. Diabetes Care 2003; 26: 1251–7.

52. Wang J, Ruotsalainen S, Moilanen L, et al. The metabolic syndrome predicts cardiovascular mortality: a 13-year follow up study in elderly non-diabetic Finns. Euro Heart J 2007, 28: 857–64.

53. Sattar N, McConnachie A, Shaper AG, et al. Can metabolic syndrome usefully predict cardiovascular disease and diabetes? Outcome data from two prospective studies. Lancet 2008; 371: 1927–35.

54. Casiglia E, Mazza A, Tikhonoff V, et al. Total cholesterol and mortality in the elderly. J Intern Med 2003; 254: 353–62.

55. Volpato S, Zuliani G, Guralnik JM, et al. The inverse association between age and cholesterol levels among older patients: the role of poor health status. Gerontology 2001; 47: 36–45.

56. Psaty BM, Anderson M, Kronmal RA, et al. The association between lipid levels and the risks of incident myocardial infarction, stroke, and total mortality: the Cardiovascular Health Study. J Am Geriatr Soc. 2004; 52: 1639–47.

57. Aronow WS and Ahn C. Incidence of new coronary events in older persons with prior myocardial infarction and serum low-density lipoprotein cholesterol $\geq$125 mg/dl treated with statins versus no lipid-lowering drug. Am J Cardiol. 2002; 89: 67–9.

58. Aronow WS, Ahn C and Gutstein H. Incidence of new atherothrombotic brain infarction in older persons with prior myocardial infarction and serum low-density lipoprotein cholesterol $\geq$125 mg/dl treated with statins versus no lipid-lowering drug. J Gerontol A Biol Sci Med Sci. 2002; 57: M333–5.

59. Foody JM, Rathore SS, Galusha D, et al. Hydroxymethylglutaryl-CoA reductase inhibitors in older persons with acute myocardial infarction: evidence for an age statin interaction. J Am Geriatr Soc. 2006; 54: 421–30.

60. Anum EA and Adera T. Hypercholesterolemia and coronary heart disease in the elderly: a meta-analysis. Ann Epidemiol. 2004; 14: 705–21.

61. Baigent C, Keech A, Kearney PM, *et al.* The Cholesterol Treatment Trialists' (CTT) Collaborators: Efficacy and safety of cholesterol-lowering treatment: prospective meta-analysis of data from 90,056 participants in 14 randomised trials of statins. Lancet 2005; 366: 1267–78.

62. Heart Protection Study Collaborative Group (2002) Heart Protection Study of cholesterol lowering with simvastatin in 20 536 high-risk individuals: a randomised placebo-controlled trial. Lancet, 360, 7–22.

63. Heart Protection Study Collaborative Group (2003) Heart Protection Study of cholesterol lowering with simvastatin in 5963 people with diabetes: a randomised placebo-controlled trial. Lancet, 361, 2005–16.

64. Costa J, Borges M, David C, *et al.* Efficacy of lipid lowering drug treatment for diabetic and non-diabetic patients: meta-analysis of randomised controlled trials. Br Med J 2006; 332; 1115–24.

65. Neil HAW, DeMicco DA, Luo D, *et al.* Analysis of efficacy and safety in patients aged 65–75 years at randomisation. Diabetes Care 2006; 29: 2378–84.

66. Mihaylova B, Briggs A, Armitage J, *et al.* The Heart Protection Study Collaborative Group: Cost-effectiveness of simvastatin in people at different levels of vascular risk: economic analysis of a randomised trial in 20,536 individuals. Lancet 2005; 365: 1779–85.

67. Sowers JR, Epstein M, Frohlich ED. Diabetes, hypertension, and cardiovascular disease: an update. Hypertension 2001; 37: 1053–9.

68. Cowie, C. C. and Harris, M. I. (1995) Physical and Metabolic Characteristics of Persons with Diabetes. 2nd edition. National Institutes of Health, National Institute of Diabetes and Digestive and Kidney Diseases, Bethesda, MD, pp. 117–64.

69. Gress TW, Nieto FJ, Shahar E, *et al.* Hypertension and antihypertensive therapy as risk factors for type 2 diabetes mellitus: Atherosclerosis Risk in Communities Study. N Engl J Med. 2000; 342: 905–12.

70. Chobanian AV, Bakris GL, Black HR, *et al.* The Seventh Report of the Joint National Committee on Prevention, Detection, Evaluation, and Treatment of High Blood Pressure: the JNC 7 Report. JAMA. 2003; 289: 2560–71.

71. UK Prospective Diabetes Study Group. Tight blood pressure control and risk of macrovascular and microvascular complications in type 2 diabetes: UKPDS 38. Br Med J. 1998; 317: 703–13.

72. Hansson L, Zanchetti A, Carruthers SG, *et al.* and the HOT Study Group. Effects of intensive blood pressure lowering and low dose aspirin in patients with hypertension: principal results of the Hypertension Optimal Treatment (HOT) randomised trial. Lancet 1998; 351: 1755–62.

73. Tuomilehto J, Rastenyte D, Birkenhager WH, *et al.* Systolic Hypertension in Europe Trial Investigators. Effects of calcium-channel blockade in older patients with diabetes and systolic hypertension. N Engl J Med. 1999; 340: 677–84.

74. Curb JD, Pressel SL, Cutler JA, *et al.* Systolic Hypertension in the Elderly Program Cooperative Research Group. Effect of diuretic based antihypertensive treatment on cardiovascular disease risk in older diabetic patients with isolated systolic hypertension. JAMA. 1996; 276: 1886–92.

75. McFarlane SI, Jacober SJ, Winer N, *et al.* Control of cardiovascular risk factors in patients with diabetes and hypertension at urban academic medical centers. Diabetes Care 2002; 25: 718–23.

76. Gianni M, Bosch J, Pogue J, *et al.* Effect of long-term ACE-inhibitor therapy in elderly vascular disease patients Eur Heart J 2007; 28: 1382–8.

77. Ravid M, Brosh D, Levi Z, *et al.* Use of enalapril to attenuate decline in renal function in normotensive, normoalbuminuric patients with type 2 diabetes mellitus. A randomized, controlled trial. Ann Intern Med. 1998; 128: 982–8.

78. Ahmad J, Siddiqui MA and Ahmad H. Effective postponement of diabetic nephropathy with enalapril in normotensive type 2 diabetic patients with microalbuminuria. Diabetes Care 1997; 20: 1576–81.

79. Bangalore S, Parkar S, Grossman E, *et al.* A meta-analysis of 94,492 patients with hypertension treated with beta blockers to determine the risk of new-onset diabetes mellitus. Am J Cardiol 2007; 100: 1254–62.

80. Elliott WJ and Meyer PM. Incident diabetes in clinical trials of antihypertensive drugs: a network meta-analysis. Lancet 2007; 369: 201–7.

81. Lithell H, Pollare T and Vessby B. Metabolic effects of pindolol and propranolol in a double-blind cross-over study in hypertensive patients. Blood Press 1992; 1: 92–101.

82. Bakris GL, Fonseca V, Katholi RE, *et al.* Metabolic effects of carvedilol vs metoprolol in patients with type 2 diabetes mellitus and hypertension: a randomized controlled trial. JAMA 2004; 292: 2227–36.

83. ALLHAT Officers and Coordinators for the ALLHAT Collaborative Research Group. (2002) Major outcomes in high-risk hypertensive patients randomized to angiotensin converting enzyme inhibitor or calcium channel blocker vs diuretic: The Antihypertensive and Lipid-Lowering Treatment to Prevent Heart Attack Trial (ALLHAT). JAMA, 288, 2981–97.

84. Brenner BM, Cooper ME, de Zeeuw D, *et al.* Effects of losartan on renal and cardiovascular outcomes in

patients with type 2 diabetes and nephropathy. N Engl J Med. 2001; 345: 861–9.

85. Parving HH, Lehnert H, Brochner-Mortensen J, *et al*. The effect of irbesartan on the development of diabetic nephropathy in patients with type 2 diabetes. N Engl J Med. 2001; 345: 870–8.

86. Lewis EJ, Hunsicker LG, Clarke WR, *et al*. Renoprotective effect of the angiotensin receptor antagonist irbesartan in patients with nephropathy due to type 2 diabetes. N Engl J Med. 2001; 345: 851–60.

87. Lindholm LH, Ibsen H, Dahlöf B, *et al*. Cardiovascular morbidity and mortality in patients with diabetes in the Losartan Intervention For Endpoint reduction in hypertension study (LIFE): a randomised trial against atenolol. Lancet 2002; 359: 1004–10.

88. Matchar DB, McCrory DC, Orlando LA, *et al*. Systematic Review: Comparative effectiveness of angiotensin converting enzyme inhibitors and angiotensin II receptor blockers for treating essential hypertension. Ann Intern Med. 2008; 148: 16–29.

89. Beckett NS, Peters R, Fletcher AE, *et al*. Treatment of hypertension in patients 80 years of age or older. N Engl J Med 2008; 358: 1887–98.

90. Langford HG, Cutter G, Oberman A, *et al*. The effect of thiazide therapy on glucose, insulin and cholesterol metabolism and of glucose on potassium: results of a cross-sectional study in patients from the Hypertension Detection and Follow-up Program. J Hum Hypertens. 1990; 4: 491–500.

91. Morigi M, Angioletti S, Imberti B, *et al*. Leukocyte-endothelial interaction is augmented by high glucose concentrations and hyperglycemia in a NF-kB dependent fashion. J Clin Invest 1998; 101: 1905–15.

92. Turner RC, Millns H, Neil HAW, *et al*. Risk factors for coronary artery disease in non-insulin dependent diabetes mellitus: United Kingdom prospective diabetes study (UKPDS:23). Br Med J 1998; 316: 823–8.

93. Letho S, Ronnemaa T, Pyorala K, *et al*. Poor glycaemic control predicts coronary heart disease events in patients with type 1 diabetes without nephropathy. Arterioscler Thromb Vasc Biol 1999; 13: 1014–19.

94. Turner RC, Cull CA, Frighi V, *et al*. Glycemic control with diet, sulfonylurea, metformin, or insulin in patients with type 2 diabetes mellitus: progressive requirement for multiple therapies (UKPDS 49): UK Prospective Diabetes Study (UKPDS) Group. JAMA 1999; 281: 2005–12.

95. DECODE Study Group. (2003) European Diabetes Epidemiology Group: Is the current definition for diabetes relevant to mortality risk from all causes and cardiovascular and noncardiovascular diseases? Diabetes Care, 26: 688–96.

96. DECODE Study Group. (2001) European Diabetes Epidemiology Group: Glucose tolerance and cardiovascular mortality: comparison of fasting and 2-hour diagnostic criteria. Arch Intern Med., 161: 397–405.

97. Selvin E, Marinopoulos S, Berkenblit G, *et al*. Meta-analysis: glycosylated hemoglobin and cardiovascular disease in diabetes mellitus. Ann Intern Med 2004; 141: 421–31.

98. Milicevic Z, Raz I, Beattie SD, *et al*. Natural history of cardiovascular disease in patients with diabetes. Diabetes Care 2008; 31 (Suppl. 2): S155–60.

99. Hanefeld M, Cagatay M, Petrowitsch T, *et al*. Acarbose reduces the risk for myocardial infarction in type 2 diabetic patients: meta-analysis of seven long-term studies. Eur Heart J 2004; 25: 10–16.

100. Carmassi F, Morale M and Puccetti R. Coagulation and fibrinolytic system impairment in insulin dependent diabetes mellitus. Thromb Res 1992; 67: 643–54.

101. Walsh MF, Dominguez LJ and Sowers JR. Metabolic abnormalities in cardiac ischaemia. Cardiol Clin 1995; 13: 529–38.

102. Beckman JA, Creager MA and Libby P. Diabetes and atherosclerosis. JAMA 2002; 287: 2570–81.

103. Gupta OP and Phatak S. Pandemic trends in prevalence of diabetes mellitus and associated coronary heart disease in India - their causes and prevention. Int J Diab 2003; 23: 37–50.

104. Kodali VRR. (2002) Epidemiology of diabetes mellitus in migrant populations, in: M. M. S. Ahuja, B. B. Tripathi, S. G. P. Moses, H. B. Chandalia, A. K. Das, P. V. Rao and S. V. Madhu (eds), RSSDI Textbook of Diabetes Mellitus, National Book Depot, India, pp. 113–19.

105. Mohan V, Deepa R, Shanthirani S, *et al*. Prevalence of coronary artery disease and its relationship to lipids in a selected population in south India. J. Am. Coll Cardiol 2001; 38: 687–97.

106. Mohan V, Deepa R, Harath SP, *et al*. Lipoprotein (a) is an independent risk factor for coronary artery disease in NIDDIM patients in south India. Diabetes Care, 1998; 21: 1819–23.

107. Saaddine JB, Engelgau MM, Beckles GL, *et al*. A diabetes report card for the United States: quality of care in the 1990s. Ann Intern Med 2002; 136: 565–74.

108. Kirk JK, Bell RA, Bertoni AG, *et al*. Qualitative review of studies of diabetes preventive care among minority patients in the United States, 1993–2003 (Review). Am J Manag Care 2005; 11: 349–60.

109. Ness J, Aronow WS. Prevalence of coronary artery disease, ischemic stroke, peripheral arterial disease, and coronary revascularization in older

African-Americans, Asians, Hispanics, whites, men, and women. Am J Cardiol 1999; 84: 932–3.

110. Gillum RF, Mussolino ME and Madans JH. Diabetes mellitus, coronary heart disease incidence, and death from all causes in African American and European American women: the NHANES I epidemiologic follow-up study. J Clin Epidemiol 2000; 53: 511–18.

111. Karter AJ, Ferrara A, Liu JY, et al. Ethnic disparities in diabetic complications in an insured population. JAMA 2002; 287: 2519–27.

112. Young BA, Maynard C and Boyko EJ. Racial differences in diabetic nephropathy, cardiovascular disease, and mortality in a national population of veterans. Diabetes Care 2003; 26: 2392–9.

113. Chaturvedi N, Jarrett J, Morrish N, et al. Differences in mortality and morbidity in African Caribbean and European people with non-insulin dependent diabetes mellitus. Br Med J 1996; 313: 848–52.

114. Bertoni AG, Kirk JK, Case LD, et al. The effects of race and region on cardiovascular morbidity among elderly Americans with diabetes. Diabetes Care 2005; 28: 2620–5.

115. Fein F and Scheuer J. (1990) Heart disease in diabetes mellitus: theory and practice. In: H. Rifkin and D. Porte, Jr (eds), Ellenberg and Rifkin's Diabetes Mellitus: Theory and Practice. 4th edition. Elsevier Science, Inc., New York, pp. 812–23.

116. Miettinen H, Lehto S, Salomaa V, et al. Impact of diabetes on mortality after the first myocardial infarction. Diabetes Care 1998; 21: 69–75.

117. Booth GL, Kapral MK, Fung K, et al. Relation between age and cardiovascular disease in men and women with diabetes compared with non-diabetic people: a population-based retrospective cohort study. Lancet 2006; 368: 29–36.

118. Chiariello M, Indolfi C, Cotecchia MR, et al. Asymptomatic transient changes during ambulatory ECG monitoring in diabetic patients. Am Heart J. 1985; 110: 529–34.

119. Marshall SM and Flyvbjerg A. Prevention and early detection of vascular complications of diabetes. Br Med J 2006; 333: 475–80.

120. Lee WL, Cheung AM, Cape D, et al. Impact of diabetes on coronary artery disease in women and men: a meta-analysis of prospective studies. Diabetes Care 2000; 23: 962–8.

121. Huxley R, Barzi F and Woodward M. Excess risk of fatal coronary heart disease associated with diabetes in men and women: meta-analysis of 37 prospective cohort studies. Br Med J 2006; 332: 73–8.

122. Becker A, Bos G, de Vegt F, et al. Cardiovascular events in type 2 diabetes: comparison with nondiabetic individuals without and with prior cardiovascular disease. 10 year follow-up of the Hoorn Study. Eur Heart J. 2003; 24: 1406–13.

123. Kronmal RA, Barzilay JI, Smith NL, et al. Mortality in pharmacologically treated older adults with diabetes: the Cardiovascular Health Study 1989–2001. PLoS Med. 2006; 3: e400.

124. Fox CS, Sullivan L, D'Agostino RB, Sr, et al. The significant effect of diabetes duration on coronary heart disease mortality: the Framingham Heart Study. Diabetes Care 2004; 27: 704–8.

125. Hu FB, Stampfer MJ, Haffner SM, et al. Elevated risk of cardiovascular disease prior to clinical diagnosis of type 2 diabetes. Diabetes Care 2002; 25: 1129–34.

126. Chen J, Marciniak TA, Radford MJ, et al. Beta-blocker therapy for secondary prevention of myocardial infarction in elderly diabetic patients. Results from the national cooperative cardiovascular project. J Am Coll Cardiol 1999; 34: 1388–94.

127. Chyun D, Vaccarino V, Murillo J, et al. Cardiac outcomes after myocardial infarction in elderly patients with diabetes mellitus. Am J Critical Care 2002; 11: 504–19.

128. Kosiborod M, Rathore SS, Inzucchi SE, et al. Admission glucose and mortality in elderly patients hospitalized with acute myocardial infarction implications for patients with and without recognized diabetes. Circulation 2005; 111: 3078–86.

129. Mehta RH, Ruane TJ, McCargar PA, et al. The treatment of elderly diabetic patients with acute myocardial infarction insight from Michigan's Cooperative Cardiovascular Project. Arch Intern Med. 2000; 160: 1301–6.

130. Donahue RP, Goldberg RJ, Chen Z, et al. The influence of sex and diabetes mellitus on survival following acute myocardial infarction: a communitywide perspective. J Clin Epidemiol. 1993; 46: 245–52.

131. Woodfield S, Ludergan C, Reiner J, et al. Angiographic findings and outcome in diabetic patients treated with thrombolytic therapy for acute myocardial infarction: the GUSTO-I experience. J Am Coll Cardiol. 1996; 28: 1661–9.

132. Malmberg K, Ryden L, Efendic S, et al. Randomized trial of insulin-glucose infusion followed by subcutaneous insulin treatment in diabetic patients with acute myocardial infarction (DIGAMI study): effects on mortality at one year. J Am Coll Cardiol. 1995; 26: 57–65.

133. Malmberg K. DIGAMI (Diabetes Mellitus, Insulin Glucose Infusion in Acute Myocardial Infarction) Study Group. Prospective randomised study of intensive insulin treatment on long term survival after acute myocardial infarction in patients with diabetes mellitus. Br Med J. 1997; 314: 1512–15.

134. Malmberg K, Ryden L, Wedel H, *et al.* DIGAMI 2 Investigators. Intense metabolic control by means of insulin in patients with diabetes mellitus and acute myocardial infarction (DIGAMI 2): effects on mortality and morbidity. Eur Heart J. 2005; 26: 650–61.

135. Fath-Ordoubadi F and Beatt KJ. Glucose-insulin-potassium therapy for treatment of acute myocardial infarction: an overview of randomized placebo-controlled trials. Circulation 1997; 96: 1152–6.

136. Kloner RA and Nesto RW. Glucose-insulin-potassium for acute myocardial infarction continuing controversy over cardioprotection. Circulation 2008; 117: 2523–33.

137. Nichols GA, Gullion CM, Koro CE, *et al.* The incidence of congestive heart failure in type 2 diabetes: an update. Diabetes Care 2004; 27: 1879–84.

138. Carr AA, Kowey PR, Devereux RB, *et al.* Hospitalisations for new heart failure among subjects with diabetes mellitus in the RENAAL and LIFE studies. Am J Cardiol 2005; 96: 1530–6.

139. Stratton IM, Adler AI, Neil HA, *et al.* Association of glycaemia with macrovascular and microvascular complications of type-2 diabetes (UKPDS 35): prospective observational study. Br Med J 2000; 321: 405–12.

140. Wong TY, Rosamond W, Chang PP, *et al.* Retinopathy and risk of congestive heart failure. JAMA 2005; 293: 63–9.

141. Yip GWK, Ho PPY, Woo KS, *et al.* Comparison of frequencies of left ventricular systolic and diastolic heart failure in Chinese living in Hong Kong. Am J Cardiol 1999; 84: 563–7.

142. Bell DS. Heart failure: the frequent, forgotten, and often fatal complication of diabetes. Diabetes Care 2003; 26: 2433–41.

143. Heart Outcomes Prevention Evaluation Study Investigators: Effects of ramipril on cardiovascular and microvascular outcomes in people with diabetes mellitus: results of the HOPE study and MICROHOPE substudy. Lancet 2000; 355: 253–9.

144. Nichols GA, Hillier TA, Erbey JR, *et al.* Congestive heart failure in type 2 diabetes: prevalence, incidence, and risk factors. Diabetes Care 2001; 24: 1614–19.

145. Davis RC, Hobbs FD, Kenkre JE, *et al.* Prevalence of left ventricular systolic dysfunction and heart failure in high risk patients: community based epidemiological study. Br Med J 2002; 325: 1156.

146. Aronow WS and Ahn C. Incidence of heart failure in 2,737 older persons with and without diabetes mellitus. Chest 1999; 115: 867–8.

147. UK Prospective Diabetes Study (UKPDS). Intensive blood glucose control with sulphonylureas or insulin compared with conventional treatment and risk of complications in patients with type 2 diabetes (UKPDS 33). Lancet 1998; 352: 837–53.

148. Heart Outcomes Prevention Evaluation (HOPE) Study Investigators. Effects of ramipril on cardiovascular and microvascular outcomes in people with diabetes mellitus: results of the HOPE study and MICRO-HOPE substudy. Lancet 2000; 355: 253–9.

149. Shepherd J, Barter P, Carmena R, *et al.* for the Treating to New Targets Investigators. (2006) Effect of lowering LDL cholesterol substantially below currently recommended levels in patients with coronary heart disease and diabetes: the Treating to New Targets (TNT) study. Diabetes Care, 29, 1220–6.

150. Bertoni AG, Hundley WG, Massing MW, *et al.* Heart failure prevalence, incidence, and mortality in the elderly with diabetes. Diabetes Care 2004; 27: 699–703.

151. Vaur L, Gueret P, Lievre M, *et al.* Development of congestive heart failure in type 2 diabetic patients with microalbuminuria or proteinuria: observations from the DIABHYCAR (type 2 DIABetes Hypertension CArdiovascular Events and Ramipril) study. Diabetes Care 2003; 26: 855–60.

152. Epshteyn V, Morrison K, Krishnaswamy P, *et al.* Utility of B-Type Natriuretic Peptide (BNP) as a screen for left ventricular dysfunction in patients with diabetes. Diabetes Care 2003; 26: 2081–7.

153. Banerjee P, Clark AL, Nikitin N, *et al.* Diastolic heart failure: paroxysmal or chronic? Eur J Heart Fail 2004; 6: 427–31.

154. Haas SJ, Vos T, Gilbert RE, *et al.* Are beta-blockers as efficacious in patients with diabetes mellitus as in patients without diabetes mellitus who have chronic heart failure? A meta-analysis of large-scale clinical trials. Am Heart J 2003; 146: 848–53.

155. Deedwania PC, Giles TD, Klibaner M, *et al.* Efficacy, safety and tolerability of metoprolol CR/XL in patients with diabetes and chronic heart failure: experiences from MERIT-HF. Am Heart J 2005; 149: 159–67.

156. Wlodarczyk JH, Keogh A, Smith K, *et al.* CHART: congestive cardiac failure in hospitals, an Australian review of treatment. Heart Lung Circ 2003; 12: 94–102.

157. Del Sindaco DA, Pulignano GB, Cioffi GC, *et al.* Safety and efficacy of carvedilol in very elderly diabetic patients with heart failure. J Cardiovasc Med 2007; 8: 675–82.

158. Shekelle PG, Rich MW, Morton SC, *et al.* Efficacy of angiotensin converting enzyme inhibitors and beta-blockers in the management of left ventricular systolic dysfunction according to race, gender, and diabetic status: a meta-analysis of major clinical trials. J Am Coll Cardiol 2003; 41: 1529–38.

159. Young JB, Dunlap ME, Pfeffer MA, *et al.*, for the Candesartan in Heart Failure Assessment of Reduction in Mortality morbidity (CHARM) Investigators. (2004) Mortality and morbidity reduction with candesartan in patients with chronic heart failure and left ventricular systolic dysfunction: results of the CHARM low-left ventricular ejection fraction trials. Circulation, 110: 2618–26.

160. Cohn JN and Tognoni G. The Valsartan Heart Failure Trial Investigators. A randomized trial of the angiotensin-receptor blocker valsartan in chronic heart failure. N Engl J Med 2001; 345: 1667–75.

161. Fernandez HM, Leipzig RM, Larkin RJ, *et al.* The Randomized Aldactone Evaluation Study Investigators. Spironolactone in patients with heart failure. N Engl J Med 2000; 342: 132–4.

162. Huxley R, Barzi F and Woodward M. Excess risk of fatal coronary heart disease associated with diabetes in men and women: meta-analysis of 37 prospective cohort studies. Br Med J 2006; 332: 73–8.

163. Ahmed A, Aban IB, Vaccarino V, *et al.* A propensity-matched study of the effect of diabetes on the natural history of heart failure: variations by sex and age Heart 2007; 93: 1584–90.

164. Klimt CR, Knatterud GI, Meinert CL, *et al.* University Group Diabetes Program. A study of the effects of hypoglycaemic agents on vascular complications in patients with adult-onset diabetes, II: mortality results. Diabetes 1970; 19 (Suppl.): S789–830.

165. Karter AJ, Ahmed AT, Liu J, *et al.* Pioglitazone initiation and subsequent hospitalisation for congestive heart failure. Diabet Med 2005; 22: 986–93.

166. Masoudi FA, Inzucchi SE, Wang Y, *et al.* Thiazolidinediones, metformin, and outcomes in Relation between chronic heart failure and diabetes mellitus 1237 older patients with diabetes and heart failure: an observational study. Circulation 2005; 111: 583–90.

167. Domanski M, Krause-Steinrauf H, Deedwania, P. *et al.* The effect of diabetes on outcomes of patients with advanced heart failure in the BEST trial. J Am Coll Cardiol 2003; 42: 914–22.

168. Smooke S, Horwich TB and Fonarow GC. Insulin-treated diabetes is associated with a marked increase in mortality in patients with advanced heart failure. Am Heart J 2005; 149: 168–74.

169. UK Prospective Diabetes Study (UKPDS) Group. Effect of intensive blood-glucose control with metformin on complications in overweight patients with type 2 diabetes (UKPDS 34). Lancet 1998; 352: 854–65.

170. Eurich DT, Majumdar SR, McAlister FA, *et al.* Improved clinical outcomes associated with metformin in patients with diabetes and heart failure. Diabetes Care 2005; 28: 2345–51.

171. Kahn SE, Haffner SM, Heise MA, *et al.* Glycaemic durability of rosiglitazone, metformin, or glyburide monotherapy. N Engl J Med. 2006; 355: 2427–43.

172. Stettler C, Allemann S, Juni P, *et al.* Glycemic control and macrovascular disease in types 1 and 2 diabetes mellitus: meta-analysis of randomized trials. Am Heart J. 2006; 152: 27–38.

173. Lincoff AM, Wolski K, Nicholls SJ, *et al.* Pioglitazone and risk of cardiovascular events in patients with type 2 diabetes mellitus: a metaanalysis of randomized trials. JAMA. 2007; 298: 1180–8.

174. Berlie HD, Kalus JS and Jaber LA. Thiazolidinediones and the risk of edema: a meta-analysis. Diabetes Res Clin Pract. 2007; 76: 279–89.

175. Karalliedde J and Buckingham RE. Thiazolidinediones and their fluid-related adverse effects: facts, fiction and putative management strategies. Drug Safety 2007; 30: 741–53.

176. Nissen SE and Wolski K. Effect of rosiglitazone on the risk of myocardial infarction and death from cardiovascular causes. N Engl J Med. 2007; 356: 2457–71.

177. Singh S, Loke YK and Furberg CD. Long-term risk of cardiovascular events with rosiglitazone: a meta-analysis. JAMA. 2007; 298: 1189–95.

178. Singh S, Loke YK and Furberg CD. Thiazolidinediones and heart failure: a teleo-analysis. Diabetes Care 2007; 30: 2148–53.

179. Lipscombe LL, Gomes T, Le'vesque LE, *et al.* Thiazolidinediones and cardiovascular outcomes in older patients with diabetes. JAMA 2007; 298: 2634–43.

180. Derosa G, Cicero AF, D'Angelo A, *et al.* Effects of 1 year of treatment with pioglitazone or rosiglitazone added to glimepiride on lipoprotein(a) and homocysteine concentrations in patients with type 2 diabetes mellitus and metabolic syndrome: a multicenter, randomized, double-blind, controlled clinical trial. Clin Ther. 2006; 28: 679–88.

6

Stroke and Diabetes

Janice E. O'Connell and Christopher S. Gray

Department of Geriatric Medicine, University of Newcastle, Sunderland Royal Hospital, Sunderland, UK

Key messages

- Type 2 diabetes mellitus is the predominant form in stroke patients. It is not only a risk factor for cerebrovascular disease but also increases the likelihood of a poor clinical outcome following acute stroke.
- Hyperglycaemia after acute stroke is associated with a poor prognosis, both in diabetic and non-diabetic individuals.
- Acute treatment of post-stroke hyperglycaemia with insulin has not been shown to be beneficial in recent clinical trials.
- Primary and secondary stroke prevention in patients with type 2 diabetes requires good diabetic control, plus management of all other vascular risk factors.

6.1 Introduction

The spectrum of cerebrovascular disease ranges from reversible neurological symptoms and signs due to transient cerebral ischaemia to permanent neurological deficit consequent on brain infarction or primary intracerebral haemorrhage. Furthermore, cerebrovascular disease is now recognized as a major cause of cognitive decline, not only due to vascular dementia but also as a contributor to Alzheimer's disease through a mixed vascular and Alzheimer's-type pathology. Both type 1 diabetes mellitus (T1DM) and type 2 diabetes melli-

tus (T2DM) are known to be important risk factors for stroke [1, 2]. However, this association is primarily for ischaemic stroke, and there is no proven link between diabetes and primary intracerebral haemorrhage. The predominant form of diabetes in older people is T2DM, and in this chapter we will focus on the relationship between T2DM, ischaemic stroke and transient ischaemic attack (TIA).

6.1.1 Definitions

The World Health Organization (WHO) diagnostic criteria make an arbitrary time distinction at 24 h from symptom onset between TIAs, where transient neurological dysfunction lasts less than 24 h, and the completed stroke, with symptoms and signs persisting beyond this time [3]. However, more recent evidence shows that most TIAs resolve within 1 h and, moreover, TIA patients with symptoms lasting more than 6 h have neuroradiological evidence of ischaemic change on magnetic resonance imaging (MRI) brain scan. A new definition for TIA has therefore been proposed: '...a brief episode of neurological dysfunction with symptoms lasting less than one hour and without evidence of acute infarction' [4].

Within the group of patients with ischaemic stroke, there are several potential pathophysiological mechanisms. Approximately 29–44% will be due to thrombosis *in situ*, 20–25% to cardioembolism, 13–21% to small-artery disease (lacunar stroke) and 15–17% to mixed or undetermined aetiologies [5]. In diabetes and

Diabetes in Old Age. Third Edition. Edited by Alan J. Sinclair
© 2009 John Wiley & Sons, Ltd

impaired glucose tolerance, atherosclerotic changes in the vasculature are accelerated, with a threefold increased risk for asymptomatic carotid artery stenosis seen in T2DM [6]. There remains conflicting evidence as to the clinical and pathological type of ischaemic stroke that predominates in diabetic individuals. Large-artery atherosclerotic disease was previously felt to be more severe in patients with diabetes mellitus (DM), but more recent evidence suggested an association between DM and small-vessel lacunar events [7, 8]. A meta-analysis of population-based studies however, failed to demonstrate any association between DM and small-vessel disease (OR 1.1 95% CI: 0.8–1.4, p = 0.82) [9].

6.1.2 Epidemiology of stroke

In both the UK and USA, cerebrovascular disease is the third major cause of death, and the most important cause of severe adult disability in the community [10]. Stroke is also the single most expensive medical disorder, consuming up to 6% of the total clinical budget [11]. Against this background of the high costs of medical and social care, the major risk factors for cerebrovascular disease have been well defined and the management of modifiable risk factors outlined in national guidelines and service frameworks [12, 13]. Until recently, the burden of stroke on health and social services has been relatively under-recognized in comparison with other diseases such as cancer and coronary heart disease (CHD). However, with the recent publication of the Department of Health National Stroke Strategy comes the recognition of the importance of stroke as a major cause of morbidity and mortality in the UK [14]. There are likely to be major changes in the organization and delivery of stroke services in England and Wales in the next decade.

Stroke is primarily a disorder of old age, with its peak incidence seen in those over 75 years of age. Nevertheless, a significant proportion of patients is younger and has potentially modifiable risk factors, including T2DM. Over the past few decades, we have witnessed demographic shifts in our population towards the extremes of old age, with maximal population expansion in those aged over 75 years. Despite guidance-based interventions for the detection and early management of vascular risk factors, some (including T2DM) remain under-recognized, especially in the elderly. It seems likely therefore that the incidence of stroke in our ageing population will continue to rise.

6.2 Diabetes, hyperglycaemia and stroke risk in older people

Both T1DM and T2DM are important risk factors for cerebrovascular disease, conferring a two- to three-fold increased risk of first and recurrent stroke [1, 2]. In older people, the prevalent form is T2DM, seen in up to 7% of individuals. Glucose tolerance is known to decline with ageing, with estimates that a further 7.7–14.8% of older adults will have unrecognized T2DM according to 1997 American Diabetes Association and 1985 World Health Organisation criteria, respectively [15]. The prevalence of T2DM in an elderly Caucasian population may be as high as 20%, with even higher rates in other ethnic groups such as south Asians living in Britain [16]. Although most diabetic patients have multiple risk factors for vascular disease, diabetes remains an independent risk factor for stroke across all age groups. Furthermore, as a marker of arteriosclerotic vascular disease, it is estimated that the prevalence of carotid artery disease in elderly diabetics is 20% [17]. The increased likelihood of suffering cardiovascular disease (CVD) is not confined to people with diabetes, but also includes those with impaired glucose tolerance, asymptomatic non-fasting hyperglycaemia and hyperinsulinaemia [18].

Since most strokes occur in older people, it follows that the majority of diabetic stroke patients will have T2DM. Published estimates of the actual stroke risk in diabetics vary, due to differences in the populations studied, the diagnostic criteria employed or the use of indirect measures such as glycated haemoglobin (HbA_{1C}) concentration. A fairly reliable risk estimate for stroke risk in T2DM may be obtained from a recent cohort study of all known T2DM cases on the UK General Practice Research Database [19]. Here, 41 799 patients with T2DM aged 35–89 years at outset were followed for 7 years, during which the absolute rate of stroke was 11.91 per 1000 person-years, compared to 5.55 per 1000 person-years for non-diabetic matched controls. The age-adjusted hazard ratio for stroke in T2DM compared with controls was 2.19 (95% CI: 2.09–2.32). Additional stroke risk factors in T2DM included the duration of diabetes, smoking, obesity, atrial fibrillation and hypertension. The Nurses' Health Study, a female-only cohort, also confirmed the relationship between T2DM and ischaemic stroke, with a relative risk of 2.3 (95% CI: 2.0–2.6) [20]. In this study, the risk of stroke was associated with the duration of T2DM, and similar risks for large-artery and lacunar infarction were observed. The incidence and risk factors for stroke in T2DM were also examined in another recent cohort study of 14 432 patients attending 201 Italian diabetes centres, which found 296 incident strokes over a 4-year follow-up period [21]. Pre-existing cardiovascular disease was identified as an important risk factor, with an age-standardized incidence of stroke in men of 13.7 per 1000 patient-years in those with known CVD versus 5.5 per 1000 patient-years in diabetics with no previous CVD.

In general, such epidemiological studies classify patients as diabetic if the diagnosis were known to their health care provider prior to the incident event. Given that the prevalence of unrecognized T2DM in the older population may be as high as 14.8%, the impact of DM on stroke incidence is likely to be underestimated.

6.2.1 Control of DM and stroke risk

Epidemiological studies provide conflicting evidence regarding the association between chronic hyperglycaemia and stroke risk [22]. However, there appears to be a relationship between hyperglycaemia as measured by HbA_{1C} and incident stroke, with a threshold $\geq 7\%$ [23]. Most interventional studies have shown that improved glucose control in both T1DM and T2DM can delay only the development and progression of microvascular complications such as retinopathy, nephropathy and neuropathy. It is, therefore, important to emphasize that patients with T2DM are more likely to develop macrovascular complications of

their disease. Data from the United Kingdom Prospective Diabetes Study (UKPDS) confirmed that over a 9-year period, 20% of individuals with T2DM would experience macrovascular complications, including ischaemic stroke, whilst only 9% would have microvascular problems [24]. A recent inception cohort study in Saskatchewan, Canada confirmed that macrovascular complications such as stroke occur early after the diagnosis of T2DM [25]. Here, during the five years following the initiation of oral hypoglycaemic therapy, 9.1% of 12 272 diabetic patients had a stroke, representing a twofold risk compared to the general population (Figure 6.1).

The intensive treatment of T2DM can be shown to result in an improved maintenance of euglycaemia, but the clinical benefits of such a strategy are largely confined to the prevention of microvascular complications. The UKPDS was a randomized controlled trial that examined the effect of intensive blood glucose control with either sulphonylureas or insulin compared with conventional care upon the risk of both microvascular and macrovascular complications [26]. Intensive treatment resulted in a significant 11% reduction in HbA_{1C} that was maintained throughout 10 years of follow-up. However, this improvement in glucose control was not associated with a reduction in the rate of stroke, with 5.6% of patients in the intensive treatment group and 5.2% in the conventional treatment group having a fatal or non-fatal stroke. In the intensive treatment group there was a non-significant reduction in myocardial infarction (MI) (Figure 6.2). In addition, within the intensive treatment group there was a non-significant trend (p = 0.07) towards an increase in stroke risk

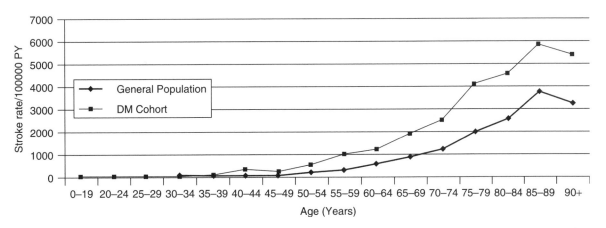

Figure 6.1 Age-standardized stroke hospitalization rates for the cohort with newly treated type 2 diabetes mellitus (DM) and the 1996 general population of Saskatchewan. PY = patient-years. Reprinted with permission from Ref. [25].

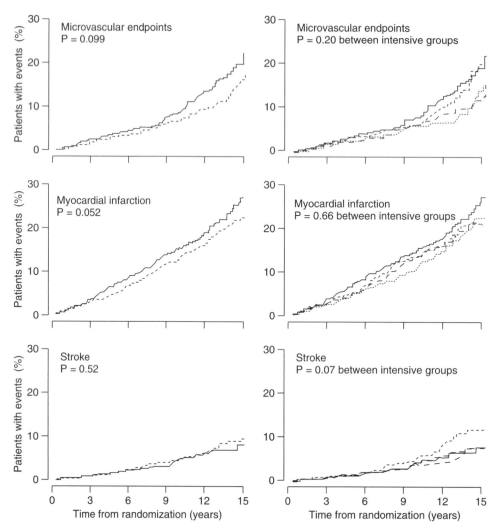

Figure 6.2 Kaplan-Meier plots of aggregate end points: microvascular disease, myocardial infarction and stroke for intensive and conventional treatment and by individual intensive therapy in UKPDS 33. Reprinted with permission from Ref. [26].

with glibenclamide (7.3%) compared to either chlorpropamide (5.3%) or insulin (4.6%) therapy.

The question is, therefore, as the intensive treatment of T2DM with either insulin or a sulphonylurea does not reduce the risk of cerebrovascular disease, is there a role for monotherapy with metformin? Evidence from the UKPDS indicates that whilst treatment with insulin, chlorpropamide or glibenclamide achieves similar degrees of diabetic control, there is the attendant risk of weight gain. In patients with T2DM who are overweight, the use of metformin can achieve equivalent levels of glycaemic control, without affecting weight or

increasing the risk of hypoglycaemia [27]. In fact, during the long-term follow-up of overweight participants in UKPDS, who were randomized to diet alone versus intensive treatment with metformin, insulin or sulphonylurea, additional clinical benefits were observed with metformin therapy [28]. When compared with dietary management alone, metformin treatment decreased not only the risk of all-cause mortality by 36%, but also the combined risk of MI, sudden death, angina, peripheral vascular disease and stroke by 30%. Furthermore, in comparison with sulphonylurea or insulin, metformin was associated with significantly greater reductions in any diabetes-related end point, including all-cause mortality and stroke. Although the results of UKPDS 34 suggested that the addition of metformin to sulphonylurea therapy might actually increase mortality, it is likely that the need for such combined treatment identified those patients whose prognosis was already poor due to factors such as age and poor glycaemic control.

Since the publication of the UKPDS results, additional oral antidiabetic drugs have been introduced that are used as either monotherapy or in combination with sulphonylureas or metformin. These include meglitinides, alpha-glucosidase inhibitors and thiazolidinediones. The PROspective pioglitAzone Clinical Trial In macroVascular Events (PROactive) was a randomized controlled trial involving 5238 patients with T2DM who received the thiazolidinedione drug pioglitazone, or placebo, in addition to their usual cardiovascular and diabetic medications [29]. A pre-specified subgroup analysis was undertaken of all participants in PROactive with a previous history of stroke; this involved 486 subjects in the treatment arm and 498 in the placebo group. The use of pioglitazone was associated with a trend towards benefit for the primary end point of all-cause mortality, major vascular events or intervention (p = 0.0670). In this subgroup analysis, active treatment also reduced the rate of fatal and non-fatal stroke (5.6% versus placebo 10.2%, p = 0.0085). There was some early evidence that the use of another drug in the same class, rosiglitazone, may be associated with a reduction in the progression of carotid intima-media thickness in T2DM [30]. However, further trials are required to establish the role of this class of drugs in the prevention of cerebrovascular events in T2DM, particularly given recent concerns about the safety of thiazolidinediones in patients with cardiac disease [31]. With respect to the other new oral hypoglycaemic agents, in the STOP-NIDDM trial using the alpha-glucosidase inhibitor acarbose in patients with impaired glucose tolerance, there were very low stroke rates in both active and placebo-treated groups [32]. At present, there is no evidence available regarding the effect of meglitinide analogues on the long-term outcomes of T2DM, including macrovascular complications such as stroke [33].

Individuals with T2DM have a higher prevalence of hypertension, central obesity and atherogenic dyslipidaemia [34]. These factors, when clustered together, are termed the *metabolic syndrome* or *syndrome X*. Whilst diabetes alone increases the risk of stroke, the presence of T2DM as a component of the metabolic syndrome leads to a further rise in stroke risk. In the Framingham Offspring Study, diabetes was associated with a 2.47-fold increased risk of stroke compared to a 3.28-fold increase for diabetes plus the metabolic syndrome [35]. Among 14 000 patients with CHD followed prospectively for 4.8 to 8.1 years, those with the metabolic syndrome had a 1.49 increased odds for ischaemic stroke or TIA [36]. Insulin resistance is a precursor to impaired glucose tolerance, and is seen in both T2DM and the metabolic syndrome. Most epidemiological studies describe a significant association between insulin resistance and stroke risk [22]. The recent British Women's Heart and Health Study included a prospective cohort of 3246 women aged between 60 and 79 years, who were free of diabetes, stroke or CHD at baseline. Fasting insulin and a homeostasis model assessment for insulin sensitivity were associated with stroke and CHD, while fasting blood glucose and HbA_{1C} were not, indicating a role for insulin resistance as a vascular risk factor [37]. The link between T2DM, insulin resistance and the metabolic syndrome must be taken into account in any strategies for vascular risk reduction in older diabetics. Specific therapies for the prevention of cerebrovascular disease in T2DM will be considered later in the chapter.

6.3 Diabetes, post-stroke hyperglycaemia and prognosis after acute stroke

Beyond increasing the risk of first or recurrent stroke, diabetes is also associated with a poor prognosis following the acute event, increasing both mortality and dependency [38, 39]. This association also extends to the finding of hyperglycaemia in the immediate aftermath of stroke – the so-called post-stroke hyperglycaemia (PSH) [40–42]. PSH may reflect the metabolic stress of the acute event, and/or impaired glucose metabolism (impaired glucose tolerance or diabetes) previously manifest or otherwise. In one series of UK stroke patients, it was estimated that up to 68% had PSH, defined by a plasma glucose concentration $>6.0\,mmol\,l^{-1}$ [43]. The connection between PSH and poor outcome after acute stroke has now been identified in a number of clinical studies, and overall it is estimated to be associated with a two- to sixfold increased risk of mortality. In contrast to early reports that PSH and a poor prognosis was confined to patients with the most severe strokes, other studies have now demonstrated that this risk extends across all clinical subtypes of stroke [44].

Table 6.1   Admission glycaemic status and stress hyperglycaemia in acute stroke.*

	Admission plasma glucose	Admission glycated haemoglobin (HbA$_{1c}$)
Stress hyperglycaemia	↑	→
Impaired glucose tolerance/diabetes with stress hyperglycaemia	↑	↑
Impaired glucose tolerance/diabetes without stress hyperglycaemia	→	↑
Normal glucose tolerance without stress hyperglycaemia	→	→

Within normal laboratory range   →
Above normal laboratory range   ↑
*Adapted from Ref. [40].

PSH may occur due to a number of different mechanisms, which may influence – either independently or in combination – the subsequent clinical outcome. PSH was previously thought to be largely due to an acute stress response occurring in association with elevations in plasma cortisol, glucagon, catecholamines and often also leukocytosis [45]. Although these acute physiological responses may be contributory, more recent clinical data suggest that much of this response is associated with an impaired glucose metabolism, with the prevalence of previously unrecognized diabetes or impaired glucose tolerance preceding stroke being as high as 42%. On the basis of an acute stroke patient's admission plasma glucose and HbA$_{1C}$ level, it is possible to determine whether or not stress is a major component of their hyperglycaemia (Table 6.1).

In patients with PSH and no previous history of dysglycaemia, the diagnosis of DM or impaired glucose tolerance should ideally be made after the stress of the acute ictus has dissipated. In one cohort study, oral glucose tolerance tests (GTTs) were performed 3 months after acute stroke in patients presenting with PSH (admission plasma glucose >6.0 mmol l^{-1}) [46]. Diabetes or impaired glucose tolerance were found in 58% of subjects, with an estimated prevalence of previously unrecognized diabetes of 16–24%. The finding of an admission plasma glucose >6.0 mmol l^{-1} plus HbA$_{1C}$ >6.2% was highly predictive of diabetes at 3 months after stroke (positive predictive value 80%, negative predictive value 96%).

While associations between PSH and clinical outcome are seen both in the presence and absence of impaired glucose tolerance or diabetes, the combination of stress hyperglycaemia and impaired glucose metabolism is likely to be associated with the worst prognosis [40]. However, while demonstrating an association between hyperglycaemia and stroke outcome does not prove cause and effect, the totality of the clinical evidence tends to support a direct relationship.

6.4   Diabetes, hyperglycaemia and acute stroke treatment

There is still no safe, simple and effective medical therapy that can be given to the majority of acute stroke patients. Even in the absence of a simple medical treatment, the benefits of organized and coordinated stroke care have been recognized in terms of reduced mortality, dependency and institutionalization, leading to the widespread introduction of specialist stroke services [47, 48]. Thrombolysis with alteplase (recombinant tissue plasminogen activator, rt-PA) is the only approved medical therapy for patients with ischaemic stroke. Intravenous thrombolysis of acute ischaemic stroke with alteplase within 3 h of symptom onset has been shown in randomized controlled trials to improve functional outcome [49]. More recent data from the European SITS-MOST study of the use of alteplase in routine clinical practice confirms similar outcomes to the clinical trials: 11.3% mortality and 54.8% independent at 3 months, as estimated by a modified Rankin score of 0–2. Concerns remain, however, regarding the risks and benefits of alteplase, with a rate of symptomatic intracerebral haemorrhage at 7 days of 7.3% [50]. Furthermore, the routine use of alteplase in the UK at present is minimal, with <1% of stroke patients receiving this treatment in 2006 [51]. Even in experienced North American stroke centres, less than 20% of potentially eligible patients receive such treatment [52]. The target of the recent Department of Health Stroke Strategy is for 10% of acute stroke patients to receive treatment with rt-PA [14]. The problem with thrombolytic therapy for acute stroke is the identification of those patients most likely to benefit, and those in whom an increased risk may be conferred. Factors such as increasing age, stroke severity, raised blood pressure and extensive cerebral infarction on baseline computed tomography (CT) have been shown to increase the risk of complications. There is also evidence that hyperglycaemia (>11.2 mmol l^{-1}) may increase the risk of intracerebral haemorrhage fivefold following routine thrombolysis. In addition, clinical outcome following thrombolysis is worse in hyperglycaemic patients, even after the successful restoration of blood flow [53, 54]. There is some evidence that hyperglycaemia at the time of acute stroke may predict non-recanalization following thrombolysis. In one study, the finding of a blood glucose concentration >8.8 mmol l^{-1} at more than 2 h after thrombolysis was an independent predictor of failure to recanalize (OR 7.3, 95% CI: 1.3–42.3) [55].

In the absence of a simple early medical therapy applicable to the majority of stroke patients, an essential part of acute stroke unit care is the intensive monitoring of physiological variables (hydration, blood glucose, temperature, blood pressure, oxygen saturation). The RCP National Clinical Guidelines for Stroke emphasize the need to consider the early management of hyperglycaemia, hypertension, hydration and pyrexia [12]. Whilst there is accumulating evidence for a link between hyperglycaemia, diabetes and enhanced cerebral ischaemic damage, until recently intervention to modulate hyperglycaemia in acute stroke had not been examined in a randomized controlled trial.

Early clinical trials in acute MI and critically ill patients in the intensive care unit support the concept of treating hyperglycaemia and maintaining euglycaemia with insulin. A variety of methods for insulin administration is available in these settings, and both sliding-scale insulin and glucose-potassium-insulin (GKI) regimes have potential disadvantages [56]. An early overview of trials in acute MI has shown that treatment with a GKI-based regimen reduces in-patient mortality by 28% [57]. In addition, the use of insulin after acute MI may confer survival benefits, even in the absence of initial hyperglycaemia [58]. Consistent with these findings is evidence from a recent meta-analysis of 35 randomized controlled trials concerning the effects of insulin in 8478 critically ill patients with hyperglycaemia. In the majority of these studies, insulin was administered as a GKI infusion. Treatment with insulin decreased mortality by 15%, with the greatest benefit seen

in the surgical intensive care patients [59]. In the first DIGAMI study, patients presenting with acute MI and admission plasma glucose >11.0 mmol l^{-1} (with or without a previous history of diabetes) were randomized to an insulin infusion for >24 h, followed by subcutaneous insulin four times daily for more than 3 months [60]. Such treatment conferred a significant 52% relative reduction in mortality up to 12 months after the acute event. In view of the uncertainty regarding the relative contributions of the acute GKI infusion or subsequent insulin-based metabolic control to the overall outcome, the DIGAMI 2 study was undertaken. This trial randomized 1253 patients with T2DM and acute MI to one of three treatment arms: 24 h GKI followed by long-term subcutaneous insulin; 24 h GKI then conventional glucose control; or routine care [61]. Although DIGAMI 2 failed to replicate the results of the earlier trial, with no benefit being seen in either of the GKI treatment limbs, the trial included only those patients with T2DM in whom the baseline glucose was much lower than the original DIGAMI cohort, and the degree of glucose lowering achieved was less. This may partially explain the differing results obtained from the two studies.

Such a prolonged insulin treatment regimen is not feasible in the majority of acute stroke units, where the complexity of clinical care combined with the practical difficulties in maintaining hydration and nutrition may make routine treatment with insulin beyond 24 h unsafe. Furthermore, whilst hyperglycaemia may be seen in the majority of acute stroke patients, this is usually mild with mean plasma glucose concentrations of 8–9 mmol l^{-1} [62]. Glucose control following stroke is further complicated by the fact that up to one-third of patients have dysphagia in the immediate aftermath of the acute event. In two-thirds of cases, these swallowing difficulties usually resolve within the first week; however, nutritional support and supplementation may be fraught with practical and ethical problems. There is accumulating evidence that PSH is maximal in the initial 12–18 h after stroke, and that glucose levels will decline spontaneously without specific intervention [62].

Treatment with a variable-dose GKI infusion can safely induce and maintain euglycaemia during the first 24 h in hospital. The United Kingdom Glucose Insulin in Stroke Trial (GIST-UK) was a pragmatic multicentre, randomized controlled trial that sought to determine whether outcome from acute stroke could be favourably influenced by GKI-induced and maintained euglycaemia when delivered as part of routine stroke unit care [63]. Patients presenting within 24 h of symptom onset of ischaemic stroke or primary intracerebral haemorrhage were randomized to receive either variable-dose GKI or saline as a continuous intravenous infusion for 24 h. The purpose of the GKI treatment was to maintain capillary glucose levels at 4–7 mmol l^{-1}, with no glucose-lowering intervention in the control group. Patients with insulin-treated DM were excluded from the trial, and participants had only modest degrees of PSH (median baseline glucose 7.6 mmol l^{-1}, IQR 6.7–9.0). The primary outcome for the trial was mortality at 90 days, with a secondary outcome of avoidance of death or severe disability.

Recruitment into the GIST-UK study was halted due to slow enrolment, at which time 933 patients had been included. There was no significant reduction in mortality at 90 days (GKI versus control OR 1.14, 95% CI: 0.86–1.51, p = 0.37), nor any significant differences for secondary functional outcomes, as measured using the modified Rankin scale and Barthel index (Figure 6.3). In the GKI treatment group, both overall mean plasma glucose and mean systolic blood pressure were significantly lower than in the control arm (mean difference in glucose 0.57 mmol l^{-1}, p < 0.001; mean difference in blood pressure 9.0 mmHg, p < 0.0001) (Figure 6.4). The hypotensive effect of GKI treatment was unexpected, and might in part have been due to the potassium component of the infusion or, conversely, the result of a relative pressor effect of intravenous saline. The results of GIST-UK were at variance with the results of trials of glucose-lowering in coronary care and intensive care unit settings. It

should be remembered, however, that the glucose intervention in GIST-UK was short-term, whereas in DIGAMI the treatment was continued for a minimum of 12 weeks [60]. Furthermore, GIST-UK was a pragmatic trial designed to be carried out in NHS acute stroke units, where the much more intensive glucose intervention and monitoring seen in ICCU trials could not be achieved [64]. One criticism of GIST-UK when compared to DIGAMI was that the intensity of glucose-lowering was insufficient to influence the outcome. A *post hoc* analysis of the GIST population found that intensive lowering of glucose (>2 mmol l^{-1}) between baseline and 24 h with GKI was associated with a 34% excess mortality when compared to patients with a glucose reduction <2 mmol l^{-1}. Although this finding was reported with caution, recent evidence obtained with positron emission tomography (PET) scanning suggested that hyperglycaemia might not be directly harmful to the ischaemic brain, and in the presence of cerebral ischaemia lactate derived from anaerobic metabolism may be the preferred energy supply [65]. Thus, an intensive reduction of glucose may in fact reduce glucose load to the brain and attenuate lactate production.

As the first clinical trial of glucose modulation in acute stroke, GIST-UK was planned during the 1990s, and it is encouraging that other clinical trials are currently being undertaken in this area (GRASP trial, www.grasptrial.org; IRIS trial, www.iristrial.org; NICE and SUGAR study) Alternative methods of insulin administration were examined in the recently published Treatment of Hyperglycaemia in Ischaemic

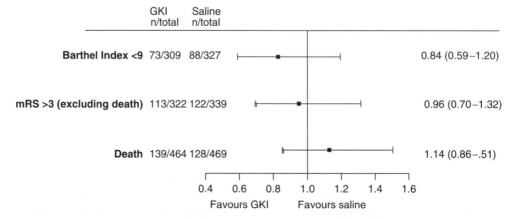

Figure 6.3 Glucose insulin in stroke trial (GIST-UK). Common odds ratios (ORs) for primary and secondary outcomes with 95% CIs in the intention-to-treat data set. GKI = glucose-potassium-insulin. Reprinted with permission from Ref. [63].

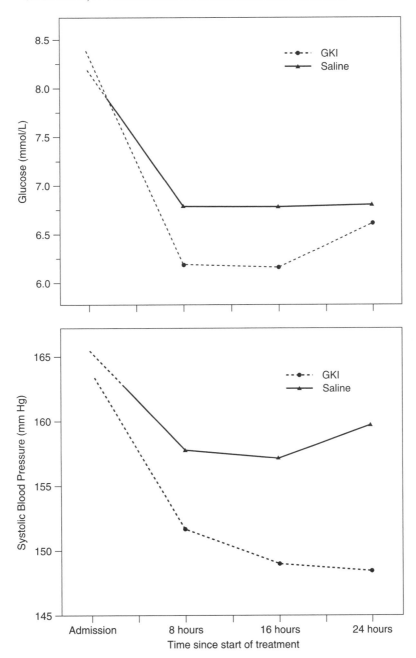

Figure 6.4 Glucose insulin in stroke trial (GIST-UK). Mean plasma glucose concentration and systolic blood pressure at baseline, 8 h, 16 h and 24 h. Reprinted with permission from Ref. [63].

Stroke (THIS) trial [66]. In this pilot study, 46 patients were randomized within 12 h of cerebral infarction to receive either aggressive treatment with continuous intravenous insulin (target glucose <7.2 mmol l^{-1}) or usual treatment with subcutaneous insulin four times daily (target <11.1 mmol l^{-1}). The glucose levels were seen to be significantly lower in the aggressive treatment group (7.4 versus 10.5 mmol l^{-1}, $p < 0.001$), with hypoglycaemia occurring in 35% of these patients. Unfortunately, the small number of patients included in this pilot study precluded any assessment of the clinical efficacy of this treatment strategy.

Clinical guidelines emphasize the role of physiological monitoring and intervention in acute stroke care [12]. However, thresholds for the routine treatment of hyperglycaemia vary across centres and between clinicians, with varying local policies for the management of PSH. The physiological effect of interventions such as saline hydration or glucose modulation is poorly understood, and requires further investigation. In GIST-UK, a simple saline infusion, which is part of routine stroke unit care, was associated with a significant reduction in plasma glucose. However, the small reduction in glucose concentration achieved with GKI was not associated with a net clinical improvement, and any benefit from such reductions may be offset by a greater decrease in blood pressure. The challenge for future trials in acute stroke will be to determine the safety and efficacy of glucose-lowering in an appropriate high-dependency environment, while maintaining other physiological variables such as blood pressure within a satisfactory range. Despite the absence of conclusive clinical trial evidence, in patients for whom thrombolysis is contemplated, it would seem prudent to attempt the correction of hyperglycaemia, although the therapeutic time window for thrombolytic therapy is so short that effective glycaemic control may actually follow rather than precede such treatment.

6.5 Stroke prevention in type 2 diabetes

Diabetes and hyperglycaemia are not only major risk factors for stroke but also important prognostic factors for clinical outcome. After the initial phase of the illness, the intensive management of vascular risk factors confers major benefits for stroke patients. Until a safe, simple and effective acute therapy is developed for the majority of stroke patients, however, the priority must be to reduce mortality, disability and dependency through the implementation of proven primary and secondary preventive strategies.

The latest guidelines on the management of CVD in diabetes emphasize that stroke prevention should be based on a multifactorial strategy, including the treatment of hypertension, hyperglycaemia, microalbuminuria, hyperlipidaemia, and also the use of antiplatelet medication [67].

6.5.1 Hypertension

Hypertension is the single most important potentially reversible risk factor for cerebrovascular disease in both diabetic and non-diabetic individuals. The results of epidemiological studies have shown that usual systolic and diastolic blood pressure levels are directly and continuously associated with a risk of both cerebral infarction and primary intracerebral haemorrhage in patients with and without a history of hypertension [68, 69]. Furthermore, a similar linear relationship exists between systolic and diastolic blood pressure and the risk of recurrent cerebrovascular events following stroke or TIA [70]. Reducing diastolic blood pressure by 5–6 mmHg in people with hypertension and no history of cerebrovascular disease decreases their risk of stroke by approximately one-third, with all major classes of antihypertensive agents appearing equally effective [71]. In addition, pharmacological intervention to lower blood pressure has been shown to reduce the risk of stroke recurrence in hypertensive stroke survivors [72]. Although hypertension is a major determinant of stroke risk in diabetics, most patients have other risk factors such as dyslipidaemia and ischaemic heart disease that may influence the choice of antihypertensive therapy.

Embedded within the United Kingdom Prospective Diabetes Study was a randomized controlled trial (UKPDS 38) to establish if the tight control of blood pressure (<150/85 mmHg) decreased morbidity and mortality in patients with T2DM [73]. Treated hypertensive diabetics whose blood pressure was above this target level and those who were previously untreated (≥160/≥90 mmHg) received either intensive or less-intensive blood pressure-lowering therapy. The intensive treatment comprised an angiotensin-converting enzyme (ACE) inhibitor (captopril) or a β-blocker (atenolol), with a target blood pressure of <150/85 mmHg. The purpose of the other treatment limb was a less tight control of blood pressure (<180/105 mmHg), avoiding ACE inhibitors and β-blockers. Almost one-third (29%) of patients randomized to the tight control group needed three or more agents to control their blood pressure, compared to only 11% in the less-intensive treatment group. A tight control resulted in a significantly lower blood pressure; the mean blood pressure over 9 years of follow-up was 144/82 mmHg in the intensive treatment group compared to 154/87 mmHg in the other limb. After a median follow-up period of 8.4 years, the intensive management of hypertension in these UKPDS patients resulted in a 24% relative risk reduction for the development of any diabetes-related end point. There was no significant difference in diabetic control between the two blood pressure treatment groups (mean

HbA$_{1C}$ 7.2% for both). Intensive treatment resulted in a significant 44% relative reduction in fatal or non-fatal stroke, but no significant decrease in MI. These results were similar to those seen with other trials of blood pressure-lowering treatment in older people [74, 75]. Thus, intensive glycaemic control alone in T2DM is not sufficient to reduce risk of stroke; simultaneous management of hypertension is also necessary.

UKPDS 38 also showed that intensive blood pressure treatment necessitated combination therapy. It should be noted that even in the UKPDS 38 tight control group, the mean level of blood pressure achieved was still higher than the current UK recommended target of <130/80 mmHg for clinic readings [76]. However, this trial did demonstrate that the lowest risk of complications due to diabetes was seen in patients with a systolic blood pressure <120 mmHg, in line with current recommendations [77]. The choice of antihypertensive therapy for patients with T2DM will also be influenced by the results of more recent clinical trials. In the ASCOT study, 19 257 patients with hypertension and three other cardiovascular risk factors were randomized to receive amlodipine (plus perindopril if required) or atenolol (plus a thiazide diuretic) [78]. The amlodipine-based regime prevented more cardiovascular events and induced less diabetes than the atenolol-based regime. In the ASCOT study, it is possible that differing effects of the two treatment arms on variables other than blood pressure contributed to the different event rates, particularly for stroke [79].

There is accumulating evidence from ASCOT and other studies that, for patients at high risk of vascular disease, the benefits of antihypertensive therapy may extend beyond blood pressure lowering. In the HOPE study, 9297 high-risk vascular patients aged ≥55 years, including 3577 (38%) with diabetes plus one additional risk factor (including stroke or TIA), received treatment with the ACE inhibitor ramipril or placebo [80]. Ramipril resulted in modest reductions in office blood pressure compared to placebo (3.8/2.8 mmHg). Nevertheless, the overall results confirmed that the relative risk of any stroke or fatal stroke was decreased by 32% and 61%, respectively. Ramipril was beneficial even in those who were normotensive at baseline. A further analysis of the results for the 3577 diabetic participants showed a significant 33% reduction in stroke risk, again irrespective of baseline blood pressure [81]. Thus, as in the UKPDS, the benefits observed with fairly modest reductions in office blood pressure were greater than might be predicted from epidemiological data [82]. Explanations for this observation include a

protective effect on the vasculature of drugs such as ACE inhibitors, or an enhanced control of ambulatory blood pressure levels compared with clinic readings [83].

Further evidence for the beneficial effect of ACE inhibitors in reducing the risk of recurrent stroke comes from the PROGRESS trial [84]. This study recruited 6105 hypertensive and normotensive patients with a history of cerebrovascular disease, of whom 13% were diabetic. The maximum beneficial effect was seen in patients on combined therapy with the ACE inhibitor perindopril plus the diuretic, indapamide. Mean blood pressure lowering on combined therapy was 12/5 mmHg compared with perindopril monotherapy (mean 5/3 mmHg). Treatment with perindopril plus indapamide resulted in a relative risk reduction for recurrent stroke of 43%, compared to a non-significant 5% decrease with perindopril alone. However, no subgroup analysis was performed for the diabetic patients enrolled in this study. Additional data to support the use of ACE inhibitors in T2DM derive from the ADVANCE trial [85], where 11 140 patients with T2DM were randomized to receive perindopril plus indapamide along with their usual treatment, irrespective of their initial blood pressure. A modest reduction in blood pressure of 5.6/2.2 mmHg was seen with perindopril/indapamide, but there was a 9% reduction in risk of all major macrovascular or microvascular events as well as a decrease in all-cause mortality.

In hypertensive diabetic patients, the intensity of blood pressure therapy is important in order to maximally decrease their risk of stroke and other vascular events. In order to further investigate the intensity of blood pressure lowering, the HOT study examined the optimum treatment level for diastolic blood pressure. The study found that there was a twofold increase in the incidence of cardiovascular events in hypertensive diabetic patients, and that in these individuals an intensive treatment to reduce the diastolic blood pressure to <80 mmHg resulted in a 30% reduction in the risk of stroke compared with more modest reductions in blood pressure to <90 mmHg [86]. Treatment in the HOT study was with a calcium channel blocker-based regime, but for many patients this was combined with a β-blocker or ACE inhibitor.

Intensive blood pressure-lowering in T2DM is being evaluated as part of the on-going Action to Control Cardiovascular Risk in Diabetes (ACCORD) trial [87]. The blood pressure limb of ACCORD is comparing target systolic pressures of <120 mmHg versus <140 mmHg.

Current international management guidelines recommend a target systolic blood pressure of <130 mmHg for diabetic patients [67]. However, accumulating evidence infers that high-risk vascular patients such as diabetics should be treated even more aggressively, irrespective of baseline blood pressure, in order to reduce the risk of cerebrovascular events. The management of hypertension immediately after acute stroke is more contentious [88]. Most acute stroke patients are hypertensive on admission to hospital, and in many cases the blood pressure falls spontaneously over the first 7–10 days. The cerebral autoregulation of blood flow is impaired early after stroke, and cerebral perfusion may become dependent upon systemic blood pressure levels. Thus, lowering the blood pressure in the acute phase after stroke could be potentially harmful, and on-going clinical trials are addressing this issue. In the PROGRESS and HOPE trials, ACE inhibitor therapy was delayed for 2–4 weeks after stroke. Based on current evidence, it would seem prudent to withhold antihypertensive therapy until stroke patients are clinically and neurologically stable, except for specific clinical circumstances such as accelerated hypertension where immediate blood pressure-lowering is mandatory [89].

6.5.2   Dyslipidaemia

The relationship between dyslipidaemia and CVD is qualitatively similar in diabetic and non-diabetic patients, but for any given level of cholesterol the absolute risk is higher for diabetics. The evidence that dyslipidaemia is a risk factor for stroke is conflicting, with a recent meta-analysis showing no apparent association [68]. Many studies, however, do not distinguish between cerebral infarction and primary intracerebral haemorrhage. Evidence from Caucasian and Asian population studies shows a positive association between total cholesterol levels and the risk of cerebral infarction, possibly offset by a negative correlation between cholesterol and risk of intracerebral haemorrhage [90, 91].

It should be remembered that the majority of diabetic patients at risk of stroke are older and have T2DM. In these individuals, the predominant lipid abnormalities are raised triglycerides and reduced HDL-cholesterol. In contrast to the evidence linking dyslipidaemia to ischaemic heart disease, it is only more recently that statin therapy has also been shown to be effective in reducing cerebrovascular disease. A meta-analysis of the early statin trials confirmed that, in patients with

known ischaemic heart disease, cholesterol-lowering therapy was associated with a 30% reduction in the risk of stroke [92]. The beneficial effects of statins were observed in people with only moderately raised cholesterol levels. Furthermore, statins did not seem to increase the risk of haemorrhagic stroke, despite the epidemiological evidence for an association between low cholesterol and intracerebral haemorrhage.

The Cholesterol Treatment Trialists' Collaboration has recently published a meta-analysis focusing on the use of statins in diabetic patients [93].

Data from 14 randomized controlled trials were used in this meta-analysis, which included 18 686 diabetics, 17 220 of whom had T2DM. The analysis was undertaken in the context of the 71 370 non-diabetic participants in the same studies. Over a mean follow-up period of 4.3 years, a total of 3247 vascular events occurred in the diabetic patients. A 9% proportional reduction in all-cause mortality per mmol l^{-1} decrease in LDL-cholesterol was observed, similar to the 13% reduction seen in non-diabetic individuals. Among diabetics, there was a significant decrease in vascular deaths (rate ratio 0.87, p = 0.008), with no effect seen on non-vascular mortality. Furthermore, in people with diabetes there was a significant decrease in stroke (rate ratio 0.79, p = 0.0002), with significant reductions also seen for MI and coronary death or revascularisation (Figure 6.5). Among diabetics, the proportional effects of statins were similar, irrespective of any past history of vascular disease or other baseline characteristics. These findings strengthen the evidence for the use of statin therapy in all diabetic patients at high risk of vascular disease. The lipid limb of the on-going ACCORD trial includes 5518 participants with T2DM who are receiving either fenofibrate or placebo to determine whether the use of a fibrate to increase HDL-cholesterol and lower triglycerides, together with a statin to lower LDL-cholesterol, will reduce the risk of vascular events [87].

6.5.3   Antiplatelet therapy

Antiplatelet therapy is an important part of secondary prevention in patients with TIA or stroke. The Antiplatelet Trialists' Collaboration meta-analysis confirmed a significant reduction in vascular events (non-fatal MI, non-fatal stroke, vascular death) in diabetic patients with vascular disease who were treated with antiplatelet agents [94]. The results of the recent ESPRIT trial, in combination with those of previous trials, provide evidence for the use of

Major vascular event and prior diabetes	Events (%)			RR(CI)
	Treatment	Control		
Major coronary event				
Diabetes	776(8.3%)	979(10.5%)		0.78(0.69–0.87)
No diabetes	2561(7.2%)	3441(9.6%)		0.77(0.73–0.81)
Any major coronary event	**3337(7.4%)**	**4420(9.8%)**		**0.77(0.74–0.80)**
Test for heterogeneity within subgroup: $\chi^2_1 = 0.1$; p = 0.8				
Coronary revascularisation				
Diabetes	491(5.2%)	627(6.7%)		0.75(0.64–0.88)
No diabetes	2129(6.0%)	2807(7.9%)		0.76(0.72–0.81)
Any coronary revascularisation	**2620(5.8%)**	**3434(7.6%)**		**0.76(0.73–0.80)**
Test for heterogeneity within subgroup: $\chi^2_1 = 0.1$; p = 0.8				
Stroke				
Diabetes	407(4.4%)	501(5.4%)		0.79(0.67–0.93)
No diabetes	933(2.7%)	1116(3.2%)		0.84(0.76–0.93)
Any stroke	**1340(3.0%)**	**1617(3.7%)**		**0.83(0.77–0.88)**
Test for heterogeneity within subgroup: $\chi^2_1 = 0.8$; p = 0.4				
Major vascular event				
Diabetes	1465(15.6%)	1782(19.2%)		0.79(0.72–0.86)
No diabetes	4889(13.7%)	6212(17.4%)		0.79(0.76–0.82)
Any major vascular event	**6354(14.1%)**	**7994(17.8%)**		**0.79(0.77–0.81)**
Test for heterogeneity within subgroup: $\chi^2_1 = 0.0$; p = 0.9				

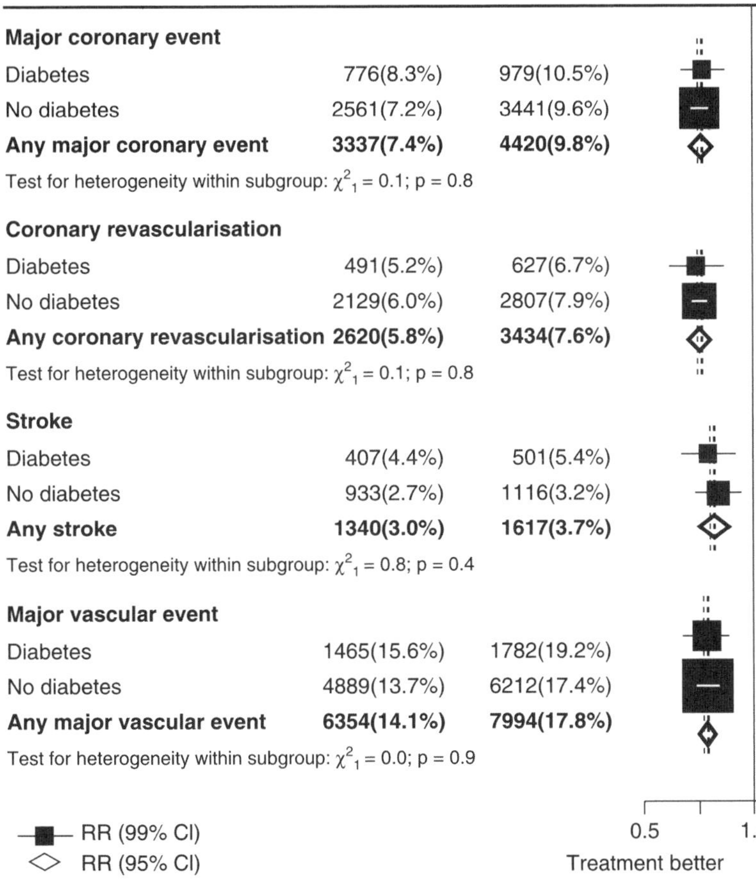

RR (99% CI)
RR (95% CI)

0.5 1.0 1.5
Treatment better   Control better

Figure 6.5 Cholesterol treatment trialists' collaboration. Proportional effects on major vascular events per mmol l^{-1} reduction in LDL-cholesterol in participants with or without diabetes. RR = relative risk. Reprinted with permission from Ref. [93].

aspirin plus dipyridamole after ischaemic stroke in preference to aspirin alone [95]. Current clinical guidelines therefore recommend the use of aspirin plus modified-release dipyridamole for the secondary prevention of occlusive vascular events following ischaemic stroke or TIA [12, 96]. The MATCH trial assessed the role of combined antiplatelet therapy with aspirin plus clopidogrel in patients with ischaemic cerebrovascular disease, with a combined vascular end point of ischaemic stroke and rehospitalization for TIA [97]. The combination of aspirin plus clopidogrel produced a marginally increased relative risk reduction when compared to aspirin, which did not achieve statistical significance and was offset by a higher risk of bleeding in this population. Among the 68% of the

MATCH study population who were diabetic, aspirin plus clopidogrel produced a slightly higher relative risk reduction than in the remainder of the study population, but this again was not significant and was associated with increased bleeding.

6.6 Conclusions

Older patients with T2DM are at high risk of macrovascular complications, including stroke and TIA. In addition, cerebrovascular disease is a major contributor to cognitive decline in this population. A reduction in cerebrovascular disease can be achieved by a comprehensive strategy of vascular risk reduction aimed at multiple risk factors [98]. On-going clinical trials such as ACCORD should clarify the risks and benefits of a strategy of intensive glucose and blood pressure control plus management of lipids with statins and fibrates; the glucose-lowering limb of this study was recently stopped 18 months early due to an increased mortality when blood glucose concentrations were lowered below current recommended levels [87]. Based on the available evidence, treatment of the older person with T2DM should encompass lifestyle changes, a tight control of glycaemia and hypertension, and targeted specific drug therapies such as ACE inhibitors, statins and antiplatelet agents.

References

1. Kannel, W. B. and McGee, D. L. (1979) Diabetes and cardiovascular disease. The Framingham study. *JAMA*, 241, 2035–8.

2. Fuller, J. H., Shipley, M. J., Rose, G., Jarrett, R. J. and Keen, H. (1983) Mortality from coronary heart disease and stroke in relation to degree of glycaemia: the Whitehall study. *Br Med J (Clin Res Ed.)*, 287, 867–70.

3. World Health Organization (1971) Cerebrovascular Diseases: Prevention, Treatment and Rehabilitation. Report of a WHO meeting. *World Health Organ Tech Rep Ser*, 469, 1–57.

4. Albers, G. W., Caplan, L. R., Easton, J. D., Fayad, P. B., Mohr, J. P., Saver, J. L. and Sherman, D. G. (2002) Transient ischemic attack - proposal for a new definition. *N Engl J Med*, 347, 1713–6.

5. Adams, H. P., Jr., Bendixen, B. H., Kappelle, L. J., Biller, J., Love, B. B., Gordon, D. L. and Marsh, E. E., 3rd (1993) Classification of subtype of acute ischemic stroke. Definitions for use in a multicenter clinical trial. TOAST. Trial of Org 10172 in Acute Stroke Treatment. *Stroke*, 24, 35–41.

6. De Angelis, M. (2003) Prevalence of carotid stenosis in type 2 diabetic patients asymptomatic for cerebrovascular disease. *Diabetes Nutrition and Metabolism*, 16, 48–55.

7. You, R., McNeil, J. J., O'Malley, H. M., Davis, S. M. and Donnan, G. A. (1995) Risk factors for lacunar infarction syndromes. *Neurology*, 45, 1483–7.

8. Karapanayiotides, T., Piechowski-Jozwiak, B., Van Melle, G., Bogousslavsky, J. and Devuyst, G. (2004) Stroke patterns, etiology, and prognosis in patients with diabetes mellitus. *Neurology*, 62, 1558–62.

9. Schulz, U. G. and Rothwell, P. M. (2003) Differences in vascular risk factors between etiological subtypes of ischemic stroke: importance of population-based studies. *Stroke*, 34, 2050–9.

10. Isarol, P. A. and Forbes, J. F. (1992) The cost of stroke to the National Health Service in Scotland. *Cerebrovasc Dis*, 1, 47–50.

11. Macdonald, B. K., Cockerell, O. C., Sander, J. W. and Shorvon, S. D. (2000) The incidence and lifetime prevalence of neurological disorders in a prospective community-based study in the UK. *Brain*, 123 (Pt 4), 665–76.

12. Intercollegiate Stroke Working Party. (2008) National Clinical Guidelines for Stroke, 3rd edition. London, Royal College of Physicians.

13. Department Of Health (2001) National Service Framework for Older People. Department of Health, London.

14. Department Of Health (2007) National Stroke Strategy. Department of Health, London.

15. Wahl, P. W., Savage, P. J., Psaty, B. M., Orchard, T. J., Robbins, J. A. and Tracy, R. P. (1998) Diabetes in older adults: comparison of 1997 American Diabetes Association classification of diabetes mellitus with 1985 WHO classification. *Lancet*, 352, 1012–15.

16. Gunarathne, A., Patel, J. V., Potluri, R., Gammon, B., Jessani, S., Hughes, E. A. and Lip, G. Y. (2008) Increased 5-year mortality in the migrant South Asian stroke patients with diabetes mellitus in the United Kingdom: The West Birmingham Stroke Project. *Int J Clin Pract.*, 62 (2), 197–201.

17. Laakso, M. (1999) Hyperglycaemia and cardiovascular disease in Type 2 diabetes. *Diabetes*, 48, 937–42.

18. Coutinho, M., Gerstein, H. C., Wang, Y. and Yusuf, S. (1999) The relationship between glucose and incident cardiovascular events. A metaregression analysis of published data from 20 studies of 95,783 individuals followed for 12.4 years. *Diabetes Care*, 22, 233–40.

19. Mulnier, H. E., Seaman, H. E., Raleigh, V. S., Soedamah-Muthu, S. S., Colhoun, H. M., Lawrenson, R. A. and De Vries, C. S. (2006) Risk of stroke in people with type 2 diabetes in the UK: a study using the General Practice Research Database. *Diabetologia*, 49, 2859–65.

20. Janghorbani, M., Hu, F. B., Willett, W. C., Li, T. Y., Manson, J. E., Logroscino, G. and Rexrode, K. M. (2007) Prospective study of type 1 and type 2 diabetes and risk of stroke subtypes: the Nurses' Health Study. *Diabetes Care*, 30, 1730–5.

21. Giorda, C. B., Avogaro, A., Maggini, M., Lombardo, F., Mannucci, E., Turco, S., Alegiani, S. S., Raschetti, R., Velussi, M. and Ferrannini, E. (2007) Incidence and risk factors for stroke in type 2 diabetic patients: the DAI study. *Stroke*, 38, 1154–60.

22. Air, E. L. and Kissela, B. M. (2007) Diabetes, the metabolic syndrome, and ischemic stroke: epidemiology and possible mechanisms. *Diabetes Care*, 30, 3131–40.

23. Myint, P. K., Sinha, S., Wareham, N. J., Bingham, S. A., Luben, R. N., Welch, A. A. and Khaw, K. T. (2007) Glycated hemoglobin and risk of stroke in people without known diabetes in the European Prospective Investigation into Cancer (EPIC)-Norfolk prospective population study: a threshold relationship? *Stroke*, 38, 271–5.

24. Turner, R., Cull, C. and Holman, R. (1996) United Kingdom Prospective Diabetes Study 17: a 9-year update of a randomized, controlled trial on the effect of improved metabolic control on complications in non-insulin-dependent diabetes mellitus. *Ann Intern Med*, 124, 136–45.

25. Jeerakathil, T., Johnson, J. A., Simpson, S. H. and Majumdar, S. R. (2007) Short-term risk for stroke is doubled in persons with newly treated type 2 diabetes compared with persons without diabetes: a population-based cohort study. *Stroke*, 38, 1739–43.

26. United Kingdom Prospective Diabetes Study Group. (1998) Intensive blood glucose control with sulphonylureas or insulin compared with conventional treatment and risk of complications in patients with type 2 diabetes (UKPDS 33). *Lancet*, 352, 837–53.

27. United Kingdom Prospective Diabetes Study Group. (1995) United Kingdom Prospective Diabetes Study (UKPDS) 13: Relative efficacy of randomly allocated diet, sulphonylurea, insulin or metformin in patients with newly diagnosed non-insulin dependent diabetes followed for three years. *Br Med J*, 310, 83–8.

28. United Kingdom Prospective Diabetes Study Group. (1998) Effect of intensive blood glucose control with metformin on complications in overweight patients with type 2 diabetes. (UKPDS 34). *Lancet*, 352, 854–65.

29. Wilcox, R., Bousser, M. G., Betteridge, D. J., Schernthaner, G., Pirags, V., Kupfer, S. and Dormandy, J. (2007) Effects of pioglitazone in patients with type 2 diabetes with or without previous stroke: results from PROactive (PROspective pioglitAzone Clinical Trial In macroVascular Events 04). *Stroke*, 38, 865–73.

30. Hedblad, B., Zambanini, A., Nilsson, P., Janzon, L. and Berglund, G. (2007) Rosiglitazone and carotid IMT progression rate in a mixed cohort of patients with type 2 diabetes and the insulin resistance syndrome: main results from the Rosiglitazone Atherosclerosis Study. *J Intern Med*, 261, 293–305.

31. Macfarlane, D. P. and Fisher, M. (2006) Thiazolidinediones in patients with diabetes mellitus and heart failure: implications of emerging data. *Am J Cardiovasc Drugs*, 6, 297–304.

32. Chiasson, J. L., Josse, R. G., Gomis, R., Hanefeld, M., Karasik, A. and Laakso, M. (2003) Acarbose treatment and the risk of cardiovascular disease and hypertension in patients with impaired glucose tolerance: the STOP-NIDDM trial. *JAMA*, 290, 486–94.

33. Black, C., Donnelly, P., McIntyre, L., Royle, P. L., Shepherd, J. P. and Thomas, S. (2007) Meglitinide analogues for type 2 diabetes mellitus. *Cochrane Database Syst Rev*, CD004654.

34. Gil-Nunez, A. (2007) The metabolic syndrome and cerebrovascular disease: suspicion and evidence. *Cerebrovasc Dis*, 24 (Suppl. 1), 64–75.

35. Najarian, R. M., Sullivan, L. M., Kannel, W. B., Wilson, P. W., D'Agostino, R. B. and Wolf, P. A. (2006) Metabolic syndrome compared with type 2 diabetes mellitus as a risk factor for stroke: the Framingham Offspring Study. *Arch Intern Med*, 166, 106–11.

36. Koren-Morag, N., Goldbourt, U. and Tanne, D. (2005) Relation between the metabolic syndrome and ischemic stroke or transient ischemic attack: a prospective cohort study in patients with atherosclerotic cardiovascular disease. *Stroke*, 36, 1366–71.

37. Lawlor, D. A., Fraser, A., Ebrahim, S. and Smith, G. D. (2007) Independent associations of fasting insulin, glucose, and glycated haemoglobin with stroke and coronary heart disease in older women. *PLoS Med*, 4, e263.

38. Pulsinelli, W. A., Levy, D. E., Sigsbee, B., Scherer, P. and Plum, F. (1983) Increased damage after ischemic stroke in patients with hyperglycemia with or without established diabetes mellitus. *Am J Med*, 74, 540–4.

39. Oppenheimer, S. M., Hoffbrand, B. I., Oswald, G. A. and Yudkin, J. S. (1985) Diabetes mellitus and early mortality from stroke. *Br Med J (Clin Res Ed)*, 291, 1014–15.

40. Gray, C. S., Taylor, R., French, J. M., Alberti, K. G., Venables, G. S., James, O. F., Shaw, D. A., Cartlidge, N. E. and Bates, D. (1987) The prognostic value of stress hyperglycaemia and previously unrecognized diabetes in acute stroke. *Diabet Med*, 4, 237–40.

41. Weir, C. J., Murray, G. D., Dyker, A. G. and Lees, K. R. (1997) Is hyperglycaemia an independent predictor of poor outcome after acute stroke? Results of a long-term follow up study. *Br Med J*, 314, 1303–6.

42. Power, M. J., Fullerton, K. J. and Stout, R. W. (1988) Blood glucose and prognosis of acute stroke. *Age Ageing*, 17, 164–70.

43. Scott, J. F., Robinson, G. M., French, J. M., O'Connell, J. E., Alberti, K. G. and Gray, C. S. (1999) Prevalence of admission hyperglycaemia across clinical subtypes of acute stroke. *Lancet*, 353, 376–7.

44. Gray, C. S., O'Connell, J. E. and Lloyd, H. (2001) Diabetes, hyperglycaemia and recovery from stroke. *Geriatrics and Gerontology International*, 1, 2–7.

45. O'Connell, J. E. and Gray, C. S. (1991) The stress response to acute stroke. *Stress Medicine*, 7, 239–43.

46. Gray, C. S., Scott, J. F., French, J. M., Alberti, K. G. and O'Connell, J. E. (2004) Prevalence and prediction of unrecognised diabetes mellitus and impaired glucose tolerance following acute stroke. *Age Ageing*, 33, 71–7.

47. Stroke Unit Trialists' Collaboration (1997) Collaborative systematic review of the randomised trials of organised inpatient (stroke unit) care after stroke. *Br Med J*, 314, 1151–9.

48. Seenan, P., Long, M. and Langhorne, P. (2007) Stroke units in their natural habitat: systematic review of observational studies. *Stroke*, 38, 1886–92.

49. Hacke, W., Donnan, G., Fieschi, C., Kaste, M., Von Kummer, R., Broderick, J. P., Brott, T., Frankel, M., Grotta, J. C., Haley, E. C., Jr., Kwiatkowski, T., Levine, S. R., Lewandowski, C., Lu, M., Lyden, P., Marler, J. R., Patel, S., Tilley, B. C., Albers, G., Bluhmki, E., Wilhelm, M. and Hamilton, S. (2004) Association of outcome with early stroke treatment: pooled analysis of ATLANTIS, ECASS, and NINDS rt-PA stroke trials. *Lancet*, 363, 768–74.

50. Wahlgren, N., Ahmed, N., Davalos, A., Ford, G. A., Grond, M., Hacke, W., Hennerici, M. G., Kaste, M., Kuelkens, S., Larrue, V., Lees, K. R., Roine, R. O., Soinne, L., Toni, D. and Vanhooren, G. (2007) Thrombolysis with alteplase for acute ischaemic stroke in the Safe Implementation of Thrombolysis in Stroke-Monitoring Study (SITS-MOST): an observational study. *Lancet*, 369, 275–82.

51. Clinical Effectiveness Evaluation Unit. (2006) National Sentinel Audit of Stroke, 2006. Royal College of Physicians, London.

52. Johnston, S. C., Fung, L. H., Gillum, L. A., Smith, W. S., Brass, L. M., Lichtman, J. H. and Brown, A. N. (2001) Utilization of intravenous tissue-type plasminogen activator for ischemic stroke at academic medical centers: the influence of ethnicity. *Stroke*, 32, 1061–8.

53. Els, T., Klisch, J., Orszagh, M., Hetzel, A., Schulte-Monting, J., Schumacher, M. and Lucking, C. H. (2002) Hyperglycemia in patients with focal cerebral ischemia after intravenous thrombolysis: influence on clinical outcome and infarct size. *Cerebrovasc Dis*, 13, 89–94.

54. Bruno, A., Levine, S. R., Frankel, M. R., Brott, T. G., Lin, Y., Tilley, B. C., Lyden, P. D., Broderick, J. P., Kwiatkowski, T. G. and Fineberg, S. E. (2002) Admission glucose level and clinical outcomes in the NINDS rt-PA Stroke Trial. *Neurology*, 59, 669–74.

55. Ribo, M., Molina, C., Montaner, J., Rubiera, M., Delgado-Mederos, R., Arenillas, J. F., Quintana, M. and Alvarez-Sabin, J. (2005) Acute hyperglycemia state is associated with lower tPA-induced recanalization rates in stroke patients. *Stroke*, 36, 1705–9.

56. Sawin, C. T. (1997) Action without benefit. The sliding scale of insulin use. *Arch Intern Med*, 157, 489.

57. Fath-Ordoubadi, F. and Beatt, K. J. (1997) Glucose-insulin-potassium therapy for treatment of acute myocardial infarction: an overview of randomized placebo-controlled trials. *Circulation*, 96, 1152–6.

58. Diaz, R., Paolasso, E. A., Piegas, L. S., Tajer, C. D., Moreno, M. G., Corvalan, R., Isea, J. E. and Romero, G. (1998) Metabolic modulation of acute myocardial infarction. The ECLA (Estudios Cardiologicos Latinoamerica) Collaborative Group. *Circulation*, 98, 2227–34.

59. Pittas, A. G., Siegel, R. D. and Lau, J. (2004) Insulin therapy for critically ill hospitalized patients: a meta-analysis of randomized controlled trials. *Arch Intern Med*, 164, 2005–11.

60. Malmberg, K., Ryden, L., Efendic, S., Herlitz, J., Nicol, P., Waldenstrom, A., Wedel, H. and Welin, L. (1995) Randomized trial of insulin-glucose infusion followed by subcutaneous insulin treatment in diabetic patients with acute myocardial infarction (DIGAMI study): effects on mortality at 1 year. *J Am Coll Cardiol*, 26, 57–65.

61. Malmberg, K., Ryden, L., Wedel, H., Birkeland, K., Bootsma, A., Dickstein, K., Efendic, S., Fisher, M., Hamsten, A., Herlitz, J., Hildebrandt, P., Macleod, K., Laakso, M., Torp-Pedersen, C. and Waldenstrom, A. (2005) Intense metabolic control by means of insulin in patients with diabetes mellitus and acute myocardial infarction (DIGAMI 2): effects on mortality and morbidity. *Eur Heart J*, 26, 650–61.

62. Gray, C. S., Hildreth, A. J., Alberti, G. K. and O'Connell, J. E. (2004) Poststroke hyperglycemia: natural history and immediate management. *Stroke*, 35, 122–6.

63. Gray, C. S., Hildreth, A. J., Sandercock, P. A., O'Connell, J. E., Johnston, D. E., Cartlidge, N. E., Bamford, J. M., James, O. F. and Alberti, K. G. (2007) Glucose-potassium-insulin infusions in the management of post-stroke hyperglycaemia: the UK Glucose Insulin in Stroke Trial (GIST-UK). *Lancet Neurol*, 6, 397–406.

64. Van Den Berghe, G., Wouters, P., Weekers, F., Verwaest, C., Bruyninckx, F., Schetz, M., Vlasselaers, D., Ferdinande, P., Lauwers, P. and Bouillon, R. (2001) Intensive insulin therapy in the critically ill patients. *N Engl J Med*, 345, 1359–67.

65. Smith, D., Pernet, A., Hallett, W. A., Bingham, E., Marsden, P. K. and Amiel, S. A. (2003) Lactate: a preferred fuel for human brain metabolism in vivo. *J Cereb Blood Flow Metab*, 23, 658–64.

66. Bruno, A., Kent, T. A., Coull, B. M., Shankar, R. R., Saha, C., Becker, K. J., Kissela, B. M. and Williams, L. S. (2008) Treatment of Hyperglycemia In Ischemic Stroke (THIS). A randomized pilot trial. *Stroke*, 39, 384–9.

67. Ryden, L., Standl, E., Bartnik, M., Van Den Berghe, G., Betteridge, J., De Boer, M. J., Cosentino, F., Jonsson, B., Laakso, M., Malmberg, K., Priori, S., Ostergren, J., Tuomilehto, J., Thrainsdottir, I., Vanhorebeek, I., Stramba-Badiale, M., Lindgren, P., Qiao, Q., Priori, S. G., Blanc, J. J., Budaj, A., Camm, J., Dean, V., Deckers, J., Dickstein, K., Lekakis, J., McGregor, K., Metra, M., Morais, J., Osterspey, A., Tamargo, J., Zamorano, J. L., Deckers, J. W., Bertrand, M., Charbonnel, B., Erdmann, E., Ferrannini, E., Flyvbjerg, A., Gohlke, H., Juanatey, J. R., Graham, I., Monteiro, P. F., Parhofer, K., Pyorala, K., Raz, I., Schernthaner, G., Volpe, M. and Wood, D. (2007) Guidelines on diabetes, pre-diabetes, and cardiovascular diseases: executive summary. The Task Force on Diabetes and Cardiovascular Diseases of the European Society of Cardiology (ESC) and of the European Association for the Study of Diabetes (EASD). *Eur Heart J*, 28, 88–136.

68. Prospective Studies Collaboration. (1995) Cholesterol, diastolic blood pressure and stroke: 13,000 strokes in 450,000 people in 45 prospective cohorts. *Lancet*, 346, 1647–53.

69. Eastern Stroke and Coronary Heart Disease Collaborative Research Group. (1998) Blood pressure, cholesterol and stroke in eastern Asia. *Lancet*, 352, 1801–7.

70. Rodgers, A., MacMahon, S., Gamble, G., Slattery, J., Sandercock, P. and Warlow, C. (1996) Blood pressure and risk of stroke in patients with cerebrovascular disease. The United Kingdom Transient Ischaemic Attack Collaborative Group. *Br Med J*, 313, 147.

71. Neal, B., MacMahon, S. and Chapman, S. (2000) Blood pressure lowering treatment trialists' collaboration. Effects of ACE inhibitors, calcium antagonists and other blood pressure lowering drugs: results of prospectively designed overviews of randomised controlled trials. *Lancet*, 356, 1955–64.

72. Gueyffier, F., Boissel, J. P., Boutitie, F., Pocock, S., Coope, J., Cutler, J., Ekbom, T., Fagard, R., Friedman, L., Kerlikowske, K., Perry, M., Prineas, R. and Schron, E. (1997) Effect of antihypertensive treatment in patients having already suffered from stroke. Gathering the evidence. The INDANA (INdividual Data ANalysis of Antihypertensive intervention trials) Project Collaborators. *Stroke*, 28, 2557–62.

73. United Kingdom Prospective Diabetes Study Group. (1998) Tight blood pressure control and risk of macrovascular and microvascular complications in type 2 diabetes: UKPDS 38. *Br Med J*, 317, 703–13.

74. Dahlof, B., Lindholm, L. H., Hansson, L., Schersten, B., Ekbom, T. and Wester, P. O. (1991) Morbidity and mortality in the Swedish Trial in Old Patients with Hypertension (STOP-Hypertension). *Lancet*, 338, 1281–5.

75. SHEP Co-Operative Research Group. (1991) Prevention of stroke by antihypertensive drug treatment in older persons with isolated systolic hypertension. Final results of the Systolic Hypertension in the Elderly Program (SHEP). *JAMA*, 265, 3255–64.

76. Williams, B., Poulter, N. R., Brown, M. J., Davis, M., McInnes, G. T., Potter, J. F., Sever, P. S. and McInnes, G. T. (2004) Guidelines for management of hypertension: report of the fourth working party of the British Hypertension Society, 2004-BHS IV. *J Hum Hypertens*, 18, 139–85.

77. Adler, A. I., Stratton, I. M., Neil, H. A., Yudkin, J. S., Matthews, D. R., Cull, C. A., Wright, A. D., Turner, R. C. and Holman, R. R. (2000) Association of systolic blood pressure with macrovascular and microvascular complications of type 2 diabetes (UKPDS 36): prospective observational study. *Br Med J*, 321, 412–19.

78. Dahlof, B., Sever, P. S., Poulter, N. R., Wedel, H., Beevers, D. G., Caulfield, M., Collins, R., Kjeldsen, S. E., Kristinsson, A., McInnes, G. T., Mehlsen, J., Nieminen, M., O'Brien, E. and Ostergren, J. (2005) Prevention of cardiovascular events with an antihypertensive regimen of amlodipine adding perindopril as required versus atenolol adding bendroflumethiazide as required, in the Anglo-Scandinavian Cardiac Outcomes Trial-Blood Pressure Lowering Arm (ASCOT-BPLA): a multicentre randomised controlled trial. *Lancet*, 366, 895–906.

79. Poulter, N. R., Wedel, H., Dahlof, B., Sever, P. S., Beevers, D. G., Caulfield, M., Kjeldsen, S. E., Kristinsson, A., McInnes, G. T., Mehlsen, J., Nieminen, M., O'Brien, E., Ostergren, J. and Pocock, S. (2005) Role of blood pressure and other variables in the differential cardiovascular event rates noted in the Anglo-Scandinavian Cardiac Outcomes Trial-Blood Pressure Lowering Arm (ASCOT-BPLA). *Lancet*, 366, 907–13.

80. Hope Study Investigators. (2000) Effects of an angiotensin-converting enzyme inhibitor, ramipril, on cardiovascular events in high-risk patients. *N Engl J Med*, 342, 145–53.

81. Hope Study Investigators. (2000) Effects of ramipril on cardiovascular and microvascular outcomes in people with diabetes mellitus: results of the HOPE study and MICRO-HOPE. *Lancet*, 358, 1033–41.

82. Bosch, J., Yusuf, S., Pogue, J., Sleight, P., Lonn, E., Rangoonwala, B., Davies, R., Ostergren, J. and Probstfield, J. (2002) Use of ramipril in preventing

stroke: double blind randomised trial. *Br Med J*, 324, 699–702.

83. Svensson, P., De Faire, U., Sleight, P., Yusuf, S. and Ostergren, J. (2001) Comparative effects of ramipril on ambulatory and office blood pressures: a HOPE Substudy. *Hypertension*, 38, E28–32.

84. Progress Collaborative Group. (2001) Randomised trial of a perindopril-based blood pressure-lowering regimen among 6,105 individuals with previous stroke or transient ischaemic attack. *Lancet*, 358, 1033–41.

85. Patel, A., MacMahon, S., Chalmers, J., Neal, B., Woodward, M., Billot, L., Harrap, S., Poulter, N., Marre, M., Cooper, M., Glasziou, P., Grobbee, D. E., Hamet, P., Heller, S., Liu, L. S., Mancia, G., Mogensen, C. E., Pan, C. Y., Rodgers, A. and Williams, B. (2007) Effects of a fixed combination of perindopril and indapamide on macrovascular and microvascular outcomes in patients with type 2 diabetes mellitus (the ADVANCE trial): a randomised controlled trial. *Lancet*, 370, 829–40.

86. Hansson, L., Zanchetti, A., Carruthers, S. G., Dahlof, B., Elmfeldt, D., Julius, S., Menard, J., Rahn, K. H., Wedel, H. and Westerling, S. (1998) Effects of intensive blood-pressure lowering and low-dose aspirin in patients with hypertension: principal results of the Hypertension Optimal Treatment (HOT) randomised trial. HOT Study Group. *Lancet*, 351, 1755–62.

87. Buse, J. B., Bigger, J. T., Byington, R. P., Cooper, L. S., Cushman, W. C., Friedewald, W. T., Genuth, S., Gerstein, H. C., Ginsberg, H. N., Goff, D. C., Jr., Grimm, R. H., Jr., Margolis, K. L., Probstfield, J. L., Simons-Morton, D. G. and Sullivan, M. D. (2007) Action to Control Cardiovascular Risk in Diabetes (ACCORD) trial: design and methods. *Am J Cardiol*, 99, 21i–33i.

88. O'Connell, J. E. and Gray, C. S. (1996) Treatment of post-stroke hypertension. A practical guide. *Drugs Aging*, 8, 408–15.

89. Robinson, T. G. and Potter, J. F. (2004) Blood pressure in acute stroke. *Age Ageing*, 33, 6–12.

90. Iso, H., Jacobs, D. R., Jr., Wentworth, D., Neaton, J. D. and Cohen, J. D. (1989) Serum cholesterol levels and six-year mortality from stroke in 350,977 men screened for the multiple risk factor intervention trial. *N Engl J Med*, 320, 904–10.

91. Yano, K., Reed, D. M. and Maclean, C. J. (1989) Serum cholesterol and hemorrhagic stroke in the Honolulu Heart Program. *Stroke*, 20, 1460–5.

92. Bucher, H. C., Griffith, L. E. and Guyatt, G. H. (1998) Effect of HMGcoA reductase inhibitors on stroke. A meta-analysis of randomized, controlled trials. *Ann Intern Med*, 128, 89–95.

93. Kearney, P. M., Blackwell, L., Collins, R., Keech, A., Simes, J., Peto, R., Armitage, J. and Baigent, C. (2008) Efficacy of cholesterol-lowering therapy in 18,686 people with diabetes in 14 randomised trials of statins: a meta-analysis. *Lancet*, 371, 117–25.

94. Antiplatelet Trialists' Collaboration. (1994) Collaborative overview of randomised trials of antiplatelet therapy - I: Prevention of death, myocardial infarction and stroke by prolonged antiplatelet therapy in various categories of patients. *Br Med J*, 308, 81–106.

95. Halkes, P. H., Van Gijn, J., Kappelle, L. J., Koudstaal, P. J. and Algra, A. (2006) Aspirin plus dipyridamole versus aspirin alone after cerebral ischaemia of arterial origin (ESPRIT): randomised controlled trial. *Lancet*, 367, 1665–73.

96. National Institute for Health and Clinical Excellence. (2005) Technology Appraisal 90. Clopidogrel and modified release dipyridamole in the prevention of occlusive vascular events. NICE, London.

97. Diener, H. C., Bogousslavsky, J., Brass, L. M., Cimminiello, C., Csiba, L., Kaste, M., Leys, D., Matias-Guiu, J. and Rupprecht, H. J. (2004) Aspirin and clopidogrel compared with clopidogrel alone after recent ischaemic stroke or transient ischaemic attack in high-risk patients (MATCH): randomised, double-blind, placebo-controlled trial. *Lancet*, 364, 331–7.

98. Gaede, P., Vedel, P., Larsen, N., Jensen, G. V., Parving, H. H. and Pedersen, O. (2003) Multifactorial intervention and cardiovascular disease in patients with type 2 diabetes. *N Engl J Med*, 348, 383–93.

7

Diabetes-Related Renal Disease in Older People

Latana A. Munang[1] and John M. Starr[2]

[1] *Liberton Hospital, 113 Lasswade Road, Edinburgh, UK*
[2] *University of Edinburgh, Royal Victoria Hospital, Edinburgh, UK*

Key messages

- Diabetic renal disease is associated with increased cardiovascular mortality and progression to end-stage renal failure.
- Early identification of renal disease through regular screening, good management of cardiovascular risk factors, tight blood pressure and glycaemic control are key treatment goals.
- Appropriate patients should be referred promptly to the nephrologist.

7.1 Introduction

Diabetes mellitus (DM) is the leading cause of chronic kidney disease in Western countries, with approximately 40% of patients with type 1 and type 2 DM eventually developing diabetes-related renal disease [1]. In addition, up to 20% of patients newly diagnosed with type 2 DM will already have diabetic renal disease, and a further 30–40% will develop the condition, mostly within 10 years [2].

Diabetic nephropathy is independently associated with increased cardiovascular mortality [3] as well as with a higher risk of progression to end-stage renal failure. In the United Kingdom, diabetic renal disease accounts for 20% of people commencing renal replacement therapy [4]. In the USA, the incidence of diabetic end-stage renal failure is 153 cases per million population [5].

7.2 Changes in the diabetic kidney

Injury in the diabetic kidney was initially thought to be due to haemodynamic changes of hyperperfusion and hyperfiltration, but it is increasingly clear that these changes are only one part of complex pathophysiological interactions. The results of recent studies have suggested that genetic influences and metabolic pathways involving oxidative stress, endothelial dysfunction, cytokines and growth factors are equally important [6–8]. Although previously debated as separate entities, it is now acknowledged that the basic pathophysiological mechanisms underlying diabetic nephropathy are similar in both type 1 and type 2 DM. However, many people with type 2 DM have the additional factors of hypertension, obesity, dyslipidaemia and ischaemic renal disease of arteriosclerosis, all of which can contribute to kidney damage, producing complex patterns of nephropathy [7].

Structurally, microscopic changes in the diabetic kidney include a thickening of the glomerular basement membrane and an increase in the mesangial matrix and mesangial cell proliferation, giving rise to diffuse *glomerulosclerosis*. Nodular glomerulosclerosis is

Diabetes in Old Age. Third Edition. Edited by Alan J. Sinclair
© 2009 John Wiley & Sons, Ltd

characterized by Kimmelstiel–Wilson lesions, which are distinctive ball-like areas of mesangial expansion with halos of glomerular capillary loops around the nodule. There is also podocyte effacement and loss. In the tubulointerstitium, the tubular basement membrane is also thickened, accompanied by tubular atrophy, interstitial fibrosis and arteriosclerosis.

The earliest indicator of renal disease in diabetes is *microalbuminuria*. This refers to albumin values in the urine that, although low, are above normal levels. Next, proteins appear non-selectively in the urine, and this is followed by decline in glomerular filtration function and ultimately, established renal failure. Approximately one-third of people with microalbuminuria will progress to proteinuria, one-third will remain microalbuminuric, and one-third will revert to normal albumin excretion [9]. Of those who become proteinuric, almost all will develop end-stage renal disease or die prematurely of cardiovascular disease [6]. It is therefore crucial that diabetic renal disease is detected as early as possible so as to allow prompt intervention.

7.3 Screening for diabetic renal disease

Current guidelines recommend annual screening for microalbuminuria and proteinuria [10–12], preferably using an early morning urine sample to avoid postural proteinuria and calculating the albumin: creatinine ratio (ACR), using a laboratory method as albumin concentration alone can be unreliable. Daily (24 h) urine collections are cumbersome and unnecessary, as spot ACR measurements have demonstrated an excellent correlation with these [13]. If protein is detected, any underlying urinary tract infection, intercurrent acute illness, congestive heart failure, severe hypertension and haematuria should be excluded as potential causes. Three positive tests are required over a period of less than 6 months in order to make a firm diagnosis of persistent microalbuminuria or proteinuria. Current UK guidelines define microalbuminuria as an ACR of $>2.5\,\mathrm{mg\,mmol^{-1}}$ in men and $>3.5\,\mathrm{mg\,mmol^{-1}}$ in women, while proteinuria is defined as an ACR of $\geq 30\,\mathrm{mg\,mmol^{-1}}$ [10, 11]. ACR values in women are higher for the equivalent level of urinary albumin excretion in men, mainly because women normally have lower urinary creatinine concentrations. In the USA, guidelines define microalbuminuria as an ACR between 30 and $300\,\mathrm{mg\,g^{-1}}$, while proteinuria is an ACR of $>300\,\mathrm{mg\,g^{-1}}$ [12].

Microalbuminuria or proteinuria does not automatically confirm diabetic nephropathy. Hence, it is important to exclude other causes of renal disease by taking a full clinical history and examination. However, in patients with at least a 10-year history of type 1 DM with retinopathy, increasing albuminuria and blood pressure, as well as a declining renal function in keeping with the natural history of diabetic nephropathy, no further investigations are needed [6]. The association between renal disease, retinopathy, albuminuria and duration of diabetes is less clear-cut in type 2 DM, but in the absence of any other suspicious features the deteriorating renal function can be assumed to be diabetic renal disease, without the need for further investigations. Serological autoantibodies, renal imaging and kidney biopsy may be indicated when the diagnosis is in doubt. However, the risk:benefit ratio of undertaking these investigations must be carefully considered as these tests carry a substantial risk, particularly for older people. Complications of renal biopsy include bleeding and perinephric haematomas, while radiological studies using contrast agents may precipitate an acute decline in renal function.

Screening for diabetic renal disease also includes the regular measurement of serum creatinine levels, at least annually. Serum creatinine is, however, a crude measure of renal function, as levels may vary depending on age, gender, muscle mass and diet. In older people with a relatively lower muscle mass, serum creatinine levels are often within the normal range, even when their renal function has declined significantly, leading to under-detection [14].

Because of the insensitivity of serum creatinine, current guidelines now recommend using the four-variable Modification of Diet in Renal Disease (MDRD) formula to estimate the glomerular filtration rate (GFR) (Table 7.1) [15]. Although less accurate in early chronic kidney disease, this is the preferred method in older people [16, 17]. It is also important to note that the development of the MDRD formula did not include patients with diabetes [18], and consequently potential accuracy problems persist when using this formula in this patient population. Cystatin C, a low-molecular-weight cysteine protease inhibitor which is freely filtered by the kidney, can also be measured in the serum as a marker of kidney function, but this has yet to achieve routine clinical use. Cystatin C has been shown to be more accurate than creatinine in detecting early kidney disease in patients with diabetes [19] and in older people, in addition to serving

Table 7.1 Estimation of the glomerular filtration rate using the four-variable MDRD equation.

$$GFR \ (ml\,min^{-1} \ per \ 1.73\,m^2) = 186 \times \{[serum \ creatinine \ (\mu mol\,l^{-1})/88.4]^{-1.154}\}$$
$$\times \ age \ (years)^{-0.023}$$
$$\times \ 0.742 \ if \ female, \ and$$
$$\times \ 1.21 \ if \ African-American$$

as a strong prognostic indicator of death and cardiovascular disease (CVD) [20].

7.4 Chronic kidney disease

Chronic kidney disease (CKD) is defined as either kidney damage or a decreased GFR of $<60\,ml\,min^{-1}$ per $1.73\,m^2$ persisting for at least 3 months, regardless of the underlying aetiology. Kidney damage may be indicated by persistent microalbuminuria or proteinuria or haematuria, by radiologically demonstrable structural abnormalities, or by biopsy-proven chronic glomerulonephritis. The level of kidney function determines the stage of CKD (Table 7.2) [15, 21].

Early CKD causes few, if any, symptoms – which is why an initial recognition through regular screening of patients with diabetes is essential. Patients may present with a poor appetite, nausea and vomiting, tiredness, breathlessness, peripheral oedema, itch, cramps or restless legs, but they may often be asymptomatic, even at CKD Stage 5.

Kidney function tests should be carried out at least annually to monitor progression of the disease, and more frequently in the latter stages of CKD. Ideally, patients with CKD Stage 3 should be assessed every 6 months, and those with CKD Stage 4 or 5 every 3 months. The GFR of patients with diabetes and proteinuria can decline as rapidly as $1.2\,ml\,min^{-1}$ per month if left untreated, although in some patients the GFR may remain stable for a long time [1]. The rate of GFR decline can be estimated by plotting the reciprocal of creatinine concentration against time; a change in the gradient of the curve, indicating an acceleration of the rate of decline, should trigger investigations to determine the causes of worsening renal function, which may potentially be reversible. UK guidelines for referral to a nephrologist are outlined in Table 7.3 [15].

7.5 Management of diabetic renal disease

7.5.1 Primary prevention

The ultimate aim is to intervene early enough to prevent the development of diabetic renal disease. The results of several studies have shown that, the better the glucose control, the lower the risk of developing microalbuminuria [22, 23]. Thus, the lowest possible HbA1c should be the target, generally below 6.5–7.5%, adjusted to suit each individual. Good blood pressure control also reduces the risk of developing diabetic renal disease [2], with the upper limit of acceptable blood pressure generally 140/80 mmHg.

It is important to remember that the intensive management of older patients may be hazardous because hypotension and hypoglycaemia occur more frequently than in younger people. Both conditions can be controlled using the usual medications, but lower starting doses should be used with careful titration and monitoring for side effects.

Table 7.2 Classification of chronic kidney disease [15, 21].

Stage	GFR (ml min^{-1} per 1.73 m^2)	Description
1	>90	Normal kidney function but with evidence of kidney damage
2	60–89	Mildly reduced kidney function with evidence of kidney damage
3	30–59	Moderately reduced kidney function
4	15–29	Severely reduced kidney function
5	<15 or on dialysis	Established renal failure

Table 7.3 Criteria for referral to specialist nephrology services [15].

Stage of CKD	Referral to nephrologists
1 and 2	Not required unless other problems occur (see below)
3	Routine referral if: Progressive fall in GFR Microscopic haematuria Urinary protein/creatinine ratio >45 mg mmol^{-1} Unexplained anaemia, abnormal potassium, calcium or phosphate Suspected systemic illness, e.g., systemic lupus erythematosus Uncontrolled blood pressure (>150/90 mmHg while receiving three antihypertensive agents)
4	Urgent referral or routine referral if stable (<2 ml min^{-1} per 1.73 m^2 change in GFR over $\geq$ 6 months)
5	Immediate referral
Renal problems irrespective of GFR	Immediate referral Malignant hypertension Hyperkalaemia (K$^+$>7 mmol l^{-1}) Urgent referral Nephrotic syndrome Routine referral Dipstick proteinuria and urine protein/creatinine ratio >100 mg mmol^{-1} Dipstick proteinuria and microscopic haematuria Macroscopic haematuria, but urological tests negative

7.5.2 Management of microalbuminuria and proteinuria

Although it may not be possible to completely prevent the development of diabetic renal disease, the process can be delayed significantly. The rate of change of albuminuria has been shown to be an independent predictor of death and cardiovascular events in these patients [3]. Therefore, the main goals of treatment concentrate on preventing progression from microalbuminuria to proteinuria, slowing down the decline of renal function in patients with proteinuria, and preventing cardiovascular events.

7.5.3 Glycaemic control

Good glycaemic control is important. On the other hand, the lower the HbA1c goal and the tighter the glycaemic control, the higher the risk of more frequent and more severe hypoglycaemic episodes, particularly in older patients.

While there are currently no evidence-based guidelines in recommending which types of insulin to use, it is important to note that the effect of insulin may be impaired in patients with renal disease, resulting in higher insulin doses being required [24]. However, impaired kidney function also means that the half-life of insulin is prolonged because of decreased degradation, and this will result in more hypoglycaemic episodes. Consequently, insulin doses must be titrated cautiously.

Similarly, the clearance of most oral agents is also decreased, giving rise to a higher risk of adverse side effects. In patients with CKD Stage 3–5, long-acting sulphonylureas such as chlorpropamide and glibenclamide should be avoided because of the risk of profound hypoglycaemia. Glipizide can be used without dose adjustment as its metabolites are inactive, while α-glucosidase inhibitors should also be avoided because of potential hepatic damage. Although there is a lower risk of hypoglycaemia with metformin, it is contraindicated in patients with serum creatinine concentrations $\geq$ 1.5 mg dl^{-1} in men and $\geq$ 1.4 mg dl^{-1} in women, because potential accumulation even in mild renal disease places patients at risk of lactic acidosis [12]. Recent studies have suggested that thiazolidinediones such as roziglitazone and pioglitazone may have a protective effect in slowing down the progression of diabetic renal disease [25], and as these drugs are metabolized by the liver they are safe to use in patients with CKD, without any dose adjustment.

In advanced renal disease, although good glycaemic control may no longer be necessary to prevent further deterioration in kidney function, it is still important for preventing the progression of retinopathy, neuropathy and macrovascular disease.

7.5.4 Blood pressure and renin–angiotensin system blockade

The importance of reducing systemic blood pressure in delaying the progression of diabetic renal disease is well recognized. Additionally, blocking the renin–angiotensin system (RAS) with angiotensin-converting enzyme (ACE) inhibitors or angiotensin receptor blockers (ARBs) is renoprotective, independent of its blood pressure-reducing effect [26]. Therefore, all diabetic patients with microalbuminuria and proteinuria should be commenced on an ACE inhibitor or ARB. It is important to re-check serum creatinine and potassium at 1–2 weeks after commencing these agents, and also after each increase in dose. While a small rise in serum creatinine is common, a creatinine increase of $>20\%$ or a fall in GFR of $>15\%$ should prompt consideration of withdrawal and further investigation for renal artery stenosis.

The systemic blood pressure will often remain elevated, despite the maximum tolerated dose of ACE inhibitor or ARB, and it is not uncommon for patients with advancing renal disease to require four or five antihypertensive agents, including calcium-channel blockers, beta-blockers, alpha-blockers and diuretics. Loop diuretics are preferred to thiazides in the later stages of CKD, as the diuretic efficacy of thiazides tends to decrease with deteriorating renal function and the potential for electrolyte disturbances becomes higher. The target blood pressure varies between guidelines, but range from 120/70 to 140/80 mmHg [6, 10–12].

7.5.5 Diet and nutrition

The reduction of dietary protein intake to $0.8\,\mathrm{g\,kg^{-1}}$ body weight is recommended in CKD Stages 1–4, in order to reduce proteinuria and slow the rate of renal function decline [12]. However, patients with CKD are already subject to dietary restrictions because of hyperkalaemia, hyperphosphataemia and hypertension, in addition to the restrictions already required because of diabetes. Malnutrition may occur as a consequence of these imposed restrictions, and this can lead to progressive muscle weakness, poor exercise tolerance, an increased susceptibility to infection and high mortality. It is therefore important that each patient is interviewed by a dietician for individual dietary assessment and advice.

7.6 Managing cardiovascular risk

Cardiovascular disease is the leading cause of death in CKD, with most patients more likely to die from a cardiovascular event before reaching end-stage renal failure. Aggressive risk management is therefore important and will also delay the progression of renal disease. Patients should be advised on smoking cessation, weight loss, exercise, and limiting both alcohol and sodium intake. Aspirin is also recommended for primary and secondary prevention.

7.6.1 Dyslipidaemia

The management of dyslipidaemia is important in reducing the cardiovascular risk of all patients with diabetic renal disease. It is suggested that lipid levels be measured annually, aiming for a target LDL-cholesterol of $<100\,\mathrm{mg\,dl^{-1}}$ for CKD Stages 1–4 [12]. In addition to lifestyle measures such as diet, exercise and weight loss, the use of statins are recommended as the agents of choice, although combination therapies may be required to achieve target levels [27].

7.7 Management of CKD and its complications

Most patients up to CKD Stage 3 can be managed safely by general practitioners in the community. The main complications of CKD involve the bones, anaemia and metabolic acidosis [28]. In addition to the above-described measures, all patients should undergo at least annual monitoring of their haemoglobin (Hb), potassium, calcium and phosphate. Renal ultrasonography may be indicated in patients with lower urinary tract symptoms, persistent hypertension and unexpected progressive declining renal function.

Renal bone disease starts at Stage 3, causing an impaired renal production of active 1,25-dihydroxy vitamin D. This is very important in older people, as a large proportion will have coexisting osteoporosis. Both, hypocalcaemia and hyperphosphataemia cause secondary hyperparathyroidism, and treatment with ergocalciferol or cholecalciferol with calcium supplement may be indicated. Phosphate binders can also be used for treating hyperphosphataemia.

Anaemia of CKD begins at Stage 3 and, if left untreated, may cause left ventricular hypertrophy and failure, a poor quality of life and impaired cognition. Anaemic patients with Hb $<11\,g\,dl^{-1}$ should be considered for treatment with erythropoiesis-stimulating agents and intravenous iron [29]. A stable Hb between 10.5 and $12.5\,g\,dl^{-1}$ is recommended, depending on the individual's functional needs. Blood transfusions should be avoided if possible in those patients where renal transplantation is a treatment option.

Metabolic acidosis is uncommon before CKD Stage 4, but can contribute to bone disease, muscle wasting, anorexia, hypoalbuminaemia and a progressive deterioration of renal function. It should be corrected with supplementary sodium bicarbonate, aiming to maintain plasma bicarbonate at $\geq 20\,mmol\,l^{-1}$.

All patients who reach CKD Stage 4 or 5 should be discussed with a nephrologist, because they must be adequately informed about their treatment options as they approach end-stage renal failure. Most patients need at least one year to prepare for renal replacement therapy (RRT) [30], and a prompt referral is associated with better outcomes [31]. Most patients who reach end-stage renal failure have progressed from earlier stages of CKD, yet up to one-third are referred late and will only be examined by a nephrologist less than one month before requiring RRT. Delays in these referrals occur more frequently in older people, contributing to excess mortality [32].

7.7.1 End-stage renal disease and RRT

Today, increasing numbers of older people are undergoing RRT. In the UK, the median age of patients starting dialysis has risen from 63.9 years in 1998 to 65.5 years in 2005, and at present 25% of dialysis patients are aged >75 years [4]. The guidelines recommend starting RRT when the GFR falls below $15\,ml\,min^{-1}$ per $1.73\,m^2$ and there are problems of symptomatic uraemia, uncontrollable fluid balance, blood pressure or malnutrition. Even when asymptomatic, RRT should be started when the GFR falls to $<6\,ml\,min^{-1}$ per $1.73\,m^2$ [33].

7.7.2 Haemodialysis

Haemodialysis is the most common form of RRT employed in older people. This involves passing the patient's blood into a dialyzer, where molecules diffuse across a semi-permeable membrane and fluid is removed by ultrafiltration. Anticoagulation with heparin and good vascular access are required for haemodialysis. Ideally, a subcutaneous arteriovenous fistula should be formed 6 months before starting dialysis, but synthetic grafts, central venous catheters and semi-permanent tunnelled central catheters may be also be used in the short to intermediate term. Generally, patients undergo three haemodialysis sessions per week, each lasting 3–5 h. The procedure is normally carried out in hospital units, although home haemodialysis may be possible for appropriate patients, with good outcomes [34].

7.7.3 Peritoneal dialysis

Peritoneal dialysis is normally carried out at home, thus allowing much greater patient independence. However, because it uses the peritoneum as the semi-permeable membrane for dialyzing, it is contraindicated in patients who have had major abdominal surgery or peritoneal adhesions, unrepaired inguinal hernias or compromised respiratory function; thus, a large number of older people are excluded. Common problems include infection (hence, good personal hygiene is essential) and fluid overload due to inadequate ultrafiltration.

7.7.4 Renal transplantation

Renal transplantation is clearly preferable to dialysis as it offers CKD patients a return to normality. However, the scarcity of donor organs means that many older patients are not considered for transplantation because of their comorbidity and shorter life expectancy. There is currently no age limit to transplantation in the UK, but only 14% of renal transplant recipients are over the age of 60 [35], despite increasing evidence showing transplantation to be worthwhile in older patients if they are selected carefully and their immunosuppression tailored sensibly [36, 37]. The main complications are graft rejection, infection and malignancy, but CVD remains the leading cause of death.

7.8 Conservative management of renal disease

Although life-prolonging, RRT may not be the best treatment for all patients. Survival after dialysis for older, heavily dependent patients with more comorbidity is not significantly longer than those treated palliatively [38]. Neither is the patient's quality of life necessarily better, as many older patients receiving RRT spend a considerable proportion of their time in hospital with a higher risk of developing multiple complications [39]. Conservative or non-dialytic management aims to relieve the symptoms of end-stage renal failure, including the treatment of anaemia with erythropoiesis-stimulating agents and the control of nausea and pruritus with appropriate drugs. End of life care is equally important, and requires a close collaboration with palliative services and primary care.

Today, conservative care specialist nurses are available at many renal units to facilitate this treatment option for patients.

7.9 Conclusions

The current aging population and global epidemic of diabetes means that the number of people with diabetic renal disease will continue to increase. Early recognition, aggressive management of cardiovascular risk factors and tight control of both blood pressure and

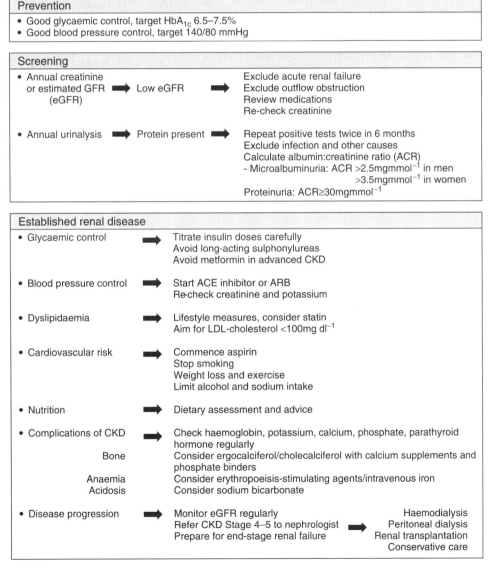

Figure 7.1 Approach to management of diabetic renal disease.

glycaemia are key strategies in reducing mortality and delaying progression to end-stage renal failure (Figure 7.1). Patients should be informed at an early stage regarding the likely course of their disease, and their prognosis. Appropriate patients should be referred to nephrology services promptly, so that they may be adequately prepared to make informed choices about their treatment options.

References

1. Gross JL, de Azevedo MJ, Silveiro SP, Canani LH, Caramori ML and Zelmanovitz T. Diabetic nephropathy: diagnosis, prevention, and treatment. *Diabetes Care* 2005; **28** (**1**): 164–76.

2. Thomas MC and Atkins RC. Blood pressure lowering for the prevention and treatment of diabetic kidney disease. *Drugs* 2006; **66** (**17**): 2213–34.

3. Yuyun MF, Dinneen SF, Edwards OM, Wood E and Wareham NJ. Absolute level and rate of change of albuminuria over 1 year independently predict mortality and cardiovascular events in patients with diabetic nephropathy. *Diabet Med* 2003; **20**: 277–82.

4. Ansell D, Feest TG, Tomson C, Williams AJ and Warwick G. UK Renal Registry Ninth Annual Report, December. The Renal Association, Petersfield, Hampshire; 2006.

5. U.S. Renal Data System. *Annual Data Report: Atlas of Chronic Kidney Disease and End-Stage Renal Disease in the United States*. National Institutes of Health, National Institute of Diabetes and Digestive and Kidney Diseases, Bethesda; 2007.

6. Marshall SM. Recent advances in diabetic nephropathy. *Postgrad Med J* 2004; **80**: 624–33.

7. Wolf G. New insights into the pathophysiology of diabetic nephropathy: from haemodynamics to molecular pathology. *European Journal of Clinical Investigation* 2004; **34**: 785–96.

8. Caramori ML and Mauer M. Diabetes and nephropathy. *Curr Opin Nephrol Hypertens* 2003; **12**: 273–82.

9. Marshall SM and Flyvbjerg A. Prevention and early detection of vascular complications of diabetes. *Br Med J* 2006; **333**: 475–80.

10. National Institute for Clinical Excellence. *Management of Type 2 diabetes: the prevention and early management of renal disease*. National Institute for Clinical Excellence, London; 2002.

11. Scottish Intercollegiate Guidelines Network. *Management of diabetes*. SIGN Publication No. 55, November 2001.

12. National Kidney Foundation. KDOQI Clinical Practice Guidelines and Clinical Practice Recommendations for Diabetes and Chronic Kidney Disease. *Am J Kidney Dis* 2007; **49** (Suppl. 2): S1–S180.

13. Gansevoort RT, Verhave JC, Hillege HL, Burgerhof JG, Bakker SJ, de Zeeuw D and de Jong PE. The validity of screening based on spot morning urine samples to detect subjects with microalbuminuria in the general population. *Kidney Int* 2005; **98** (Suppl.): S28–35.

14. Swedko PJ, Clark HD, Paramsothy K and Akbari A. Serum creatinine is an inadequate screening test for renal failure in elderly patients. *Arch Intern Med* 2003; **163**: 356–60.

15. Royal College of Physicians. *Chronic kidney disease in adults: UK guidelines for identification, management and referral*. Royal College of Physicians, London; 2005.

16. Burkhardt H, Hahn T, Gretz N and Gladisch R. Bedside estimation of the glomerular filtration rate in hospitalized elderly patients. *Nephron* 2005; **101**: c1–8.

17. Cirillo M, Anastasio P and De Santo NG. Relationship of gender, age and body mass index to errors in predicted kidney function. *Nephrol Dial Transplant* 2005; **20**: 1791–8.

18. Poggio ED, Wang X, Greene T, Van Lente F and Hall PM. Performance of the modification of diet in renal disease and Cockcroft-Gault equations in the estimation of GFR in health and in chronic kidney disease *J Am Soc Nephrol* 2005; **16**: 459–66.

19. MacIsaac RJ, Tsalamandris C, Thomas MC, Premaratne E, Panagiotopoulos S, Smith TJ, Poon A, Jenkins MA, Ratnaike SI, Power DA and Jerums G. The accuracy of cystatin C and commonly used creatinine-based methods for detecting moderate and mild chronic kidney disease in diabetes *Diabet Med* 2007; **24**: 443–8.

20. Shlipak MG, Wassel Fyr CL, Chertow GM, Harris TB, Kritchevsky SB, Tylavsky FA, Satterfield S, Cummings SR, Newman AB and Fried LF. Cystatin C and mortality risk in the elderly: the health, aging, and body composition study. *J Am Soc Nephrol* 2006; **17** (**1**): 254–61.

21. Levey AS, Coresh J, Balk E, Kausz AT, Levin A, Steffes MW, Hogg RJ, Perrone RD, Lau J and Eknoyan G. National Kidney Foundation practice guidelines for chronic kidney disease: Evaluation, classification and stratification. *Ann Intern Med* 2003; **139** (**2**): 137–47.

22. Diabetes Control and Complications Trial (DCCT) Research Group. The effect of intensive treatment of diabetes on the development and progression of long term complications in insulin-dependent diabetics. *N Engl J Med* 1993; **329**: 977–86.

23. UK Prospective Diabetes Study. Intensive blood glucose control with sulphonylureas or insulin compared with conventional treatment and risk of complications

in patients with type 2 diabetes. *Lancet* 1998; **352**: 837–53.

24. Cavanaugh KL. Diabetes management issues for patients with chronic kidney disease. *Clinical Diabetes* 2007; **25** (**3**), 90–7.

25. Sarafidis PA and Bakris GL. Protection of the kidneys by thiazolidinediones: an assessment from bench to bedside. *Kidney Int* 2006; **70**: 1223–33.

26. Strippoli GFM, Bonifati C, Craig M, Navaneethan SD and Craig JC. Angiotensin converting enzyme inhibitors and angiotensin II receptor antagonists for preventing the progression of diabetic kidney disease. *Cochrane Database of Systematic Reviews* 2006; (**4**), CD006257.

27. Solano MP and Goldberg RB. Management of dyslipidemia in diabetes. *Cardiology in Review* 2006; **14** (**3**); 125–35.

28. Lederer E and Ouseph R. Chronic kidney disease. *Am J Kidney Dis* 2007; **49** (**1**): 162–71.

29. National Collaborating Centre for Chronic Conditions. *Anaemia management in chronic kidney disease: national clinical guideline for management in adults and children*. Royal College of Physicians, London, 2006.

30. Department of Health. *National Service Framework for Renal Services: Part 2 - Chronic kidney disease, acute renal failure and end of life care*. Department of Health, London; 2005.

31. Stack AG. Impact of timing of nephrology referral and pre-ESRD care on mortality risk among new patients in the United States. *Am J Kidney Dis* 2003; **41**: 310–18.

32. Schwenger V, Morath C, Hofmann A, Hoffmann O, Zeier M and Ritz E. Late referral – a major cause of poor outcome in the very elderly dialysis patient. *Nephrol Dial Transplant* 2006; **21**: 962–7.

33. European Renal Association. European Best Practice Guidelines. Section I: Measurement of renal function, when to refer and when to start dialysis: I.3 When to start dialysis. *Nephrol Dial Transplant* 2002; **17**, 10–11.

34. Saner E, Nitsch D, Descoeudres C, Frey FJ and Uehlinger DE. Outcome of home haemodialysis patients: a case cohort study. *Nephrol Dial Transplant* 2005; **20** (**3**): 604–10.

35. NHS Blood and Transplant. *UK Transplant Activity Report 2006-2007*. NHS, Bristol, UK; 2007

36. Segoloni GP, Messina M, Giraudi R, Leonardi G, Torta E, Gabrielli D, Ferrari A, Pellu V, Tattoli F and Fop F. Renal transplantation in patients over 65 years of age: no more a contraindication but a growing indication. *Transplantation Proceedings* 2005; **37** (**2**): 721–5.

37. Otero-Raviña F, Rodríguez-Martínez M, Gude F, Gonzalez-Juanatey JR, Valdes F and Sanchez-Guisande D. Renal transplantation in the elderly: does patient age determine the results? *Age and Ageing* 2005; **34**: 583–7.

38. Smith C, Da Silva-Gane M, Chadna S, Warwicker P, Greenwood R and Farrington K. Choosing not to dialyse: evaluation of planned non-dialytic management in a cohort of patients with end-stage renal failure. *Nephron Clin Pract* 2003; **95**: c40–6.

39. Munshi SK, Vijayakumar N, Taub NA, Bhullar H, Lo TCN and Warwick G. Outcome of renal replacement therapy in the very elderly. *Nephrol Dial Transplant* 2001; **16**: 128–33.

8

Management of Eye Disease and Visual Loss

Nina Tumosa

Geriatrics Research, Education and Clinical Center, St Louis VAMC, and Division of Geriatrics, Saint Louis University, St Louis MO, USA

Key messages

- The management of diabetic retinopathy requires good communication between the patient and his/her health care providers.
- Diabetic retinopathy can result in blindness or severe visual impairment if diabetes mellitus (DM) is left untreated.
- While new treatments such as the use of antibodies, cytokines and fusion proteins to prevent diabetic retinopathy show promise, at present the best way to prevent diabetic retinopathy is strict control of DM through the use of nutritional therapy, exercise and pharmacological agents.

8.1 Introduction

Diabetes mellitus (DM) is a chronic disease with a long-term risk for visual and neurological impairments. Diabetic retinopathy (retinal changes that occur in patients with DM) is characterized by microaneurysms, exudates, haemorrhages and, less commonly, neovascularization, and is more common than other microvascular complications of DM. Diabetic patients with poorer long-term glycemic control are more vulnerable to diabetic retinopathy than are those with better glycemic control. Retinopathy and other microvascular complications are attributed to chronic hyperglycemia, vascular damage and leakage, oedema, capillary basement membrane thickening, neovascularization, haemorrhage and ischaemia. Diabetic retinopathy is believed to be a leading cause of blindness in the industrialized world in people between the ages of 25 and 74 [1], and the fourth leading cause of blindness in people of all ages in developing countries [2]. The prevalence of DM for all age-groups worldwide was estimated to be 2.8% in 2000 and 4.4% in 2030. The total number of people with DM is projected to rise from 171 million in 2000 to 366 million in 2030. The most important demographic change to DM prevalence across the world appears to be the increase in the proportion of people aged over 65 years [3]. Diabetic retinopathy causes considerable morbidity and mortality, and has a large economic impact [4]; consequently, its prevention and successful treatment are desirable public health goals [5].

8.2 Risk factors

Many risk factors may affect the rate at which diabetic retinopathy progresses (see Table 8.1). It is incumbent upon the health care team to educate the diabetic patient about these risk factors and to develop a care plan that addresses those factors that are modifiable

Diabetes in Old Age. Third Edition. Edited by Alan J. Sinclair
© 2009 John Wiley & Sons, Ltd

Table 8.1 Risk factors for diabetic retinopathy.

Risk factor	Reference(s)
Age	[6, 7]
Race	[8–10]
Obesity	[8]
Smoking	[11]
Proteinuria	[12]
Depression	[13, 14]
Dyslipidaemia	[11]
Duration of DM	[6, 7, 9, 10]
Eating disorders	[15]
Gestational diabetes	[16]
Poor glycemic control	[6, 17]
Parental history of DM	[8]
Cardiovascular disease	[18, 19]
Uncontrolled systemic hypertension	[9, 11, 12]
Rapid pre-cataract surgery glycemic control	[20]

in an effort to prevent or slow down the onset or progression of diabetic retinopathy.

There are many clinical signs that are indicative of the presence of diabetic retinopathy. Optometrists and ophthalmologists are the most likely providers to first find or confirm the diagnosis of diabetic retinopathy to their diabetic patients. These providers perform thorough ocular assessments on patients who report a history of having been diagnosed with DM or who are suspected of having DM because of the presence of multiple risk factors listed above, or because of specific visual complaints such as fluctuating vision or 'seeing red' (which is a sign of a vitreous haemorrhage). The American Diabetes Association's Clinical Practice Guidelines [21] for examining a patient with diabetic retinopathy include performing:

- Comprehensive eye examinations within 3–5 years of the onset of DM (type 1 diabetics) and immediately after initial diagnosis (type 2 diabetics).

- Subsequent annual dilated fundus examinations.

- Comprehensive eye examinations for pregnant women in the first trimester with close follow-up and counselling throughout pregnancy and in the first year post-partum.

- Prompt referral to a retinal specialist of patients with macular oedema, severe non-proliferative diabetic retinopathy or proliferative diabetic retinopathy.

- Strict control of elevated blood pressure.

The ocular assessment that optometrists or ophthalmologists perform may include tests for visual acuity, pupil function assessment, extraocular muscle motilities, visual field distortions (Amsler Grid), colour vision changes, tear film break-up time and contrast sensitivity changes, as well as the performance of biomicroscopy, tonometry, gonioscopy, dilated stereoscopic fundus examination and fundus photography [22]. The clinical signs that are indicative of the presence of diabetic retinopathy, and which can be confirmed during this thorough visual assessment of the retina include any of the following items:

- Cotton wool spots

- Arteriolar narrowing

- Fibrotic proliferation

- Decreased visual acuity

- Hard exudates (Figure 8.1)

- Colour vision abnormalities

- Blot haemorrhages (Figures 8.2 and 8.3)

- Flame-shaped haemorrhages (Figure 8.2)

- Venous tortuosity and beading

- Metamorphosia and/or scotomas

- Dot haemorrhages and microaneurysms

- Intraretinal microvascular abnormalities

Macular changes that are secondary to the presence of diabetic retinopathy and can best be confirmed during a dilated fundus examination include:

Retinal detachment
Vitreous haemorrhage
Preretinal haemorrhage
Disc neovascularization (Figure 8.4)
Neovascularization elsewhere (Figure 8.5).

8.3 Management of diabetic retinopathy

The management of diabetic retinopathy requires the attention of all members of the health care team. The team should include the primary care physician, nurse, social worker, nutritionist, exercise therapist, optometrist, ophthalmologist, endocrinologist, health educator and geriatrician, as well as the family caregiver

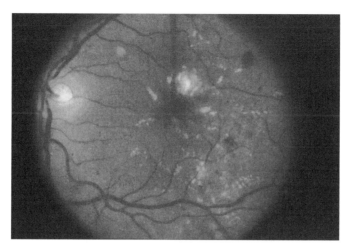

Figure 8.1 Maculopathy. Certain pathological changes occur in the macula as a result of early diabetes mellitus. These changes include leakage of blood vessels around the macula (black space in the middle of the picture). Remnants of blood products show as white spots (hard exudates) arrayed around the macula.

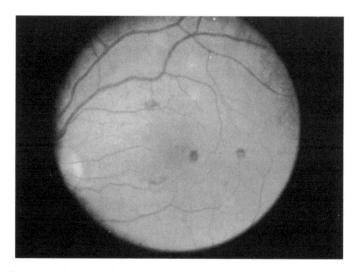

Figure 8.2 Background retinopathy. Pathological changes that occur early in diabetes mellitus elsewhere in the retina (other than the macula, as shown in Figure 8.1) include haemorrhages at the ends of the blood vessels. These appear either as dark circles to the left of the centrally located macula (blot haemorrhages) or as a more diffuse pooling of blood (flame haemorrhages) in the superior and inferior quadrants, just to the right of the macula.

and patient. A good management strategy is easier to implement if the patient and all family caregivers are aware of possible signs and symptoms that are commonly found in diabetic patients. Because diabetic retinopathy does not hurt (the only nerve in the eye is the sensory optic nerve which has no pain receptors), the patient must be educated about common vision changes that are harbingers of diabetic retinopathy and the vision-threatening progression of the disease. There is no point in having excellent prevention and

treatment protocols for diabetic retinopathy if the patient ignores them because of the painless, insidious nature and progression of the condition. The common ocular and periocular manifestations of DM are listed in Table 8.2.

There is great incentive for aggressively treating and managing diabetic retinopathy. Blindness or severe visual impairment can result from a number of DM-caused conditions including, in order of decreasing frequency, vitreous or preretinal haemorrhage,

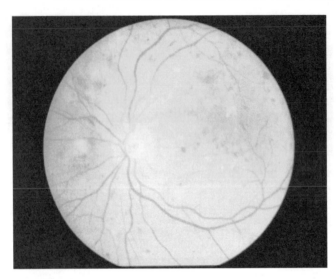

Figure 8.3 Pre-proliferative retinopathy. More extensive pathological retinal changes are characteristic of chronic diabetes mellitus. In the early stages of the disease, the haemorrhages are small but can be seen in all quadrants of the image.

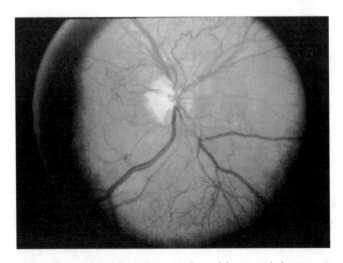

Figure 8.4 Proliferative retinopathy of the disk (NVD). With proliferative diabetic retinopathy, some areas of the retina lose their capillary vessels and become non-perfused. This image shows the resulting new blood vessels on the disk. The new blood vessels are tortuous and numerous.

macular oedema or related pigmentary change, macular or retinal detachment and neovascular glaucoma [25, 26]. Diabetic retinopathy typically begins as a series of non-proliferative abnormalities, and then progresses to proliferative diabetic retinopathy. Macular oedema can develop at any time during the progression of diabetic retinopathy. Macular ischemia, retinal and vitreous haemorrhage, and retinal detachment are the primary causes of blindness in patients with diabetic retinopathy.

8.4 Treatments of diabetic retinopathy

The key to preventing diabetic retinopathy is the strict control of DM through the use of nutritional therapy, exercise and drug treatment. This means that education of people with DM plays a critical role in the management and treatment of DM and, therefore, of diabetic retinopathy. For the past 25 years, the

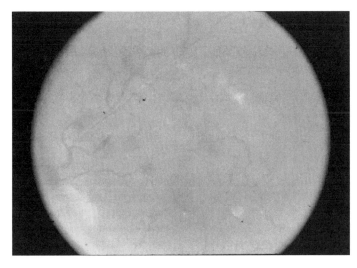

Figure 8.5 Proliferative retinopathy elsewhere in the retina (NVE). With proliferative diabetic retinopathy, some areas of the retina lose their capillary vessels and become non-perfused. This image shows the resulting, tortuous new blood vessels in other areas of the retina, away from the disk.

treatment of diabetic retinopathy has been replete with ever-improving surgery within the eyeball, using lasers and other surgical procedures (e.g., pars plana vitrectomy) that remove the scar tissue and debris resulting from haemorrhages. Currently, promising new treatments using antibodies, growth factors and steroids to decrease the progressive effects of diabetic retinopathy are being widely investigated.

8.4.1 Nutritional treatment

Nutritional therapy is an integral component in maintaining normal blood glucose levels and in treating the chronic complications of DM. Tobacco use and diet – in particular the consumption of fatty acids and dietary fibre – are significantly associated with the rate of progression of diabetic retinopathy and retinopathy-related risk factors [27]. Diets created with the aim of achieving good metabolic control have resulted in the excellent control of diabetic retinopathy [28]. The American Diabetes Association [29] recommends that such diets be based on individual assessment and treatment goals and outcomes. The diets should take into consideration usual eating habits and other lifestyle factors. This personalized approach requires that ongoing nutrition self-management education and care be provided by the health care team for individuals with DM. Although a diet prescribed by a registered dietician should form the basis for the nutritional treatment, all members of the medical team must have updated nutritional knowledge (preferably provided by a dietician) in order to support the patient in adopting a healthy lifestyle [30]. The team members must be aware of the purpose and importance of the nutritional therapy. They must also understand the role of dietary fat in controlling diabetes, know the definition of the glycaemic index and be able to identify foods containing carbohydrates/mono-unsaturated fats in order to be able to assess the value and appropriateness of reported diets [31].

8.4.2 Exercise therapy

Physical activity is a powerful tool for helping persons with DM to achieve metabolic goals [32]. Because intensive glycaemic and blood pressure control has been shown to delay both the onset and progression of diabetic retinopathy, exercise protocols that help reduce glycaemia and blood pressure should delay the progression of diabetic retinopathy. Longitudinal studies have indicated significant improvements in glucose metabolism with aerobic exercise training, and also with resistance training in middle-aged and older men and women [33]. Because older adults with type 2 DM have mobility impairment and reduced fitness, a number of investigations are ongoing which aim to optimize exercise programmes, albeit with only limited success. For example, a specially developed form of Tai Chi, while developed specifically for diabetic patients, may not have been of sufficient intensity,

Table 8.2 Visual problems resulting from diabetes mellitus.

Site or condition	Visual system consequences
Refraction	Fluctuations in refractive error Distorted vision Blurred vision
Tear films	Dry eyes
Pupil	Rubeosis
Cornea	Ulcers Abrasions Hypoesthesia Poor epithelial healing
Iris	Neovascularization Neovascular glaucoma
Lens	Premature cortical cataracts Posterior subcapsular cataracts [23]
Ciliary body	Premature presbyopia
Extraocular muscles	Cranial nerve palsies Nerve III Nerve IV (diplopia) Nerve VI (diplopia)
Eyelids	Cranial nerve VII palsy (Bell's palsy)
Vitreous	Detachments
Optic nerve	Ischaemic optic neuropathy Neovascularization of the disc
Macula	Maculopathy • Oedematous • Exudative • Ischaemic Macula oedema
Retina	Detachments Soft exudates Hard exudates Retinal oedema Vein occlusions Microaneurysms Artery occlusions Neovascularizations Intraretinal haemorrhages
Trabecular network (Ganglion cell apoptosis)	Increased incidence of open-angle glaucoma [24]

frequency or duration to effect any positive changes in many aspects of physiology or health status relevant to older people with DM [34]. Further research is clearly necessary before specific exercise protocols can be identified for slowing the progression of diabetic retinopathy.

8.4.3 Surgical treatment

Until very recently, no pharmacological agent has demonstrated the ability to slow the progression of diabetic retinopathy. Since the advent of laser technology during the 1980s, pan retinal photocoagulation laser surgery has been used with great success in the treatment of macular edema [35] and vitreous haemorrhage [36, 37] that accompany proliferative diabetic retinopathy. While focal laser photocoagulation reduces the risk of moderate visual loss by 50–70% in eyes with macular oedema, the downside of these procedures is a lack of efficacy in some patients, patient discomfort, the need for repeated treatment, constriction of peripheral visual fields, decreased night vision, reduced near vision, loss of acuity, and the risk of retinal damage and scarring. Early vitrectomy improves visual recovery in patients with proliferative retinopathy with accompanying severe vitreous haemorrhage. The intravitreal injection of steroids can be used when conventional treatments have failed in eyes, when there is a persistent loss of vision. Nonetheless, laser photocoagulation and vitrectomy remain the conventional management protocols for diabetic retinopathy [38].

8.4.4 Pharmacological approaches

The ultimate goal of any treatment of diabetic retinopathy is the prevention of vision loss. Traditionally, the pharmacological methods to achieve this goal have been limited to strict metabolic control and tight blood pressure control, and these have been used successfully to reduce the risk of moderate and severe visual loss by 50% of patients with severe non-proliferative and proliferative diabetic retinopathy [39]. However, to better address the 50% of patients who have been unable to control diabetic retinopathy using these methods, there is an active research agenda to develop new pharmaceuticals that will better protect visual acuity, macular thickness and, therefore, patient quality of life.

A growing number of biological agents such as cytokines, monoclonal antibodies and fusion proteins have become available for the treatment of various autoimmune, neoplastic, cardiovascular, infectious, allergic and other conditions. Their introduction has resulted in marked clinical improvements for many patients in a variety of conditions. Many new studies on the treatment of diabetic retinopathy have been initiated based on the observations that microvascular damage to patients with chronic hyperglycaemia is mediated by interrelated pathways involving aldose reductase, advanced glycation end products, protein kinase C (PKC) and vascular endothelial growth factor (VEGF). Thus, a variety of promising new therapies for diabetic retinopathy-targeting pathways that cause microvascular damage are under investigation [39, 40]. Many of these therapies involve direct growth factor modulators, including VEGF inhibitors, PKC inhibitors and steroids. Several investigations involving human subjects are currently under way, including a combination of pan retinal photocoagulation and intravitreal injections of triamcinolone acetonide (IVTA) [41, 42] to treat proliferative diabetic retinopathy; intravitreal injections of antibodies against VEGF to treat diabetic oedema [43, 44]; and the use of antibodies against VEGF, growth factors and steroids to treat neovascularization [45]. All of these studies currently are under way, but no specific treatment recommendations have yet been made. Each of the investigating groups has emphasized the need for a more comprehensive evaluation in a multicenter randomized controlled clinical trial with longer follow-up before clinical guidelines can be developed.

8.5 Conclusions

Relatively recent improvements in the understanding of a need for tight glycaemic and blood pressure control have focused the treatment of DM into four main strategies, namely exercise, diet, surgery and pharmaceuticals. Each of these strategies plays an important role in reducing the incidence of blindness caused by diabetic retinopathy. However, this broad front of treatment options relies on excellent patient education for its success.

Patient knowledge of actual and target HbA1c values is needed for effective patient involvement in dia-

betes control. Better diabetes self-care understanding, self-efficacy and behaviors related to glycaemic control can be achieved through educational strategies that provide information to patients, thus motivating them to effectively manage their DM [46, 47]. Educational tools such as reminder cards, informational brochures, self-care assessments, lists of available diabetes services and daily recording sheets all enhance patient health literacy and compliance. Personal control over one's own health care has been shown to improve DM control among patients who were taught to self-monitor their blood glucose in France [48], Turkey [49] and the United States [50]. Clear and concise patient education material that is culturally competent is critical. In addition, all interdisciplinary team members providing care to the diabetic patient must give consistent and similar advice and information, which in turn means that there must be a coordination of educational materials and of the message given to the patient (Table 8.3).

This consistent, culturally sensitive, educational approach is particularly important for the elderly patient with diabetic retinopathy [51], as this condition is often just one of many 'geriatric diseases' that a patient might have. Other common conditions or diseases might include cataracts, arthritis, cancer, cardiac disease, pulmonary disease, incontinence, cognitive decline and sleep deprivation, to mention a few. Some of those diseases/conditions have a direct effect on the health of the eye, and must be considered when developing treatment plans for diabetic retinopathy (see Table 8.3). Today, the management and treatment of a single disease is no longer sufficient for elderly patients, who tend to become a 'treatment unit' rather than a particular disease. That said, the active management of diabetic retinopathy does need to be addressed because it has the potential to progress to visual disability and/or blindness. Visual loss has a major impact on quality of life of an older person because it contributes not only to morbidity but also to mortality [52, 19, 4, 53]. If the patient wishes to actively address the DM then the health care team should provide the educational materials that will assist in that goal. Yet, if the loss of sight is not a priority, then the team must also respect that decision. The interdisciplinary health care team, when developing educational interventions, must avoid two pitfalls that are particularly apropos to the geriatric diabetic patient:

Table 8.3 The importance of maintaining healthy eyes.

Medical conditions or diseases	Effect on healthy eyes
Poor glycaemic control	Fluctuation in visual acuity
	Distorted vision
	Cataracts
High blood pressure	Retinal arteriolar narrowing
	Blurred vision
	Glaucoma
Cardiovascular disease/stroke	Central retinal artery occlusions
	Central retinal vein occlusions
	Peripheral visual field loss
	Glaucoma
Peripheral vascular disease	Anterior ischemic optic neuropathy
	Central retinal artery occlusions
	Central retinal vein occlusions
	Retinal haemorrhaging
	Glaucoma
Atherosclerosis	Increased frequency and extent of retinal haemorrhages
	Increased microaneurysms and ischaemic areas
	Retinal venous occlusions
	Macular degeneration
	Poor blood flow
	Retinal oedema

- The team must not project an attitude of fear of vision loss, nor of defeatism, which might indicate a lack of faith in the patient's ability to manage diabetic retinopathy along with other coexisting conditions and diseases.

- The team must also provide support for the patient's health care priorities, which may or may not rate the prevention of diabetic retinopathy as highly as does the team. In other words, the team must not practice excessive interventionism that might be inappropriate to the patient's wishes.

Only through education and communication can the entire health care team – which includes not only the patient but also the family and the healthcare providers – make the appropriate decisions to treat the entire patient, and not just a single disease.

References

1. NIH www.nei.nih.gov/eyedata (last accessed 13 October 2007).
2. World Health Organization. http://www.who.int/mediacentre/factsheets/fs282/en/ (last accessed 25 November 2007).
3. Wild S, Roglic G, Green A, Sicree R and King H. (2004) Global prevalence of diabetes: estimates for the year 2000 and projections for 2030. *Diabetes Care* 27 (5): 1047–53.
4. Morello CM. (2007) Etiology and natural history of diabetic retinopathy: an overview. *Am J Health Syst Pharm*, 64 (17 Suppl. 12): S3–7.
5. Healthy People 2020. http://www.healthypeople.gov/ (last accessed 1 October 2007).
6. Cikamatana L, Mitchell P, Rochtchina E, Foran S and Wang JJ. (2007) Five-year incidence and progression of diabetic retinopathy in a defined older population: the Blue Mountains Eye Study. *Eye* 21 (4): 465–71.
7. Roy, MS. (2000) Diabetic retinopathy in African Americans with type 1 diabetes: The New Jersey 725: I. Methodology, population, frequency of retinopathy, and visual impairment. *Arch Ophthalmol* 118 (1): 97–104.
8. Harris MI, Hadden WC, Knowler WC and Bennett PH. (1987) Prevalence of diabetes and impaired glucose tolerance and plasma glucose levels in U.S. population aged 20-74 yr. *Diabetes* 36 (4): 524–34.
9. Roy MS and Affouf M. (2006) Six-year progression of retinopathy and associated risk factors in African American patients with type 1 diabetes mellitus: the New Jersey 725. *Arch Ophthalmol*, 124 (9): 1297–306.

10. Varma R, Torres M, Pena F, Klein R and Azen SP. (2004) Prevalence of diabetic retinopathy in adult Latinos: the Los Angeles Latino eye study. *Ophthalmology* 111 (7): 1298–306.

11. Bloomgarden ZT. (2007) Screening for and managing diabetic retinopathy: current approaches. *Am J Health Syst Pharm.* 64 (12 Suppl. 12): S8–14.

12. Klein R, Klein BE, Moss SE and Cruickshanks KJ. (1998) The Wisconsin Epidemiologic Study of Diabetic Retinopathy: XVII. The 14-year incidence and progression of diabetic retinopathy and associated risk factors in type I diabetes. *Ophthalmology* 105 (10): 1801–15.

13. Anderson D, Horton C and O'Toole M. (2007) Integrating depression care with diabetes care in real-world settings: Lessons from the Robert Wood Johnson Foundation Diabetes Initiative. *Diabetes Spectrum* 20: 10–16.

14. Roy MS, Roy A and Affouf M. (2007) Depression is a risk factor for poor glycemic control and retinopathy in African-Americans with type 1 diabetes. *Psychosom Med* 69 (6): 537–42.

15. Rodin G, Olmsted MP, Rydall AC, Maharaj SI, Colton PA, Jones JM, Biancucci LA and Daneman D. (2002) Eating disorders in young women with type 1 diabetes mellitus. *J Psychosom Res* 53 (4): 943–9.

16. Steinhart JR, Sugarman JR and Connell FA. (1997) Gestational diabetes is a herald of NIDDM in Navajo women. High rate of abnormal glucose tolerance after GDM. *Diabetes Care* 20 (6): 943–7.

17. Mitchell P, Smith W, Wang JJ and Attebo K. (1998) Prevalence of diabetic retinopathy in an older community. The Blue Mountain Study. *Ophthalmology* 105 (3): 406–11.

18. Juutilainen A, Lehto S, Ronnemaa T, Pyorala K and Laakso M. (2007) Retinopathy predicts cardiovascular mortality in type 2 diabetic men and women. *Diabetes Care* 30 (2): 292–9.

19. Lovestam-Adrian M, Hansson-Lundblad C and Torffvit O. (2007) Sight-threatening retinopathy is associated with lower mortality in type 2 diabetic subjects: a 10-year observation study. *Diabetes Res Clin Pract.* 77 (1): 141–7.

20. Suto C, Hori S, Kato S, Muraoka K and Kitano S. (2006) Effect of perioperative glycemic control in progression of diabetic retinopathy and maculopathy. *Arch Ophthalmol* 124 (1): 38–45.

21. The American Diabetes Association's Clinical Practice Guidelines (http://diabetes.org/for-health-professionals-and-scientists/cpr.jsp (last accessed 27 October 2007).

22. Onofrey BE, Skorin L, Jr and Holdeman NR. (eds) (2005) *Ocular Therapeutics Handbook - A Clinical Manual*, 2nd edition. Lippincott Williams and Wilkins, Philadelphia.

23. Klein BE, Klein R and Lee KE. (1998) Diabetes, cardiovascular disease, selected cardiovascular disease risk factors, and the 5-year incidence of age-related cataract and progression of lens opacities: the Beaver Dam Eye Study. *Am J Ophthalmol* 126 (6): 782–90.

24. Nakamura M, Kanamori A and Negi A. (2005) Diabetes mellitus as a risk factor for glaucomatous optic neuropathy. *Ophthalmologica* 219 (1): 1–10.

25. Fong DS, Ferris FL, III, Davis MD and Chew EY. (1999) Causes of severe visual loss in the early treatment diabetic retinopathy study: ETDRS Report no. 24. Early Treatment Diabetic Retinopathy Study Research Group. *Am J Ophthalmol* 127 (2): 137–41.

26. Fong DS, Sharza M, Chen W, Paschal JF, Ariyasu RG and Lee PP. (2002) Vision loss among diabetics in a group model health maintenance organization (HMO). *Am J Ophthalmol* 133 (2): 236–41.

27. Cundiff DK and Nigg CR. (2005) Diet and diabetic retinopathy: insights from the Diabetes Control and Complications Trial (DCCT). *MedGenMed* 7 (1): 3.

28. Hansson-Lundblad C, Agardh E and Agardh CD. (1997) Retinal examination internals in diabetic patients on diet treatment only. *Acta Ophthalmol Scand* 75 (3): 244–8.

29. The American Diabetes Association. (2004) Nutrition recommendations and principles for people with diabetes mellitus. *Diabetes Care* 23 (Suppl. 2): S43–6.

30. Koura MR, Khairy AE, Abdel-Aal NM, Mohamed HF, Amin GA and Sabra AY. (2001) The role of primary health care in patient education for diabetes control. *Egypt Public Health Assoc* 76 (3-4): 241–64.

31. Heller T, Maisios M and Shahar D. (2007) Physicians' and nurses' knowledge and attitude towards nutritional therapy in diabetes. *Harefuah*, 146 (9): 670–4.

32. Franz MJ. (1997) Lifestyle modifications for diabetes management. *Endocrinol Metab Clin North Am* 26 (3): 499–510.

33. Ryan, AS. (2000) Insulin resistance with aging: effects of diet and exercise. *Sports Med* 30 (5): 327–46.

34. Tsang T, Orr R, Lam P, Comino EJ and Singh MF. (2007) Health benefits of Tai Chi for older patients with type 2 diabetes: the "Move It For Diabetes study" – a randomized controlled trial. *Clin Interv Aging* 2 (3): 429–39.

35. Fong DS, Strauber SF, Aiello LP, Beck RW, Callanan DG, Danis RP, David MD, Feman SS, Ferris F, Friedman SM, Garcia CA, Glassman AR, Han DP, Le D, Kollman C, Lauer AK, Recchia FM and Solomon SD. (2007) Writing Committee for the Diabetic Retinopathy Clinical Research Network. *Arch Ophthalmol* 125 (4): 469–80.

36. Lovestam-Adrian M, Agardh CD, Torffvit O and Agardh E. (2003) Type 1 diabetes patients with severe non-proliferative retinopathy may benefit from

panretinal photocoagulation. *Acta Ophthalmol Scand* 81 (3): 221–5.

37. Luttrull JK, Musch DC and Spink CA. (2007) Subthreshold diode micropulse panretinal photocoagulation for proliferative diabetic retinopathy. *Eye*, 22 (5), 607–12.

38. Mohamed Q, Gillies MC and Wong TY. (2007) Management of diabetic retinopathy: a systematic review. *JAMA* 298 (8): 902–16.

39. Yam JC and Kwok AK. (2007) Update on the treatment of diabetic retinopathy. *Hong Kong Med J* 13 (1): 46–60.

40. Ryan GJ. (2007) New pharmacologic approaches to treating diabetic retinopathy. *Am J Health Syst Pharm* 64 (17 Suppl. 12): S15–21.

41. Choi KS, Chung JK and Lin SH. (2007) Laser photocoagulation combined with intravitreal triamcinolone acetonide injection in proliferative diabetic retinopathy with macular edema. *Korean J Ophthalmol* 21 (1): 11–17.

42. Zein WM, Noureddin BN, Jurdi FA, Schakal A and Bashshur ZF. (2006) Panretinal photocoagulation and intravitreal triamcinolone acetonide for the management of proliferative diabetic retinopathy with macular edema. *Retina* 26 (2): 137–42.

43. Arevalo JF, Fromow-Guerra J, Quiroz-Mercado H, Sanchez JG, Wu L, Maia M, Berrocal MH, Solis-Vivanco A, Farah ME and the Pan-American Collaborative Retina Study Group. (2007) Primary intravitreal bevacizumab (Avastin) for diabetic macular edema: results from the Pan-American Collaborative Retina Study Group at 6-month follow-up. *Ophthalmology* 114 (4): 743–50.

44. Haritoglou C, Kook D, Neubauer A, Wold A, Prigliner S, Strauss R, Gandorfer A, Ulbig M and Kampik A. (2006) Intravitreal bevacizumab (Avastin) therapy for persistent diffuse diabetic macular edema. *Retina* 26 (9): 999–1005.

45. Emerson MV and Lauer AK. (2007) Emerging therapies for the treatment of neovascular age-related macular degeneration and diabetic macular edema. *BioDrugs* 21 (4): 245–57.

46. Heisler M, Smith DM, Hayward RA, Krein SL and Kerr EA. (2003) How well do patients' assessments of their diabetes self-management correlate with actual glycemic control and receipt of recommended diabetes services? *Diabetes Care* 26 (3): 738–43.

47. Heisler M, Piette JD, Spencer M, Kieffer E and Vijan S. (2005) The relationship between knowledge of recent HbA1c values and diabetes care understanding and self-management. *Diabetes Care* 28 (4): 816–22.

48. Guerci B, Drouin P, Grange V, Bougneres P, Fontaine P, Kerlan V, Passa P, Thivolet CH, Vialettes B and Charbonnel B, for the ASIA Group. (2003) Self-monitoring of blood glucose significantly improves metabolic control in patients with type 2 diabetes mellitus: the Auto-Surveillance Intervention Active (ASIA) study. *Diabetes Metabol* 29 (6): 587–94.

49. Ozmen B and Boyvada S. (2003) The relationship between self-monitoring of blood glucose control and glycosylated haemoglobin in patients with type 2 diabetes with and without diabetic retinopathy. *J Diabetes Complications* 17 (3): 128–34.

50. Murata GH, Shah JH, Hoffman RM, Wendel CS, Adam KD, Solvas PA, Bokhari SU and Duckworth WC. (2003) Intensified blood glucose monitoring improves glycemic control in stable, insulin-treated veterans with type 2 diabetes: the Diabetes Outcomes in Veterans Study (DOVES). *Diabetes Care* 26 (6): 1759–63.

51. Massin P and Kaloustian E. (2007) The elderly diabetic's eyes. *Diabetes Metab* 33 (Suppl. 1): S4–9.

52. Hirari FE, Moss SE, Klein BE and Klein R. (2008) Relationship of glycemic control, exogenous insulin, and C-peptide levels to ischemic heart disease mortality over a 16-year period in persons with older-onset diabetes: The Wisconsin Epidemiologic Study of Diabetic Retinopathy (WESDR). *Diabetes Care*, 31 (3), 493–7.

53. West SK, Munoz B, Istre J, Rubin GS, Friedman SM, Fried LP, Bandeen-Roche K and Schein OD. (2000) Mixed lens opacities and subsequent mortality. *Arch Ophthalmol* 118 (3): 393–7.

9

The Diabetic Foot

Andrew J. M. Boulton[1] and Matthew J. Young[2]
[1]*Manchester Royal Infirmary, Manchester, UK*
[2]*Edinburgh Royal Infirmary, Edinburgh, UK*

Key messages

- All patients with diabetes should be screened annually for risk of foot ulceration; those with significant risk factors require more frequent review and education in self-foot care.
- Neuropathic foot ulcers under pressure areas will heal if the ulcer is adequately off-loaded; this is frequently neglected in clinical practice.
- Most diabetic foot ulcers will heal if the arterial inflow is sufficient, any infection is treated aggressively, and the pressure is removed from the ulcer area.
- Any patient presenting with a unilateral, warm swollen foot in the presence of neuropathy should be assumed to have an acute Charcot joint, until proven otherwise.

9.1 Introduction

The St Vincent timescale [1] to reduce the number of amputations for diabetes in Europe by 50% within 3 years seems a dim and distant memory to those who work with the diabetic foot. The publication of BDA (=RCP) guidelines in England and Wales, and SIGN guidelines in Scotland, have demonstrated that there is still a lack of good evidence-based randomized controlled trials on which to base diabetic foot care [2, 3]. More recently, the National Institute of Clinical

Excellence (NICE) has published guidelines of foot care for patients with type 2 diabetes [4]. However, evidence is at last beginning to appear that structured diabetic foot care, when performed in a multidisciplinary team, does eventually result in significant improvements in amputation rates among people with diabetes [5].

Foot problems in diabetes can develop from a number of component causes. The main contributing factors include sensorimotor and autonomic neuropathy, peripheral vascular disease (PVD), limited joint mobility and high foot pressures. The existence of other long-term complications of diabetes (particularly end-stage renal disease as a consequence of nephropathy) also influence the development of foot ulceration. Clearly, general practitioners, geriatricians and diabetologists must all pay particular attention to the feet of older patients to prevent significant avoidable morbidity and mortality in this vulnerable group.

Lower-limb amputation is more common in older, usually type 2, diabetic patients [6]; indeed, the average age of diabetic foot clinic attendees is over 60 years, which clearly shows that the elderly are at particular risk of foot ulceration. Reduced mobility (particularly at the hip) in patients aged over 60 impairs their ability to inspect the feet, and leads to the continued progression of foot lesions that are often beyond the point of repair even before they are discovered [7]. Very often, patients with severely impaired vision depend on other people to inspect their feet, but when this is not

Diabetes in Old Age. Third Edition. Edited by Alan J. Sinclair
© 2009 John Wiley & Sons, Ltd

possible it may be very difficult for the patient to ensure that their foot care is adequate.

Diabetes alone probably does not add to the prevalence of bunions, clawed toes and medial arterial calcification that is seen in the elderly [8, 9]. Neuropathy, however, is more prevalent in the elderly, and increases with both age and the duration of diabetes. Once this is superimposed on the normal aging process, then skeletal abnormalities (including spontaneous fractures) become significantly more common [9]. If the increased prevalence of PVD in older type 2 diabetic patients is added to the increase in neuropathy then, together with difficulties in personal foot care, this fully explains the particular predilection for foot problems that exists in older diabetic patients. The demographic changes, increasing numbers of elderly people, the increasing proportion of those who live alone, and increasing levels of obesity – all of which are currently occurring within the United Kingdom – will only serve to add to the already substantial numbers of type 2 diabetic patients who develop foot ulceration and peripheral ischaemia. The challenge, therefore, is to reduce this excess burden of risk to a minimum by accurate detection and the amelioration of risk.

9.2   Peripheral sensorimotor neuropathy

Peripheral sensorimotor neuropathy is a major contributory cause in 80% of diabetic foot ulceration [10]. The incidence of diabetic peripheral sensorimotor neuropathy increases with the duration of diabetes; however, as the prevalence depends on the diagnostic criteria used, the prevalence rates reported from different epidemiological studies will vary considerably [11]. A large UK multicentre study which screened a large hospital-treated diabetic population found that the overall prevalence of neuropathy was 28.5% [12], with more than half of all patients with type 2 diabetes, and aged over 60 years, being found to have neuropathy. Therefore, the majority of the elderly population with diabetes is at an increased risk of foot ulceration.

The most common symptoms of sensory neuropathy are numbness, lancinating pain, 'pins and needles', burning pain and hyperaesthesiae, typically with nocturnal exacerbation. The clinical signs are usually sensory loss in a glove-and-stocking distribution (see Figure 9.1). Whilst loss of pain, fine touch and temperature sensation are related to small (often unmyelinated) fibre involvement, a loss of vibration perception and proprioception is believed to be related to large (usually myelinated) fibre damage. Painful symptoms are found in approximately 11% of all diabetic patients, and can be particularly distressing.

The therapies for painful diabetic neuropathy vary from non-pharmacological interventions such as transcutaneous nerve stimulation or complementary therapies to drugs with potentially major side effects. In each case there is often a clear placebo effect, and it is often better to start with low doses and build up to an effective dose of any drug therapy. None of the non-analgesic pharmacological agents, tricyclics or anti-arrhythmics is currently licensed for this use, and the use of such agents should therefore be explained to the patient, in detail, including their often significant side-effect profiles, prior to their use. Particular care with these agents is needed in the elderly population, in view of their frequent adverse side effects [13]. The most commonly used drugs are tricyclic antidepressants and anti-epileptics, such as gabapentin and pregabalin. Both, gabapentin and pregabalin are licensed for the treatment of painful neuropathy on the basis of promising clinical trials: similarly, the dual reuptake inhibitor duloxetine, also has demonstrated proven efficacy in large, randomized controlled trials. Although such therapies are useful, like all adjuvant analgesics they require careful titration in order to minimize the side effects [11, 13]. Capsaicin 0.075% cream has been licensed for the treatment of post-herpetic neuralgia for many years, and more recently was licensed for the treatment of painful peripheral neuropathy. In addition to monotherapy, it can also be safely added to any existing, partially effective oral agent. Unfortunately, its usefulness is often limited by a poor understanding of the need to use it little and often, and to persevere beyond the initial first week or two, during which time it may even make the symptoms a little worse [14].

It must be remembered that in some patients the presenting feature of peripheral neuropathy, and indeed of diabetes itself, may be *foot ulceration*, as the progression to an insensitive foot may occur without any positive symptoms. It is not uncommon for neuropathic diabetic patients to present because of the smell caused by purulent discharge. Thus, the absence of symptoms must never be equated with an absence of risk of ulceration.

The diagnosis of diabetic peripheral neuropathy for clinical purposes is a complex issue [11, 15]. The diagnosis of the 'at-risk' neuropathic foot during routine screening at the annual review requires

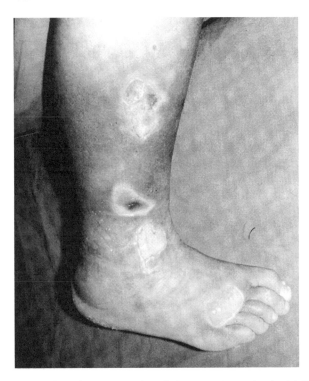

Figure 9.1 Extensive burns on the leg of a neuropathic diabetic patient who had fallen asleep in front of the gas fire, to be woken by the smell of burning.

a less-sophisticated clinical examination than the differential diagnosis of diabetic peripheral neuropathy in secondary care, which often demands a more detailed investigation. For routine screening purposes, clinical examination using 10 g monofilaments and, for example, a 128 Hz tuning fork will suffice. The requirements for the comprehensive diabetic foot examination to identify the high-risk foot were the subject of a recent task force of the American Diabetes Association [16]. The vibration perception threshold (VPT) can be measured quantitatively using a Neurothesiometer (Arnold Horwell, UK). Such measurements have shown to be increased in association with other measurements of diabetic peripheral neuropathy, but also increase with normal aging; therefore the use of age-related normal values have been recommended. Other authors have claimed that the increased coefficient of variation in older patients makes the measurement of vibration perception threshold unreliable, and that it should be supplemented by other tests of neuropathy [17]. For screening purposes, however, this may not be necessary. A VPT >25 V has been shown in cross-sectional and prospective studies to be strongly

predictive of subsequent foot ulceration [18]. In the latter study, patients with a VPT >25 V were sevenfold more likely to develop a foot ulcer than a patient with a VPT <25 V over a 4-year period. This increased to 11-fold when recurrent ulceration was considered, as no patient with a VPT <25 V developed a second ulcer. This study also revealed a relationship between foot ulceration and increasing age although, even after correcting for this, the VPT remained a strong predictor of foot ulceration risk.

Monofilaments represent a quick method for assessing the at-risk foot in diabetes, and currently are used extensively in the United Kingdom. There is some doubt as to the reliability of manufacture of monofilaments, and widely varying rates of ulcer incidence have been reported in studies that have used monofilaments as a screening tool [19]. In general a 10 g monofilament should be used in a variety of sites on the foot, with a clearly defined pass/fail criterion. Monofilament remain relatively cheap to buy and easy to use, and therefore are very popular with many foot clinics [16].

Diabetologists. however, still tend to diagnose peripheral neuropathy on clinical grounds, and this approach can be improved by use of a neuropathy disability score (NDS) [12]. The NDS is derived from an examination of the ankle reflex vibration sensation, using a 128 Hz tuning fork, a pin-prick sensation and temperature (with a cold tuning fork) sensation at the great toe. Each sensory modality is scored as either normal = 0 or reduced = absent = 1 for each side, and the ankle reflexes as normal = 0, present with reinforcement = 1 or absent = 2 per side. Thus, while the total maximum abnormal score is 10, a score ≥ 6 can be regarded as indicative of significant peripheral neuropathy. Such a score correlates well with the VPT measurements which, as described above, predict foot ulceration in diabetic patients. The NDS was confirmed as being the best predictor for the risk of foot ulceration in a large prospective community study conducted in the UK [20]. If a Neurothesiometer is available, then a VPT >25 V in both feet will predict that up to 84% of such patients will develop foot ulceration over the next four years [18].

Motor fibre loss is another significant result of peripheral neuropathy leading to small muscle atrophy in the foot. As a consequence, there is an imbalance between flexor and extensor muscle function that results in clawing of the toes, prominent metatarsal heads and anterior displacement of the metatarsal footpads (Figure 9.2). Abnormally high foot pressures usually develop under these areas and, as discussed below, can lead to foot ulceration in the susceptible foot.

In addition, the gait pattern is significantly altered in patients with diabetic neuropathy [21]; this may alter the foot pressure distribution and make the foot more prone to the effects of high pressure. Gait problems, with increasing falls, and the risks of injury to the feet, are increased in neuropathic diabetic patients. Such problems are more pronounced in elderly neuropathic patients, and even worse in those with visual handicap, increasing the risk of foot ulceration.

9.3 Autonomic neuropathy

Autonomic neuropathy results in a wide spectrum of problems in the cardiovascular, gastrointestinal and genitourinary systems, and is known to be associated with the development of foot ulceration in diabetic patients [22]. In the foot, denervation of the sweat glands leads to dry, atrophic skin and callus formation. Severe cracking of the skin often occurs under these circumstances, and facilitates microbial infections. The regular use of emollient creams or ointments, often

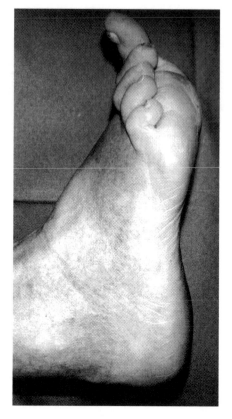

Figure 9.2 At-risk foot, showing prominent metatarsal heads and clawed toes.

twice a day, is required to keep the skin supple and reduce the risk of such fissures.

A loss of sympathetic tone in small vessels also leads to a reduced resistance and increased arteriovenous shunting. The venous PO_2 and pressure is raised in the neuropathic limb to a level approaching that of arterial blood, and has been measured at higher levels than in the endoneurium [23]. Thus, in a diabetic patient with autonomic neuropathy, but without coexisting vascular disease, the blood flow is increased at rest and the distended dorsal foot veins can be seen. Initially, the overall increase in blood flow increases capillary pressure; however, over time this leads to microvascular sclerosis and, when taken in conjunction with the increased shunting in the diabetic neuropathic foot, it may lead to inadequate nutritional flow and subsequent tissue ischaemia, greatly increasing the risk of ulceration [24]. The coexistence of autonomic neuropathy and macrovascular disease may cause a further deterioration in the level of tissue oxygenation.

9.4 Peripheral vascular disease

Both, the micro- and macrocirculation in the lower extremities are affected by diabetes. In the microcirculation, the skin capillary pressure is increased in patients with type 1 diabetes (of either recent onset or of long duration), and this abnormality reverses when the diabetes control is improved [25]. This increase in the capillary pressure is most likely responsible for the loss of the blood flow autoregulation, increased arteriovenous shunting, impaired hyperaemic response, changes in capillary blood flow and basement membrane thickening seen in diabetic patients. This microvascular sclerosis may contribute to nephropathy, retinopathy and probably also neuropathy, but the direct role in the development of foot ulceration remains unclear.

Macrovascular disease is more common in diabetic patients. Peripheral vascular disease is estimated to occur at least twice as commonly in diabetic than in non-diabetic patients [26]. Lipid disorders, platelet dysfunction, increased coagulation and endothelial cell dysfunction have been implicated in the pathogenesis of the atherosclerosis. Peripheral vascular disease usually has the same clinical presentation as that seen in non-diabetic patients, with intermittent claudication, rest pain, ulceration and gangrene being the main clinical features [26]. However, the symptoms may be masked by coexisting peripheral neuropathy, and significant ischaemia may develop in the absence of pain.

Although the femoropopliteal segments are most often affected, small vessels below the knee, such as the tibial and peroneal arteries, are more severely affected in diabetic than in non-diabetic patients [27]. This means, overall, that vascular disease in diabetic patients is more likely to lead to amputation even though, level for level, the outcome of revascularization is similar to that in the non-diabetic population. In addition, the presence of simultaneous cardiac and cerebrovascular disease means that the long-term survival after such procedures is often shorter. Medial arterial calcification is another common finding in diabetic patients, and can be recognized on X-ray films by its 'pipe-stem' appearance. Medial arterial calcification is reported to be associated with diabetic peripheral somatosensory and autonomic neuropathy.

Previous studies of the quantitative distribution of medial arterial calcification within the diabetic foot have shown the condition to be significantly associated with an increased prevalence of cardiovascular mortality [28], although this may also be related to the increase in medial arterial calcification associated with diabetic nephropathy, which is an independent marker of increased mortality in diabetes [29]. Diabetes alone does not increase the prevalence of medial arterial calcification in matched groups of controls and non-neuropathic subjects, although there is significantly heavier arterial calcification in the feet of neuropathic diabetic patients [9]. The VPT, duration of diabetes and serum creatinine are all independent predictors of the degree of medial arterial calcification which, when present, is known to alter the pulse waveform and falsely elevate ankle pressures in diabetic patients [30]. Therefore, it has been suggested that toe systolic pressure measurements might replace ankle pressure measurements as an index of arterial inflow to the diabetic foot, as the ankle pressure index (measured with Doppler ultrasound) may be misleadingly high despite the presence of occlusive PVD. If the ankle systolic pressure is more than 75 mmHg above the brachial systolic pressure, then this is highly indicative of medial arterial calcification and the poor reliability of the ankle pressure to indicate lower extremity arterial disease [31]. Since it is also possible that medial arterial calcification will falsely elevate the ankle pressure into the normal range in some neuropathic patients, a normal ankle pressure should be interpreted with caution, and perhaps be complemented with plain radiography of the foot, particularly in elderly and neuropathic diabetic patients. A low ankle pressure, together with an ankle pressure index <0.9, suggests the presence of arterial occlusive disease and the need for further investigation [31]. However, despite all of the problems associated with ankle pressure measurements, foot pulses remain the best clinical guide to the presence of PVD in diabetes. Nonetheless, the American Diabetes Association has recommended that all diabetic patients aged >50 years should undergo an annual ankle brachial index check [32]. Diabetic patients with neuropathy may have significant ischaemia with no pain because of the loss of pain sensation. The absence of foot pulses indicates the presence of vascular disease, even if the popliteal pulse is present and there is no complaint of claudication or rest pain. Any areas of cyanosis or peripheral necrosis are also indicative of arterial insufficiency.

Diabetic patients with evidence of PVD should be referred for vascular assessment with arterial reconstruction or angioplasty where appropriate [26]. The best advice for any stable claudicant with no evidence of tissue loss is to 'stop smoking and keep walking'. Indeed, there is considerable evidence that, in order to be effective, the patient should walk to the point of claudicating, and even for some distance with claudication. It is believed that this might encourage the proliferation of collateral circulation [33].

Although the long-term benefits of reconstructive surgery for diabetic patients with claudication remain the subject of dispute among vascular surgeons, this approach should be considered if the walking distance is reduced, even before the onset of tissue loss. A reducing claudication distance is a sign of impending critical ischaemia in diabetic patients, who have a greater tendency towards an early and more aggressive progression of arterial disease. Most vascular teams will not consider patients with stable claudication for surgery, and will generally wait for the development of critical limb ischaemia prior to intervention. However, diabetic patients also have a higher amputation rate than non-diabetic patients for similar initial grades of arterial disease [34]. With such clear evidence that tissue loss has a significantly adverse effect on limb prognosis, surgery before the onset of critical ischaemia has its advocates in many centres, and should be encouraged.

As an additional consideration, peripheral autonomic neuropathy is usually present in patients with foot ulceration; the patients can therefore be said to have performed *auto-sympathectomy*. Surgical sympathectomy is still occasionally attempted in a number of diabetic patients but, because of the pre-existing peripheral autonomic changes and associated medial arterial calcification, it is unlikely to produce any substantial benefit.

9.5   Limited joint mobility

Diffuse collagen abnormalities are common in diabetic patients [35]. The main pathogenic mechanism for these abnormalities is a glycation of collagen, which results in the thickening and increased crosslinking of collagen bundles [36]. One of the clinical manifestations of this change is a thick, tight and waxy skin, leading to a restriction of joint movements. Patients with such limited joint mobility are unable to oppose the palms of their hands (the 'prayer sign'; see Figure 9.3). The term 'cheiroarthropathy' has been used to describe this condition, although as other joints – including those in the shoulder, hip and foot – can also be affected a more appropriate term is 'limited joint mobility', and this is now in general use [37, 38]. Limited joint mobility in the foot mainly involves the subtalar joint, which provides the foot with

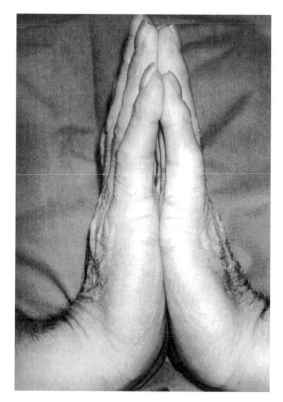

Figure 9.3   The 'prayer sign'.

shock-absorbing capacity during walking [39]. This results in increased plantar foot pressures and, in the neuropathic foot, may be a contributory factor to the development of foot ulceration [40]. Limited extension of the great toe, known as 'hallux rigidus', can also predispose to ulceration by limiting the adaptive extension of the toe during the final 'toe-off' phase of walking, thus increasing the vertical and shear forces on the toe.

9.6   Foot pressure abnormalities

The two main factors responsible for the development of high foot pressures, motor neuropathy and limited joint mobility, have already been discussed. *Callus formation*, which itself is a result of high foot pressures and dry skin, may also act as a foreign body and result in further increases of these pressures [41]. In contrast, the patient's age and bodyweight do not significantly influence the foot pressure, most likely because the foot contact surface area also increases with weight [42, 43].

Intermittent moderate stress on healthy tissue for an excessive time – as in the case of abnormal pressures applied on the plantar surface of the foot during excessive walking – can lead to tissue inflammation and, finally, to ulceration. At the microscopic level, it is believed that pressure overcomes the nutritive capillary blood flow of the skin, and this leads to a localized tissue necrosis and breakdown [44]. The demonstration of increased arteriovenous shunting in the diabetic foot, and the reports of an impaired hyperaemic injury response in neuropathic patients [45, 46] may also contribute to the increased risk of ulceration. Studies in dogs have shown that repetitive moderate trauma leads to the eventual breakdown of the skin and ulceration [44]. Thermography of the feet of patients with diabetic neuropathy has shown hot spots of inflammation in areas of high foot pressures and repetitive trauma [47]. Sensory dysfunction is crucial for the development of neuropathic ulceration. In a non-neuropathic subject, the pain which accompanies the inflammation will usually force the individual to rest the foot before it progresses to ulceration, whereas a patient with a loss of pain awareness will continue to walk long after an ulcer has developed. Therefore, high foot pressures alone, in the absence of sensory neuropathy, do not result in foot ulceration. This can be illustrated in patients with rheumatoid arthritis, in whom joint involvement in the feet results in high foot pressures comparable to those found in diabetic patients, but not in ulceration [48].

The measurement of foot pressures is not routine in most clinics. A careful visual inspection, with palpation of the foot, can detect most high-pressure areas, and accommodative insoles can therefore be made to redistribute pressure away from vulnerable areas, without the need for expensive foot pressure measuring systems. A simple foot pressure map, the Podotrack or PressureStat, has been shown to be accurate when compared to complex optical foot pressure systems, and may also be used in patient education as the high-pressure areas are a dark grey or black colour, which emphasize to the patient which particular areas under the foot are at greatest risk [49].

9.7 Other risk factors

9.7.1 History of previous foot problems

A history of previous foot problems in a diabetic patient strongly suggests that they are at high risk for future problems, especially lower-limb amputation.

Studies of patients with traumatic or diabetic amputations have shown that amputation alone does not cause an increase in the loads under the remaining foot. However, in a neuropathic diabetic patient amputation is associated with high pressure under the remaining foot, probably related to neuropathy and limited joint mobility in that foot [50].

In a prospective study of the prediction of foot ulceration using VPTs, recurrent ulceration was common, affecting over 50% of the patients. In addition, in an audit of dressing policy at the Manchester Foot Hospital, the median number of ulcers per patient was two (range 1 to 12) [51]), again suggesting that over half the patients re-ulcerated despite preventive care and advice. The likely causes for this are unknown, but it appears that those patients who do not wear their recommended shoes (which are usually supplied), or do not follow the appropriate advice, are those who subsequently re-ulcerate. Strategies to increase footwear acceptability and compliance can reduce re-ulceration rates.

9.7.2 Reduced resistance to infection

There are many reasons for impaired resistance to infection in a diabetic ulcer. Diabetes is associated with impaired neutrophil function, particularly in the presence of a high blood glucose, and both macrocirculatory and microcirculatory abnormalities lead to relative hypoxia in the wound [52]. Multiple microbes (often a mixture of aerobic and anaerobic bacteria) are usually found in cultures from foot ulcers. The most common pathogenic organisms in diabetic foot ulcers are *Staphylococcus* and *Streptococcus* sp.; the streptococci are often faecal in origin. The clinical relevance of organisms grown from superficial swabs is variable, as other organisms may colonize the wound surface and the quality of the sample and method of transport and culture may markedly influence the reliability of the result [53]. The treatment of infections associated with foot ulceration is detailed further in the management of foot ulceration (see below).

9.7.3 Smoking and alcohol

Smoking is known to be associated with foot ulceration, probably by increasing the prevalence of vascular disease [54]. Recurrent neuropathic foot ulceration has been reported as being more common in patients with high alcohol consumption [55].

9.7.4   Other complications of diabetes

Foot pressures in patients with nephropathy are higher than in diabetic patients without renal impairment. In combination with neuropathy, which is also more common in such patients, this imposes a serious risk for foot ulceration [56].

9.8   The classification of ulceration

The most widely used and validated foot ulcer classification systems are the Wagner [57], the University of Texas (UT) [58, 59] and the PEDIS [60] systems.

The best known system – the Wagner – labels patients with risk factors but no ulcer 'grade 0', the 'at-risk' foot. The classification divides foot ulcers into five categories.

- Grade 1 are superficial ulcers limited to the dermis.

- Grade 2 are transdermal ulcers with exposed tendon or bone, without osteomyelitis or abscess.

- Grade 3 are deep ulcers with osteomyelitis or abscess formation.

- Grade 4 is applied to the feet, with localized gangrene confined to the toes or forefoot.

- Grade 5 applies to feet with extensive gangrene.

The UT system uses the Wagner grades 1 to 3, but to each adds a stage: A = no infection or ischaemia; B = infection, no ischaemia; C = ischaemia no infection; and D = both infection and ischaemia.

A significant problem with the Wagner classification is that it does not differentiate between those grade 1–3 ulcers which are associated with arterial insufficiency. Such ulcers might be expected to heal less well. Neither does it differentiate those grade 1 and 4 ulcers which are significantly infected, and which might also be expected to have a poorer prognosis. Despite this, the Wagner classification has been shown to provide an accurate guide to the risk of amputation in a number of studies, and remains the standard by which other classifications have to be judged. The most successful recent system is the UT, which uses depth and ischaemia as its main classification criteria, and therefore is able to predict the progression from ulceration to amputation with some accuracy [58]. In a comparative study, the Texas system demonstrated some advantages over the Wagner, although both were good predictors of outcome [59].

There are, however, a number of classification systems currently in use at different centres, and with such a variety available it is clear that no one scheme can offer an ideal compromise between comprehensive applicability and simplicity. The reviewers of classification systems usually require each system to include their own particular facet. For example, when the UT system was reviewed by Levin [61], he noted that the site of ulceration was missing, despite the fact that this has been shown to be an uncertain predictor of outcome. A good classification system would seem to require some allowance for patient factors and the inclusion of a deformity index, particularly in relation to ulceration in association with Charcot feet (see Section 9.14). At present, most of the current classifications force the user to become totally foot-centred at the expense of the patient as a whole. Whilst this is not likely to create problems in multidisciplinary practice, it is a possible cause of fragmented care where the foot clinic is separate from diabetology and other support. Addressing the social and diabetes factors of patients is likely to improve foot ulcer outcomes [6], and this is particularly true of the elderly living alone.

9.9   The At-risk foot

The mainstay of risk reduction must lie with foot care education and the amelioration of other risk factors, if present (see Table 9.1). Footcare education should be concise and repeated regularly in order to have the maximum effect on patient behaviour [62]. Video presentations have been shown to be effective at imparting knowledge about foot care [63], but should not supplant one-to-one or small-group education. The main aspects of foot care education include the need for regular, at least once-daily, inspection of the feet for new lesions, and the need to have shoes measured each time they are acquired. These are two aspects which appear, from experience, to be regularly overlooked in the majority of patients with ulcers. Although education is the potential saviour of the diabetic foot, there is a considerable body of evidence to suggest that whilst knowledge about diabetic foot problems may increase, attitudes to – and compliance with – the necessary care may remain unchanged [64].

The limitations of current education and preventive methods are highlighted by the number of patients who have recurrent ulceration, even in specialist clinics

Table 9.1 At-risk groups for diabetic foot ulceration.

Patients with:

- a history of previous ulceration
- peripheral neuropathy
- peripheral vascular disease
- limited joint mobility
- bony deformities
- diabetic nephropathy (especially on dialysis)
- visual impairment
- a history of alcohol excess
- patients who live alone
- elderly patients

Table 9.2 General principles of foot care education.

1. Target the level of information to the needs of the patient. Those not at risk may require only general advice about foot hygiene and shoes.

2. Assess the ability of the patient to understand and perform the necessary components of footcare. If this is limited, then the spouse or carer should be involved at the beginning of the process.

3. Suggest a positive approach to foot care with 'dos' rather than 'don'ts' as the principle of active rather than passive foot care is more likely to be successful and acceptable to the patient:
   - Inspect the feet daily
   - Report any problems immediately
   - Have your feet measured every time new shoes are brought
   - Buy shoes with a square toe box and laces
   - Inspect the inside of shoes for foreign objects every day before putting them on
   - Attend a fully trained podiatrist regularly
   - Cut your nails straight across, and not 'rounded'
   - Keep your feet away from heat (fires, radiators and hot water bottles) and check the bathwater before stepping into it
   - Always wear something on your feet to protect them and never walk barefoot

4. Repeat the advice at regular intervals and check that it is being followed.

5. Disseminate advice to other family members and other health care professionals involved in the care of the patient.

(see Table 9.2). The lack of perceived vulnerability in neuropathic patients has been highlighted as one reason for this [65, 66]. Until this point is addressed effectively, education programmes may be limited in their success.

Hospital shoes are the second line of risk reduction for those patients with deformity which increases foot ulcer risk. The attendance of a dedicated orthotist as part of the diabetic foot care team can significantly improve shoe acceptability and compliance among patients, and reduce recurrence rates in those with healed ulcers.

As mentioned repeatedly in this text, the elderly pose particular problems when trying to impart effective foot care advice and strategies. Many are unable to perform routine foot care because of poor eyesight and reduced mobility which make it difficult to inspect the foot, and so a spouse or carer should be taught how to provide foot care. There is a particular problem when the patient lives alone, especially if they are partially sighted, and this may be insoluble, despite home support services.

9.10 Superficial ulcers: Wagner/UT Grade 1

Superficial plantar ulcers are predominantly neuropathic in origin, and form at sites of pressure such as metatarsal heads or plantar prominences, including the rocker bottom of advanced midfoot Charcot neuroarthropathy (see Section 9.14). Ulceration of the dorsum of clawed toes in shoes that are too shallow at the toe-box or the lateral and medial aspects of toes are more commonly seen in neuroischaemic patients, but any pressure point can ulcerate in any patient, particularly callused plantar areas [67]. Superficial ulcers are believed to form when pressure leads to a reduction in skin blood flow, to autolysis, and to a breakdown in the dermal layer which results in the formation of an ulcer (Figures 9.4 and 9.5).

Neuropathy allows diabetic patients to continue to stress the skin, by walking or continuing to wear the same tight shoes even after the ulcer has formed. Continued walking inevitably leads to deterioration in the foot. The causative factor, which may be unknown to the patient, may be deduced from the site or nature of the ulcer. In particular, any assessment of the patient with a foot ulcer should pay careful attention to their shoes. Bedrest causing heel ulcers, and trauma,

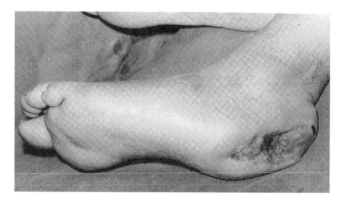

Figure 9.4   Heel ulcer due to pressure from resting on unprotected heels in a neuropathic patient.

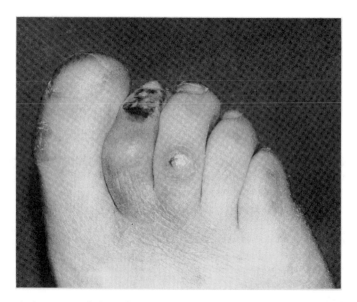

Figure 9.5   Shoe-induced ulceration of clawed toes in a neuropathic diabetic patient.

including the heat of hot-water bottles or inappropriate 'self-chiropody', are easily recognized causes of ulceration [68].

The relief of pressure is the principal mode of management of superficial ulcers, regardless of origin. Metatarsal head ulceration can be unloaded in a variety of ways. Bed rest, with adequate heel protection, is theoretically the most effective, but is difficult to enforce, carries its own risks and, especially if in hospital, is expensive. For this reason a number of ambulatory methods of off-loading ulcer sites have been devised: these include the total contact cast (TCC: 'gold standard') and the more often used removable cast walkers (RCW) or Scotch-cast boot [69]. Research has shown that patients frequently fail to wear the

RCW [70]; however, if the RCW is rendered irremovable by, for example, wrapping it with Scotchcast, then the efficacy of the device in healing ulcers is equivalent to that of the TCC [71]. It must be stressed to the patient that such devices are supplied only for minimal walking, such as to the toilet indoors, and not for 'trips to the shops'. There is often a problem in the patient group of elderly men or women who live alone, especially if they abuse alcohol or have no carers. In such patients the advice to stop excess walking may not always be followed.

Shoe-induced dorsal and digital ulcers can be easily unloaded by the provision of, or by recommending the wearing of, appropriately fitting wide and extra-depth

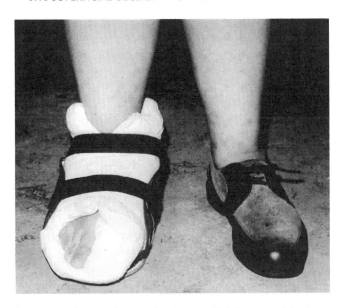

Figure 9.6 'Scotch-cast' boot (right foot) and extra-depth shoe (left foot) used in the prevention and treatment of diabetic foot ulceration reduction system, including whether it is being used and whether the patient is able to rest sufficiently at home [72].

shoes with or without insoles and toe spacers or props as required (Figure 9.6).

Callus should be debrided at every clinic visit [69, 70], as this not only unloads the plantar ulcer but also encourages healing. The formation of excessive callus is a sign that the patient is still walking. Low levels of callus formation are also seen in neuroischaemic patients, and this too may be debrided with care. Whilst *bleeding* is a sign that viable tissue has been reached during the debridement of neuropathic ulcers, the neuroischaemic ulcer should not be traumatized if possible.

The presence or absence of *infection* is difficult to determine in a diabetic foot ulcer. Necrosis, slough and erythema are not universal and systemic features are rare; however, the diagnosis remains a clinical one [73]. Culture from the ulcer surface is likely to produce a mixed growth of dubious significance. Culture from ulcer scrapings during debridement, or better, deep surgical debridement, may provide a more reliable guide to the principal organism responsible for the infection; however, this too may be misleading and broad-spectrum antibiotics are first choice in the treatment of infected ulcers. The provision of 'prophylactic' antibiotics has few advocates, and the case for their use is not clear from the currently available published evidence: it is not recommended [73]. Neuropathic ulcers which are not overtly infected (UT grade 1A) are best

managed by aggressive debridement and appropriate offloading. In neuroischaemic ulceration (UT grade 1C or D), the additional ischaemic risk and potential for foot-threatening infections should encourage the use of long-term antibiotics [74].

The choice of antibiotics for those with clinically infected ulcers is also difficult, but in general most opinion seems to support the use of broad-spectrum monotherapy; co-amoxiclav is regularly used in the authors' and many other units, as is clindamycin, which is also a useful antibiotic for foot infections. These can be started until the results of cultures are known; this should be followed by targeted narrow-spectrum antibiotics prescribed according to the results of cultures.

X-radiography of the foot is recommended to detect osteomyelitis in the majority of patients with ulcers which are either deeper than grade 1 on inspection, have a history of penetrative trauma, are associated with swelling and redness, are not healing after a month, or probe to bone.

It is important to measure the size of the ulcer in order to gauge the progress of healing. The minimum measurement should be the diameter of the ulcer in two planes at right-angles. Tracing the perimeter and/or photographs are also useful to measure progress. Failure of the ulcer to heal should prompt an investigation as to the effectiveness of any pressure-relieving modality.

If all of these aspects are satisfactory, then the question of vascular insufficiency should be addressed. Even in apparently purely neuropathic ulcers there may be an underlying element of vascular impairment which, without correction, might significantly impede the healing of recalcitrant ulceration. The successful treatment of vascular insufficiency can dramatically improve healing rates.

Dressings alone will not heal an ulcer without adequate pressure relief. Although the dry dressing is still in common use, a moist wound environment encourages granulation tissue formation [75]. Sadly, a good evidence base for the efficacy of almost any dressing is lacking [76].

The use of wound-healing factors and biosynthetic skin replacements has not, to date, lived up to initial expectations. Autologous, blood-derived, wound-healing factor has been used for many years, particularly in the United States, but adequate controlled studies in diabetic patients are uncommon [77]. Platelet-derived growth factor has been shown to increase the healing rate and total percentage of healed ulcers compared to placebo [78]. The biosynthetic dermal replacement Dermagraft (Smith and Nephew, UK) has shown some promise in clinical trials of patients with neuropathic diabetic foot ulcers [79]. The main market for these products must, however, remain the difficult-to-heal ulcer, and in most cases appropriate care and pressure relief will achieve healing of superficial ulcers of neuropathic and neuroischaemic origins.

9.10.1 The myth of the non-healing ulcer?

Many reports have tried to categorize ulcers as healing and non-healing. It is important to be able to identify those patients in whom treatment is failing and for whom a new approach should be used. If no objective measure of ulcer healing is used, then there is no possibility that such patients will be detected, and once again the need for measurement and standardized descriptions of ulcers cannot be stressed too highly.

It is clear that the primary reasons for failure of the neuropathic plantar diabetic foot ulcer to heal are inadequate or inappropriate pressure relief, inadequate debridement and infection control, failure to recognize or treat vascular insufficiency, or patient non-compliance. It is only when all of these factors have been addressed, including angiography and reconstruction where necessary, or by the use of irremovable off-loading casts that an ulcer can truly be described as non-healing. Such ulcers will be rare [72].

Once an ulcer is healed, that patient is left in the highest category of all for predicting future ulcer risk. Education, footcare, chiropody, footwear and careful follow-up are all necessary in an attempt to prevent the recurrence of foot ulceration.

9.11 Deep ulcers: Wagner/UT Grades 2 and 3

Deep ulcers are usually superficial ulcers that have continued to be traumatized by an insensate patient. Continued walking on plantar ulcers or the wearing of inappropriate shoes advances the cycle of tissue destruction and enlarges the ulcer cavity. If this process continues, it may lead to the involvement of underlying tendons (Wagner/UT grade 2) and eventually to bone, causing osteomyelitis (grade 3). Occasionally, penetrating injuries will cause the primary formation of a deep abscess.

X-radiography of the feet should be performed routinely in all patients with deep ulcers. If osteomyelitis is suspected, but is not apparent on initial plain radiographs, then further investigations with ^{99m}Tc radioisotopes and labelled white cell scanning should be performed. Computed tomography (CT) and magnetic resonance imaging scans are also used in centres with ready access to such facilities. If the ulcer can be probed to bone, then this is likely to be complicated by osteomyelitis in all cases, and therefore empirical treatment has been advocated: however, an inability to probe to bone probably excludes osteomyelitis [80].

As with superficial ulcers, pressure relief remains the mainstay of treatment of deep ulceration, but the treatment of sepsis and aggressive surgical debridement is increasingly important. If the patient is systemically well, and there is no evidence of spreading infection, then he or she can often be managed as an outpatient. The use of total contact casts is, however, contraindicated in patients with oedema secondary to deep infection, owing to the risk of swelling within the cast, leading to cast trauma. Regular debridement down to the ulcer base is required. Bleeding points demonstrate adequate debridement in the neuropathic foot. In the foot with coexisting ischaemia, debridement should be less aggressive, and the patient may require admission for investigation and the treatment of osteomyelitis, surgical debridement or intravenous antibiotics.

Diabetes control should be optimized if possible, as there is evidence to suggest that healing is impaired with poor blood glucose control, although this

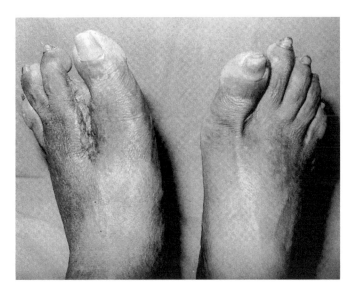

Figure 9.7   Ray amputation of second toe and associated metatarsal.

does not necessarily mean a need for insulin in a non-insulin-dependent patient.

Podiatric debridement and conservative care will lead to the healing of over 60% of such ulcers [81]. If surgical debridement is required then it should aim to remove all the infected tissue in one operation. This may necessitate a partial amputation, commonly of a metatarsal and associated toe (the 'ray amputation'; see Figure 9.7), which should then heal well if the blood supply is adequate (Wagner Grade 3, UT 3B) [82]. The removal of all the infected and/or necrotic tissue should produce an improvement in the patient's metabolic state and, in neuropathic patients with adequate blood supply, even extensive tissue loss will heal. Local operations in neuroischaemic patients can lead to larger non-healing wounds, so it is important to ensure the vascular status of the patient prior to forefoot and other surgery. If vascular disease is suspected from the absence of pulses (UT 3D), the site of the ulcer, failure to heal despite adequate therapy or the presence of local gangrene, then a vascular opinion should be obtained before any decision to operate. Where indicated, the restoration of an impaired blood flow may remove the need for amputation, or at least markedly reduce its scope.

Previous concerns about the long-term patency of arterial grafts in diabetic patients should be discounted. There is evidence to show that a successful arterial bypass operation has the same graft survival rate in diabetic patients as in those without diabetes [83]. Once

healing has been achieved, subsequent graft failure may not lead to loss of the limb as the vascular requirements of healed tissue seem to be lower than that of healing ulcers.

Slough is commonly seen in neuroischaemic ulcers, and impedes healing by blocking the formation of granulation tissue. Chemical debridement with desloughing agents such as hydrogels or hydrofoams seems to help in the early stages of healing if there is adherent slough. Necrotic eschar is probably best removed mechanically. An alternative is larval debridement, which has been effective in removing slough and necrotic debris from wounds in a number of case reports. This method is usually used in neuroischaemic ulcers to debride recalcitrant slough. If larvae are used it may take more than one application to clear the ulcer of slough. Recent observations suggest that larvae might even be helpful in eradicating MRSA from foot ulcers [84].

Antibiotic use should be universal in all deep ulcers and again should, at least initially, be broad-spectrum in nature until a definitive pathogen is isolated. The average number of potential pathogens isolated from a wound swab is more than two organisms [85]. The deeper the tissue that is cultured, or the growth of an organism from the bloodstream, increases the reliability of the pathogenicity of the isolate. Combination therapy for initial blind treatment has traditionally been ampicillin, flucloxacillin and metronidazole intravenously, or ciprofloxacin and metronidazole. Clinical trial evidence has shown that the use of ciprofloxacin and clindamycin as combination therapy in oral or intravenous dosing also seems to be effective. Outpatient treatment might be with these antibiotics or clindamycin alone, which is a useful oral antibiotic for the treatment of mild to moderate infections, and in the long-term treatment of osteomyelitis.

Dressings should conform to the cavity left by a deep ulcer. Deep ulcers often have tendons at their bases and should not be allowed to become too dry. Once again, the choice of dressing is rarely based upon any clinical trial. Theoretical concepts would point to the use of a moist wound-healing environment with enough absorbency to deal with wound exudation. Foam dressings are the authors' current choice as a primary or secondary dressing for such ulcers.

If the patient has been admitted, then once the initial infection has been controlled the outpatient care, using off-loading casts or similar, can be restarted. Although the clinical progress of these ulcers is slow, eventually complete healing can be achieved. Regular measurement of the ulcer is important to gauge progress above the usual; 'It looks better = the same = worse' notes are commonplace in most clinical records. Failure to improve should again prompt a search for the reasons behind the lack of appropriate healing.

9.12   Localized gangrene: Wagner Grade 4

Localized gangrene is commonly seen at the ends of toes (Figure 9.8) and at the apex of the heel. These are regions where there are endarteries with little collateral circulation if a feeder branch artery fails. As well as being a sign of global arterial insufficiency in the foot, and therefore of neuroischaemia, digital necrosis can occur as a result of infection in a purely neuropathic foot, leading to an infective vasculitis and digital artery closure [86].

Vascular assessment is mandatory for all patients with localized gangrene. No clinical arterial insufficiency may be found in patients with toe gangrene alone, but if treatable arterial insufficiency is found then correction will significantly reduce the amount of tissue loss. Angioplasty and proximal reconstructive surgery is as effective in diabetic patients as non-diabetic patients. However, the vascular disease of diabetic patients is often below the trifurcation of the popliteal artery.

Interventional radiology with angioplasty can now be used to tackle tibial and peroneal disease. Today,

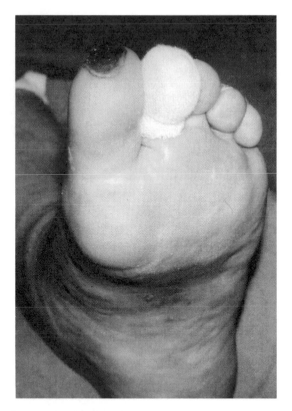

Figure 9.8   Localized gangrene at the end of the great toe.

the technique of percutaneous transluminal angioplasty using an inflatable balloon is increasingly used, even in distal obstructions [87]. Positioned at the site of an atheromatous narrowing within an artery, the balloon stretches the vessel, thus splitting the plaque and restoring the luminal area. Re-endothelialization must then occur over the fissured plaque, and it is usual to use intravenous heparin to prevent thrombotic occlusion during the first 24 h after angioplasty. In general, the success rate for the recanalization of an arterial occlusion by angioplasty is proportionate to the length of stenosis or thrombosis. Recanalization can usually be achieved in over 90% of short stenoses in appropriately skilled hands [88]. However, even a good technical result with total recanalization of an occluded vessel does not always lead to clinical improvement in the limb if the distal run-off is poor, and this may require further treatment to the distal vessels. Angioplasty has been performed at the level of the tibial and peroneal arteries since 1982, and may be the therapy of first line in elderly diabetic patients with other medical conditions, or in whom a vein is not available for distal bypass.

Arterial tears and early thrombotic occlusion are the main adverse events associated with angioplasty, but fortunately the incidence of these problems is low.

There remains a problem with long-term reocclusion. Even in technically successful angioplasties with good run-off, intimal hyperplasia or recurrence of native disease lead to reocclusion rates which approach 50% overall, depending on the duration of the follow-up. However, these rates are similar in diabetic and non-diabetic patients. Re-angioplasty may be possible, and, even if a vessel does re-stenose or occlude, there may have been sufficient duration of improved circulation to facilitate healing or to allow a plane of tissue viability to establish or even close the lesion (Figure 9.9). Once a lesion is closed, the blood supply requirements may be lower than those for an ulcerated limb, and limb salvage rates are usually higher than patency rates in most series.

There is evidence that in iliac vessels, or in situations where re-stenosis is likely, stenting the artery wall can prevent re-occlusion [89]. Iliac angioplasty with or without stenting can also be employed to increase arterial inflow to the limb and improve the chances of a lower bypass remaining patent. Reconstructive surgery, particularly with *in situ* or reversed saphenous vein as a conduit, can now be performed at the level of the dorsalis pedis artery to restore pulsatile flow below the tibial arteries [90]. The availability of such techniques is often limited to regional centres, and indeed this may be appropriate in order to achieve the best limb salvage rates from what are highly specialized surgery and angioplasty.

9.12.1 Indications for revascularization

Many surgeons speak of an aggressive limb salvage approach in the management of the ischaemic diabetic limb [91]. Such an approach is often – and probably should always be – based on appropriate patient selection. If the patient is expected to have a reasonable life expectancy, then it should be remembered that concomitant cardiac and cerebrovascular disease is likely to result in death in over 50% of vascular disease patients within 5 years, regardless of whether they have diabetes [92]. It is the practice of many American surgeons to attend to these vascular beds at the same time as, or prior to, revascularization of the lower limbs, but such a policy requires greater resources than are likely to be available in most state-funded health care systems. In general, the patient must be able to undergo what is usually a lengthy operation, particularly for distal bypass, and any pre-existing lung or cardiac pathology may limit their ability to withstand the operation, or may limit its effectiveness. If the patient has a low functional capacity with a poor potential for rehabilitation beyond a wheelchair, then such an approach is not tenable. Similarly, if the patient is neither able nor motivated to walk, or will not stop smoking, then the graft patency will be jeopardized.

If surgery to vessels below the knee is required, then this must be performed with a vein as the conduit.

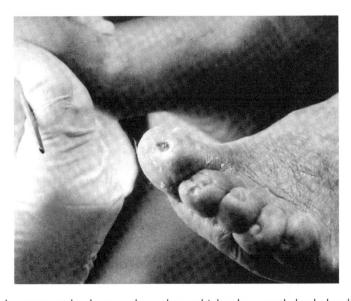

Figure 9.9 Gangrene has separated to leave a clean ulcer, which subsequently healed well.

Synthetic grafts, even with vein cuffs, have such low patency rates as to render attempts at below-knee reconstructive surgery using such materials pointless [93]. If the leg veins are varicosed, or have been harvested for coronary grafting, then an arm vein can be used, but this adds to the technical aspects and duration of the operation. If a short length of vein can be found, a popliteal artery to foot bypass may be almost as successful as a femoral artery to distal bypass [94]. Similarly, the patient must have suitable anatomy with adequate inflow and a patent foot vessel on which to graft. If the nature and extent of infection and necrosis is such that it encroaches upon the potential graft site, then again the likelihood is that the graft will fail. This once again highlights the need for control of infection.

Any centre wishing to offer reconstructive surgery, and particularly distal surgery, must operate a graft surveillance programme in order to assess the clinical progress of patients and to audit the results. During the follow-up period the other vascular trees, coronaries, carotids and the other limb may need attention to reduce the coexisting morbidity and mortality and to improve patient outcome.

The nature of diabetes as a systemic disorder usually implies that, in those patients requiring reconstructive surgery, there are other associated complications. This is particularly true of the elderly patient with diabetes. Typically, the intensive care stay is often longer in diabetic patients, and the perioperative management of diabetes control, cardiac and renal impairment and radiological investigation require a team approach to the management of surgery in such patients [95].

9.12.2 Proximal arterial reconstruction

These operations are divided into inflow procedures, usually aorto-iliac surgery, where synthetic graft materials are normally used, and where, because of high flow rates, the graft patency is excellent. For aorto-bifemoral grafts the 5-year patency rate is commonly over 85%. The patency of aorto-bifemoral grafts is the same in both diabetic and non-diabetic patients, although because of associated cardiovascular disease the overall patient survival rates are lower in diabetic patients, but not usually significantly so [92].

Reconstructive surgery below the inguinal ligament is usually referred to as an *outflow procedure*; the usual operation is the femoro-popliteal bypass graft around a superficial femoral occlusion. Synthetic graft materials can be used for these operations, but vein grafts have

better secondary patency rates. Regardless of the conduit used, the long-term patency depends on the flow rate through the graft, which in turn is influenced by the run-off vessels. In most series the 5-year patency averages 70%, although reoperation and redo angioplasty rates are higher in diabetic patients in some series [96]. Despite the predilection for vascular disease to be multi-level and to affect the infra-popliteal vessels in diabetes, there appears to be no significant difference in patency rates between diabetic and non-diabetic patients. This may be due to patient selection, but there also is some evidence that femoral disease and distal disease do not always coexist in diabetic patients. In addition, owing to a high coexisting mortality, graft patency may exceed the life expectancy of the patient [96].

9.12.3 Distal reconstructive operations

These operations are all outflow procedures performed to vessels below the popliteal artery. As outlined above, autologous vein is the only suitable conduit for these procedures, which can limit the suitability of many patients for surgery. In general, these are operations performed for limb salvage. The flow rate may mean that in many cases the graft may have failed by one year; however, the limb be saved if the lesion has closed. In selected centres, the 5-year limb salvage rates approach 85% despite a graft patency of only 68%, and are at least 50% in unselected British centres [26, 92]. Infection should be treated promptly to prevent rapidly spreading gangrene and systemic infection leading to a severely ill and toxic patient. The antibiotic regimens outlined above under deep ulcers should also be appropriate for these patients. Well-circumscribed, localized, usually digital, necrosis with viable tissue borders can often be left to separate undisturbed; this is usually termed 'auto-amputation'. The wound left behind should then be treated as a neuroischaemic ulcer in the usual manner, and will usually heal well.

More extensive or spreading necrosis in a toxic patient, particularly if there is no reversible arterial lesion, may require primary amputation. This decision should be taken only after review by a vascular surgeon, as arterial reconstruction or angioplasty can markedly improve the level at which the amputation stump is viable.

The remaining foot of an amputee is at an exceedingly high risk of ulceration and further surgery. General aftercare should be as for other ulcers, but with particular attention to the intact foot. A partial amputation of a toe or ray leads to biomechanical changes within the foot which are often very different from normal and frequently produces new pressure points at risk of ulceration. Transmetatarsal or Lisfranc amputations are often very poorly functioning amputations in diabetic patients. Amputation, at whatever level, results in special orthotic needs that must be addressed by the footcare team. Insoles and orthoses all require careful and regular review to ensure that they are functioning correctly in order to reduce the significant reulceration and amputation rate of diabetic amputees.

9.13 Extensive gangrene: Wagner Grade 5

Extensive necrosis of the foot is due to arterial occlusion and failure of arterial inflow, and usually presents with multiple areas of necrosis, generally in the context of the neuroischaemic foot. Primary amputation is the usual treatment for extensive gangrene; however, the extent of amputation can sometimes be reduced by pre-amputation arterial reconstructive surgery. For this reason, the counsel of perfection is that a vascular assessment should be performed in all patients prior to amputation. Either femoropopliteal or similar bypass operations might improve the viability of a distal stump, or convert an above-knee to a below-knee amputation. Again, this may not always be possible in diabetic patients, because the arterial disease is often below the popliteal trifurcation, and if the necrosis extends beyond the dorsalis pedis artery it will preclude distal bypass.

Metabolic and infection control should be attended to as a priority, as these patients are often very ill owing to the toxic effects of the necrotic tissue burden. In addition, coexistent coronary and cerebral vascular disease often makes the anaesthetic choice difficult, and regional anaesthesia is commonly used for amputation surgery in diabetic patients. Close cooperation between the medical, surgical and anaesthetic teams is likely to produce the best survival outcomes for these patients.

If the patient survives the immediate perioperative period, then the mortality rate in patients following major amputation is >50% at one year. Care of the remaining foot is particularly important to prevent further amputation, and this usually results in confinement to a wheelchair. Significant improvements in preservation of the remaining limb can be achieved if the patient returns to the diabetic foot clinic for follow-up after amputation [97]. The patient is likely to die from other major vessel problems, particularly coronary artery

and cerebrovascular disease, and treatment for these conditions – including aspirin, lipid modification and blood pressure control – should also be addressed during the follow-up period.

9.14 The diabetic Charcot foot

The devastating effects of Charcot neuroarthropathy in the diabetic foot, including mortality, have been well described [98–101]. Diabetes is now believed to be the leading cause of Charcot neuroarthropathy in the developed world [102], with 80% of patients who develop Charcot neuroarthropathy having a known duration of diabetes of over 10 years. The long duration of diabetes prior to the initiation of the Charcot process probably reflects the degree of neuropathy that is usually present in these patients. Autonomic neuropathy appears to be a universal finding in diabetic Charcot patients [103]. The duration of diabetes appears to be more important than age alone, but this is compounded in type 2 diabetic patients, who frequently have a long prodromal disease duration prior to diagnosis.

The initiating event of the Charcot process is often a seemingly trivial injury, which may result in a minor periarticular fracture or in a major fracture, despite the inability of the patient to recall the injury in many cases. Following this there is a rapid onset of swelling, an increase in temperature in the foot, and often an ache or discomfort. The patient may have noticed a change in the shape of the foot; others have described the sensation, or the sound, of the bones crunching as they walk. The blood supply to the Charcot foot is always good; indeed, there are case reports of the Charcot process starting in patients following arterial bypass surgery [104]. It is assumed that autonomic neuropathy plays a part in the increased vascularity of bone, possibly by increased arteriovenous shunting [105], and this increases osteoclastic activity, resulting in the destruction, fragmentation and remodelling of bone. It is these processes which, if left untreated, lead to the characteristic patterns of deformity in the Charcot foot, including the collapse of the longitudinal and transverse arches leading to a rocker bottom foot (see Figures 9.10 and 9.11). Recent research into the pathogenesis of this condition has focused on the potential role if inflammation and pro-inflammatory cytokines [102, 106].

Charcot neuroarthropathy passes from this acute phase of development through a stage of coalescence, in which the bone fragments are reabsorbed, the

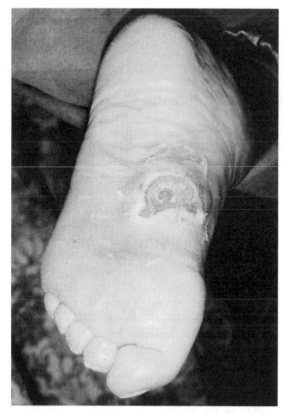

Figure 9.10 Anteroposterior view of sole of a Charcot foot, showing a plantar prominence which has ulcerated.

oedema lessens, and the foot cools. It then enters the stage of reconstruction, in which the final repair and regenerative modelling of bone takes place to leave a stable, chronic Charcot foot [107]. The time course of these events is variable but is often up to a year.

Intervention must be made in the earliest phase to prevent subsequent deformity and to reduce the risk of amputation [108].

Radiographs of the foot should be performed to make the initial diagnosis (Figure 9.12). The characteristic appearances of bone destruction, fragmentation, loss of joint architecture and new bone formation should be determined. The confirmation of Charcot neuroarthropathy can be made through bone scans, and CT or MRI scans, but this is usually not required in the majority of clinical settings.

Management of the Charcot foot has always been difficult, and varies from the expectant to the markedly interventional [109]. The first principles of management are rest and freedom from weight-bearing. Non-weight-bearing is useful to reduce the activity, but weight-bearing frequently restarts when walking is recommenced. In the United States, in particular, the practice of prolonged (one year or more) immobilization in a plaster of Paris cast is the usual treatment. The total-contact cast is usually the method employed, but this requires frequent changes as the oedema reduces. Plaster casting will stabilize the foot but, again, whilst casting reduces activity initially, when the plaster is finally removed after 6–12 months the acute destructive process may restart. Surgical fusion of the joints of the foot in their anatomical positions has usually met with little success during the active phase.

Surgery may still be used, for example to remove a plantar prominence once the process has finally settled [78, 110]. The end of the active phase can be assessed by following skin temperature and radiographic change [111]. In the United Kingdom, total-contact casting is

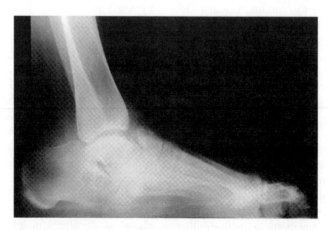

Figure 9.11 Charcot neuroarthropathy: lateral X-radiograph showing destruction of the talus and mid-foot.

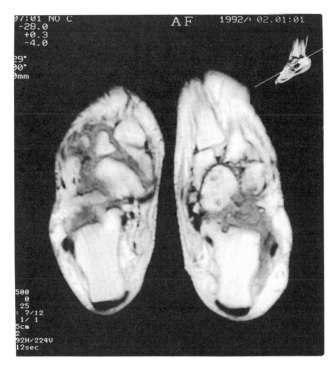

Figure 9.12 Magnetic resonance image of the talus and mid-foot of the patient in Figure 9.11. Note the bilateral Charcot changes. Such changes are often difficult to interpret, even by experienced radiologists.

still the mainstay of treatment in the active phase. The Scotch-cast boot (see Figure 9.6) can also be used to rest the active Charcot foot, and is particularly useful to provide pressure redistribution of a rocker bottom foot with an ulcer at its apex. Casting is usually continued for several weeks after the temperature differential between the active and contralateral foot is below 1.5°C. The overall role of surgery in the quiescent Charcot foot was reviewed by Salamon and Saltzman [112].

As yet, there is no definitive treatment aimed at the underlying inflammation or overactivity of osteoclasts in the active destructive phase of Charcot neuroarthropathy. Two clinical studies, including a randomized placebo-controlled trial, of the use of intravenous pamidronate have now been performed in acute Charcot neuroarthropathy. In patients with acute destructive-phase Charcot neuroarthropathy, treatment with intravenous bisphosphonate caused a rapid resolution of symptoms and signs, including foot temperature, and a marked improvement in the biochemical markers of bone turnover, particularly alkaline phosphatase concentrations [113, 114]. Such therapy should, therefore, be considered in addition to the use of rest and casting outlined above.

9.15 Conclusions

The diabetic foot syndrome is a significant cause of morbidity and mortality in elderly diabetic patients. However, by recognizing the known risk associations, and taking measures to reduce their effect, the incidence of foot ulceration can be significantly reduced. If, in turn, foot ulceration is managed in a systematic and appropriate manner then the incidence of amputations because of ulceration can be significantly reduced. This is the ultimate goal in treating diabetic foot problems. Clear evidence of the success of a multidisciplinary approach should lead to its adoption more widely than is currently the case.

References

1. WHO=IDF (1990) Diabetes care and research in Europe: the St Vincent Declaration. *Diabetic Medicine*, **7**, 360.
2. Specialist UK Workgroup Reports (1996) St Vincent and improving diabetes care: report of the Diabetic Foot and Amputation Subgroup. *Diabetic Medicine*, **13** (Suppl. 4): S27–42.

3. SIGN (1997) *Management of Diabetic Foot Disease*. Scottish Intercollegiate Network Guideline, Edinburgh.

4. McIntosh A, Peters J, Young R *et al.* (2003) Prevention and Management of Foot Problems in Type 2 diabetes: Clinical Guidelines and Evidence. Sheffield, University of Sheffield. (See also www.nice.org.uk/guidance/index ref CG10.)

5. Krishhan S, Nash F, Baker N, Fowler D and Rayman G (2008) Reduction in diabetic amputations over 11 years in a defined UK population: benefits of multi-disciplinary team work and continuous prospective audits. *Diabetes Care*, **31**, 99–101.

6. Boulton AJM, Vileikyte L, Ragnarson-Tennvall G and Apelqvist J (2005) The global burden of diabetic foot disease. *Lancet*, **366**, 1719–24.

7. Thomson FJ and Masson EA (1992) Can elderly diabetic patients co-operate with routine foot care? *Age and Aging*, **21**, 333–7.

8. Cavanagh PR, Young MJ, Adams JE, Vickers KL and Boulton AJM (1994) Radiographic abnormalities in the feet of neuropathic diabetic patients. *Diabetes Care*, **17**, 201–9.

9. Young MJ, Adams JE, Anderson GF, Boulton AJM and Cavanagh PR (1993) Medial arterial calcification in the feet of diabetic patients and matched non-diabetic control subjects. *Diabetologia*, **36**, 615–21.

10. Reiber GE, Pecararo RE and Koepsell TD (1992) Risk factors for amputation in patients with diabetes mellitus. *Annals of Internal Medicine*, **117**, 97–105.

11. Boulton AJM, Malik RA, Arezzo JC and Sosenko JM (2004) Diabetic somatic neuropathies. *Diabetes Care*, **27**, 1458–86.

12. Young MJ, Boulton AJM, Macleod AF, Williams DRR and Sonksen PH (1993) A multicentre study of the prevalence of diabetic peripheral neuropathy in the United Kingdom hospital clinic population. *Diabetologia*, **36**, 150–4

13. Boulton AJM, Vinik AI, Arezzo JC *et al.* (2005) Diabetic neuropathies: a statement by the American Diabetes Association. *Diabetes Care*, **28**, 956–62.

14. Young MJ (1998) Capsaicin as topical therapy for painful diabetic neuropathy. *The Diabetic Foot*, **1**, 147–50.

15. Young MJ and Matthews CF (1998) Screening for neuropathy – can we achieve our ideals? *The Diabetic Foot*, **1**, 22–5.

16. Boulton AJM, Armstrong DG, Albert SF *et al.* (2008) Comprehensive foot examination and risk assessment: a report of the task force of the foot care interest group of the American Diabetes Association, with endorsement by the American Association of Clinical Endocrinologists. *Diabetes Care*, **31**, 1679–85.

17. Thomson FJ, Masson EA and Boulton AJM (1992) Quantitative vibration perception testing in elderly people: an assessment of variability. *Age and Aging*, **21**, 171–4.

18. Young MJ, Breddy JL, Veves A and Boulton AJM (1994) The use of vibration perception to predict diabetic neuropathic foot ulceration: a prospective study. *Diabetes Care*, **17**, 557–60.

19. Booth J and Young MJ (2000) Differences in performance of commercially available 10 g monofilaments. *Diabetes Care*, **23**, 984–8.

20. Abbott CA, Carrington AL, Ashe H *et al.* (2002) The North West Diabetes Foot Care Study: incidence of, and risk factors for, new diabetic foot ulceration in a community based patient cohort. *Diabetic Med*, **19**, 377–84.

21. Cavanagh PR and Ulbrecht JS (2008) The biomechanics of the foot in diabetes mellitus. In: JS Bowker and MA Pfeifer (eds) *Levin and O'Neal's The Diabetic Foot*. Mosby, Philadelphia, 7th edition, pp. 115–84.

22. Vinik AI, Maser RE, Mitchell BD and Freeman R (2003) Diabetic autonomic neuropathy. *Diabetes Care*, **26**, 1553–79.

23. Purewal TS, Goss DE, Watkins PJ and Edmonds ME (1995) Lower limb venous pressure in diabetic neuropathy. *Diabetes Care*, **18**, 377–81.

24. Flynn MD and Tooke JE (1992) Aetiology of diabetic foot ulceration: a role for the microcirculation? *Diabetic Medicine*, **9**, 320–9.

25. Sandeman DD, Shore AC and Tooke JE (1992) Relation of skin capillary pressure in patients with insulin-dependent diabetes mellitus to complications and metabolic control. *New England Journal of Medicine*, **327**, 760–4.

26. Simms M (2006) Peripheral vascular disease and reconstruction. In: AJM Boulton, PR Cavanagh and G Rayman (eds) *The Foot in Diabetes*. John Wiley and Sons, Chichester, 4th edn, pp. 250–64.

27. Van derFeen C, Neijens FS, Kanters SD *et al.* (2002) Angiographic distribution of lower extremity atherosclerosis in patients with and without diabetes. *Diabetic Med*, **19**, 366–70.

28. Janka HU, Stadl E and Mehnert H (1980) Peripheral vascular disease in diabetes mellitus and its relation to cardiovascular risk factors: screening with Doppler ultrasonic technique. *Diabetes Care*, **3**, 207–13.

29. Jensen T, Borch-Johnsen K, Kofoed-Enevoldsen A and Deckert T (1987) Coronary heart disease in young Type 1 (insulin-dependent) diabetic patients with and without diabetic nephropathy: incidence and risk factors. *Diabetologia*, **30**, 144–8.

30. Gibbons GW and Freeman D (1987) Vascular evaluation and treatment of the diabetic. *Clinics in Podiatric Medicine and Surgery*, **4**, 377–81.

31. Orchard TJ and Strandness DE (1993) Assessment of peripheral vascular disease in diabetes. *Diabetes Care*, **16**, 1199–209.

32. American Diabetes Association (2003) Peripheral arterial disease in people with diabetes (Consensus Statement). *Diabetes Care*, **26**, 3333–41.

33. Hiatt WR, Regensteiner JG, Hargaten ME *et al.* (1990) Benefit of exercise conditioning for patients with peripheral arterial disease. *Circulation*, **81**, 602–9.

34. McAllister FF (1976) The fate of patients with intermittent claudication managed conservatively. *American Journal of Surgery*, **132**, 593–5.

35. Larkin JG and Frier BM (1986) Limited joint mobility and Dupuytrens contracture in diabetic, hypertensive and normal populations. *British Medical Journal*, **292**, 1494.

36. Goodfield MJB and Millard LG (1988) The skin in diabetes mellitus. *Diabetologia*, **31**, 567–75.

37. Rosenbloom AL, Silverstain JM, Lezotte DC, Richardon K and McCallum M (1981) Limited joint mobility in childhood diabetes indicates increased risk for microvascular disease. *New England Journal of Medicine*, **305**, 191–4.

38. Campbell RR, Hawkins SJ, Maddison PJ and Reckless JPD (1988) Limited joint mobility in the diabetes mellitus. *Annals of the Rheumatic Disease*, **44**, 93–7.

39. Delbridge L, Perry P, Marr S, Arnold N, Yue DK, Turtle JR and Reeve TS (1988) Limited joint mobility in the diabetic foot: relationship to neuropathic ulceration. *Diabetic Medicine*, **5**, 333–7.

40. Fernando DJS, Masson EA, Veves A and Boulton AJM (1991) Relationship of limited joint mobility to abnormal foot pressures and diabetic foot ulceration. *Diabetes Care*, **14**, 8–11.

41. Young MJ, Cavanagh PR, Thomas G, Johnson MM, Murray H and Boulton AJM (1992) The effect of callus removal on dynamic plantar foot pressures in diabetic patients. *Diabetic Medicine*, **9**, 55–7.

42. Veves A, Fernando DJS, Walewski P and Boulton AJM (1991) A study of plantar pressures in a diabetic clinic population. *The Foot*, **1**, 89–92.

43. Cavanagh PR, Sims DS, Jr and Sanders LJ (1991) Body mass is a poor predictor of peak plantar pressure in diabetic men. *Diabetes Care*, **14**, 750–5.

44. Boulton AJM (2004) The diabetic foot: from art to science. *Diabetologia*, **47**, 1343–53.

45. Rayman G, Willams SA, Spencer PD, Smaje LH, Wise PH and Tooke JE (1986) Impaired microvascular response to minor skin trauma in Type 1 diabetes. *British Medicine Journal*, **292**, 1295–8.

46. Walmsley D, Wales JK and Wiles PG (1989) Reduced hyperaemia following skin trauma: evidence for an impaired microvascular response to injury in the diabetic foot. *Diabetologia*, **32**, 736–9.

47. MacFarlane IA, Benbow SJ, Chan AW, Bowsher D and Williams G (1993) Diabetic peripheral neuropathy: the significance of plantar foot temperatures as demonstrated by liquid crystal contact thermography. *Diabetic Medicine*, **10** (Suppl. 1), P104.

48. Masson EA, Hay EM, Stockley I, Veves A, Betts RP and Boulton AJM (1989) Abnormal foot pressures alone may not cause ulceration. *Diabetic Medicine*, **6**, 426–8.

49. Van Schie CH, Abbott CA, Vileikyte L, Shaw JE, Hollis S and Boulton AJM. (2000) A comparative study of the podotrack, a simple semi-quantitative plantar pressure measuring device, and the optical pedobarograph in the assessment of pressures under the diabetic foot. *Diabetic Med*, **16**, 154–9.

50. Veves A, Van Ross ERE and Boulton AJM (1992) Foot pressure measurements in diabetic and non-diabetic amputees. *Diabetes Care*, **15**, 905–7.

51. Knowles A, Westwood B, Young MJ and Boulton AJM (1993) A retrospective study to assess the outcome of diabetic ulcers that have been dressed with Granuflex and other dressings. In: *Proceedings of the Joint Meeting of the Wound Healing Society and the European Tissue Repair Society*, Amsterdam, August 1993, P 68.

52. Pecoraro RE, Ahroni JH, Boyko EJ and Stensel VL (1991) Chronology and determinants of tissue repair in diabetic lower-extremity ulcers. *Diabetes*, **40**, 1305–13.

53. Louie TJ, Gartlett JG and Tally FP (1976) Aerobic and anaerobic bacteria in diabetic foot ulcers. *Annals of Internal Medicine*, **85**, 461–3.

54. Delbridge L, Appleberg M and Reeves TS (1983) Factors associated with the development of foot lesions in the diabetic. *Surgery*, **93**, 78–82.

55. Young RJ, Zhou YQ, Rodriguez E, Prescott RJ, Ewing DJ and Clark BF (1986) Variable relationship between peripheral somatic and autonomic neuropathy in patients with different syndromes of diabetic polyneuropathy. *Diabetes*, **35**, 192–7.

56. Fernando DJS, Hutchison A, Veves A, Gokal R and Boulton AJM (1991) Risk factors for non-ischaemic foot ulceration in diabetic nephropathy. *Diabetic Medicine*, **8**, 223–5.

57. Young MJ (2000) Classification of ulcers and its relevance to management. In: AJM Boulton, PR Cavanagh and H Connor (eds) *The Foot in Diabetes*, 3rd edn. John Wiley & Sons, Chichester.

58. Lavery LA, Armstrong DG and Harkless LB (1996) Classification of diabetic foot wounds. *Journal of Foot and Ankle Surgery*, **35**, 528–31.

59. Oyibo S, Jude EB, Tarawneh I *et al.* (2001) The effects of ulcer size and site, patient age, sex and type and duration of diabetes on the outcome of diabetic foot ulcer. *Diabetic Med*, **18**, 133–8.

60. Schaper NC (2004) Diabetic foot ulceration classification system for research purposes: a progress report on criteria for including patients in research studies. *Diabete Metab Res Rev*, **20** (Suppl. 1), S90–5.

61. Levin ME (1998) Classification of diabetic foot wounds. *Diabetes Care*, **21**, 681.

62. Barth R, Campbell LV, Allen S, Jupp JJ and Chisholm DJ (1991) Intensive education improves knowledge, compliance, and foot problems in Type 2 diabetes. *Diabetic Medicine*, **8**, 111–17.

63. Knowles EA, Kumar S, Veves A, Young MJ, Fernando DJS and Boulton AJM (1992) Essential elements of footcare education are retained for at least a year. *Diabetic Medicine*, **9** (Suppl. 2), S6.

64. Vileikyte L (2006) Psychological and behavioural issues in diabetic foot ulceration. In: AJM Boulton, PR Cavanagh and G Rayman (eds) *The Foot in Diabetes*, John Wiley & Sons, Chichester, 4th edn, pp. 132–42.

65. Stuart L and Wiles PJ (1993) Knowledge and beliefs towards footcare among diabetic patients: a comparison of qualitative and quantitative methodologies. *Diabetic Medicine*, **9** (Suppl. 2), S3.

66. Stuart L and Wiles PJ (1993) The influence of a learning contract on levels of footcare. *Diabetic Medicine*, **10** (Suppl 3), S3.

67. Murray HJ, Young MJ, Hollis S and Boulton AJM (1996) The association between callus formation, high pressures and neuropathy in diabetic foot ulceration. *Diabetic Medicine*, **13**, 979–82.

68. Boulton AJM (1990) Diabetic foot. Neuropathic in origin? *Diabetic Medicine*, **7**, 852–8.

69. Armstrong DG, Lavery LA, Kimbriel HR, Nixon BP and Boulton AJM (2003) Activity patterns of patients with diabetic foot ulceration: patients with active ulceration may not adhere to a standard pressure off-loading regimen. *Diabetes Care*, **26**, 2595–2597.

70. Armstrong DG, Lavery LA, Nixon BP and Boulton AJM. (2004) It's not what you put on, but what you take off: Techniques for debriding and off-loading the diabetic foot wound. *Clin Infect Dis*, **39** (Suppl. 2), S92–9.

71. Katz IA, Harlan A, Miranda-Palma B *et al.* (2005) A randomized trial of two irremovable off-loading devices in the management of plantar, neuropathic diabetic foot ulcers. *Diabetes Care*, **28**, 555–9.

72. Cavanagh PR, Ulbrecht JS and Caputo GM (1998) The non-healing diabetic foot wound: fact or fiction? *Ostomy Wound Management*, **44** (3A Suppl.), 6S–12S.

73. Lipsky BA (2008) New developments in diagnosing and treating diabetic foot infections. *Diabete Metab Res Rev*, **24** (Suppl. 1): S66–71.

74. Foster A, McColgan M and Edmonds M (1989) Should oral antibiotics be given to 'clean' foot ulcers with no cellulites? *Diabetic Medicine*, **15** (Suppl. 2), A27 (abstract).

75. Porter M. (1999) Making sense of dressings. *Wound Management*, **2**, 10–12.

76. Knowles EA (2006) Dressings: is that an evidenced-base? In: AJM Boulton, PR Cavanagh and G Rayman (eds) *The Foot in Diabetes*. John Wiley & Sons, Chichester, 4th edn, pp. 186–97.

77. Krupski WC, Reilly LM, Perez S, Moss KM, Crombleholme PA and Rapp JH (1991) A prospective randomized trial of autologous platelet-derived wound healing factors for the treatment of chronic nonhealing wounds: A preliminary report. *Journal of Vascular Surgery*, **14**, 526–36.

78. Young MJ (1999) Becaplermin and its role in healing neuropathic diabetic foot ulcers. *The Diabetic Foot*, **2**, 105–7.

79. Gentzkow GD, Iwasaki SD, Hershon KS *et al.* (1996) Use of Dermagraft, a cultured human dermis, to treat diabetic foot ulcers. *Diabetes Care*, **19**, 350–2.

80. Lavery LA, Armstrong DG, Peters EJ and Lipsky BA (2007) Probe to bone tests for diagnosing diabetic foot osteomyelitis: reliable or relic? *Diabetes Care*, **30**, 270–4.

81. Pittet D, Wyssa B, Clavel C, Kursteiner K, Vaucher J and Lew PD (1999) Outcome of diabetic foot infections treated conservatively; a retrospective cohort study with long term follow up. *Archives of Internal Medicine*, **159**, 851–6.

82. McKeown KC (1994) The history of the diabetic foot. In: AJM Boulton, H Connor and PR Cavanagh (eds) *The Foot in Diabetes*, 2nd edn. John Wiley & Sons, Chichester, pp. 5–14.

83. Wolfle KB, Bruijnen H, Loeprecht H *et al.* (2003). Graft patency in clinical outcome of femoro-distal arterial reconstruction in diabetic and non-diabetic patients: results of a multicentre comparative analysis. *Eur J Vasc Endovasc Surg*, **25**, 229–34.

84. Bowling FL, Salgami EV and Boulton AJM (2007) Larval therapy: a novel treatment in eliminating methacillin-resistant *Staphylococcus aureus* from diabetic foot ulcers. *Diabetes Care*, **30**, 370–1.

85. Hunt JA (1992) Foot infections are rarely due to a single microorganism. *Diabetic Medicine*, **9**, 749–52.

86. Edmonds M, Foster A, Greenhill M, Sinha J, Philpott-Howard J and Salisbury J (1992) Acute septic vasculitis not diabetic microangiopathy leads to digital necrosis in the neuropathic foot. *Diabetic Medicine*, **9** (Suppl. 1), 85.

87. Bolia A (2006) Interventional radiology in the diabetic foot. In: AJM Boulton, PR Cavanagh and G Rayman (eds) *The Foot in Diabetes*, 4th edition, John Wiley & Sons, Chichester, pp. 238–49.

88. Mansell PI, Gregson R and Allison SP (1992) An audit of lower limb angioplasty in diabetic patients. *Diabetic Medicine*, **9**, 84–90.

89. Palmaz JC, Laborde JC and Rivera FJ (1992) Stenting of the iliac arteries with the Palmaz stent: experience from a multicentre trial. *Cardiovascular Interventional Radiology*, **15**, 291–7.

90. Estes JM and Pomposelli FB (1996) Lower extremity arterial reconstruction in patients with diabetes mellitus. *Diabetic Medicine*, **13** (Suppl. 1), S43–57.

91. Gibbons GW (1994) Vascular surgery: its role in foot salvage. In: AJM Boulton, H Connor and PR Cavanagh (eds) *The Foot in Diabetes*. John Wiley & Sons, Chichester, pp. 177–90.

92. Sigurdsson HH, Macaulay EM, McHardy KC and Cooper GG (1999) Long-term outcome of infra-inguinal bypass for limb salvage: are we giving diabetic patients a fair deal? *Practical Diabetes International*, **16**, 204–6.

93. Cheshire NJW, Wolfe JHN, Noone MA, Davies BA and Drummond M (1992) The economics of femoro-crural reconstruction for critical leg ischaemia with and without autologous vein. *Journal of Vascular Surgery*, **15**, 167–75.

94. Pomposelli JB, Jepson SJ, Gibbons GW, Campbell DR, Freeman DV, Miller A and LoGerfo FW (1991) A flexible approach to infra-popliteal vein grafts in patients with diabetes mellitus. *Archives of Surgery*, **126**, 724–9.

95. Hirsch IB and White PF (1988) Medical management of surgical patients with diabetes. In: ME Levin and LW O'Neal (eds) *The Diabetic Foot*. CV Mosby, St Louis, pp. 423–32.

96. Bartlett FF, Gibbons GW and Wheelcock FC (1986) Aortic reconstruction for occlusive disease: comparable results in diabetics. *Archives of Surgery*, **121**, 1150–3.

97. Abbott CA, Carrington AL and Boulton AJM (1996) Reduced bilateral amputation rate in diabetic patients: effect of a foot care clinic. *Diabetic Medicine*, **13** (Suppl. 7), S45.

98. Sinha S, Munichoodappa CS and Kozak GP. Neuroarthropathy (Charcot joints) in diabetes mellitus. *Medicine (Baltimore)*, **51**, 191–210.

99. Cofield RH, Morrison MJ and Beabout JW (1983) Diabetic neuroarthropathy in the foot: patient characteristics and patterns of radiographic change. *Foot and Ankle*, **4**, 15–22.

100. Sammarco GJ (1991) Diabetic arthropathy. In: GJ Sammarco (ed.) *The Foot In Diabetes*. Lea & Febiger, Philadelphia.

101. Gazis A, Pound N, Macfarlane RM *et al.* (2004) Mortality in patients with diabetic neuropathic osteoarthropathy (Charcot foot). *Diabetic Med*, **21**, 1243–6.

102. Jeffcoate WJ (2008) Charcot neuroarthropathy. *Diabete Metab Res Rev*, **24** (Suppl. 1): S58–61.

103. Marshall A, Young MJ and Boulton AJM (1993) The neuropathy of patients with Charcot feet: is there a specific deficit? *Diabetic Medicine*, **10** (Suppl. 1), 101.

104. Edelman SV, Kosofsky EM, Paul RA and Kozak GP (1987) Neuro-osteoarthropathy (Charcot's joints) in diabetes mellitus following revascularisation surgery: three case reports and a review of the literature. *Archives of Internal Medicine*, **147**, 1504–8.

105. Edmonds ME, Clarke MB, Newton S, Barrett J and Watkins PJ (1985) Increased uptake of bone radiopharmaceutical in diabetic neuropathy. *Quarterly Journal of Medicine*, **57**, 843–55.

106. Jeffcoate WJ, Game F and Cavanagh PR (2005). The role of pro-inflammatory cytokines in the cause of neuropathic osteoarthropathy (acute Charcot foot) in diabetes. *Lancet*, **366**, 2058–61.

107. Eichenholtz SN (1966) *Charcot Joints*. Charles C. Thomas, Springfield, IL.

108. Gazis A, Macfarlane RM and Jeffcoate WJ (2000) Delay in diagnosis of the Charcot foot. *Diabetic Medicine*, **17** (Suppl. 1), 80.

109. Lesko P and Maurer RC (1989) Talonavicular dislocations and midfoot arthropathy in neuropathic diabetic feet: natural course and principles of treatment. *Clinical Orthopaedics*, **240**, 226.

110. Young MJ (1999) The management of neurogenic arthropathy – A tale of two Charcots. *Diabetes Metabolism Research and Reviews*, **15**, 59–64.

111. Sanders LJ and Frykberg RG (1991) Diabetic neuropathic osteo- arthropathy: the Charcot foot. In: RG Frykberg (ed.) *The High Risk Foot in Diabetes*. Churchill Livingstone, New York, pp. 297–338.

112. Salamon M and Saltzman CL (2006) The operative treatment of Charcot neuroarthropathy of the foot and ankle. In: AJM Boulton (ed.) *The Foot in Diabetes*. John Wiley & Sons, Chichester, pp. 274–84.

113. Selby PL, Young MJ and Boulton AJM (1994) Pamidronate in the treatment of diabetic Charcot neuroarthropathy. *Diabetic Medicine*, **11**, 28–31.

114. Jude EB, Selby PL, Burgess J *et al.* (2001). Bisphosphonates in the treatment of Charcot neuroarthropathy: a double-blind randomised controlled trial. *Diabetologia*, **44**, 2032–7.

10

Diabetic Neuropathy

Solomon Tesfaye

University of Sheffield, Royal Hallamshire Hospital, Sheffield Teaching Hospitals
NHS Foundation Trust, Sheffield, UK

Key messages

- Diabetic neuropathy may affect up to 30% of all people with diabetes, and is the main initiating factor for foot ulceration and amputation.
- The detection of neuropathy in a patient with diabetes should not prevent the usual screening for other causes of neuropathy.

10.1 Introduction

Diabetic neuropathy is a common complication of diabetes and a cause of considerable morbidity and increased mortality. Diabetic neuropathy encompasses several neuropathic syndromes, the most common of which is diabetic peripheral neuropathy (DPN), the main initiating factor for foot ulceration. Some patients with peripheral neuropathy may experience troublesome neuropathic pain that is difficult to treat. DPN is also associated with autonomic neuropathy that can involve almost all the systems of the body and may have devastating consequences, such as sudden death.

10.2 Epidemiology

Both, clinic- and population-based studies show surprisingly similar prevalence rates for DPN, as affecting approximately 30% of all diabetic people [1]. The EURODIAB Prospective Complications Study, which involved the examination of 3250 type 1 diabetes patients, from 16 European countries, found a prevalence rate of 28% for DPN at baseline [2]. The study also showed that, over a 7-year period, about one-quarter of type 1 diabetic patients developed DPN, with age, duration of diabetes and poor glycaemic control being major factors [3]. The development of neuropathy was also associated with potentially modifiable cardiovascular risk factors such as hypertension, hyperlipidaemia, obesity and cigarette smoking [3]. Based on recent epidemiological studies, correlates of DPN include increasing age, increasing duration of diabetes, poor glycaemic control, retinopathy, albuminuria and vascular risk factors [3].

10.3 Classification of diabetic polyneuropathy

Figure 10.1 shows a modified clinical classification of diabetic polyneuropathy originally suggested by Thomas [4]. Attempts at classification stimulate thought as to the aetiology of the various syndromes, and also assist in the planning of management strategy for the patient.

10.4 Diabetic peripheral neuropathy (DPN)

This is by far the most common neuropathic syndrome encountered in clinical practice. The sensory symptoms

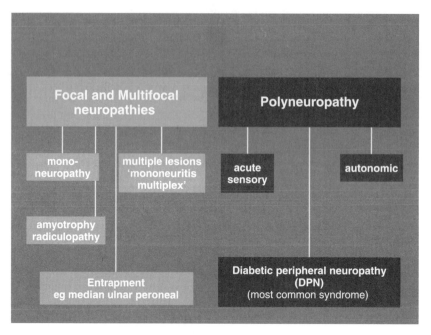

Figure 10.1   Classification of diabetic polyneuropathy [4].

start in the toes and then extend to involve the feet and legs in a stocking distribution. Once the disease is established in the lower limbs, the upper limbs also become involved, with a similar progression that starts in the fingers. There is an associated autonomic neuropathy that is often detectable by autonomic function tests; however, clinically overt autonomic neuropathy is less common.

The main clinical presentation of DPN is a sensory loss which the patient may not be aware of; it may be described as 'numbness' or 'dead feeling'. As the disease advances, motor manifestations such as wasting of the small muscles of the hands and limb weakness become apparent. Some patients may experience a progressive build-up of unpleasant sensory symptoms [5] in the lower limbs, including tingling (paraesthesiae), burning pain; shooting pains, lancinating pains, contact pain (allodynia) and aching pain. Occasionally, the pain can extend above the feet and may involve the whole of the legs, and when this is the case there is usually involvement also of the upper limbs.

Painful diabetic neuropathy is characteristically more severe at night, and often disturbs sleep [6]. It also has a major impact on functionality (e.g., ability to maintain work), mood and the quality of life. Depressive symptoms as a result of the unremitting pain are common [7].

It is a great paradox that subjects with painful neuropathy may at the same time have a severe absence of sensation, the so-called 'painful-painless foot' [8]. DPN is indeed the main initiating risk factor for foot ulceration and amputation. This underpins the need for careful examination and screening of the feet of all diabetic people, in order to identify those at risk of developing foot ulceration. This is particularly important in the elderly, as many live alone (are socially isolated), are immobile and have poor vision. The insensate foot is at risk of developing mechanical and thermal injuries, and patients must therefore be warned about these and given appropriate advice with regard to foot care. In those with advanced neuropathy, there may be *sensory ataxia*. The unfortunate sufferer is affected by unsteadiness on walking and even falls, particularly in the elderly and those with poor vision.

DPN is usually easily detected by a simple, bed-side peripheral neurological examination [9]. For this, the shoes and socks should be removed and the feet examined at least annually, but more often if neuropathy is present. The most common presenting abnormality is a reduction or absence of vibration sense in the toes. As the disease progresses there is sensory loss in a 'stocking' and sometimes in a 'glove' distribution involving all modalities. When there is severe sensory loss, proprioception may also be impaired, leading to a positive Romberg's sign. Ankle tendon reflexes are lost, and with a more advanced neuropathy the knee reflexes are often reduced or absent. Many of these sensory modalities, including ankle reflexes, are also decreased with advancing age; consequently, a good discriminator for the presence of DPN in old age is the loss of any 'pin prick' sensation.

Muscle strength is usually normal early during the course of the DPN. However, with progressive disease there may be generalized muscular wasting, especially in the small muscles of the hands and feet. Affected patients may have problems with the fine movements of fingers and in handling small objects. The typical clawing of the toes seen in advanced DPN is due to unopposed (because of wasting of the small muscles of the foot) pulling of the long extensor and flexor tendons. This results in elevated plantar pressure points at the metatarsal heads that are prone to *callus formation* and *foot ulceration*. Deformities such as a *bunion* can form the focus of ulceration and with more extreme deformities, such as those associated with Charcot arthropathy [10], the risk is further increased. As inappropriate footwear is the most common form of trauma to the neuropathic foot, any clinical assessment should also include an examination of the shoes for poor fit, abnormal wear, and internal pressure areas or foreign bodies. A summary of the clinical assessment of the diabetic patient for DPN is shown in Table 10.1.

Autonomic neuropathy affecting the feet can cause a reduction in sweating and consequent dry skin that is likely to crack easily, thus predisposing the patient to the risk of infection. The neuropathic foot without peripheral vascular disease is also warm, due to the presence of arteriovenous shunting and distended veins [11].

Table 10.2 Differential diagnosis of DPN.

Metabolic
- Diabetes
- Amyloidosis
- Uraemia
- Myxoedema
- Porphyria
- Vitamin deficiency (thiamine, B_{12}, B_6, pyridoxine)

Drugs and chemicals
- Alcohol
- Cytotoxic drugs (e.g. vincristine)
- Chlorambucil
- Nitrofurantoin
- Isoniazid

Neoplastic disorders
- Bronchial or gastric carcinoma
- Lymphoma

Infective or inflammatory
- Leprosy
- Guillain–Barré syndrome
- Lyme borreliosis
- Chronic inflammatory demyelinating polyneuropathy
- Polyarteritis nodosa

Genetic
- Charcot–Marie–Tooth disease
- Hereditary sensory neuropathies

10.4.1 Differential diagnosis of DPN

Before attributing the neuropathy to diabetes, other common causes of neuropathy must first be excluded. The absence of other complications of diabetes, rapid weight loss, excessive alcohol intake and other atypical features in either the history or clinical examination should direct the physician to search for other causes of neuropathy (Table 10.2).

10.4.2 Acute painful neuropathies

Acute painful neuropathies are transient neuropathic syndromes characterized by an acute onset of pain

Table 10.1 Clinical assessment for DPN.

History	Signs
• *Sensory symptoms*	*Inspection*
• *Motor symptoms*	*Reflexes (ankle reflex unreliable in the elderly)*
• *Assessment of disability*	*Sensory*
• *Exclude other causes of neuropathy*	• vibration
	• light touch
	• Pinprick *(good discriminator in the elderly)*
	• 10 g Monofilament
	Assess footwear

(within weeks) in the lower limbs, and are relatively uncommon. Marked neuropathic pain involving both limbs is invariably present, and often distressing to the patient. There are two distinct syndromes, the first of which occurs within the context of poor glycaemic control, and the second with rapid improvement in glycaemic control.

Acute painful neuropathy of poor glycaemic control

This occurs usually in type 1 or type 2 diabetic subjects with poor glycaemic control, and there is often an associated severe weight loss [12]. Ellenberg coined the description of this condition as 'neuropathic cachexia' [13]. Patients typically experience a persistent burning pain associated with *allodynia* (contact pain). Although the pain is most marked in the feet, it often affects the whole of the lower extremities. As in chronic DPN, the pain is typically worse at night, although unremitting pain during day time is also common. The acute-onset distressing pain often results in depression.

In acute painful neuropathies the sensory loss is usually surprisingly mild, or even absent. There are usually no motor signs, although ankle jerks may be absent. Nerve conduction studies are also usually normal or mildly abnormal. The temperature discrimination threshold (small fibre function) is however, affected more commonly than the vibration perception threshold (large fibre function). There is complete resolution of symptoms within 12 months, and weight gain is usual with continued improvement in glycaemic control with the use of insulin.

Acute painful neuropathy of rapid glycaemic control (insulin neuritis)

The term 'insulin neuritis' is a misnomer, as the condition can follow rapid improvement in glycaemic control with oral hypoglycaemic agents. The author has therefore recommended that the term 'acute painful neuropathy of rapid glycaemic control' be used to describe this condition [14]. The natural history of acute painful neuropathies is an almost guaranteed improvement [14], in contrast to chronic DPN. The patient presents with burning pain, paraesthesiae, allodynia, often with a nocturnal exacerbation of symptoms; depression may also be a feature. There is no associated weight loss, unlike acute painful neuropathy of poor glycaemic control. Sensory loss is often mild or absent, and there are no motor signs. There is little or no abnormality on nerve conduction studies. The

prognosis is good, with usually complete resolution of symptoms within 12 months. The management of painful symptoms is as used to treat chronic DPN.

10.5   Asymmetrical neuropathies

Focal or asymmetrical neuropathies have a relatively rapid onset, and complete recovery is usual. This contrasts with chronic DPN, where there is usually no improvement in symptoms for several years after onset. Unlike chronic distal symmetrical neuropathy, asymmetrical neuropathies are often unrelated to the presence of other diabetic complications. Asymmetrical neuropathies predominantly affect middle-aged/older patients and are more common in men [15]. A careful history is therefore essential in order to identify any associated symptoms that might point to another cause for the neuropathy.

10.6   Diabetic amyotrophy

This syndrome was first described by Garland [16], who noted the presence of progressive, asymmetrical proximal leg weakness and atrophy. Consequently, Garland coined the term '*diabetic amyotrophy*', although this condition has also been named '*proximal motor neuropathy*', '*femoral neuropathy*' or '*plexopathy*'. Both, type 1 and type 2 diabetic patients aged over 50 years are affected.

The patient presents with severe pain which is felt deep in the thigh, but can sometimes be of burning quality and extend below the knee. The pain is usually continuous and often causes insomnia and depression [17]. There is an associated weight loss which can sometimes be very severe, and can raise the possibility of an occult malignancy. On examination, there is profound wasting of the quadriceps, with marked weakness in these muscle groups, although the hip flexors and hip abductors can also be affected. The thigh adductors, glutei and hamstring muscles may also be involved, and the knee jerk is usually reduced or absent. Such profound weakness can lead to difficulty in rising from a low chair or climbing stairs. Sensory loss is unusual, but if it is present it indicates a coexistent DPN.

Other causes of quadriceps wasting, such as nerve root and cauda equina lesions and occult malignancy causing proximal myopathy syndromes (e.g. polymyocytis), should be excluded. Today, MR imaging of the lumbosacral spine is mandatory in order to exclude focal nerve root entrapment and other pathologies. An erythrocyte sedimentation rate (ESR), X-radiography of the lumbar/sacral spine and chest X-radiography and ultrasound of the abdomen may also be required. Electrophysiological studies may demonstrate an increased femoral nerve latency and active denervation of the affected muscles. Levels of cerebrospinal fluid (CSF) protein are often elevated.

The natural history of diabetic amyotrophy is that of gradual recovery, although there is paucity of prospective studies. Coppack and Watkins [17] have reported that pain usually starts to settle after about 3 months, and usually settles by 1 year, while the knee jerk is restored in 50% of the patients after 2 years. Recurrence, on the other hand, is a rare event. Management is largely symptomatic and supportive; patients should be encouraged and reassured that this condition is likely to resolve. Controversy persists as to whether the use of insulin therapy influences the natural history of this syndrome. Some patients benefit from physiotherapy that involves extension exercises aimed at strengthening the quadriceps. The management of pain in proximal motor neuropathy is similar to that of chronic painful DPN.

10.7 Cranial mononeuropathies

Third cranial nerve palsy is the most common cranial mononeuropathy. Typically, the patient will present with pain in the orbit, or occasionally with a frontal headache [18]. Frequently, ptosis and ophthalmoplegia is also evident, although the pupil is usually spared [19]. Recovery occurs usually over 3–6 months. The clinical onset and time scale for recovery, and the focal nature of the lesions on the third cranial nerve identified at post-mortem examination, suggested an ischaemic aetiology [20]. It is important to exclude any other cause of third cranial nerve palsy (aneurysm or tumour) by the use of CT or MR scanning, where the diagnosis is in doubt. Fourth, sixth and seventh cranial nerve palsies have also been described in diabetic subjects.

10.8 Thoracoabdominal neuropathy

Diabetic thoracoabdominal neuropathy (also known as *truncal radiculopathy*) is characterized by an acute onset pain in a dermatomal distribution over the thorax or the abdomen [21]. The pain is usually asymmetrical, and can cause local bulging of the muscle [22]. There may also be patchy sensory loss, and other causes of nerve root compression should be excluded. Recovery is usually the rule within several months, although symptoms can sometimes persist for a few years. Some patients presenting with abdominal pain have undergone unnecessary investigations such as barium enema, colonoscopy and even laparotomy, when the diagnosis could easily have been made via a careful clinical history and examination.

10.9 Pressure palsies

10.9.1 Carpal tunnel syndrome

The patient typically has pain and paraesthesia in the hands, but this sometimes radiates to the forearm and is particularly marked at night. In severe cases a clinical examination may reveal a reduction in sensation in the median territory in the hands, and wasting of the muscle bulk in the thenar eminence. The clinical diagnosis is easily confirmed by median nerve conduction studies, while treatment involves surgical decompression at the carpel tunnel in the wrist. There is generally a good response to surgery, although painful symptoms may relapse more commonly than in the non-diabetic population.

10.9.2 Ulnar nerve and other isolated nerve entrapments

The ulnar nerve is also vulnerable to pressure damage at the elbow, and this results in a wasting of the dorsal interossei, particularly the first dorsal interossius. This is easily confirmed by ulnar electrophysiological studies.

Rarely, the patient may present with wrist drop due to radial nerve palsy after prolonged sitting (with pressure over the radial nerve in the back of the arms), while unconscious during hypoglycaemia, or asleep after excessive alcohol intake.

In the lower limbs the common peroneal (lateral popliteal) is the most commonly affected nerve, and this results in foot drop. Unfortunately, complete recovery is not usual. The lateral coetaneous nerve of the thigh is occasionally also affected with entrapment neuropathy in diabetes. Phrenic nerve involvement in association with diabetes has also been described.

10.10 Pathogenesis of diabetic peripheral neuropathy

Historically, there have been two distinct views with regards to the pathogenesis of DPN. The first view involves the metabolic factors [23] that are primarily important in the pathogenesis of DPN, while the second view contends that vascular factors [24] determine the etiological factors for neuropathy (Table 10.3). Today, however, most authorities agree that the truth most likely lies between the two cases, and that both metabolic and vascular factors are important.

10.11 Autonomic neuropathy

Autonomic neuropathy can affect many systems and result in significant morbidity (Table 10.4) and mortality. Autonomic involvement usually has a gradual onset and is slowly progressive. In the EURODIAB study, the prevalence of autonomic neuropathy (defined as the presence of two abnormal cardiovascular autonomic function tests) was 23%, and the prevalence increased with age, duration of diabetes, glycaemic control and presence of cardiovascular risk factors, in particular hypertension [25].

10.11.1 Cardiovascular autonomic neuropathy

Cardiovascular autonomic neuropathy is a serious complication of longstanding diabetes, and causes postural hypotension, changes in peripheral blood flow, and may also be a cause of sudden death.

Postural hypotension

It is now generally accepted that a fall in systolic blood pressure of >20 mmHg is considered abnormal [25]. Coincidental treatment with tricyclic antidepressants for neuropathic pain, and also with diuretics, may exacerbate postural hypotension, the chief symptom of which is dizziness on standing. The symptoms of postural hypotension can be disabling for some patients who may not be able to walk for more than a few minutes. Severely affected patients are prone to unsteadiness and falls. The degree of dizziness does not appear to correlate with the postural drop in blood pressure. There is increased mortality in subjects with postural hypotension, although the reasons for this are not fully clear.

Table 10.3 Proposed hypotheses of diabetic peripheral nerve damage.

- Chronic hyperglycaemia
- Nerve microvascular dysfunction
- Increased free radical formation
- Polyol pathway hyperactivity
- Protein kinase C hyperactivity
- Non-enzymatic glycation
- Abnormalities of nerve growth

Table 10.4 Clinical consequences of autonomic neuropathy.

Cardiac autonomic neuropathy

- sudden death
- silent ischaemia
- exercise intolerance
- orthostatic hypotension
- foot vein distension/arteriovenous shunting

Gastrointestinal autonomic neuropathy

- gastroparesis
- diarrhoea or constipation

Bladder hypomotility

- urinary incontinence/retention

Erectile dysfunction

Gustatory sweating

The management of subjects with postural hypotension poses major problems, and for some patients there may not be any satisfactory treatment. Current treatments include: (i) the removal of any drugs that might result in orthostatic hypotension, such as diuretics, beta-blockers, anti-anginal agents; (ii) advising patients to get up from the sitting or lying position very slowly, and to cross the legs while doing so; (iii) increasing the sodium intake to 10 g (185 mmol) per day and fluid intake to 2–2.5 l per day (note: care must be exercised in elderly patients with heart failure); (iv) the use of custom-fitted elastic stockings which extend to the waist; (v) treatment with fludrocortisone (starting at 100 μg per day) while carefully monitoring urea and electrolytes; and (vi) in severe cases the alpha-1 adrenoreceptor agonist, midodrine (or occasionally oc-treotide) may be effective.

Changes in peripheral blood flow

Autonomic neuropathy can cause arteriovenous shunting, with prominent veins in the neuropathic leg [11]. The leg vein oxygen tension and capillary pressure are increased in the neuropathic leg due to sympathetic denervation. Thus, in the absence of peripheral vascular disease the neuropathic foot is warm, and this may be one of the factors that cause osteopenia associated with the development of Charcot neuroarthropathy [10].

Cardiovascular autonomic function tests

Five cardiovascular autonomic function tests are now widely used for the assessment of autonomic function. These tests are non-invasive, and do not require sophisticated equipment. All that is required is an electrocardiogram machine, an aneroid pressure gauge attached to a mouthpiece, a hand-grip dynamometer and sphygmomanometer. Reference data for the cardiovascular autonomic function tests are listed in Table 10.5 [26].

10.11.2 Gastrointestinal autonomic neuropathy

Gastroparesis

Autonomic neuropathy can reduce oesophageal motility (dysphagia and heart-burn), and cause gastroparesis (reduced gastric emptying, vomiting, swings in blood sugar levels) [27].

The diagnosis of *gastroparesis* is often made on clinical grounds by the evaluation of symptoms, and sometimes the presence of succusion splash, while barium swallow and follow through, and also gastroscopy, may reveal a large food residue in the stomach. Gastric motility and emptying studies can sometimes be performed in specialized units, and may help with diagnosis.

Management of diabetic gastroparesis include: optimization of glycaemic control; the use of anti-emetics (metoclopramide and domperidone) and the use of a cholinergic agent that stimulates oesophageal motility (erythromycin, which may enhance the activity of the gut peptide, motilin). Gastric electrical stimulation (GES) has recently been introduced as a treatment option in patients with drug refractory gastroparesis to increase the quality of life by alleviating nausea and vomiting frequencies [28]. This service is offered at specialist units.

Severe gastroparesis causing recurrent vomiting, is associated with dehydration, swings in blood sugar levels and weight loss, and is therefore an indication for hospital admission. The patient should be adequately hydrated with intravenous fluids and the blood sugar level should be stabilized by intravenous insulin, while anti-emetics could be given intravenously. If the course of the gastroparesis is prolonged, then total parenteral nutrition or feeding through a gastrostomy tube may be required.

Autonomic diarrhoea

The patient may present with diarrhoea that tends to be worse at night, or alternatively some may present with constipation. Both, the diarrhoea and constipation, respond to conventional treatment. Diarrhoea associated with bacterial overgrowth may respond to treatment

Table 10.5 Reference values for cardiovascular function tests.

Parameter	Normal	Borderline	Abnormal
Heart rate tests			
Heart rate response to standing up (30: 15 ratio)	$\geq$1.04	1.01–1.03	$\leq$1.00
Heart rate (beats/min) response to deep breathing (maximum minus minimum heart rate)	$\geq$15	11–14	$\leq$10
Heart rate response to Valsalva manoeuvre (Valsalva ratio)	$\geq$1.21	–	$\leq$1.20
Blood pressure tests			
Blood pressure response to standing up (fall in systolic BP)	$\leq$10 mmHg	11–29 mmHg	$\geq$30 mmHg
Blood pressure response to sustained hand-grip (increase in diastolic BP)	$\geq$16 mmHg	11–15 mmHg	$\leq$10 mmHg

with a broad-spectrum antibiotic such as erythromycin, tetracycline or ampicillin.

10.11.3 Abnormalities of bladder function

Bladder dysfunction is a rare complication of autonomic neuropathy and may result in hesitancy of micturition, an increased frequency of micturition and, in serious cases, with urinary retention associated with overflow incontinence. Such a patient is prone to urinary tract infections. Ultrasound scan of the urinary tract, in addition to urodynamic studies, may be required. Treatment manoeuvres include mechanical methods of bladder emptying by applying suprapubic pressure, or the use of intermittent self-catheterization. Anti-cholinesterase drugs such as neostigmine or peridostigmine may be useful. Long-term indwelling catheterization may be required in some cases, but this unfortunately predisposes the patient to urinary tract infections and long-term antibiotic prophylaxis may be required.

10.11.4 Gustatory sweating

Increased sweating usually affecting the face, and often brought about by eating (gustatory sweating), can be very embarrassing to patients. Unfortunately there is no totally satisfactory treatment for gustatory sweating, although the anticholinergic drug poldine may be useful in a minority of patients.

10.12 Management of painful diabetic neuropathy

The treatment scenario for painful neuropathy is less than satisfactory, as currently available treatment approaches may not completely abolish the pain [29]. A careful history and examination of the patient is essential in order to exclude other possible causes of leg pain, such as peripheral vascular disease, prolapsed intervertebral discs, spinal canal stenosis and corda aquina lesions [29]. Unilateral leg pain should arouse a suspicion that the pain may be due to lumbar-sacral nerve root compression. These patients may well need to be investigated with a lumbar-sacral magnetic resonance imaging (MRI). Other causes of peripheral neuropathy include an excessive alcohol intake and vitamin B_{12} deficiency. Where pain is the predominant symptom, the quality and severity should be assessed; neuropathic pain may be disabling in some patients,

and an empathetic approach is essential. In general, patients should be allowed to express their symptoms freely without too many interruptions. The psychological support of the patient's painful neuropathy is an important aspect of the overall management of the pain.

10.12.1 Glycaemic control

Today, there is little doubt that good blood sugar control prevents/delays the onset of diabetic neuropathy [30]. In addition, painful neuropathic symptoms may also improved by improving metabolic control, if necessary with the use of insulin in type 2 diabetes, although evidence from controlled trials is missing [31]. Thus, the first step in the management of painful neuropathy is an attempt to improve glycaemic control, where appropriate. Clearly, in elderly patients where there is a significant risk of hypoglycaemia, this may not be advisable.

10.12.2 Tricyclic compounds

Tricyclic compounds are regarded as one of the first-line treatment agents for painful diabetic neuropathy [29], with a number of double-blind clinical trials having confirmed their effectiveness beyond any doubt. As these drugs have unwanted adverse side effects such as drowsiness, anticholinergic side effects such as dry mouth, and dizziness due to postural hypotension in those patients with autonomic neuropathy, all patients should be commenced on imipramine or amitriptyline at a low dose level (10–25 mg, taken before bed), with the dose gradually being titrated as necessary up to 100 mg per day. Caution should be taken in elderly patients and in those with cardiovascular disease; in general, these compounds are also best avoided in patients with documented cardiovascular disease, as an increased mortality has been reported. The mechanism of action of tricyclic compounds in improving neuropathic pain is not fully understood; however, their effect does not seem to be mediated via their antidepressant properties, as they appear to be effective even in those patients in depressed mood [32].

10.12.3 Serotonin noradrenaline reuptake inhibitors

Serotonin noradrenaline reuptake inhibitors (SNRIs), such as duloxetine, relieve pain by increasing the synaptic availability of 5-hydroxytryptamine (5-HT) and noradrenaline (norepinephrine) in the descending pathways that are inhibitory to pain impulses. Duloxetine is now also a first line-agent, and is licensed for the treatment of painful diabetic neuropathy. The efficacy of duloxetine in painful neuropathy has been investigated in three identical trials [33], from which pooled data have shown daily doses of both 60 mg and 120 mg to be effective in relieving painful symptoms. Treatment was found to be effective within a week and this was maintained for 12 weeks. Duloxetine is contraindicated in patients with liver disease. Although nausea is the most common side effect, it is usually self limiting.

10.12.4 Anticonvulsants

Older anticonvulsants, including sodium valproate and carbamazepine, are effective but tend to have more adverse side effects. Gabapentin (and more recently pregabalin) administered at 300–600 mg per day [34] have also been found effective, and can serve as first-line agents for the management of painful diabetic neuropathy. Adverse side effects include dizziness, somnolence and peripheral oedema.

10.12.5 Intravenous lignocaine

Intravenous lignocaine at a dose of 5 mg kg^{-1} bodyweight, with a further 30 min with a cardiac monitor *in situ*, has also been found to be effective in relieving neuropathic pain for up to 2 weeks [35]. This form of treatment is useful in subjects that have severe pain which will not respond to the above-described agents; however, the patient must be brought into the hospital for a few hours during treatment.

10.12.6 Alpha-lipoic acid

Infusion of the antioxidant alpha-lipoic acid, at a dose of 600 mg per day, both orally and intravenously, has also been found to be useful in reducing neuropathic pain [36].

10.12.7 Lacosamide

Lacosamide represents another promising anticonvulsant for the treatment of painful DPN. Whilst, in a phase II study, lacosamide was found to be beneficial in relieving painful DPN, phase III studies are now required to assess the situation [37].

10.12.8 Opiates

The opiate derivative tramadol (50–100 mg, four times daily) has been found effective in relieving neuropathic pain [38]. Another opioid, oxycodone slow release, has also been shown to be effective in the management of neuropathic pain [39]. Recently, combinations of morphine and gabapentin [40], and oxycodone and gabapentin [41], were found to be more effective than either drug alone on its own in the management of diabetic neuropathic pain.

10.12.9 Management of disabling painful neuropathy not responding to pharmacological treatment

Neuropathic pain can sometimes be extremely severe, and interfere significantly with the patient's sleep and daily activities. Unfortunately, those patients who are not helped by conventional pharmacological treatment may pose a major challenge, as they may become severely distressed and are occasionally

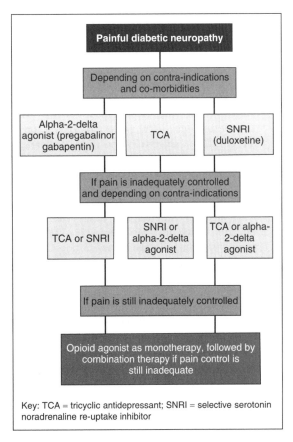

Figure 10.2 Proposed treatment algorithm for painful diabetic neuropathy. (Adapted from Ref. [43]).

wheelchair-bound. Such patients may respond to electrical spinal cord stimulation which relieves both background and peak neuropathic pain [42]. This form of treatment is particularly advantageous, as the patient does not have to take any other pain-relieving medications, with all their adverse side effects.

10.12.10   Treatment algorithm

A recent consensus meeting carefully evaluated the trial evidence for the various pharmacological treatments for painful DPN, and suggested a treatment algorithm [43] (Figure 10.2). It must be emphasized that, as all of the pharmacological agents used have adverse side effects, the drugs must be commenced at the smallest doses and gradually increased in order to minimize such problems. This is particularly important in elderly patients who are prone to falls and often live alone.

References

1. Ziegler D. Diagnosis, staging and epidemiology of diabetic peripheral neuropathy. Diab Nutr Metab 1994; 7: 342–8.
2. Tesfaye S, Stephens L, Stephenson J, Fuller J, Platter ME, Ionescu-Tirgoviste C and Ward JD. The prevalence of diabetic neuropathy and its relation to glycaemic control and potential risk factors: the EURODIAB IDDM Complications Study. Diabetologia 1996; 39: 1377–84.
3. Tesfaye S, Chaturvedi N, Eaton SEM, Witte D, Ward JD and Fuller J. Vascular risk factors and diabetic neuropathy. New Engl J Med 2005; 352: 341–50.
4. Thomas PK. Metabolic neuropathy. J Roy Coll Phys (Lond) 1973; 7: 154–74.
5. Tesfaye S. Diabetic neuropathy: achieving best practice. Br J Vasc Dis 2003; 3: 112–17.
6. Tesfaye S and Price D. (1997) Therapeutic approaches in diabetic neuropathy and neuropathic pain. In: AJM Boulton (ed). *Diabetic Neuropathy*. Marius Press, Carnforth, pp. 159–81.
7. Quattrini C and Tesfaye S. Understanding the impact of painful diabetic neuropathy. Diabetes Metab Res Rev 2003; 19 (Suppl. 1), S1–8.
8. Ward JD. The diabetic leg. Diabetologia 1982; 22: 141–7.
9. Eaton SEM and Tesfaye S. Clinical manifestations and measurement of somatic neuropathy. Diabetes Reviews 1999; 7: 312–25.
10. Rajbhandari SM, Jenkins R, Davies C and Tesfaye S. Charcot neuroarthropathy in diabetes mellitus. Diabetologia 2002; 45; 1085–96.
11. Ward JD, Simms JM, Knight G, Boulton AJM and Sandler DA. Venous distension in the diabetic neuropathic foot (physical sign of arterio-venous shunting). J Roy Soc Med 1983; 76: 1011–14.
12. Archer AG, Watkins PJ, Thomas PJ, Sharma AK and Payan J. The natural history of acute painful neuropathy in diabetes mellitus. J Neurol Neurosurg Psychiatr 1983; 46: 491–6.
13. Ellenberg M. Diabetic neuropathic cachexia. Diabetes 1974; 23: 418–23.
14. Tesfaye S, Malik R, Harris N, Jakubowski J, Mody C, Rennie IG and Ward JD. Arteriovenous shunting and proliferating new vessels in acute painful neuropathy of rapid glycaemic control (insulin neuritis). Diabetologia 1996; 39: 329–35.
15. Matikainen E and Juntunen J. Diabetic neuropathy: Epidemiological, pathogenetic, and clinical aspects with special emphasis on type 2 diabetes mellitus. Acta Endocrinol Suppl. (Copenh) 1984; 262: 89–94.
16. Garland H. Diabetic amyotrophy. Br Med J 1955; 2: 1287–90.
17. Coppack SW and Watkins PJ. The natural history of femoral neuropathy. Q J Med 1991; 79: 307–13.
18. Asbury AK, Aldredge H, Hershberg R and Fisher CM. Oculomotor palsy in diabetes mellitus: a clinicopathological study. Brain 1970; 93: 555–7.
19. Leslie RDG and Ellis C. Clinical course following diabetic ocular palsy. Postgrad Med J 1978; 54: 791–2.
20. Dreyfuss PM, Hakim S and Adams RD. Diabetic ophthalmoplegia. Archives of Neurology and Psychiatry 1957; 77: 337–49.
21. Ellenberg M. Diabetic truncal mononeuropathy - a new clinical syndrome. Diabetes Care 1978; 1: 10–13.
22. Boulton AJM, Angus E, Ayyar DR and Weiss R. Diabetic thoracic polyradiculopathy presenting as abdominal swelling. Br Med J 1984; 289: 798–9.
23. Stevens MJ, Feldman EL, Thomas T and Greene DA. (1998) Pathogenesis of diabetic neuropathy. In: A. Veves (ed.) *Contemporary Endocrinology: Clinical Management of Diabetic Neuropathy*. Humana Press, Totowa NJ, pp. 13–48.
24. Cameron NE, Eaton SE, Cotter MA and Tesfaye S. Vascular factors and metabolic interactions in the pathogenesis of diabetic neuropathy. Diabetologia 2001; 44: 1973–88.
25. Witte DR, Tesfaye S, Chaturvedi N, Eaton SEM, Kempler P, Fuller JH and the EURODIAB Prospective Complications Study Group. Risk factors for cardiac autonomic neuropathy in Type 1 diabetes mellitus. Diabetologia 2005; 48: 164–71.

26. Ewing DJ, Martyn CN, Young RJ and Clarke BF. The value of cardiovascular autonomic function tests: ten years experience in diabetes. Diabetes Care 1985; 8: 491–8.

27. Horowitz M and Fraser R. Disordered gastric motor function in diabetes mellitus. Diabetologia 1994; 37: 543–51.

28. Lin Z, Forster J, Sarosiek I and McCallum RW. Treatment of diabetic gastroparesis by high-frequency gastric electrical stimulation. Diabetes Care 2004; 27 (5): 1071–6.

29. Tesfaye S and Kempler P. Painful diabetic neuropathy. Diabetologia 2005; 48: 805–7.

30. Diabetes Control and Complications Trial Research Group. (1995) The effect of intensive diabetes therapy on the development and progression of neuropathy. Ann Int Med 122: 561–8.

31. Boulton AJM, Drury J, Clarke B and Ward JD. Continuous subcutaneous insulin infusion in the management of painful diabetic neuropathy. Diabetes Care 1982; 5: 386–90.

32. Max MB, Culnane M, Schafer SC et al. Amitriptyline relieves diabetic neuropathy pain in patients with normal or depressed mood. Neurology 1987; 37: 589–96.

33. Goldstein DJ, Lu Y, Detke MJ, Lee TC and Iyengar S. Duloxetine vs. placebo in patients with painful diabetic neuropathy. Pain 2005; 116 (1-2): 109–18.

34. Freeman R, Durso-Decruz E and Emir B. Efficacy, safety and tolerability of pregabalin treatment of painful diabetic peripheral neuropathy: findings from 7 randomized, controlled trials across a range of doses. Diabetes Care 2008 31 (7): 1448–54.

35. Kastrup J, Angelo H, Petersen P, Dejgård A and Hilsted J. (1986) Treatment of chronic painful neuropathy with intravenous lidocaine infusion. Br Med J 292: 173.

36. Zeigler D, Hanefeld M, Ruhnau KJ, et al. Treatment of symptomatic diabetic peripheral neuropathy with anti-oxidant alpha-lipoic acid: a 3-week multicentre randomised controlled trial (ALADIN Study). Diabetologia 1995; 38: 1425–33.

37. Rauck RL, Shaibani A, Biton V, Simpson J and Koch B. Lacosamide in painful diabetic peripheral neuropathy: a phase 2 double-blind placebo-controlled study. Clin J Pain 2007; 23: 150–8.

38. Harati Y, Gooch C, Swenson M, Edelman S, Greene D, Raskin P, Donofrio P, Cornblath D, Sachdeo R, Siu CO and Kamin M. Double-blind randomized trial of tramadol for the treatment of the pain of diabetic neuropathy. Neurology 1998; 50 (6): 1842–6.

39. Watson CP, Moulin D, Watt-Watson J, Gordon A and Eisenhoffer J. Controlled-release oxycodone relieves neuropathic pain: a randomized controlled trial in painful diabetic neuropathy. Pain 2003; 105 (1-2): 71–8.

40. Gilron I, Bailey JM, Tu D, Holden RR, Weaver DF and Houlden. Morphine, gabapentin, or their combination for neuropathic pain. N Engl J Med. 2005; 352 (13): 1324–34.

41. Hanna M, O'Brien C and Wilson MC. Prolonged-release oxycodone enhances the effects of existing gabapentin therapy in painful diabetic neuropathy patients. Eur J Pain 2008; 12 (6): 804–13.

42. Tesfaye S, Watt J, Benbow SJ, Pang KA, Miles J and MacFarlane IA. Electrical spinal cord stimulation for painful diabetic peripheral neuropathy. Lancet 1996; 348: 1698–701.

43. Jensen TS, Backonja MM, Hernandez Jimenez S, Tesfaye S, Valensi P and Ziegler D. New perspectives on the management of diabetic peripheral neuropathic pain. Diab Vasc Dis Res 2006; 3: 108–19.

11

Erectile Dysfunction

Tamás Várkonyi[1] and Peter Kempler[2]
[1]*I. Department of Medicine, University of Szeged, Szeged, Hungary*
[2]*I. Department of Medicine, Semmelweis University, Budapest, Hungary*

Key messages

- Several complications and concomitant conditions of diabetes are regarded as risk factors of erectile dysfunction.
- The cardiovascular risk of diabetic men with erectile dysfunction must be assessed by the application of the Princeton guidelines.
- Trials with phosphodiesterase type 5 inhibitors in diabetic patients have demonstrated an improvement of erectile dysfunction, without reporting any increased mortality or high frequency of cardiovascular adverse events.

11.1 Introduction

11.1.1 Definition of erectile dysfunction

In 1993, the idiom of impotence was replaced by the term erectile dysfunction (ED) which, according to the NIH Consensus Development Panel, is defined as the '...persistent inability to achieve or maintain an erection sufficient for satisfactory sexual intercourse' [1].

11.1.2 Prevalence of erectile dysfunction

The reported prevalence of ED among the general population ranges from 19 to 52% [2, 3], this span being due most likely to differences in the criteria used to define ED, and also to the lack of systematic stratification by age. In the Massachusetts Male Aging Study, ED to some degree was found in 52% of adult men between the ages of 40 and 70 years [4]. Approximately 35–75% of men with diabetes mellitus have ED [5], and in these cases the ED has been shown to occur 5–10 years earlier than in age-matched control subjects [6]. In a study of 541 men with diabetes conducted at a community-based clinic, the prevalence of ED was seen to increase progressively with age, from 6% in men aged 20–24 years to 52% in those aged 55–59 years [7].

Among a cohort of patients with longstanding type 1 diabetes mellitus ($\geq$10 years), ED was reported in 1.1% of men aged 21–30 years, in 55% of men aged 50–60 years, and in 75% of those aged >60 years [8]. The prevalence and risk factors of diabetic complications were assessed in 3250 type 1 diabetic subjects in 31 centers as part of the EURODIAB IDDM Complications Study; the data relating to ED are listed in Table 11.1 [9]. The range of responses given to various questions regarding ED varied enormously among centres, from 2% to 85%. The similarity of patterns of answers at some centres suggested that cultural and personal attitudes did not allow patients and their doctors to communicate in such a way that the true prevalence could be ascertained. This might indicate that, in some centres, it was not possible for patients with ED to discuss their problems [9].

Diabetes in Old Age. Third Edition. Edited by Alan J. Sinclair
© 2009 John Wiley & Sons, Ltd

Table 11.1 The prevalence of erectile dysfunction in the EURODIAB IDDM complications study.

Complication	Proportion of patients (range) (%)
Problems with intercourse	16 (2–35)
Problems obtaining an erection	16 (2–85)
Problems sustaining an erection	18 (2–83)
No erections at night or in the morning	35 (23–84)

11.2 Erectile dysfunction: An observable marker of diabetes mellitus?

Using a nationally representative managed care claims database from 51 health plans and 28 million members in the United States, a retrospective cohort study was conducted to compare the prevalence rates of diabetes mellitus between men with ED (285 436) and men without ED (1 584 230) between 1995 and 2001 [10]. Logistic regression models were used to isolate the effect of ED on the likelihood of having diabetes mellitus with adjustment for age, region and seven concurrent diseases. The diabetes mellitus prevalence rates were 20.0% in men with ED, and 7.5% in men without ED; with adjustment for age, region and concurrent diseases, the odds ratio of having diabetes mellitus between men with ED and without ED was 1.60 (p < 0.0001). With adjustment for regions and concurrent diseases, the age-specific odds ratios ranged from 2.94 (p < 0.0001, age 26–35 years) to 1.05 (p = 0.1717, age 76–85 years). In summary, men with ED were more than twice as likely to have diabetes mellitus as men without ED. The authors concluded that ED should be considered as an observable marker of diabetes mellitus, strongly so for men aged ≤45 years, and likely for men aged 46–65 years, but was not a marker for men aged ≥66 years.

11.3 Risk factors of erectile dysfunction

As part of a prospective epidemiological survey – the Rancho Bernardo Study – common coronary artery disease (CAD) risk factors (age, smoking, hyperten-

sion, diabetes mellitus, hypercholesterolaemia, hypertriglyceridaemia and obesity) were examined in 570 community-dwelling men, aged 30–69 years (mean age 46 years) [11]. After an average follow-up period of 25 years, incident ED was evaluated using the five-item International Index of Erectile Function. The results showed that age, body mass index (BMI) and hypercholesterolaemia were each significantly associated with an increased risk of ED. Overall, one in five men had three or more risk factors and were at a 2.2-fold increased risk of ED [11].

When assessing the risk factors of ED in men visiting outpatient clinics, 86% of those with ED had one or more chronic disease. ED was present in 70–3% of men with coronary heart disease, in 67.8% of those with hypertension, in 78% of those with diabetes, and in 70.5% of patients with psychiatric diseases [12].

Some aspects of the metabolic syndrome are associated with ED, although it is not clear whether the risk of ED when all components of the syndrome are present is greater than the risk associated with each of its components independently [5]. The results of cross-sectional studies have shown that men with a BMI >28.7 have a 30% higher risk for ED than those with a normal BMI (≥25) [13]. The prevalence of obesity and associated vascular risk factors in men reporting symptoms of ED is remarkably high [14, 15].

In order to study whether men with ED were more likely to have hypertension than those without ED, hypertension prevalence rates were assessed among 285 436 men with ED, and also in 1 584 230 men without ED [16]. The prevalence of hypertension was seen to be 41.2% in men with ED, and 19.2% in those without ED. After controlling for subject age, census region and nine concurrent diseases, the odds ratio (OR) was 1.383 (p < 0.0001), which implied that the odds for men with ED to have hypertension were 38.3% higher than the odds for men without ED.

Longitudinal data from the Massachusetts Male Aging Study (MMAS) showed that smoking at baseline doubled the likelihood of moderate or complete ED occurring 8 years later (24% for smokers versus 14% in non-smokers) [17].

Overall, epidemiologic studies have provided powerful support for the role of cardiovascular risk factors in ED [17, 18], with diabetes, hypertension and treated heart disease each having been demonstrated as major independent risk factors for ED and cardiovascular disease [17, 18].

11.4 Pathophysiology of ED in diabetes mellitus

Among all chronic diseases, diabetes mellitus appears to have the most substantiated and characterized association with ED (Figure 11.1).

Data obtained from a recent study suggested that ED occurs at a young age in diabetic men compared to non-diabetic individuals. Nicolosi *et al.* found that the frequency of ED in diabetic men (aged 45–49 years) was similar to that in non-diabetic men (aged 70+ years). ED in patients with diabetes has a multifactorial aetiology [19], the main contributory factors being summarized as:

- Hyperglycaemia and increasing age, leading to glycation of the elastic fibres and failure of relaxation of the corpora cavernosa [20].

- Multiple drug treatments associated with ED, including diuretics and beta-blockers.

- Dyslipidaemia.

- Endothelial dysfunction of the sinusoidal endothelial cells, resulting in decreased nitric oxide (NO) release and impaired vasodilatation.

- Peripheral vascular disease resulting in reduced arterial and arteriolar inflow [21].

- Advanced glycation end products, leading to increased amounts of reactive oxidizing substances and reduced NO production [22, 23].

- Failed neural transmission from the spinal cord due to diabetic neuropathy and a reduced production of neuronal NO synthase-reduced levels of neuronal NO release to the cavernosal smooth muscle [24].

- Hypogonadotrophic hypogonadism [25].

11.5 Erectile dysfunction: A first sign of cardiovascular disease?

Evidence is accumulating in favour of a link between ED and coronary artery disease. As noted above, the common risk factors for atherosclerosis are prevalent in patients with ED, and the extent of ED has been related to the number and severity of the risk factors themselves [26]. The prevalence of ED is increased in patients with vascular diseases, such as CAD [27], diabetes [28], cardiovascular disease [29], hypertension [16] and peripheral artery disease [30]. Consequently,

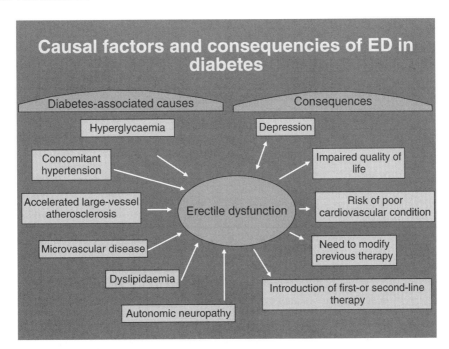

Figure 11.1 Causal factors and consequences of ED in diabetes.

a new onset or a progressive decline in erectile function represent a 'red flag' for possible cardiovascular problems, with ED serving as a 'barometer' of overall vascular fitness. Questions concerning ED should be included in the review of systems for men aged over 30 years, with ED being used as a 'hook' to gain compliance regarding the aggressive management of existing cardiovascular disease. A proportion of men will care more about their current ED than about a future risk of myocardial infarction or stroke. ED is not a clinically silent condition; rather, it may become manifest before other cardiovascular conditions do, and yet appear 'silent' to the health care provider, with many men remaining silent about the symptom unless they are asked.

11.6   The artery size hypothesis: A macrovascular link between ED and CAD

Currently, evidence is accumulating that ED should be considered a vascular disorder. Common risk factors for atherosclerosis are frequently found in association with ED, and the latter is frequently reported in vascular syndromes. Finally, a similar early impairment of endothelium-dependent vasodilatation and late obstructive vascular changes has been reported in both ED and other vascular diseases. Recently, a pathophysiological mechanism has been proposed to explain the link between ED and coronary disease, termed the 'artery size hypothesis' [31]. Given the systemic nature of atherosclerosis, all major vascular beds should be affected to the same extent; however, symptoms rarely become evident at the same time. This difference in the rate of occurrence of different symptoms has been suggested to result from the different sizes of the arteries which supply the different vascular beds that allow a larger vessel to better tolerate the same extent of plaque compared to a smaller vessel. According to this hypothesis, because the penile arteries are smaller in diameter than the coronary arteries, patients with ED will seldom have concomitant symptoms of CAD, whereas those with coronary disease will frequently complain of ED. Available clinical evidence appears to support this hypothesis [31].

11.7   Other causes of erectile dysfunction

Although the vascular diseases and other factors listed above should be considered as the most important aetiological factors of ED, certain other causes should perhaps also be mentioned.

11.7.1   Erectile dysfunction and depression

Quite often, depression will accompany aging, and indeed an association has been identified between diabetic neuropathy and depressive symptoms among diabetic patients [32]. The treatment of ED in depressed patients has been shown to improve the depressive symptoms.

Neurogenic causes of ED include:

* Radical pelvic surgery

* Pelvic/spinal cord injury

* Multiple sclerosis or demyelinating conditions

* Neuropathies

* Pudendal nerve injury

* Stroke, Alzheimer's and Parkinson's disease

The role of afferent and efferent neuropathies is shown in Table 11.2.

Table 11.2   Erectile dysfunction: the role of efferent and afferent neuropathies.

Efferent neuropathy	Afferent (somatosensory) neuropathy
• A result of disruption or dysfunction of parasympathetic efferent neural pathways	• Also called 'dorsal nerve impotence'
• Causes include spinal cord injury, multiple sclerosis, radical prostatectomy, peripheral neuropathy, other neurological diseases	• Caused by polysensory neuropathies secondary to diabetes, vitamin B_{12} deficiency and lead poisoning

11.7.2 Erectile dysfunction and drug use

Erectile dysfunction is very frequently associated with drug use; typical drugs responsible for ED include: antihypertensives [thiazide diuretics, beta-blockers, calcium-channel blockers, angiotensin-converting enzyme (ACE) inhibitors], antidepressants [tricyclic antidepressants, selective serotonin reuptake inhibitors (SSRIs)], anti-arrhythmics (e.g. digoxin), anti-androgens, H_2 receptor antagonists (e.g. cimetidine), recreational/abuse agents, cigarette smoking and cocaine or marijuana.

11.8 Differentiation between organic and psychogenic erectile dysfunction

Psychogenic ED is common is diabetic patients, the aetiology of the condition including anxiety, depression, sexual phobias, stress, direct inhibition of spinal centers and excessive sympathetic outflow. The key differences between psychogenic and organic ED are detailed in Table 11.3.

11.8.1 Diagnostic testing

The prognosis of ED is very important, as ED is considered as one of the most neglected complications of diabetes. According to the findings of a detailed review of 428 charts of male diabetic patients from 10 general practices in the UK, the prevalence of ED was 53%. However, ED was documented only in 8% of cases, while the patient had been informed about possible treatment options in only 1% of cases.

The most important diagnostic tests to be performed in men with ED are summarized in Table 11.4. A comprehensive assessment of the patient's sexual and medical history is of utmost importance; the key components are listed in Table 11.5.

11.9 Treatment of erectile dysfunction in diabetic patients

The unmet need for the treatment of ED in Europe is very high, according to the observations of The Erectile Dysfunction Observational Study. In fact, 66% of patients in nine European countries had experienced ED symptoms for one year or longer when seeking treatment [33]. Diabetic patients seeking treatment for ED have a greater severity of disease, a less-impaired sexual desire, and a more organic than functional origin, which suggests that the need for medical care among diabetic patients with ED could be even greater than in their non-diabetic counterparts [34]. Hence, those doctors participating in diabetes care have an important role to motivate their patients in this behaviour:

Table 11.3 The classification of erectile dysfunction: psychogenic or organic?

Aetiology	Psychogenic	Organic
• Onset	• Sudden onset	• Gradual onset
• Initiation	• Complete immediate loss	• Incremental progression
• Morning erection	• Morning erections present	• Lack of morning erections
• Presence or absence under certain circumstances	• Varies with partner and circumstance	• Lack of erections under most sexually stimulating circumstances

Table 11.4 Erectile dysfunction: diagnostic testing.

Mandatory or routine tests	Recommended tests	Specialized tests
• Comprehensive history (sexual, medical, drug, and psychosocial)	• Testosterone (total, free or bioavailable)	• Nocturnal penile tumescence
• Focused physical examination	• Fasting glucose and serum lipids	• Vascular studies

Table 11.5 Diagnosis of erectile dysfunction: a comprehensive history.

Sexual history	Medical history
• Erectile insufficiency	• Rule out comorbid conditions
• Altered patient or partner sexual desire	
• Ejaculation	• Atherosclerotic risk factors and vascular disease
• Orgasm	• Use of medications/recreational drugs or smoking
• Partner sexual function	• History of surgeries or pelvic/perineal trauma
• Sexually induced genital pain	• Depressive symptoms

in a recent survey, just over half of all men (50.3%) with diabetes considered that their doctor should routinely ask about their sexual health [19]. The therapy of ED in diabetic patients should be approached as first-, second- and third-line options.

11.9.1 First-Line therapy

A crucial part of the first-line therapy is the modification of lifestyle and concomitant drug therapy. The lifestyle should be modified by smoking cessation, limitation or avoidance of alcohol, the application of carbohydrate and fat restrictions in the diet, the achievement of weight loss, an initiation of regular physical exercise and an insurance of an adequate sleep [35, 36]. As diabetic patients take a high number of drugs, the consideration of any potential associations between current treatments and ED should be applied among the first-line interventions. Among antihypertensive drugs, beta-blockers, thiazide diuretics, spironolactones and clonidine should be avoided [37] or replaced (if possible) by ACE inhibitors or angiotensin receptor blockers, as these drugs have no harmful effect on erectile function. Some of centrally acting drugs, such as SSRIs or tricyclic antidepressants, are frequently administered to diabetic patients – particularly to treat chronic painful neuropathy. The detrimental influence of this therapy on ED must be taken into account [38]. Drugs which interfere with the endocrine system may alter sexual function; consequently, histamine H_2 receptor antagonists and metoclopramide must be carefully recommended for diabetic men [39].

Psychosocial counselling and education should be considered as parts of any first-line treatment, as psychological problems such as anxiety, depression and social phobias play an important role in the pathogenesis of ED [40]. It is important to note that this treatment option is not efficient in all diabetic men because there are several severe organic aetiological factors involved in the pathogenesis of ED.

As hypogonadism is a frequent cause of ED in diabetes and obesity, the replacement of androgens is a possible first-line option in these patients. Besides monotherapy in many cases, this treatment is recommended as a combination for those patients who failed phosphodiesterase type 5 (PDE5) therapy alone [41]. The route of testosterone administration can be different [42]; for example, transdermal application involves the use of a gel or scrotal and non-scrotal patches. The intramuscular injection of testosterone cyprionate or enanthate ensures a long-acting effect on ED. Implantable pellets are also available, but these have not yet been used in a high number of patients. Orally administered testosterone is quickly metabolized by the liver, which prevents the achievement of sufficiently high blood levels. The alkylated androgen preparations that are currently available in the United States are generally not recommended because of poor androgen effects, adverse lipid changes and hepatic side effects. In Europe, testosterone undecanoate has also a limited use. Concerns regarding an increased incidence of prostatic cancer, together with cardiovascular risks of testosterone replacement therapy, have led to a cautious consideration of indication and a strict follow-up of the patients because no long-term safety data have been available until very recently [43].

PDE5 Inhibitors

One of the most important first-line therapeutic approaches for ED is an inhibition of the PDE5 enzyme. This results in an amplification of the natural release of intracavernosal endothelial and neuronal nitric oxide in response to sexual stimulation. An abnormally low level of cGMP is increased by delaying the degradation of this molecule; this in turn leads to decreased intracellular Ca levels, producing smooth muscle relaxation in the corpus cavernosum and an increased blood flow [44]. As ED is closely associated with cardiac risk factors in diabetic patients, PDE5 inhibitors should be very carefully considered among those patients with cardiac risk. Notably, the risk categories of patients must be taken into account before these drugs are administered. On this basis, two international consensus conferences on sexual activity and cardiac risk were convened at Princeton University in 1999 and

Table 11.6 The risk categories of the Princeton guidelines.

Low-risk patient	Indeterminate-risk patient	High-risk patient
Asymptomatic, <3 cardiac risk factors	≥3 major cardiac risk factors	Unstable or refractory angina
Controlled hypertension	Moderate, stable angina	Uncontrolled hypertension
Mild, stable angina	Recent myocardial infarction (>2 weeks, <6 weeks)	Recent myocardial infarction (<2 weeks)
Post-successful state of coronary revascularization	Left ventricular dysfunction (NYHA class II)	Left ventricular dysfunction (NYHA class III-IV)
Uncomplicated past myocardial infarction	Non-cardiac sequelae of atherosclerotic diseases	High-risk arrhythmias
Mild valvular disease		Hypertrophic obstructive and other cardiomyopathies
Left ventricular dysfunction (NYHA class I)		Moderate/severe valvular disease

2004, mainly in order to categorize these patients [45, 46]. Three risk categories of patient were identified, based on several very important reports of the consensus panels:

- Patients in the low-risk group included: asymptomatic patients with fewer than three cardiac risk factors; patients in whom the blood pressure is well controlled with more than one antihypertensive medication; patients with mild, stable angina or past revascularization or past myocardial infarction. Patients with a presence of mild valvular disease and left ventricular dysfunction (NYHA functional class I) also belonged to this category.

- Patients at indeterminate risk would require further testing or evaluation before resuming sexual activity. These patients had more than three cardiac risk factors, moderate, stable angina, a history of myocardial infarction of more than 2 weeks but less than 6 weeks, a heart failure (NYHA class II) or non-cardiac sequelae of atherosclerotic diseases.

- The high-risk category consisted of patients whose cardiac conditions were sufficiently severe and/or unstable that sexual activity might pose a significant risk. These conditions included: unstable or refractory angina pectoris, uncontrolled hypertension, congestive heart failure (NYHA class III or IV), recent myocardial infarction (<2 weeks), high-risk, malignant arrhythmias, hypertrophic obstructive and other cardiomyopathies, and moderate to severe valvular disease.

Following the categorization of patients, an algorithm should be followed to create the individualized risk stratification. As a first step of this process, an assessment of sexual function and initial cardiovascular evaluation is recommended. The second step is to initiate or resume sexual activity or to indicate treatment for ED in those patients at low risk. At this phase, the patients at high risk should be stabilized by cardiologic treatment before sexual activity is considered, or the treatment of sexual dysfunction is recommended. Patient follow-up and reassessment at regular intervals are recommended in all cases. The third step involves seeking all risk factors of atherosclerosis in the presence of ED, as this could be the first sign of this diffuse vascular disorder. The risk categories of Princeton guidelines are listed in Table 11.6.

The overall analysis of all randomized controlled trials, in which treatment with PDE5 inhibitors was compared to controls in diabetic patients, demonstrated the improvement of ED in diabetic men without reporting any increased mortality or high frequency of cardiovascular adverse events. The use of PDE5 inhibitors in the presence of oral nitrates is absolutely contraindicated in diabetic men, as in non-diabetic subjects.

Sildenafil Sildenafil was the first PDE5 inhibitor to be developed for the treatment of ED. Sildenafil is rapidly absorbed following oral administration, and has an onset of action within 25–60 min [47]. The plasma half life is approximately 4 h. This action profile provides a spontaneity for patients, since in most of the cases successful intercourse will occur as early as 36 min. The first study in 268 men with both types of diabetes was conducted in 1999, thus establishing the efficacy and safety of sildenafil in this population [47]. The mean scores of the self-administered International Index of Erectile Function reflected significant improvements, and successful attempts at sexual intercourse were fourfold higher in comparison to placebo. Erections were improved by 56% in the sildenafil group, and by 10% in the placebo group, and the frequency of cardiovascular events in sildenafil-treated men was comparable to that in controls.

The first study in type 2 diabetic men included patients with a disease duration of at least 2 years, with similar efficacy data to the previously described study [48]. These investigations showed a more pronounced effect on erection than the previous trial on mixed diabetic men: sildenafil was better in 65% of treated patients and in 11% of placebo-receiving subjects. In addition, the treatment was well tolerated and independent of the degree of glycaemia and presence of neuropathy or vascular disease; this suggested would also be effective in diabetic patients with complications. A study in type 1 diabetic patients [49] also established better mean scores of questionnaires and an improved erection in the sildenafil group, by 66%. The rate of adverse events was low and the sildenafil was effective, irrespective of the severity of the ED. A further study [50] found that men with both types of diabetes had a lower response rate to sildenafil than had been previously reported in large, non-diabetic populations; moreover, a higher rate of cardiovascular adverse events was found than in other trials (7% versus 0%; in comparison with placebo).

Tadalafil   The mean half-life of tadalafil is 17.5 h, and a dose of 10 or 20 mg is well tolerated for up to 36 h. This duration permits once-a-day dosing, such that patients are highly compliant with this regimen [51]. Up to once daily, on-demand dosing was tested for 12 weeks in 191 type 1 and type 2 diabetic men in 2002 [52]. Therapy with tadalafil in this group consistently enhanced erectile function, and also significantly improved the patients' ability to achieve and maintain an erection. The percentage of men reporting improved erections in this study was 56% (10 mg/day) and 64% (20 mg/day). Similar increases in the proportions of positive responses to questionnaires were proven, and tadalafil was seen to be well tolerated in men with diabetes and ED, regardless of the HbA$_{1c}$ level. Interestingly, in this study, those patients taking concomitant antihypertensive medications had greater improvements in erectile function with tadalafil at 20 mg than those not taking antihypertensives. This suggested

that diabetic patients with more severe endothelial dysfunction might derive a greater benefit from the NO-potentiating effect of tadalafil.

A retrospective analysis of the data from 637 diabetic men from 12 placebo-controlled trials provided several conclusions on the effect of tadalafil on ED in diabetes [53]. First, the baseline severity of ED was more pronounced in diabetic men than in controls. Despite the more severe ED, tadalafil efficiently improved all parameters recorded in questionnaires and diaries. This improvement was slightly lower in diabetic men than in non-diabetic individuals, as a similar result was found in studies with the two further PDE5 inhibitors. Neither glycaemic control nor the applied antidiabetic therapy influenced the effect of tadalafil. The sustained efficacy for up to 36 h was evident in diabetic men treated with tadalafil. The adverse event profile observed in diabetic patients was similar to that in non-diabetic patients. An absence of the more frequent serious events of myocardial ischaemia in diabetic patients treated with tadalafil strengthened the previous observation that PDE5 inhibition is safe if patients are categorized by their cardiovascular risk before the indication. Recently, two regimens of tadalafil dosing were compared in 752 diabetic men [54], namely an on-demand treatment and a regular treatment (three times weekly). Although the efficacy measures and treatment satisfaction data reflected therapeutic success for both dosing schedules, the treatment preferences differed, this being 57.2% for on-demand regimen compared to 42.8% for three-times daily regimen.

Vardenafil   Single doses of vardenafil (10–40 mg) are rapidly absorbed following oral administration, with maximum plasma concentrations being achieved in some men within 15 min [55]. A high-fat meal, however, reduces the rate of absorption (similarly with sildenafil), such that the time to maximum plasma concentration is increased to 1 hour. A prospective study in which a large number of diabetic patients (n = 452) was enrolled analyzed the efficacy of the fixed dosing (10 or 20 mg) of vardenafil on ED in Canada and the US [56]. A dose-dependent, clinically meaningful, statistically significant improvement was found in all three primary efficacy measures of erectile function. The success rates were independent of baseline ED severity, the level of glycaemic control, and irrespective of whether patients had type 1 or type 2 diabetes. A study in Germany was designed to evaluate the efficacy of flexible dosing (5–20 mg) of tadalafil in diabetic men [57]. This method of treatment also achieved a significant improvement in several diary questions of the Sexual Encounter Profile. A similar beneficial effect was found in patients with poor, moderate or good glycaemic control. In a study on 778 Japanese diabetic men with ED, it became clear that although both 10 and 20 mg vardenafil doses were effective in improving erectile function, the 20 mg dose demonstrated a superior efficacy compared to 10 mg, which suggested an incremental clinical benefit of using the higher dose in this difficult-to-treat population [58].

As a conclusion of the experience with PDE5 inhibitors in diabetic men, it can be stated that these drugs have improved erectile function for all efficacy variables, to a significantly greater extent than the placebo control [59]. Moreover, this treatment is well tolerated and safe, when following the considerations of the cardiovascular risk stratifications of the Princeton guidelines. As the higher dose results in a greater response in these patients, the higher available dose should be used in these cases. The efficacy is independent of the type of the metabolic disease or the glycaemic control. The differences in clinical applications between PDE5 inhibitors in diabetic men – other than dosage regimens and their efficacy in patients with severe retinopathy or autonomic neuropathy – will hopefully be proven by further studies. The advantages and disadvantages of PDE5 inhibitors in diabetic patients are summarized in Table 11.7.

11.9.2 Second-line therapy

Second-line therapy is considered only in those conditions when the first-line therapy is ineffective or is contraindicated, and involves the intracavernosal, transurethral or intraurethral and topical administration of vasoactive drugs.

Intracavernosal therapy

For the intracavernosal procedure, *alprostadil* or a mixture of drugs are administered. Alprostadil has the same effect with prostaglandin E_1; thus the α_1-blocking properties mediated through a membrane receptor relax the cavernous and arteriolar smooth muscle [60]. Alprostadil produces full erections at doses as low as 2.5 µg. An open-label, flexible dose-escalating study involving 336 men was designed to evaluate the efficacy of this intracavernosal treatment in diabetes [61]. All men were fully trained in the self-injection technique before entry into the home phase, during which a satisfactory erectile response was achieved after 99% of injections, while the median alprostadil dose remained unchanged. Unfortunately, however, 24% of the study group reported penile pain and/or injection-site pain. The concept of the administration of multiple vasoactive drugs is based on the possible synergistic effect derived from the different mechanisms of action that produce the erectogenic effects. In addition, a lower frequency of adverse events is expected as it is not necessary to administer the total dose of the separate drugs. The most frequently used preparation is a three-drug mixture composed of papaverine, phentolamine and alprostadil [62]. Although the response rate to these multidrug mixtures is high, most are not approved by national health care authorities [60].

Intraurethral therapy

The efficacy of intraurethral treatment is explained by a transfer of drug from the urethra directly into the corpora cavernosa. Alprostadil is applied intraurethrally via a special applicator, the Medicated Urethral System for Erection (MUSE). The results demonstrated a successful penetration which occurred at least once during a trial, in 65–70% of patients with MUSE compared to 10–20% with placebo [63]. Although MUSE is more comfortable for most patients than intracavernosal injections, alprostadil is significantly less effective when applied in this way [64]. Both treatment modalities require that the patients be trained at the doctor's surgery before home administration.

Topical therapy

Topical drug delivery represents a simple, reversible, non-invasive, spontaneous second-line treatment option for erectile dysfunction, but the efficacy of this

Table 11.7 Advantages and disadvantages of PDE5 inhibitors in diabetic patients.

Advantages	Disadvantages
• Oral administration	• Contraindicated in males receiving nitrate treatment
• Definitely effective in prospective studies	• Careful risk assessment is required
• Influence on a main aetiological factor	• Dose regimen is different from the general population
• Efficacy independent of glycaemic state or type of disease	• The efficacy in patients with severe diabetic complications is not proven

application must be facilitated by an enhanced degree of skin and tunica permeation [65]. Nitroglycerine, papaverine, minoxidil and alprostadil are administered in this way.

11.9.3 Third-line therapy

Third-line therapy for ED is applied when there is an intolerance or lack of response to other treatment modalities. Two types of rare invasive therapeutic intervention are recognized in this category among the general population of men with ED, namely the implantation of a *penile prosthesis* and *penile revascularization* [62].

A penile prosthesis is chosen when an irreparably damaged erectile tissue is present as a result of a permanent extensive damage of the cavernosal smooth muscle with replacement by fibrous tissue. In this case, the intracavernosal spongy tissue becomes non-compliant and non-responsive to pharmacological stimulation. While this severe organic manifestation is not directly related to diabetes, it can develop as a result of an intercurrent condition (irreversible vascular damage, chronic renal disease, priapism, Peyronie's disease, penile trauma). Both, malleable and inflatable penile prostheses are available, and a high efficacy has been reported. Preoperative psychiatric screening must be performed, however, in order to exclude those patients who will not tolerate the device.

Surgery for penile revascularization has proved not to be efficient among different special populations of patients, and thus is currently contraindicated in diabetes.

11.10 Conclusions

As diabetes represents a very serious risk factor for ED, all therapeutic options should be considered at the initiation of treatment. These most important steps to achieve an effective therapy include a careful exploration of the patient's complaints, the suggestion of a lifestyle change, and the administration of PDE5 inhibitors, assuming a lack of contraindication. One of the most important elements when considering the therapy of ED in diabetic men is to design the treatment individually, with particular attention being paid to the patient's medical, psychiatric and social conditions.

References

1. NIH Consensus Development Panel on Impotence. (1993) *JAMA*, 270: 83–90.
2. Solomon H, Man JW, Wierzbicki AS and Jackson G. Relation of erectile dysfunction to angiographic coronary artery disease. *Am J Cardiol* 2003; 91 (2): 230–1.
3. O'Kane PD and Jackson G. Erectile dysfunction: is there silent obstructive coronary artery disease? *Int J Clin Pract* 2001; 55 (3): 219–20.
4. Feldman HA, Goldstein I, Hatzichristou DG, Krane RJ and McKinlay JB. Impotence and its medical and psychosocial correlates: results of the Massachusetts Male Aging Study. *J Urol* 1994; 151: 54–61.
5. Fonseca V and Jawa A. Endothelial and erectile dysfunction, diabetes mellitus, and the metabolic syndrome: common pathways and treatments? *The American Journal of Cardiology* 2005; 96 (Suppl.): 13M–18M.
6. Romeo JH, Seftel AD, Madhun ZT and Aron DC. Sexual function in men with diabetes type 2: association with glycemic control. *J Urol* 2000; 163: 788–91.
7. McCulloch DK, Campbell IW, Wu FC, Prescott RJ and Clarke BF. The prevalence of diabetic impotence. *Diabetologia* 1980; 18: 279–83.
8. Klein R, Klein BE, Lee KE, Moss SE and Cruickshanks KJ. Prevalence of self-reported erectile dysfunction in people with long-term IDDM. *Diabetes Care* 1996; 19: 135–41.
9. Tesfaye S, Stevens LK, Stephenson JM, Fuller JH, Plater M, Ionescu-Tirgoviste C, Nuber A, Pozza G, Ward JD and the EURODIAB IDDM Study Group. Prevalence of diabetic peripheral neuropathy and its relation to glycaemic control and potential risk factors: the EURODIAB IDDM Complications Study. *Diabetologia* 1996; 39: 1377–84.
10. Sun P, Cameron A, Seftel A, Shabsigh R, Niederberger C and Guay A. Erectile dysfunction – an observable marker of diabetes mellitus? A large national epidemiological study I. *Urology* 2006; 176: 1081–5.
11. Barrett-Connor E. Heart disease risk factors predict erectile dysfunction 25 years later (The Rancho Bernardo Study). *Am J Cardiol* 2005; 96 (Suppl.): 3M–7M.
12. Haczynski J, Lew-Starowicz Z, Darewicz B, Krajka K, Piotrowicz R and Ciesielka B. The prevalence of erectile dysfunction in men visiting outpatient clinics. *International Journal of Impotence Research* 2006; 18: 359–63.
13. Bacon CG, Mittleman MA, Kawachi I, Giovannucci E, Glasser DB and Rimm EB. Sexual function in men older than 50 years of age: results from the health

professionals follow-up study. *Ann Intern Med* 2003; 139: 161–8.

14. Walczak MK, Lokhandwala N, Hodge MB and Guay AT. Prevalence of cardiovascular risk factors in erectile dysfunction. *J Gend Specif Med* 2002; 5: 19–24.

15. Chung WS, Sohn JH and Park YY. Is obesity an underlying factor in erectile dysfunction? *Eur Urol* 1999; 36: 68–70.

16. Sun P and Swindle R. Are men with erectile dysfunction more likely to have hypertension than men without erectile dysfunction? A naturalistic national cohort study. *J Urol* 2005; 174: 244–8.

17. Billups KL, Bank AJ, Padma-Nathan H, Katz S and Williams R. Erectile dysfunction is a marker for cardiovascular disease: results of the Minority Health Institute Expert Advisory Panel. *J Sex Med* 2005; 2: 40–52.

18. Burchardt M, Burchardt T, Anastasiadis AG, Kiss AJ, Shabsigh A, de La Taille A, Pawar RV, Baer L and Shabsigh R. Erectile dysfunction is a marker for cardiovascular complications and psychological functioning in men with hypertension. *Int J Impot Res* 2001; 13: 276–81.

19. Nicolosi A, Glasser DB, Brock G, Laumann E and Gingell C. Diabetes and sexual function in older adults: results of an international survey. *Br J Diabetes Vasc Dis.* 2002; 2: 336–9.

20. Jiaan DB, Seftel AD, Fogarty J, Hampel N, Cruz W, Pomerantz J, Zuik M and Monnier VM. Age-related increase in an advanced glycation end product in penile tissue. *World J Urol* 1995; 13: 369–75.

21. Jevtich MJ, Edson M, Jarman WD and Herrera HH. Vascular factor in erectile failure among diabetics. *Urology* 1982; 19: 163–8.

22. Seftel AD, Vaziri ND, Ni Z, Razmjouei K, Fogarty J, Hampel N, Polak J, Wang RZ, Ferguson K, Block C and Haas C. Advanced glycation end products in human penis: elevation in diabetic tissue, site of deposition, and possible effect through iNOS or eNOS. *Urology* 1997; 50: 1016–26.

23. Burchardt T, Burchardt M, Karden J, Buttyan R, Shabsigh A, de la Taille A, Ng PY, Anastasiadis AG and Shabsigh R. Reduction of endothelial and smooth muscle density in the corpora cavernosa of the streptozotocin induced diabetic rat. *J Urol* 2000; 164: 1807–11.

24. Vernet D, Cai L, Garban H, Babbitt ML, Murray FT, Rajfer J and Gonzalez-Cadavid NF. Reduction of penile nitric oxide synthase in diabetic BB/WORdp (type I) and BBZ/WORdp (type II) rats with erectile dysfunction. *Endocrinology* 1995; 136: 5709–17.

25. Spark RF, White RA and Connolly PB. Impotence is not always psychogenic: newer insights into hypothalamic-pituitary-gonadal dysfunction. *JAMA* 1980; 243: 750–5.

26. Montorsi P, Ravagnani PM, Galli S, Salonia A, Briganti A, Werba JP and Montorsi F. Association between erectile dysfunction and coronary artery disease: matching the right target with the right test in the right patient. *Eur Urol* 2006; 50 (4): 721–31.

27. Solomon H, Man JW, Wierzbicki AS and Jackson G. Relation of erectile dysfunction to angiographic artery disease. *Am J Cardiol* 2002; 91: 230–1.

28. Bortolotti A, Parazzini F, Colli E and Landoni M. The epidemiology of erectile dysfunction and its risk factors. *Int J Androl* 1997; 20: 323–34.

29. Gazzarusso C, Giordanetti S, De Amici E, *et al.* Relationship between erectile dysfunction and silent myocardial ischemia in apparently uncomplicated type 2 diabetic patients. *Circulation* 2004; 110: 22–6.

30. Virag R and Bouilly P. Is impotence an arterial disease? A study of arterial risk factors in 440 impotence men. *Lancet* 1985; 322: 181–4.

31. Montorsi P, Ravagnani PM, Galli S, Rotatori F, Briganti A, Salonia A, Rigatti P and Montorsi F. The artery size hypothesis: a macrovascular link between erectile dysfunction and coronary artery disease. *Am J Cardiol* 2005; 96 (Suppl.): 19M–23M.

32. Vileikyte L, Leventhal H, Gonzalez JS, Peyrot M, Rubin R, Ulbrecht J, Garrow A, Waterman C, Cavanagh P and Boulton AJM. Diabetic peripheral neuropathy and depressive symptoms: the association revisited. *Diabetic Care* 2005; 28: 2378–83.

33. Haro JM, Beardsworth A, Casariego J, Gavart S, Hatzichristou D, Martin-Morales A, Schmitt H, Mirone V, Needs N, Riley A, Varanese L, von Keitz A and Kontodimas S. Treatment-seeking behavior of erectile dysfunction patients in Europe: Results of the Erectile Dysfunction Observational Study. *J Sex Med* 2006; 3 (3): 530–40.

34. Corona G, Mannucci E, Mansani R, Petrone L, Bartolini M, Giommi R, Forti G and Maggi M. Organic, relational and psychological factors in erectile dysfunction in men with diabetes mellitus. *Eur Urol.* 2004 46 (2): 222–8.

35. Rosen RC, Friedman M and Kostis JB. Lifestyle management of erectile dysfunction: the role of cardiovascular and concomitant risk factors. *Am J Cardiol* 2005; 96 (12B): 76M–79M.

36. Jardin A, Wagner G and Khoury S. (2000) Recommendations of the 1st international consultation on erectile dysfunction. In: A Jardin, G Wagner, S Khoury, F Giuliano, H Padma-Nathan and R Rosen (eds). *Erectile Dysfunction*. Plymbridge Distributors Ltd.: Plymouth, UK, pp. 711–26.

37. Richardson D and Vinik A. Etiology and treatment of erectile failure in diabetes mellitus. *Cur Diab Rep* 2002; 2: 501–9.

38. Francis ME, Kusek JW, Nyberg LM and Eggers PW. The contribution of common medical conditions and drug exposures to erectile dysfunction in adult males. *J Urol* 2007 178 (2): 591–6.

39. Lundberg PO and Biriell C. Sexual dysfunction as a suspected drug reaction reported to WHO Collaborating Centre for International Drug Monitoring. *Therapie* 1993; 48 (5): 457–9.

40. Rosen R. Psychogenic erectile dysfunction: classification and management. *Urol Clin North Am.* 2001; 28: 269–78.

41. Shabsigh R, Rajfer J, Aversa A, Traish AM, Yassin A, Kalinchenko SY and Buvat J. The evolving role of testosterone in the treatment of erectile dysfunction. *Int J Clin Pract.* 2006; 60 (9): 1087–92.

42. American Association of Clinical Endocrinologists medical guidelines for clinical practice for the evaluation and treatment of hypogonadism in adult male patients – 2002 update. *Endocr Pract.* 2002; 8 (6): 439–56.

43. Isidori AM, Giannetta E, Gianfrilli D, Greco EA, Bonifacio V, Aversa A, Isidori A, Fabbri A and Lenzi A. Effects of testosterone on sexual function in men: results of a meta-analysis. *Clin Endocrinol (Oxf).* 2005; 63 (4): 381–94.

44. Schwarz ER, Kapur V, Rodriguez J, Rastogi S and Rosanio S. The effects of chronic phosphodiesterase-5 inhibitor use on different organ systems. *Int J Impot Res* 2007; 19 (2): 139–48.

45. DeBusk R, Drory Y, Goldstein I, Jackson G, Kaul S, Kimmel SE, Kostis JB, Kloner RA, Lakin M, Meston CM, Mittleman M, Muller JE, Padma-Nathan H, Rosen RC, Stein RA and Zusman R. Management of sexual dysfunction in patients with cardiovascular disease: recommendations of The Princeton Consensus Panel. *Am J Cardiol* 2000; 86 (2): 175–81.

46. Kostis JB, Jackson G, Rosen R, Barrett-Connor E, Billups K, Burnett AL, Carson C, III, Cheitlin M, Debusk R, Fonseca V, Ganz P, Goldstein I, Guay A, Hatzichristou D, Hollander JE, Hutter A, Katz S, Kloner RA, Mittleman M, Montorsi F, Montorsi P, Nehra A, Sadovsky R and Shabsigh R. Sexual dysfunction and cardiac risk (the Second Princeton Consensus Conference). *Am J Cardiol* 2005; 96 (2): 313–21.

47. Rendell MS, Rajfer J, Wicker PA and Smith MD. Sildenafil for treatment of erectile dysfunction in men with diabetes: a randomized controlled trial. The Sildenafil Diabetes Study Group. *JAMA* 1999; 281 (5): 421–6.

48. Boulton AJ, Selam JL, Sweeney M and Ziegler D. Sildenafil citrate for the treatment of erectile dysfunction in men with type II diabetes mellitus. *Diabetologia* 2001; 44(10): 1296–301.

49. Stuckey BG, Jadzinsky MN, Murphy LJ, Montorsi F, Kadioglu A, Fraige F, Manzano P and Deerochanawong C. Sildenafil citrate for treatment of erectile dysfunction in men with type 1 diabetes: results of a randomized controlled trial. *Diabetes Care* 2003; 26 (2): 279–84.

50. Safarinejad MR. Oral sildenafil in the treatment of erectile dysfunction in diabetic men: a randomized double-blind and placebo-controlled study. *J Diabetes Complications* 2004; 18 (4): 205–10.

51. Porst H, Giuliano F, Glina S, Ralph D, Casabe AR, Elion-Mboussa A, Shen W and Whitaker JS. Evaluation of the efficacy and safety of once-a-day dosing of tadalafil 5 mg and 10 mg in the treatment of erectile dysfunction: results of a multicenter, randomized, double-blind, placebo-controlled trial. *Eur Urol* 2006, 50 (2): 351–9.

52. Saenz de Tejada I, Anglin G, Knight JR and Emmick JT. Effects of tadalafil on erectile dysfunction in men with diabetes. *Diabetes Care* 2002; 25 (12): 2159–64.

53. Fonseca V, Seftel A, Denne J and Fredlund P. Impact of diabetes mellitus on the severity of erectile dysfunction and response to treatment: analysis of data from tadalafil clinical trials. *Diabetologia* 2004, 47 (11): 1914–23.

54. Buvat J, van Ahlen H, Schmitt H, Chan M, Kuepfer C and Varanese L. Efficacy and safety of two dosing regimens of tadalafil and patterns of sexual activity in men with diabetes mellitus and erectile dysfunction: Scheduled use vs. on-demand regimen evaluation (SURE) study in 14 European countries. *J Sex Med* 2006; 3 (3): 512–20.

55. Montorsi F, Salonia A, Briganti A, Barbieri L, Zanni G, Suardi N, Cestari A, Montorsi P and Rigatti P. Vardenafil for the treatment of erectile dysfunction: a critical review of the literature based on personal clinical experience. *Eur Urol* 2005; 47 (5): 612–21.

56. Goldstein I, Young JM, Fischer J, Bangerter K, Segerson T and Taylor T. Vardenafil, a new phosphodiesterase type 5 inhibitor in the treatment of erectile dysfunction in men with diabetes: a multicenter double-blind placebo-controlled fixed-dose study. *Diabetes Care* 2003; 26: 777–83.

57. Ziegler D, Merfort F, van Ahlen H, Yassin A, Reblin T and Neureither M. Efficacy and safety of flexible-dose vardenafil in men with type 1 diabetes and erectile dysfunction. *J Sex Med* 2006; 3 (5): 883–91.

58. Ishii N, Nagao K, Fujikawa K, Tachibana T, Iwamoto Y and Kamidono S. Vardenafil 20-mg demonstrated superior efficacy to 10-mg in Japanese men with diabetes mellitus suffering from erectile dysfunction. *Int J Urol* 2006; 3 (8): 1066–72.

59. Vickers M and Satyanarayana R. Phosphodiesterase type 5 inhibitors for the treatment of erectile dysfunction in patients with diabetes mellitus. *Int J Impot Res* 2002, 14: 466–71.

60. Montorsi F, Salonia A, Zanoni M, Pompa P, Cestari A, Guazzoni G, Barbieri L and Rigatti P. Current status of local penile therapy. *Int J Impot Res* 2002; 14 (Suppl. 1): 70–81.

61. Heaton JP, Lording D, Liu SN, Litonjua AD, Guangwei L, Kim SC, Kim JJ, Zhi-Zhou S, Israr D, Niazi D, Rajatanavin R, Suyono S, Benard F, Casey R, Brock G and Belanger A. Intracavernosal alprostadil is effective for the treatment of erectile dysfunction in diabetic men. *Int J Impot Res* 2001; 13 (6): 317–21.

62. Vickers MA and Wright EA. Erectile dysfunction in the patient with diabetes mellitus. *Am J Manag Care* 2004; 10 (Suppl. 1): 3–11.

63. Ekman P, Sjogren L, Englund G and Persson BE. Optimizing the therapeutic approach of transurethral alprostadil. *Br J Urol* 2000; 86: 68–74.

64. Shabsigh R, Padma-Nathan H, Gittleman M, McMurray J, Kaufman J and Goldstein I. Intracavernous alprostadil alfadex is more efficacious, better tolerated, and preferred over intraurethral alprostadil plus optional ACTIS: a comparative, randomised, crossover, multicenter study. *Urology* 2000; 55: 109–13.

65. Goldstein I, Payton TR and Scechter PJ A double-blind, placebo-controlled, efficacy and safety study of topical gel formulation of 1% alprostadil (Topiglan) for the in-office treatment of erectile dysfunction. *Urology* 2001; 57: 301–5.

SECTION IV
Treatment and Care Issues

12

Metabolic Risk Factors, Obesity and Cardiometabolic Syndrome

Raffaele Marfella and Giuseppe Paolisso

Department of Geriatric and Metabolic Disease, Second University Naples, Piazza Miraglia, Naples, Italy

Key messages

- Metabolic syndrome is a potent indicator of future risk of type 2 diabetes and concomitant increased potential for cardiovascular morbidity and mortality.
- Worldwide, 3.2 million deaths are attributable to diabetes every year – that is 8700 deaths each day, or six deaths each minute. At least one in 10 deaths among adults aged 35–64 years is attributable to diabetes.
- Metabolic syndrome is a common condition, and its frequency is rising dramatically worldwide. At least 45% of people aged >60 years have metabolic syndrome.
- The global increase in metabolic syndrome will occur due to population ageing and growth, and to increasing trends towards obesity, unhealthy diets and sedentary lifestyles.
- A full and healthy life is possible with metabolic syndrome. With good management, many of its components can be prevented or delayed. Medication may be used to control blood glucose, blood pressure and blood lipids. In high-risk subjects, lifestyle changes are much more effective than drugs.
- Optimal health care can substantially reduce the risk of developing cardiovascular diseases.

12.1 The definition of metabolic syndrome

The 'metabolic syndrome', introduced by Reaven in 1988 [1], has been characterized by the simultaneous presence of hypertension, a degree of glucose intolerance, high triglyceride levels and low high-density lipoprotein (HDL) concentrations. The basic abnormalities underlying these alterations have been indentified in resistance of insulin to mediate glucose utilization. In this context, the term 'insulin resistance syndrome' has often been proposed to define this aggregation of risk factors. The syndrome has also been referred to as 'metabolic syndrome', the 'plurimetabolic syndrome' and the 'deadly quartet'. Recently, the National Cholesterol Education Program's Adult Treatment Panel III report (NCEP ATP III) has underlined the central role of this syndrome in the prevention of cardiovascular disease (CVD) [2], Defining this clustering of metabolic risk factors as "metabolic syndrome". This definition suppose that insulin resistance is the primary cause of associated risk factors. However, several other metabolic abnormalities have been associated with the syndrome, including obesity (notably abdominal obesity), high apolipoprotein (apo) B levels, reduced low-density lipoprotein (LDL) levels, and also abnormalities in fibrinolysis and coagulation [3].

Diabetes in Old Age. Third Edition. Edited by Alan J. Sinclair
© 2009 John Wiley & Sons, Ltd

12.1.1 How should metabolic syndrome be defined clinically?

Three health authorities have provided practical criteria to identify patients with metabolic syndrome, however, these criteria differ between organizations [2, 4, 5]. The tools suggested by the NCEP ATP III, the World Health Organization (WHO) and the American Association of Clinical Endocrinologists (AACE) to identify, clinically the metabolic syndrome are summarized in Tables 12.1, 12.2 and 12.3, respectively.

For the NCEP ATP III, when three of the five criteria listed in Table 12.1 are present, a diagnosis of metabolic syndrome can be made. As evidenced in Table 12.1, this guideline considers waist circumference as a criteria to evaluate the level of adiposity, while an explicit demonstration of insulin resistance (IR) is not required.

In contrast, the WHO guidelines view IR, as a required component for diagnosis. In addition to IR, two other risk factors are required for a diagnosis of the metabolic syndrome. Microalbuminuria has been also added to the list as a criterion.

Finally, the AACE criteria seem to be a compromise between the NCEP ATP III and WHO guidelines. Moreover, the number of risk factors required to make the diagnosis of the metabolic syndrome is not specified and left to clinical judgement. Both, the AACE and WHO guidelines have included IR measurements that are beyond routine clinical assessment. Indeed, glycemic alterations derived from an oral glucose tolerance test are included in the risk factors useful to identify the metabolic syndrome.

Table 12.1 NCEP ATP III clinical criteria for the metabolic syndrome.

Risk factors	Defining level
Abdominal obesity, given as waist circumference	
Men	>102 cm (>40 in)
Women	>88 cm (>35 in)
Triglycerides	$\geq$150 mg/dL ($\geq$1.7 mmol l^{-1})
HDL cholesterol	
Men	<40 mg/dL (<1.0 mmol l^{-1})
Women	<50 mg/dL (<1.3 mmol l^{-1})
Blood pressure	$\geq$130/$\geq$85 mmHg
Fasting glucose	$\geq$110 mg/dL ($\geq$6.1 mmol l^{-1})

Derived from Ref. [2].

Table 12.2 WHO clinical criteria for the metabolic syndrome.

Insulin resistance, identified by ONE of the following:
- Type 2 diabetes
- Impaired fasting glucose
- Impaired glucose tolerance
- Or for those with normal fasting glucose levels (<110 mg/dL), glucose uptake below the lowest quartile for background population under investigation under hyperinsulinaemic, euglycaemic conditions

Plus any TWO of the following:
- Antihypertensive medication and/or high blood pressure ($\geq$140 mmHg systolic or $\geq$90 mmHg diastolic)
- Plasma triglycerides $\geq$150 mg/dL ($\geq$1.7 mmol l^{-1})
- HDL cholesterol <35 mg/dL (<0.9 mmol l^{-1}) in men or <39 mg/dL (1.0 mmol l^{-1}) in women
- BMI >30 kg m^{-2} and/or waist:hip ratio >0.9 in men, >0.85 in women
- Urinary albumin excretion rate $\geq$20 µg/ min or albumin:creatine ratio $\geq$30 mg g^{-1}

Derived from Ref. [4].

Table 12.3 AACE clinical criteria for the metabolic syndrome.

Risk factor components	Cutpoints for abnormality
Overweight/obesity	BMI $\geq$25 kg m^{-2}
Elevated triglycerides	$\geq$150 mg/dL (1.7 mmol l^{-1})
Low HDL choleterol	
Men	<40 mg/dL (1.0 mmol l^{-1})
Women	<50 mg/dL (1.3 mmol l^{-1})
Elevated blood pressure	$\geq$130/85 mmHg
2-Hour postglucose challenge	>140 mg/dL
Fasting glucose	Between 110 and 126 mg/dL
Other risk factors	Family history of type 2 diabetes, hypertension, or CVD, polycystic ovary syndrome, sedentary lifestyle, advancing age, ethnic groups having high risk for type 2 diabetes or CVD

Derived from Ref. [5].

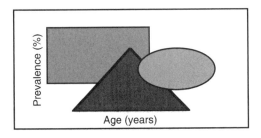

Figure 12.1 Age-specific prevalence of the metabolic syndrome among 8814 US adults aged at least 20 years, by gender. National Health and Nutrition Examination Survey III, 1988–1994. Reproduced from Ref. [6].

These definitions of the metabolic syndrome have allowed to define prevalence of this condition in the worldwide population. Overall, the unadjusted prevalence of the metabolic syndrome was approximately 22% in this US adult population. However, the prevalence increases with age, both in men and women, to reach almost 45% for subjects aged >60 years (Figure 12.1) [6]. Moreover, considering the epidemic of obesity [7], these numbers will increase in the near future. The metabolic syndrome is a rapidly growing threat to public health, and a major challenge that physicians and public health agencies must face.

12.2 Pathogenesis of the metabolic syndrome

The interactions of many susceptibility genes and many environmental exposures play a pivotal role in the pathogenesis of the metabolic syndrome. These considerations are supported by the observations that each component of the metabolic syndrome is regulated through both genetic and environmental factors. Indeed, physical inactivity, combined with an atherogenic diet (rich in saturated fat, trans fatty acids and refined sugars), are responsible for the rising prevalence of the metabolic syndrome. These lifestyle variables, determining obesity as well as insulin resistance, alter the metabolic homeostasis and lead to the multiplex risk factors.

The National Heart, Lung and Blood Institute (NHLBI), in collaboration with the American Heart Association (AHA), have identified three potential aetiological categories of the metabolic syndrome:

- Category 1 = obesity and disorders of adipose tissue.

- Category 2 = insulin resistance.

- Category 3 = a constellation of independent factors (e.g. molecules of hepatic, vascular and immunological origin) that mediate specific components of the metabolic syndrome [8].

The visceral obesity may be responsible for the clustering of risk factors. This hypothesis is supported by the fact that visceral obesity is strongly associated with all cardiovascular risk factors [9, 10]. Therefore, it is possible to define the metabolic syndrome as a cluster of the metabolic complications associated with obesity (more specifically visceral obesirty). Adipose tissue is now recognized as an endocrine organ that secretes numerous proteins which exert a variety of effects [11]. Indeed, hyperplasia and hypertrophy of adipocytes (as seen in obesity) leads to an increased production of leptin, resistin, acylation-stimulating protein and many other proteins, as well as hypertrophic adipocytes produce various proinflammatrory cytokines implicate in the IR and atherosclerotic processs such as tumor necrosis factor (TNF-alpha) and interleukin (IL) 6, and also a decreased production of adiponectin that have a protective effects on vascular health. Through these mechanisms, it is clear that obesity plays a central role in the pathogenesis of the metabolic syndrome. Moreover, this role is also accentuated by the observations that weight loss reducing proinflammatory citokines and leptin improves insulin sensitivity [12]. Indeed, there is substantial evidence that weight loss – particularly the mobilization of visceral adipose tissue – leads to simultaneous improvements of the metabolic profile. Taken together, these arguments place (visceral) obesity at the heart of the metabolic syndrome. Despite these facts, disagreement persists as to whether IR or abdominal obesity is the primary contributor to the metabolic syndrome. It is true that there is a broad range of insulin sensitivity at any given level of body fat, and a large spectrum of obesity at any given level of insulin sensitivity [13, 14]. However, this also means that not all insulin-resistant individuals are overweight, nor all overweight individuals are insulin-resistant. Some investigators place a greater priority on IR by arguing that insulin resistance/hyperinsulinaemic individuals, with or without obesity, are more likely to display the abnormalities of the metabolic syndrome [15]. They believe that IR or hyperinsulinaemia directly causes other metabolic risk factors. Finally, one point of agreement is that IR generally increases with body fat content [14]. It became also evident that central obesity is highly correlated with IR, and consequently central obesity may be a surrogate for IR. It is also clear that both factors can play an independent role in the syndrome, giving their independent effects on cardiovascular risk factors and CVD. Finally, one point is certain, however – that the rising prevalence of metabolic syndrome is a direct consequence of obesity epidemia, which in turn is driven by changeable factors such as high-calorie diets and a sedentary lifestyle.

12.3　Metabolic syndrome in older persons

As noted above, the key player in the metabolic syndrome is IR. Moreover, due to the fact that the aging process is significantly associated with an increase in IR *per se*, older persons with metabolic syndrome must be recognized as a delicate group of individuals with an increased risk of developing type 2 diabetes mellitus and CVD. The aging process is associated with impaired glucose handling, mainly due to a decline in insulin action [16–19]. There is strong evidence that an increased resistance to insulin action is one of the main components of diminished homeostatic glucose regulation in older persons. Insulin-mediated glucose uptake (measured using a glucose clamp technique) was shown to decline progressively with aging [20]. The unifying hypothesis described by Barbieri *et al.* [20], explaining the relationship between IR and age, encompasses four main pathways:

- Anthropometric changes (an increase in fat mass with a parallel decline in fat free mass).

- Environmental changes (diet habits and reduced physical activity).

- Neurohormonal variations, which may have an opposite effect of that of insulin at skeletal muscle and adipose levels.

- A rise in oxidative stress.

Consequently, any one of the individual components of the metabolic syndrome may have a greater clinical importance when present in an older person. Indeed, the management of metabolic syndrome in older persons will lead clinicians to adopt precise measures. However, this approach has not been completely translated

into clinical practice, and many geriatricians claim that the administration of any available medical treatments is still conditioned to a previous diagnosis of specific diseases. Therefore, only new clinical trials aimed at treating metabolic syndrome components in older persons will be required to focus on significant differences when treating older, middle-aged and younger persons with metabolic syndrome.

12.4　Insulin resistance and dyslipidaemia

Increased plasma triglycerides, reduced LDL-cholesterol levels and reduced HDL-cholesterol levels constitute the atherogenic dyslipidaemia of metabolic syndrome. In particular, IR is associated with: (i) hypertriglyceridaemia and a subsequent increase in very low density lipoproteins (VLDL); (ii) small and dense LDL; and (iii) lower HDL levels. Visceral fat seems to have a major role and, indeed, the quantity of visceral fat tissue [measured using computed tomography (CT)], waist circumference and IR are all significantly linked one to another [21, 23]. Visceral fat tissue and IR are known to be at the basis of an increased hepatic production of triglycerides and VLDL, as well as a reduced intravascular breakdown of VLDL and chylomicrons. Under physiological conditions, insulin will inhibit lipolysis and promote lipogenesis. Thus, by promoting the flow of intermediates through glycolysis, insulin will promote formation of the α-glycerol phosphate and fatty acids necessary for triglyceride formation. Insulin then, stimulates fatty acid synthase, thus leading to an increased fatty acid synthesis. At the same time, in the adipose tissue cell, insulin inhibits the breakdown of triglycerides by inhibiting the activity of a hormone-sensitive lipase, the enzyme required for triglyceride breakdown. This enzyme is also found on the luminal surface of the endothelium of capillaries in both adipose and skeletal muscle tissues. However, at the level of the endothelium, insulin increases the activity of lipoprotein lipase, which in turn increases the breakdown of triglycerides in VLDLs as well as chylomicrons; this is an important role in the uptake of free fatty acids (FFAs) from the bloodstream to adipose tissue. As a result, lipoproteins synthesized in the liver are taken up by adipose tissue and FFAs are ultimately stored as triglycerides. During an IR state, insulin action on adipose tissue is no longer effective in repressing the activity of such lipoprotein lipase, and a consequent rise occurs in the plasma concentrations of

FFAs [24]. On the vascular level, a reduced activity of lipoprotein lipase results in a slower catabolism of chylomicrons and VLDLs, and this is clinically expressed as hypertriglyceridaemia. Such triglycerides will be secreted by the liver as VLDL in circulation, thereby creating a vicious cycle. Fasting hypertriglyceridaemia has been identified as an independent risk factor for ischaemic heart disease (IHD) [24]; notably, these authors reported that triglyceride-rich lipoproteins have a different atherogenic potential. In addition to the direct atherogenic effect of triglyceride-rich lipoproteins, high triglyceride levels appear to be a marker of a series of other potentially atherogenic and prothrombotic changes.

The second observation seen in the atherogenic profile during IR is the presence of small, dense and highly atherosclerotic LDLs. The exact mechanisms involved in the formation of small and dense LDL is not completely understood, although the hepatic lipase (HL) enzyme found on the endoluminal surface of hepatic sinusoids appears to have an important role in lipoprotein size and density formation. Hepatic lipase acts specifically by hydrolyzing phospholipids and triglycerides found in HDLs and intermediate density lipoproteins (IDLs), and is also known to hydrolyze phospholipids and triglycerides in LDLs [25]. In particular, it has been shown that the more active the HL, the greater the release of phospholipids and triglycerides, and this results in the formation of smaller and more dense LDLs [26]. Considering that IR is associated with a significantly greater activity of HL, this alteration might explain why a greater concentration of smaller and denser LDLs are found in IR individuals. Furthermore, LDLs in the bloodstream of IR persons have higher concentrations of triglycerides due to the cholesterol ester transfer protein (CETP), an enzyme that transfers triglycerides from VLDLs to LDLs [27], thus forming the perfect substrate for highly active HL (no longer insulin-inhibited) and the formation of smaller and more dense LDLs. Small dense LDLs might be more atherogenic than normal dense LDLs due to the fact that they: (i) are more toxic to the endothelium; (ii) have a greater capability of crossing the endothelial membrane; (iii) have an increased susceptibility to oxidation; and (v) are more selective to bound to scavenger receptors on monocyte-derived macrophages [27].

The third altered lipid profile observed during metabolic syndrome is the occurrence of lower HDL concentrations. The HDL are smaller and more dense during an IR state, and their size is inversely correlated with their triglyceride content – a phenomenon due to an increased catabolism of HDL itself [28]. The higher concentrations of triglycerides in HDL is due to increased activity of CETP, which also transfers triglycerides from VLDLs to HDLs [29]. Consequently, an increased liver lipase activity (this is no longer effectively inhibited by insulin) results in a smaller core volume of HDL and the formation of smaller and more dense HDL. During this phase, apo A-I, which normally is present on the surface of HDL, becomes detached (this can be detected by significantly higher urinary concentrations) [30]. These above changes are especially active during an IR state. Hence, all three altered lipid profiles – hypertriglyceridaemia, smaller and dense LDLs and lower HDL concentrations – constitute the so-called 'atherogenic lipoprotein profile' [30].

12.5 Insulin resistance and obesity

A further component of the metabolic syndrome is obesity, notably the presence of extensive visceral fat tissue. It has been shown in many studies that increased visceral fat is a risk factor for age-related diseases such as hypertension, type 2 diabetes mellitus, CVD and reduced cognitive functioning [31–34]. It is well known that aging is associated with a decrease in lean body mass (especially muscle tissue) and a parallel rise in fat mass [35]. There is a slow, progressive redistribution of fat as the intra-abdominal fat tends to increase while the subcutaneous fat on the limbs tends to decrease. Data have repeatedly demonstrated that intra-abdominal fat is a major clinical parameter associated with IR. Although the mechanisms for the link between IR and intra-abdominal fat accumulation have not been fully elucidated, it has been suggested that a high lipolytic response of visceral adipose tissue to catecholamine exposes the liver to high FFA concentrations, which are known to play a role in IR (see above). Increased adipose tissue present in overweight and obese individuals is no longer considered to be an inert bystander, but rather as an active endocrine organ capable of regulating whole-body metabolism and other vital functions related to inflammation and immune responses [36–41]. These actions are mediated by a number of molecules that are secreted by adipocytes and act in an autocrine, paracrine or endocrine fashion. Among those identified to date are leptin, adipsin, resistin and adiponectin, all of which are believed to adapt metabolic fluxes to the amount of stored energy

[42]. It follows that an understanding of the regulation and expression of such adipokines in older individuals with different body fat density and distribution, may indicate a new target for preventive measures, especially when considering cardiovascular functioning. The deregulation of the adipokine network has been implicated in the etiology of IR and other components of the metabolic syndrome, such as glucose intolerance, obesity, dyslipidaemia and hypertension [43]. In addition, there is a growing list of adipokines involved in the control of pro-inflammatory markers (e.g. TNF-α, IL-6, IL-1p, IL-8, IL-10, transforming growth factor-p, nerve growth factor) and of acute-phase response (plasminogen activator inhibitor-1, haptoglobin, serum amyloid A) [44, 45]. The production of these proteins by adipose tissue is increased in obesity, and raised circulating levels of several acute-phase proteins (as well as of inflammatory cytokines) has led to the view that obesity, characterized by a chronic low-grade inflammatory state, is linked to IR and the metabolic syndrome. An increase in fat tissue, especially in the abdominal area, has also been associated with increased plasma levels of diverse pro-inflammatory cytokines. In particular, the increase in pro-inflammatory cytokines or adipokines include 1L-6, resistin, TNF-α and C-reactive protein (CRP) reflect the overproduction by the expanded adipose tissue. This production supports evidence that monocyte-derived macrophages reside in adipose tissue, and are at least in part the source of cytokine production locally and in the systemic circulation. The magnitude of this vicious cycle remains unknown.

In recent years, much attention has been paid to an anti-inflammatory adipokine, adiponectin, which has also been shown to be involved in the modulation of IR [46] and also to demonstrate anti-atherogeneic effects [47]. Some studies have shown that low concentrations of adiponectin are linked to myocardial infarction [48] and to the progression of subclinical coronary heart disease [48]. Previous studies have shown that the aging process itself is also associated with a deregulation of the inflammatory response [49–51]. Such deregulation is defined by presence of high plasma concentrations of pro-inflammatory cytokines such as, TNF-α, IL-6 and acute phase reactive proteins in older persons [52]. A growing body of evidence has also shown that TNF-α, IL-6 and CRP contribute to age-related IR [50]. In particular, diverse pro-inflammatory cytokine concentrations have been linked to aging, IR and the metabolic syndrome. These cytokines are most likely important in controlling the degree of IR, as their serum levels have been shown to be significantly higher in obese humans.

12.6 Insulin resistance and arterial hypertension

Arterial hypertension, which is another component of the metabolic syndrome, clusters with many metabolic diseases such as obesity, type 2 diabetes mellitus, atherosclerosis and dyslipidaemic states. The association between IR and arterial hypertension was documented some 50 years ago [53], and numerous studies have since been conducted to investigate the association in detail. In fact, one study showed specifically that a strong association existed among hypertension, hyperinsulinaemia and reduced glucose tolerance in a large population of patients ($n = 2475$) [54]. Another study evaluated the ability of hyperinsulinaemia (as a surrogate measure of IR) in predicting the development of coronary heart disease (CHD) and hypertension [55] in a healthy population. Here, it was found that 25% of the population with the highest insulin response (post glucose challenge) had a significantly higher increase in the incidence of hypertension (twofold) or CHD (threefold). Furthermore, the results were found to be independent of any differences in age, gender or body mass index (BMI). Indeed, these results indicated the importance of IR and/or hyperinsulinaemia on vascular disease development over a 15-year time frame. The mechanisms responsible for the relationship between IR and hypertension are multifactorial [56].

First, it is important to note that insulin is a vasodilator when given intravenously to normal-weight subjects [57], but has a vasoconstrictor effect in IR, aged and type 2 diabetes mellitus patients [58]. It is widely known that insulin is capable of stimulating the production of nitric oxide (NO), thus resulting in an increased blood flow, especially in skeletal muscle. Due to the fact that a common pathway exists between the insulin-dependent release of NO and the metabolic actions of the insulin, any altered activity of such a pathway would result in both decreased vasodilatation and a reduced glucose skeletal muscle uptake. In fact, these alterations would explain the presence of an increased peripheral blood flow, especially in skeletal muscle tissue, following an inadequate release of insulin-dependent NO release.

Second, insulin has a direct effect on cardiac muscle tissue [59] by increasing cardiac output and rate through the activity of the sympathetic nervous system

(SNS) [60]. During an IR state, the SNS becomes hyperactive with subsequent peripheral vasoconstriction, increased heart rate and hypertension.

Third, it is widely known that insulin has an anti-natriuretic effect by activating the renin-angiotensin-aldosterone system [57]. Studies have also highlighted a significant and inverse relationship between IR and sodium diet restriction in both normal subjects and in patients with high blood pressure [61]. Therefore, an increased volume after renal sodium retention would contribute to a state of arterial volume-dependent hypertension.

Finally, another possible explanation between IR and hypertension may also be linked to a derangement of cations. The ATPase Na/K$^+$ pump is insulin-sensitive, and thus during IR a significant increase in intracellular sodium (Na$^+$) accompanies a consequent increase in intracellular calcium (Ca^{2+}). During the metabolic syndrome an alteration in the haemostatic system occurs which results in a potentially 'pro-thrombotic state' with severe vascular complications. Three main components of the haemostatic system are activated during an array of vascular tissue injury, including blood platelets, endothelial cells and plasma coagulation factors. During an IR state, such reliability becomes less effective, which shows that insulin is intrinsically involved in the correct operation of such a system. Therefore, any alteration in the insulin signalling pathway has been shown to result in an amplified platelet activation and increased coagulation cascade activity, accompanied by a parallel reduction in fibrinolysis. Insulin receptors are normally present on the surface of blood platelets, and when insulin binds to such receptors the insulin signalling pathway is activated. Various studies have shown that insulin is capable of reducing the platelet response to adenosine diphosphate (ADP), thrombin, adrenaline (epinephrine) and platelet-activating factor, as well as angiotensin II [62, 63]. Furthermore, activation of the insulin signalling pathway also results in lower concentrations of calcium in the platelets. Therefore, a normal insulin action has an inhibitory/regulatory action on platelet aggregation. In an IR state, such equilibrium is lost and a persistent pro-thrombic condition occurs with an increased risk for vascular obstruction. Increased levels of fibrinogen have been associated with IR. Fibrinogen is not only of fundamental importance in thrombin activity regulation, but also has a predictive value for future cardiovascular events [64, 65]. In this context, it is important to underline that pro-inflammatory cytokine production from adipose tissue is known to have a marked influence on the hypercoagulable state by increasing hepatic fibrinogen production, as well as causing endothelial dysfunction towards a hypercoagulable condition. During IR, the simultaneous increase of both tissue factor (TF) and factor VII significantly enhances activation of the coagulation cascade.

12.7 Potential components of the metabolic syndrome in the elderly

12.7.1 Oxidative stress

Recent research has focused on the progressive changes that occur in DNA structure in the metabolic syndrome, and the potential consequences of such mutations. It has been suggested that excess and unopposed oxidative stress is a major cause of the increased mitochondrial DNA (mtDNA) mutations that occur with aging and metabolic syndrome. Oxidative stress is characterized by an uncontrolled production of free radicals that are derived from oxygen and produced by splitting covalent bond into atoms or molecules with an unpaired electron; this results in the formation of highly reactive oxygen species (ROS). Under normal physiological conditions, the intra-mitochondrial environment is characterized by a substantial equilibrium between the production of ROS and the activity of anti-oxidant mechanisms, such as glutathione peroxidase (GSH-Px) and superoxide dismutase (SOD). However, when the endogenous production of ROS substantially increases with a parallel decrease in anti-oxidant agents, tissue damage will occur as result of such oxidative stress. The results of various studies have suggested that the degree of unopposed oxidative stress is also predictive of mortality. In particular, the production of free radicals in the heart, kidney and liver is inversely proportional to the maximum lifespan [66], while the rate of mitochondrial oxygen radical generation is negatively associated with animal longevity. In animal models, calorie restriction also decreases mitochondrial oxygen radical production and oxidative damage to mtDNA and decreasing the rate of aging; some epidemiological studies have also suggested that dietary anti-oxidants might have a significant impact on age-related disease states [67, 68]. The benefits of supplemental anti-oxidants remain unproven in clinical trials.

Oxidative stress also adversely impacts other vulnerable targets, including the lipid and protein components of membranes. Free radicals then allow for lipid oxidation and a consequent reduction in transmembrane transportation. This mechanism of uncontrolled oxidative stress (which is already active in older persons) becomes extremely active during the metabolic syndrome, and the link between IR and endothelial dysfunction may explain, in part, the increased risk for CVD associated with metabolic syndrome. The mechanisms by which IR leads to endothelial dysfunction are certainly multiple and complex. All major abnormalities of the metabolic syndrome, such as hyperglycaemia, hypertension, dyslipidaemia and altered coagulation, are also directly linked to endothelial dysfunction. However, with regard to the link between IR and oxidative stress, it is important to underline recent observations. As noted above, insulin has a direct vasodilatory effect which is mediated through the stimulation of NO production in endothelial cells [69]. During an IR state, the ability to stimulate NO becomes limited, while at the same time an increase in ROS, such as superoxide, occurs. Pro-inflammatory cytokines (e.g. TNF-α and IL-6) function synergistically with ROS towards creating endothelial disarray and thus, an increased risk for the development of vascular disease. Therefore, it might be speculated that individuals who exhibit the metabolic syndrome may have an abnormality in their NO production by endothelial cells and a simultaneous and constant stimulation of pro-atherogenic changes in the vasculature in response to IR.

12.7.2   Homocysteine

Homocysteine, a sulphur-containing amino acid which is formed during the metabolism of methionine, has emerged as a novel independent biomarker for the development of atherosclerotic disease in coronary, cerebral and peripheral vascular beds. In fact, there is an increased risk for CVD in those with elevated fasting plasma total homocysteine levels. It has been shown that those individuals with hyperinsulinaemia (which is considered a marker of IR) had significantly higher homocysteine levels than those with normal insulin levels. The plasma levels of insulin seem to influence homocysteine metabolism, possibly through the effects on glomerular filtration or by influencing the activity of key enzymes in homocysteine metabolism. These authors also confirmed that

persons with two or more metabolic syndrome phenotypes had significantly higher homocysteine levels compared to those with one or no metabolic syndrome phenotypes [70]. Interestingly, elevated homocysteine levels increase the risk for CVD in type 2 diabetes patients to a greater extent than among non-diabetic subjects. In a large community-based population of non-diabetic individuals, a modest association was found between IR and elevated homocysteine levels [71]. These authors found that the co-occurrence of specific features of metabolic syndrome – especially hypertension and central obesity – was associated with more marked elevations in homocysteine levels. Homocysteine as a contributory factor for vascular damage remains controversial; however, the presence of high plasma levels of homocysteine may play an important role and are capable of promoting oxidative damage to the endothelium of vascular cells through an auto-oxidation, the formation of homocysteine mixed disulfides and ROS formation [72]. In particular, the oxidation of two homocysteine molecules results in the formation of oxidized disulfide, two protons and two electrons, while promoting the formation of ROS. The activation of ROS is only one of the many damaging effects of homocysteine, as it may act either alone or in concert with other multiple injurious stimuli to damage endothelial cell function. The combined effect of hypercoagulabilty and IR strengthen the processes of oxidation, glycation or homocysteinylation of LDLs necessary for the transformation in atherogenic particles. There are multiple metabolic toxicities associated with metabolic syndrome (and in particular IR) which are also associated with the production of ROS, thus creating multiple injurious stimuli and a higher risk for accelerated atherosclerosis.

12.7.3   Cognitive functioning

The aging process is associated with a significant decline in cognitive functioning. Indeed, many studies have attempted to discover the mechanisms involved with cognitive decline in vulnerable older persons. Many of the same risk factors associated with CVD have also been recognized with a higher risk for developing compromised cognitive functioning. The risk of cognitive impairment, especially in older persons with metabolic syndrome, needs to be recognized by physicians, due to the fact that its association with a lower functional status in older persons opens new public health concerns. The metabolic syndrome and its individual components have also been associated with an increased risk of developing cognitive impairment and decline over four years in high-functioning older persons, even after adjusting for comorbidities [73]. In particular, such decline was steeper in those who had high serum levels of inflammatory markers. Age-related IR has been shown to be independently associated with reduced cognitive functioning in older, non-diabetic persons [74]. Indeed, it is now well documented that insulin is a fundamental neuromodulator, contributing to neurobiological processes in particular, energy homeostasis and cognition. Interestingly, insulin and insulin receptors are selectively expressed in the brain [75]. Initially, the majority of glucose transporters in the brain were considered insulin-insensitive, but it has been shown recently that a significant element of brain glucose uptake is insulin-sensitive and essential for correct cognitive functioning [76]. Thus, an age-related reduction in glucose uptake due to altered insulin-signalling can lead to a deficiency of energetic substrate that cannot be compensated by other metabolic pathways [77]. Interestingly, a significant increase in peripheral IR develops as individuals age, thus raising the possibility that a reduced efficiency of the metabolic pathway responsible for energy production is one of the mechanisms of cognitive decline in older persons [78, 79]. Collectively, these findings suggest that: (i) insulin contributes to normal cognitive functioning; and (ii) insulin abnormalities exacerbate cognitive impairment, such as those associated with Alzheimer's disease. It is noteworthy that endothelial damage and vascular disease, when combined with IR, are also responsible for an age-related decline in cognitive function, even in the absence of dementia. Furthermore, any factors capable of lowering or increasing the risk of endothelial damage and/or affecting insulin action may have a role on cognitive function and cerebrovascular diseases.

12.7.4 Muscle functioning

In older persons, poor muscle strength and poor physical performance often coexist.

Midlife handgrip muscle strength has been recognized as an important factor that predicts old age functional ability [80]. Observational studies have consistently shown that chronic conditions such as CHD, diabetes and pulmonary obstructive disease are associated with lower muscle strength [81, 82]. It is also widely known that insulin plays a pivotal role for muscle contraction by increasing glucose uptake and promoting intracellular glucose metabolism. Thus, it is plausible that age-related IR may be a determinant of reduced muscle functioning, as seen clinically by a lower muscle strength. One cross-sectional study demonstrated a significant association between IR and muscle strength in older non-diabetic persons, independent of multiple confounders [81]. In particular, insulin may also be an important determinant of muscle function as glucose uptake is necessary for adequate muscle contraction. Another important role played by insulin is its ability to repress whole-body proteolysis, thus shifting total body metabolism towards an anabolic state. Therefore, it is plausible that an age-related IR may be a determinant of poor muscle strength in older persons with metabolic syndrome. Furthermore, a reduction of insulin peripheral activity may reduce the muscle tissue anabolic rate, leading to a relative catabolic state and, in turn, contributing to the impairment in muscle functioning. Indeed, insulin is known to play a pivotal role in muscle functioning by increasing glucose uptake and promoting intracellular glucose metabolism.

12.8 Therapeutic perspectives

The metabolic risk factors of the metabolic syndrome include atherogenic dyslipidaemia, hypertension, IR, a prothrombotic state and the pro-inflammatory state. Due to the fact that IR is the key player in the metabolic syndrome, drug interventions should be used either directly to improve insulin sensitivity, or indirectly to improve the metabolic changes associated with IR. All risk factors linked to IR must be treated in order to reduce the severity of metabolic syndrome (see Table 12.4). Both, the American Diabetes Association (ADA) [83] and the National Cholesterol Education Program (NCEP) have adopted guidelines for complications related to metabolic syndrome [2]. The cornerstones of metabolic syndrome treatment are the management of body weight, and ensuring that appropriate physical exercise is performed. In fact, education and training should be considered fundamental, due to the fact that environmental influences such as incorrect nutrition and physical inactivity are considered to be root causes of the metabolic syndrome. Interventions on the metabolic syndrome with physical activity have shown that regular and sustained physical activity will improve all of the risk factors [84, 85]. With regards to weight management, there is a general consensus that persons with metabolic syndrome should reduce their consumption of simple sugars and increase their intake

Table 12.4 Theraneutic approach to the various components of the metabolic syndrome.

| | Therapeutic approach | | | |
	Abdominal obesity	Dyslipidaemia	Hypertension	Impaired glucose tolerance
Diet	**Reduces calories**	**Reduces unsatured fat**	**Reduces sodium intake**	**Reduces glucose intake**
	– Daily activity/exercise	– Daily activity/exercise	– Daily activity/exercise	– Daily activity/exercise
	– Fruits	– Omega-3s	– Fruits	– Fibre
	– Vegetables	– MUFA	– Vegetables	– Fruits
	– Whole grains	– Sat fat	– Whole grains	– Vegetables
		– Trans fat		– Whole grains
Medication				
	– Rimonabant	– Statin		– Metformin
		– Fibrates	– Angiotensin-Converting	– Acarbose
			Enzyme Inhibitors	– Incretin?
			– Angiotensin receptor	– DPP-IV inhibitor?
			blocker	– Thiazolidinediones?

of fruits, vegetables and whole grains [86]. Although, the recommended intakes of carbohydrate and unsaturated fats remain controversial [87], it has been shown that low-fat diets promote weight reduction, while a higher monosaturated fat intake reduces postprandial glycaemia, reduces plasma triglyceride levels and also raises HDL concentrations [88]. Although modifications to diet and exercise need to be adapted in the first approach for ameliorating the metabolic syndrome, the use of pharmaceuticals is almost always necessary.

Thiazolidinediones (TZD or glitazones) represent a new class of oral antidiabetic drug which exert their insulin-sensitizing action by stimulating the nuclear transcription factor peroxisome proliferator-activated receptor gamma (PPAR-γ). At present, pioglitazone and rosiglitazone are available for clinical use. The different activation levels of PPAR-γ and of their co-factors determine the binding of PPAR-γ to distinct target genes, which in turn regulates their transcriptional activity. It is important to recall that PPARs are members of the superfamily of nuclear hormone receptors; these are transcription factors which transmit signals that originate from lipid-soluble factors to the genome. Nuclear receptors bind to DNA at specific sites or response elements, that in turn can activate or repress the expression of a target gene. Three different PPAR genes (α, γ and δ) have been identified [89] which play distinct expression patterns, and this suggests that they have important functional differences. TZDs dramatically upgrade insulin sensitivity through PPAR-γ, and are also capable of lowering blood glucose levels through more active glucose transporters

and by stimulating the insulin-signalling pathway. Various studies have also confirmed that PPAR-γ agonists are capable of improving the altered lipid metabolism associated with IR. PPAR-γ is highly expressed in adipose tissue, where it triggers adipocyte differentiation as well as inducing genes that are critical for adipogenesis. Adipose tissue serves as a major site of oxidized LDL (oxLDL) detoxification, causing it to be removed from the bloodstream and potentially inhibiting the formation of atherosclerotic lesions. Increasing clinical evidence has also shown that rosiglitazone treatment significantly improves factors associated with CVD, including endothelial activity, inflammatory processes and dyslipidaemia [90, 91]. Only future clinical trials conducted in older persons in an IR state will be able to clarify whether the protective factors from the use of TZDs are substantial. TZDs are also capable of reducing oxidized LDLs in both lean and obese diabetic animals [92]. In particular, TZDs have been shown to up-regulate the oxidized LDL receptor 1 (OLR1) in adipocytes by facilitating the exchange of coactivators for corepressors on the *OLR1* gene in cultured mouse adipocytes. TZDs markedly stimulated the uptake of oxLDL into adipocytes, which required OLR1. Increased OLR1 expression, resulting from TZD treatment, significantly increased the adipocyte cholesterol content and also enhanced FA uptake. While the physiological role of adipose tissue in cholesterol and oxLDL metabolism remains unknown, the induction of OLRI may be a potential means through which PPAR-γ ligands may regulate lipid metabolism and insulin sensitivity in adipocytes

[93]. A degree of caution should be applied when treating older persons with PPAR-γ agonists, due to the fact that these agents may cause water retention and an altered hepatic detoxifying activity; this in turn would exacerbate a potential condition of cardiac failure and an inadequate removal of toxic compounds due to an inappropriate liver metabolism. PPAR-α agonists or fibrates are used to treat dyslipidaemia, particularly in the case of high triglycerides and low HDL-cholesterol.

Fibrates (gemfibrozil, bezafibrate, fenofibrate) represent another class of lipid-lowering drugs known generally to be effective for reducing elevated plasma triglyceride and cholesterol levels. Although very few controlled clinical trials have been conducted comparing fibrates with statins (especially in older persons), the use of fibrates has been shown to include protective effects towards further vascular events in survivors of myocardial infarction [94]. The more pronounced effect of fibrates is a decrease in plasma triglyceride-rich lipoproteins after linking to PPAR-α. The latter is especially expressed in kidney, heart and muscle tissue (all of which metabolize large amounts of fatty acids). Fibrates are ligands for PPAR-α [95]; thus, their main mechanisms of action are linked to the activation of key genes involved in lipid metabolism. The hypotriglyceridaemic action of fibrates involves a combination effect of HL and apoC-III expression. HL is induced at the transcriptional level mediated by PPAR, while apoC-III is repressed. As a consequence a reduced secretion of VLDL particles occurs, together with an enhanced catabolism of triglyceride-rich particles. Fibrates are also known to increase the hepatic uptake of FFAs, to increase the removal of LDL particles, and to stimulate the production of HDL and its major constituents, apoA-I and apoA-II. Hypertriglyceridaemia, in association with an IR state, is considered the main target for the use of fibrates in the metabolic syndrome. In fact, in those persons undergoing therapy with fenofibrate, a 50% decrease in triglycerides levels was noted, together with a simultaneous 10–30% increase in basal HDL levels [96]. Fenofibrate was also found to be more effective in reducing the plasma concentrations of oxLDLs, while in individuals at high risk of CVD the impact of accelerating chylomicron and VLDL catabolism underlined the ability of fibrates to act on postprandial lipid metabolism [94]. Only large clinical studies will confirm the efficacy of fibrates in reducing coronary events and mortality in older, high-risk individuals.

A very recently introduced drug, rimonabant – a selective cannabinoid-1 (CB1) receptor blocker – decreases food intake and body weight while increasing adiponectin and insulin sensitivity. Drug interventions with rimonabant (e.g. the RIO-Europe study) addressed the effects of such therapy on weight loss, altered glucose metabolism and dyslipidaemia [97]. It was found that, at the one-year follow-up examination, those patients receiving 20 mg per day rimonabant showed significant reductions in both body weight and waist circumference, as well as significant improvements in lipid and glucose parameters. A significant increase was noted in HDL levels and a decrease in triglycerides, as well as a significant reduction in IR, as monitored using the homeostasis model assessment index (HOMA). The risk for cardiovascular events are significantly increased during an IR state, due to the latter being ameliorated by an enhanced lipid metabolism; hence, lipid-lowering agents such as statins may have an important role. It is widely known that statins (3-hydroxy-3-methylglutaryl-coenzyme A reductase inhibitors) lower the risk of CVD by reducing the production of all apo B-containing lipoproteins and VLDL. Statins are effective, in both the primary and secondary prevention of CHD, in middle-aged and older (<65 years) men and women, in both diabetics and non-diabetics with CHD [98, 99]. Statins used in the secondary prevention of CHD also significantly reduce not only the risk of stroke but also the frequency of daily attacks of myocardial ischaemia. Statins have been shown to reduce LDL levels by 20–50%, triglycerides by 10–40%, and to increase HDL levels by 5–12%. In fact, the Adult Treatment Panel III (ATP III) of the National Cholesterol Education Program have issued evidence-based guidelines of major clinical trials with statin therapy. According to the ATP III algorithm, persons may be allocated to one of three risk categories:

1. Established CVD and CVD risk equivalents.

2. Multiple (two or more risk factors).

3. Zero to one risk factor.

Here, the CVD risks include non-coronary forms of atherosclerotic disease, diabetes and multiple (two or more) CVD risk factors with a 10-year risk for CVD exceeding 20%. Therefore, all persons with CVD or CVD risk equivalents may be considered at high risk of CVD.

12.8.1 Therapy in high-risk CVD patients

The goal for LDL-lowering therapy is to achieve an LDL level $<100 \, \text{mg dl}^{-1}$ in high-risk patients; therefore, in persons with an LDL level $<100 \, \text{mg dl}^{-1}$ no further LDL-lowering therapy is recommended, whereas in high-risk patients with an LDL level $>100 \, \text{mg dl}^{-1}$ a diet-based therapy should be initiated. When the baseline LDL is $>130 \, \text{mg dl}^{-1}$, the LDL-lowering drug should be commenced simultaneously with diet-based therapy. Then, if high triglyceride or low HDL levels persist, consideration may given to the use of a fibrate.

12.8.2 Therapy in moderate-risk CVD patients

Moderate-risk persons have two or more risk factors and 10-year risk of between 10% and 20%. The recommendation in this case is to obtain an LDL level $<130 \, \text{mg dl}^{-1}$. When the LDL level is $100–129 \, \text{mg dl}^{-1}$, either at baseline or on lifestyle therapy, the initiation of an LDL-lowering drug to achieve LDL $<100 \, \text{mg dl}^{-1}$ is therapeutic option. When LDL-lowering drug treatment is initiated in high-risk or moderate-risk patients, it is advised that the goal of such therapy is to achieve at least a 30–40% reduction in LDL levels.

The question remains, however, as to how exactly statins improve IR. It has been reported in several studies that statins also have a beneficial impact on the chemical properties of lipoproteins by reducing not only oxLDLs but also small and dense VLDLs, all of which are commonly observed during an IR state [100]. In particular, small doses of atorvastatin (10 mg) have been shown to reduce postprandial concentrations of VLDLs, IDLs and apo B in persons with normal lipid profiles [101]. Furthermore, in patients with altered lipid profiles and altered glucose metabolism (reduced glucose tolerance or type 2 diabetes), treatment with atorvastatin led to reductions in both IR (confirmed using the HOMA index [102]) and small, dense atherogenic LDLs [103].

Simvastatin, rosuvastatin and fluvastatin have also been shown to reduce oxLDLs, thus generalizing the so-called 'class effect' of statins. It has been hypothesized that a reduction in HL activity during such therapy may be at the basis of such a phenomenon. With regards to arterial hypertension and IR, mild elevations of blood pressure can often be controlled by lifestyle changes, including a reduced sodium intake and weight loss. However, if the hypertension persists despite such changes, then anti-hypertensive drug treatment is usually required. It is widely known that the benefits derived from a reduction in arterial hypertension lower the risk for CVD [104]. It also has been suggested that the use of angiotensin-converting enzyme (ACE) inhibitors or angiotensin receptor blockers represent a better first-line therapy for metabolic syndrome patients [105]. The atherothrombotic state characterized by high concentrations of fibrinogen, PAI-1 and increased platelet aggregation may be treated when necessary with low-dose aspirin or other anti-platelet drugs [106]. Indeed, such drugs are universally recommended in patients with established CVD, although their efficacy in older persons with metabolic syndrome in the absence of CVD has still to be verified in clinical trials. However, the use of aspirin has been considered a prophylactic option when the risk for CVD is high [107].

12.9 Conclusions

Today, the proportion of aged subjects among the populations of industrialized countries continues to increase dramatically, thus predisposing such persons to development of the metabolic syndrome. If it is accepted that each single component of the metabolic syndrome is significantly linked to IR, then it will be vital for physicians to focus on correcting IR in order to improve each of these metabolic components.

References

1. Reaven GM. Banting lecture 1988. Role of insulin resistance in human disease. Diabetes 1988; 37: 1595–607.
2. Executive Summary of the Third Report of the National Cholesterol Education Program (NCEP) Expert Panel on Detection, Evaluation, and Treatment of High Blood Cholesterol in Adults (Adult Treatment Panel III). JAMA 2001; 285: 2486–97.
3. Isomaa B, Almgren P, Tuomi T, Forsen B, Lahti K, Nissen M, Taskinen MR and Groop L. Cardiovascular morbidity and mortality associated with the metabolic syndrome. Diabetes Care 2001; 24: 683–9.
4. WHO. (1999) Definition of metabolic syndrome in definition, diagnosis and classification of diabetes and its complications. Report of a WHO consultation. Part 1: Diagnosis and classification of diabetes

mellitus. WHO/NCD/NCS/99.2. World Health Organization, Department of Noncommunicable Disease Surveillance, Geneva.

5. Bloomgarden ZT. American Association of Clinical Endocrinologists (AACE) consensus conference on the insulin resistance syndrome: 25–26 August 2002, Washington, DC. Diabetes Care 2003; 26: 1297–303.

6. Einhorn D, Reaven GM, Cobin RH, Ford E, Ganda OP, Handelsman Y, Hellman R, Jellinger PS, Kendall D, Krauss RM, Neufeld ND, Petak SM, Rodbard HW, Seibel JA, Smith DA and Wilson PW. American College of Endocrinology position statement on the insulin resistance syndrome. Endocr Pract. 2003; 9: 237–52.

7. Yach D, Stuckler D and Brownell KD. Epidemiologic and economic consequences of the global epidemics of obesity and diabetes. Nat Med. 2006; 12: 62–6.

8. Bonadonna RC, Cucinotta D, Fedele D, Riccardi G, Tiengo A and the Metascreen Writing Committee. The metabolic syndrome is a risk indicator of microvascular and macrovascular complications in diabetes: results from Metascreen, a multicenter diabetes clinic-based survey. Diabetes Care 2006; 29: 2701–7.

9. Grundy SM. Metabolic syndrome: a multiplex cardiovascular risk factor. J Clin Endocrinol Metab. 2007; 92: 399–404.

10. Pi-Sunyer FX. The relation of adipose tissue to cardiometabolic risk. Clin Cornerstone 2006; 8 (Suppl. 4): S14–23.

11. Katagiri H, Yamada T and Oka Y. Adiposity and cardiovascular disorders: disturbance of the regulatory system consisting of humoral and neuronal signals. Circ Res. 2007; 101: 27–39.

12. Lee M and Aronne LJ. Weight management for type 2 diabetes mellitus: global cardiovascular risk reduction. Am J Cardiol. 2007; 99 (4A): 68B–79B.

13. Bloomgarden ZT. Insulin resistance concepts. Diabetes Care 2007; 30: 1320–6.

14. Rader DJ. Effect of insulin resistance, dyslipidemia, and intra-abdominal adiposity on the development of cardiovascular disease and diabetes mellitus. Am J Med. 2007; 120 (3 Suppl. 1): S12–18.

15. Sarti C and Gallagher J. The metabolic syndrome: prevalence, CHD risk, and treatment. J Diabetes Complications 2006; 20: 121–32.

16. Fink RI, Kolterman OG, Griffin J and Olefsky JM. Mechanisms of insulin resistance in aging. J din Invest. 1983: 71 (6): 1523–35.

17. Rowe JW, Minaker KL, Pallotta JA and Flier JS. Characterization of the insulin resistance of aging. J Clin Invest. 1983: 71 (6): 1581–7.

18. Gumbiner B, Thorburn AW, Ditzler TM, Bulacan F and Henry RR. Role of impaired intracellular glucose metabolism in the insulin resistance of aging. Metabolism 1992: 41 (10): 1115–21.

19. Ferrannini E, Vichi S, Beck-Nielsen H, Laakso M, Paolisso G and Smith U. Insulin action and age. European Group for the Study of Insulin Resistance (EGIR). Diabetes 1996: 45 (7): 947–53.

20. Barbieri M, Rizzo MR, Manzella D and Paolisso G. Age-related insulin resistance: is it an obligatory finding? The lesson from healthy centenarians. Diabetes Metab Res Rev. 2001; 17 (1): 19–26.

21. Banerji MA, Chaiken RL, Gordon D, Kral JG and Lebovitz HE. Does intra-abdominal adipose tissue in black men determine whether NIDDM is insulin-resistant or insulin-sensitive? Diabetes 1995; 44 (2): 141–6.

22. Fujimoto WY, Abbate SL, Kahn SE, Hokanson JE and Brunzell JD. The visceral adiposity syndrome in Japanese-American men. Obes Res 1994; 2: 364–71.

23. Laws A, Hoen HM, Selby JV, Saad MF, Haffner SM and Howard BV. Differences in insulin suppression of free fatty acid levels by gender and glucose tolerance status. Relation to plasma triglyceride and apolipoprotein B concentrations. Insulin Resistance Atherosclerosis Study (IRAS) Investigators. Arterioscler Thromb Vasc Biol. 1997; 17 (1): 64–71.

24. Jeppesen J, Hein HO, Suadicani P and Gyntelberg F. Triglyceride concentration and ischemic heart disease: an eight-year follow-up in the Copenhagen Male Study. Circulation 1998; 97 (11): 1029–36.

25. Zambon A, Austin MA, Brown BG, Hokanson JE and Brunzell JD. Effect of hepatic lipase on LDL in normal men and those with coronary artery disease. Arterioscler Thromb. 1993; 13 (2): 147–53.

26. Morton RE and Ziiversmit DB. Purification and characterization of lipid transfer protein(s) from human lipoprotein-deficient plasma. J Lipid Res. 1982; 23 (7): 1058–67.

27. Krauss RM. Dense low density lipoproteins and coronary artery disease. Am J Cardiol. 1995; 75 (6): 53B–57B.

28. Rashid S, Uffelman KD and Lewis GF. The mechanism of HDL lowering in hypertriglyceridemic, insulin-resistant states. J Diabetes Complications 2002; 16 (1): 24–8.

29. Clay MA, Newnham HH and Barter PJ. Hepatic lipase promotes a loss of apolipoprotein A-I from triglyceride-enriched human high density lipoproteins during incubation in vitro. Arterioscler Thromb. 1991; 1 (2): 415–22.

30. Austin MA, King MC, Vranizan KM and Krauss RM. Atherogenic lipoprotein phenotype. A proposed genetic marker for coronary heart disease risk. Circulation 1990; 82 (2): 495–506.

31. Pierson RN Jr. Body composition in aging: a biological perspective. Curr Opin Clin Nutr Metab Care 2003; 6 (1): 15–20.

32. Kannel WB, Cupples LA, Ramaswami R, Stokes J, III, Kreger BE and Higgins M. Regional obesity and risk of cardiovascular disease; the Framingham Study. Epidemiology 1991: 44 (2): 183–90.

33. Harris TB, Launer LJ, Madans J and Feldman JJ. Cohort study of effect of being overweight and change in weight on risk of coronary heart disease in old age. Br Med J. 1997; 314 (7097): 1791–4.

34. Elias MF, Elias PK, Sullivan LM, Wolf PA and D'Agostino RB. Lower cognitive function in the presence of obesity and hypertension: the Framingham Heart Study. Int J Obes Relat Metab Disord. 2003; 27 (2): 260–8.

35. Chumlea WC, Garry PJ, Hunt WC and Rhyne RL. Distributions of serial changes in stature and weight in a healthy elderly population. Hum Biol. 1988; 60 (6): 917–31.

36. Ahima RS and Flier JS. Adipose tissue as an endocrine organ. Trends Endocrinol Metab 2000; 11: 327–32.

37. Rajala MW and Scherer PE. Minireview: The adipocytes at the crossroads of energy homeostasis, inflammation, and atherosclerosis. Endocrinology 2003; 144 (9): 3765–73.

38. Lyon CJ and Law WA. Minireview: Adiposity, inflammation, and atherogenesis. Endocrinology 2003; 144 (6): 2195–200.

39. Fasshauer M and Paschke R. Regulation of adipocytokines and insulin resistance. Diabetologia 2003; 46 (12): 1594–603.

40. Trayhurn P and Wood IS. Adipokines: inflammation and the pleiotropic role of white adipose tissue. Br J Nutr. 2004; 92 (3): 347–55.

41. Yudkin JS, Stehouwer CD, Emeis JJ and Coppack SW. C-reactive protein in healthy subjects: associations with obesity, insulin resistance, and endothelial dysfunction. A potential role for cytokines originating from adipose tissue? Arterioscler Thromb Vasc Biol 1999; 19: 972–8.

42. Chandran M, Phillips SA, Ciaraldi T and Henry RR. Adiponectin: more than just another fat cell hormone? Diabetes Care 2003; 26 (8): 2442–50.

43. Cnop M, Havei PJ, Utzschneider KM, Carr DB, Sinha MK, Boyko EJ, Retzlaff BM, Knopp RH, Brunzell JD and Kahn SE. Relationship of adiponectin to body fat distribution, insulin sensitivity and plasma lipoproteins: evidence for independent roles of age and sex. Diabetologia 2003; 46 (4): 459–69.

44. Salmenniemi U, Ruotsalainen E, Pihiajamaki J, Vauhkonen I, Kainulainen S, Punnonen K, Vanninen E and Laakso M. Multiple abnormalities in glucose and energy metabolism and coordinated changes in levels of adiponectin, cytokines, and adhesion molecules in subjects with metabolic syndrome Circulation 2004; 110 (25): 3842–8.

45. Ouchi N, Kihara S, Arita Y, Maeda K, Kuriyama H. Okamoto Y, Hotta K, Nishida M, Takahashi M, Nakamura T, Yamashita S, Funahashi T and Matsuzawa Y. Novel modulator for endothelial adhesion molecules: adipocyte-derived plasma protein adiponectin. Circulation 1999; 100: 2473–6.

46. Okamoto Y, Arita Y and Nishida M. An adipocyte-derived plasma protein, adiponectin, adheres to injured vascular walls. Horm Metab Res 2000; 32: 47–50.

47. Pischon T, Girman CJ, Hotamisligil GS, Rifai N, Hu FB and Rimm EB. Plasma adiponectin levels and risk of myocardial infarction in men. JAMA 2004: 291: 1730–7.

48. Maahs DM, Ogden LG, Kinney GL, Wadwa P, Snell-Bergeon JK, Dabelea D, Hokanson JE, Ehriich J, Eckel RH and Rewers M. Low plasma adiponectin levels predict progression of coronary artery calcification. Circulation 2005; 11: 747–53.

49. Paolisso G, Rizzo MR, Mazziotti G, Tagliamonte MR, Gambardella A. Rotondi M, Carella C, Giugliano D, Varricchio M and D'Onofrio F. Advancing age and insulin resistance: role of plasma tumor necrosis factor-alpha. Am J Physiol 1998; 275: E294–9.

50. Abbatecola AM, Ferrucci L, Grella R, Bandinelli S, Bonafe M, Barbieri M, Corsi AM, Lauretani F, Franceschi C and Paolisso G. Diverse effect of inflammatory markers on insulin resistance and insulin-resistance syndrome in the elderly. J Am Geriatr Soc 2004; 52: 399–404.

51. Franceschi C, Bonafe M, Valensin S, Olivieri F, De Luca M, Ottaviani E and De Benedictis G. Inflamm-aging. An evolutionary perspective on immunosenescence. Ann N Y Acad Sci. 2000; 908: 244–54.

52. Hak AE, Pois HAP, Stehouwer CDA, *et al.* Markers of inflammation and cellular adhesion molecules in relation to insulin resistance in nondiabetic elderly: The Rotterdam study. J Clin Endocrinol Metab 2001; 86: 4398–405.

53. Welborn TA, Breckenridge A, Rubinstein AH, Dollery CT and Fraser TR. Serum-insulin in essential hypertension and in peripheral vascular disease. Lancet 1966; 18: 1336–7.

54. Modan M, Halkin H, Almog S, Lusky A, Eshkol A, Shefi M, Shitrit A and Fuchs Z. Hyperinsulinemia. A link between hypertension obesity and glucose intolerance. J Clin Invest. 1985; 75: 809–17.

55. Zavaroni I, Bonini L, Gasparini P, Barilli AL, Zuccarelli A, Dall'Aglio E, Del Signore R and Reaven GM. Hyperinsulinemia in a normal population as a predictor of non-insulin-dependent diabetes mellitus, hypertension, and coronary heart disease: the Barilla factory revisited. Metabolism 1999; 48: 989–94.

56. Ferrannini E, Buzzigoli G, Bonadonna R, Giorico MA, Oleggini M, Graziadei L, Pedrinelli R, Brandi L and Bevilacqua S. Insulin resistance in essential hypertension. N Engl J Med 1987; 317: 350–7.

57. Steinberg HO, Brechtel G, Johnson A, Fineberg N and Baron AD. Insulin-mediated skeletal muscle vasodilation is nitric oxide dependent. A novel action of insulin to increase nitric oxide release. J Clin Invest. 1994; 94: 1172–9.

58. Steinberg HO, Chaker H, Leaming R, Johnson A, Brechtel G and Baron AD. Obesity/insulin resistance is associated with endothelial dysfunction. Implications for the syndrome of insulin resistance. J Clin Invest. 1996; 97: 2601–10.

59. Maaten JC, Voorburg A, de Vries PM, ter Wee PM, Donker AJ and Gans RO. Relationship between insulin's haemodynamic effects and insulin-mediated glucose uptake. Eur J Clin Invest. 1998; 28: 279–84.

60. Grassi G, Seravalle G, Cattaneo BM, Bolla GB, Lanfranchi A, Colombo M, Giannattasio C, Brunani A, Cavagnini F and Mancia G. Sympathetic activation in obese normotensive subjects. Hypertension 1995; 25: 560–3.

61. DeFronzo RA, Cooke CR, Andres R, Falcona GR and Davis PJ. The effect of insulin on renal handling of sodium, potassium, calcium, and phosphate in man. J Clin Invest. 1975; 55: 845–55.

62. Zavaroni I, Coruzzi P, Bonini L, Mossini GL, Musiari L, Gasparini P, Fantuzzi M and Reaven GM. Association between salt sensitivity and insulin concentrations in patients with hypertension. Am J Hypertens. 1995; 8: 855–8.

63. Trovati M and Anfossi G. Insulin, insulin resistance and platelet function: similarities with insulin effects on cultured vascular smooth muscle cells. Diabetologia 1998; 41: 609–22.

64. Trovati M, Mularoni EM, Burzacca S, Ponziani MC, Massucco P, Mattiello L, Piretto V, Cavalot F and Anfossi G. Impaired insulin-induced platelet antiaggregating effect in obesity and in obese NIDDM patients. Diabetes 1995; 44: 1318–22.

65. Anand SS, Yi Q, Gerstein H, Lonn E, Jacobs R, Vuksan V, Teo K, Davis B, Montague P and Yusuf S. Relationship of metabolic syndrome and fibrinolytic dysfunction to cardiovascular disease. Circulation 2003; 108: 420–5.

66. Sohai RS, Svensson I, Sohai BH and Brunk UT. Superoxide anion radical production in different animal species. Mech Ageing Dev. 1989; 49: 129–35.

67. Gilgun-Sherki Y, Melamed E and Offen D. Antioxidant treatment in Alzheimer's disease: current state. J Mol Neurosci. 2003; 21: 1–12.

68. Paolini M, Sapone A, Canistro D, Chicco P and Valgimigli L. Antioxidant vitamins for prevention of cardiovascular disease. Lancet 2003; 362: 920–4.

69. Kuboki K, Jiang ZY, Takahara N, Ha SW, Igarashi M, Yamauchi T, Feener EP, Herbert TP, Rhodes CJ and King GL. Regulation of endothelial constitutive nitric oxide synthase gene expression in endothelial cells and in vivo: a specific vascular action of insulin. Circulation 2000; 101: 676–81.

70. Meigs JB, Jacques PF, Seihub J, Singer DE, Nathan DM, Rifai N, D'Agostino RB, Sr and Wilson PW. Fasting plasma homocysteine levels in the insulin resistance syndrome: the Framingham Offspring Study. Diabetes Care 2001; 24: 1403–10.

71. Hoogeveen EK, Kostense PJ, Beks PJ, Mackaay AJ, Jakobs C, Bouter LM, Heine RJ and Stehouwer CD. Hyperhomocysteinemia is associated with an increased risk of cardiovascular disease, especially in non-insulin-dependent diabetes mellitus: a population-based study. Arterioscler Thromb Vasc Biol. 1998; 18: 133–8.

72. Jakubowski H, Zhang L, Bardeguez A and Aviv A. Homocysteine thiolactone and protein homocysteinylation in human endothelial cells: implications for atherosclerosis. Circ Res. 2000; 87: 45–51.

73. Yaffe K, Kanaya A, Lindquist K, Simonsick E, Harris T, Shorr R, Tylavsky F and Newman A. The metabolic syndrome, inflammation, and risk of cognitive decline. JAMA 2004; 292: 2237–42.

74. Abbatecola AM, Paolisso G, Lamponi M, Bandinelli S, Lauretani F, Launer L and Ferrucci L Insulin resistance and executive dysfunction in older persons. J Am Geriatr Soc. 2004; 52: 1713–18.

75. Kyriaki G. Brain insulin: Regulation, mechanisms of action and functions. Cellular and Molecular Neurobiology 2003; 23: 1–25.

76. McEwen G and Reagan F. Glucose transporter expression in the central nervous system: relationship to synaptic function. European Journal of Pharmacology 2004; 490: 13–24.

77. Messier C, Awad N and Gagnon M. The relationships between atherosclerosis, heart disease, type 2 diabetes and dementia. Neurol Res. 2004; 26: 567–72.

78. Craft S, Dagogo-Jack SE, Wiethop BV, Murphy C, Nevins RT, Fleischman S, Rice V, Newcomer JW and Cryer PE. Effects of hyperglycemia on memory and hormone levels in dementia of the Alzheimer type: a longitudinal study. Behav Neurosci 1993; 107: 926–40.

79. Kalmijn S, Feskens EJM, Launer LJ, Stijnen T and Kromhout D. Glucose intolerance, hyperinsulinemia and cognitive function in a general population of elderly men. Diabetologia 1995; 38: 1096–102.

80. Rantanen T, Guralnik JM, Foley D, et al. Midlife hand grip strength as a predictor of older age disability. JAMA 1999: 10; 281: 558–60.

81. Kalirnan DA, Piato CC and Tobin JD. The role of muscle loss in the age-related decline of grip strength: cross-sectional and longitudinal perspectives. J Gerontol. 1990: 45: M82–8.

82. Abbatecola AM, Ferrucci L, Ceda G, Russo CR, Lauretani F, Bandinelli S, Barbieri M, Valenti G and Paolisso G. Insulin resistance and muscle strength in older persons. J Gerontol A Biol Sci Med Sci. 2005; 60: 1278–82.

83. Franz MJ, Bantle JP, Beebe CA, Brunzell JD, Chiasson JE, Garg A, Holzmeister LA, Hoogwerf B, Mayer-Davis E, Mooradian AD, Purnell JQ and Wheeler M. Evidence-based nutrition principles and recommendations for the treatment and prevention of diabetes and related complications. Diabetes Care 2002; 25: 148–98.

84. Cook S, Weitzman M, Auinger P, Nguyen M and Dietz WH. Prevalence of a metabolic syndrome phenotype in adolescents: findings from the third National Health and Nutrition Examination Survey, 1988-1994. Arch Pediatr Adolesc Med. 2003; 157: 821–7.

85. Lakka TA, Laaksonen DE, Lakka HM, Mannikko N, Niskanen LK, Rauramaa R and Salonen JT. Sedentary lifestyle, poor cardiorespiratory fitness, and the metabolic syndrome. Med Sci Sports Exerc. 2003; 35: 1279–86.

86. National Cholesterol Education Program (NCEP) Expert Panel on Detection, Evaluation. and Treatment of High Blood Cholesterol in Adults (Adult Treatment Panel III). Third Report of the National Cholesterol Education Program (NCEP) Expert Panel on Detection, Evaluation. and Treatment of High Blood Cholesterol in Adults (Adult Treatment Panel III) final report. Circulation 2002; 106: 3143–421.

87. Grundy SM, Abate N and Chandalia M. Diet composition and the metabolic syndrome: what is the optimal fat intake? Am J Med. 2002: 113 (Suppl. 9B): 25S–29S.

88. Klein S, Sheard NF, Pi-Sunyer X, Daly A, Wylie-Rosett J, Kulkarni K and Clark NG. Weight management through lifestyle modification for the prevention and management of type 2 diabetes: rationale and strategies. A statement of the American Diabetes Association, the North American Association for the Study of Obesity, and the American Society for Clinical Nutrition. Am J Clin Nutr. 2004: 80: 257–63.

89. Schoonjans K, Staels B and Auwerx J. Role of the peroxisome proliferator-activated receptor (PPAR) in mediating the effects of fibrates and fatty acids on gene expression. J Lipid Res. 1996; 37: 907–25.

90. Gilling E, Suwattee P, DeSouza C, Asnani S and Fonseca V. Effects of the thiazolidinediones on cardiovascular risk factors. Am J Cardiovasc Drugs 2002; 2: 149–56.

91. Sidhu JS, Cowan D and Kaski JC. The effects of rosiglitazone, a peroxisome proliferator-activated receptor-gamma agonist, on markers of endothelial cell activation. C-reactive protein, and fibrinogen levels in non-diabetic coronary artery disease patients. J Am Coll Cardiol. 2003; 42: 1757–63.

92. Buse JB, Tan MH, Prince MJ and Erickson PP. The effects of oral anti-hyperglycaemic medications on serum lipid profiles in patients with type 2 diabetes. Diabetes Obes Metab. 2004: 6: 133–56.

93. Chui PC, Guari HP, Lehrke M and Lazar MA. PPAR-gamma regulates adipocytes cholesterol metabolism via oxidized LDL receptor 1. J Clin Invest. 2005; 15: 2244–56.

94. Ericsson CG, Hamsten A, Nilsson J, Grip L. Svane B and de Faire U. Angiographic assessment of effects of bezafibrate on progression of coronary artery disease in young male post infarction patients. Lancet 1996; 347: 849–53.

95. Forman BM, Chen J and Evans RM. Hypolipidemic drugs, polyunsaturated fatty acids and eicosanoids are ligands for peroxisome proliferator-activated receptors alpha and delta. Proc Natl Acad Sci USA 1997; 94: 4312–17.

96. Guerin M, Bruckert E, Dolphin PJ, Turpin G and Chapman MJ. Fenofibrate reduces plasma cholesteryl ester transfer from HDL to VLDL and normalizes the atherogenic, dense LDL profile in combined hyperlipidemia. Arterioscler Thromb Vasc Biol. 1996; 16: 763–72.

97. Van Gaal LF, Rissanen A, Scheen A, Ziegler O and Rossner S. Effect of rimonabant on weight reduction and cardiovascular risk. Lancet 2005; 366: 369–70.

98. Miettinen TA, Pyorala K, Oisson AG, Musliner TA, Cook TJ, Faergeman O, Berg K, Pedersen T and Kjekshus J. Cholesterol-lowering therapy in women and elderly patients myocardial infarction or angina pectoris: findings from the Scandinavian Simvastatin Survival Study (4S). Circulation 1997; 96: 4211–18.

99. Colquhoun D, Keech A, Hunt D, Marschner I, Simes J, Glasziou P, White H, Barter P, Tonkin A and the LIP1D Study Investigators. Effects of pravastatin on coronary events in 2073 patients with low levels of both low-density lipoprotein cholesterol and high-density lipoprotein cholesterol: results from the LIPID study. Eur Heart J. 2004; 25: 771–7.

100. Stein DT, Devaraj S, Balis D, Adams-Huet B and Jialal I. Effect of statin therapy on remnant lipoprotein cholesterol levels in patients with combined hyperlipidemia. Arterioscler Thromb Vasc Biol. 2001; 21: 2026–31.

101. Parhofer KG, Barrett PH and Schwandt P. Atorvastatin improves postprandial lipoprotein metabolism in normolipidemic subjects. J Clin Endocrinol Metab. 2000; 85: 4224–30.

102. Paolisso G, Barbagallo M, Petrella G, Ragno E, Barbieri M, Giordano M and Varricchio M. Effects of simvastatin and atorvastatin administration on insulin resistance and respiratory quotient in aged dyslipidemic non-insulin dependent diabetic patients. Atherosclerosis 2000; 150: 121–7.

103. Pontrelli L, Parris W, Adeli K and Cheung RC. Atorvastatin treatment beneficially alters the lipoprotein profile and increases low-density lipoprotein particle diameter in patients with combined dyslipidemia and impaired fasting glucose type 2 diabetes. Metabolism 2002: 51: 334–42.

104. Chobanian AV, Bakris GL, Black HR, Cushman WC, Green LA, Izzo JL Jr, Jones DW, Materson BJ, Oparil S, Wright JT Jr and Roccella EJ. Seventh Report of the Joint National Committee on Prevention, Detection, Evaluation, and Treatment of High Blood Pressure. Hypertension 2003; 42: 1206–52.

105. Julius S, Kjeldsen SE, Brunner H. Hansson L, Platt F, Ekman S, Laragh JH, McInnes G, Schork AM, Smith B, Weber M and Zanchetti A. The VALUE trial: Long-term blood pressure trends in 13,449 patients with hypertension and high cardiovascular risk. Am J Hypertens. 2003; 16: 544–8.

106. Colwell JA. Antiplatelet agents for the prevention of cardiovascular disease in diabetes mellitus. Am J Cardiovasc Drugs 2004; 4: 87–106.

107. Pearson TA, Blair SN, Daniels SR, Eckel RH, Fair JM, Fortmann SP, Franklin BA, Goldstein LB, Greenland P, Grundy SM, Hong Y, Miller NH, Lauer RM, Ockene IS, Sacco RL, Sallis JF Jr, Smith SC Jr, Stone NJ and Taubert KA. AHA Guidelines for Primary Prevention of Cardiovascular Disease and Stroke: 2002 Update: Consensus Panel Guide to Comprehensive Risk Reduction for Adult Patients Without Coronary or Other Atherosclerotic Vascular Diseases. American Heart Association Science Advisory and Coordinating Committee. Circulation 2002; 106: 388–91.

Perspectives on Diabetes Care in Old Age: A Focus on Frailty

Andrej Zeyfang[1] and Jeremy D. Walston[2]
[1]*Bethesda Hospital Stuttgart, Department of Internal Medicine and Geriatrics, Stuttgart, Germany*
[2]*Johns Hopkins University School of Medicine, Baltimore, MD, USA*

Key messages

- Glucose intolerance and diabetes likely lead to a decline in muscle strength, which in turn influences frailty.
- The biology that underlies frailty – namely, the activation of inflammatory pathways and neuroendocrine dysregulation – influences a number of common chronic disease states in older adults.
- Diabetes and geriatric syndromes (immobility, depression, dementia) are interdependent and influence themselves reciprocally. Therefore, frailty develops more often in geriatric patients with diabetes.
- The early identification of geriatric syndromes in older diabetics through a comprehensive geriatric assessment and an organized care plan can improve the quality of life.

13.1 Introduction

Today, the prevalence of diabetes in older adults is increasing rapidly [1]. In addition to the common medical complications of diabetes, such as cardiovascular disease (CVD), stroke and renal failure, older adults are much more susceptible to late-life geriatric syndromes, including mobility disability, incontinence, depression and frailty [1]. These syndromes, when combined with diabetes and related medical complications, represent an especially great challenge to the quality of life of these older patients. Older diabetic patients with these syndromes also present a major challenge to health care providers because of the complexity of their cases, and because no clear evidence-based treatment regimens have been developed for this subset of diabetics. This is in part because evidence-based guidelines aimed at younger individuals suffering from diabetes cannot be simply extrapolated to the elderly without considering aspects such as multimorbidity, functional impairment, frailty and the need to evaluate individual goals, including life perspectives and the quality of life. For this rapidly growing group of older diabetics, there is a large demand for data to be acquired from randomized controlled trials that seek the best and safest methods to treat diabetes and its complications. The quest is also ongoing for data that focus on reducing the period of disability and increasing the quality of life.

Frailty is an important issue in geriatric medicine, as it characterizes that subset of older adults who are most vulnerable to adverse health care outcomes. This syndrome is relevant for the diabetologist who cares for an ever-growing number of frail, older patients because of the extreme vulnerability exhibited by this subset of patients to adverse health outcomes and iatrogenic

Diabetes in Old Age. Third Edition. Edited by Alan J. Sinclair
© 2009 John Wiley & Sons, Ltd

complications. In this chapter we will review the definitions and consequences of frailty, and also summarize the biology of frailty, as understood to date. A review of the interactions between diabetes and frailty, and modal pathways of how diabetes may accelerate frailty and how frailty may accelerate or worsen diabetes, will be provided. Finally, a discussion is included of how frailty may impact upon the treatment of diabetes and other geriatric syndromes.

13.2　The frailty syndrome and its biology

Frailty has long been recognized by practitioners of medicine as a syndrome of late-life, multisystem decline associated with vulnerability to adverse health outcomes, including accelerated mortality [2]. However, until very recently few investigators have attempted to identify its underlying aetiology and how it might interact with chronic diseases such as diabetes. This is in part due to the heterogeneity with which frailty and many complex diseases of late life present. Recently, several investigators have attempted to operationalize and characterize some of the clinical and biological characteristics of frailty (see Table 13.1). The definition proposed by Chin [6] is easiest to utilize because it has the fewest measurements. However, weight loss tends to be less predictive of adverse outcomes when inserted into other frailty models, and hence it is a relatively weak predictor. The Studenski model [4] offers utility in that it is all based on objective measurements, but it has not been widely tested in other populations. The Fried model [2] is currently the most widely utilized in both outcomes and biological research; this takes longer to complete because it incorporates two questionnaires, but these two criteria are more subjective. Most emerging definitions related to frailty have focused on the concept of weakness, fatigue, low levels of activity and the accumulation of deficits and incorporate performance measures into the examination [2–7].

The frailty metric outlined by Fried and coworkers, which includes measures of fatigue, grip strength, walking speed, weight loss and activity levels, has been instrumental in helping other investigators explore and characterize the biology that underlies frailty [2]. These studies have identified significant relationships between frailty status and the inflammatory mediators interleukin-6 (IL-6), C-reactive protein (CRP) and white blood cell counts; between frailty and low

Table 13.1 Components of different frailty screening tools.

Chin 1999 [6]	Studenski 2003 [4]	Fried 2001 [2]
• inactivity • weight loss	• gait speed • ability to rise from a chair • balance skills	• slow walking speed • poor hand grip • exhaustion • weight loss • low energy expenditure • (three out of five)

levels of insulin-like growth factor-1 (IGF-1) and dehydroepiandrosterone sulphate (DHEA-S) (hormones which are important in muscle mass maintenance); and between high levels of cortisol and frailty [8–11]. Other investigators have identified low levels of vitamin D as a strong correlate of frailty [12], and lower levels of red blood cells [13]. Importantly (as discussed below), hyperglycaemia and hyperinsulinaemia are strongly related to frailty [14, 15]. The apparent involvement of multiple systems has led investigators to hypothesize that frailty represents a multisystem decline in regulatory and metabolic systems, and that this decline manifests itself in declines in strength and energy as well as in a frank vulnerability to decline and death [16, 17].

13.3　Frailty and diabetes in late life

Many studies have previously demonstrated an increased prevalence between diabetes and late-life syndromes, including frailty. For example, in the Cardiovascular Health Study (CHS), a study of the evolution of CVD in over 5000 adults aged over 65 years, diabetes and many other medical conditions were found to be significantly over-represented in the frail compared to non-frail subsets of the cohort (Figure 13.1) [2]. The study results showed that 25% of the subset of that population deemed frail was diabetic, 18.2% of the pre-frail or intermediate subset was diabetic, while only 12% of the non-frail subset was diabetic. Furthermore, within the same population, it was apparent that those frail CHS participants who were not diabetic were significantly more likely to have higher glucose

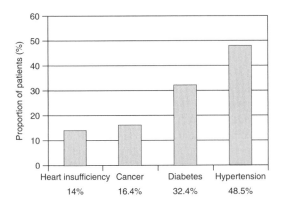

Figure 13.1 Prevalence of frailty in different medical conditions [14].

and insulin levels at baseline and after any oral glucose tolerance test than those who were not frail [14]. A more recent study in the same cohort has helped to demonstrate that insulin resistance *per se* predicts incident frailty, providing important evidence that diabetes and its underlying biology in part may drive frailty [15]. Other supportive evidence of the relationship between frailty and diabetes derives from another cohort study of older adults which showed that diabetes accelerates the loss of skeletal muscle strength – an important component of frailty [18].

Despite the fact that these studies have indicated the existence of a strong biological relationship between diabetes and frailty, or at least the strength component of frailty, many biological questions remain to be answered. Regardless of the fact that there is some evidence that incident frailty develops in the face of diabetes, it may also be true that the biology that underlies frailty may also drive the development of diabetes, or at least insulin resistance. In the following sections we will outline the biology that may contribute to late-life diabetes, and describe how diabetes, its complications and its biology may influence frailty. In the final section we will suggest how frailty and its underlying biology may drive diabetes.

13.4 The biology of late-life diabetes

Although younger and middle-aged individuals who develop diabetes generally have multiple underlying metabolic alterations, including increased hepatic gluconeogenesis, increased insulin resistance and decreased insulin secretion, data acquired from older

adults suggest that fasting hepatic glucose production is not increased [19]. Instead, there appears to be two metabolically distinct groups of older diabetics: (i) a lean subset that is insulin-deficient; and (ii) an obese subset that is mostly insulin-resistant with irregularities in glucose-stimulated pulsatile insulin secretion [20]. The older, insulin-deficient subset may be less able to respond with an appropriate glucose-triggered insulin release, in part because of an increased apoptosis of pancreatic beta cells associated with both ageing and with increased fat mass and insulin resistance [21].

There are likely several aetiologies for the age-related increases in insulin resistance represented by the second group of diabetics. First, age-related declines in skeletal muscle, combined with increased fat mass, is likely to be a major contributing factor to insulin resistance in older adults [22]. Second, age-related alterations in energy expenditure and generation, and the level of the mitochondria likely contribute to abnormalities in glucose utilization and energy expenditure and hence insulin resistance [23]. Next – although not definitively demonstrated *in vivo* – increasing numbers of senescent cells likely emerge with age. *In-vitro* models have suggested that these cells secrete inflammatory cytokines, which in turn contributes to insulin resistance via the down-regulation of *adiponectin*, a potent regulator of glucose uptake in adipose cells and a potent anti-inflammatory agent [24, 25]. Finally, multiple gene variants, including those in mitochondrial DNA, are known to influence the development of insulin resistance [26]. Many of these variants likely remain subclinical or undetectable until later in life, when other age-related changes in body composition or environmental changes, such as decreased activity, leads to the expression of the phenotype. In addition to the multiple age-related biological aetiologies of insulin resistance, there are also important environmental and disease-related aetiologies that impact insulin resistance with aging. First, multiple chronic disease states trigger chronic inflammatory responses, which in turn exacerbate insulin resistance in older adults [27]. Further, corticosteroids given to treat chronic inflammatory conditions worsen insulin resistance. Chronic disease states and functional decline leads to decreased activity levels, which in turn contributes to insulin resistance. In summary, one dominant biological aetiology of insulin resistance related to aging *per se* likely does not predominate in any given older diabetic. Rather, it is likely that multiple aetiologies coexist in each individual with insulin resistance, and that many of these age-related abnormalities increase with age.

13.4.1 How might diabetes and its underlying biology impact frailty?

Although it is clear that diabetes and frailty are closely associated in clinical studies of older adults, to date only minimal evidence has been acquired from longitudinal studies which suggests that one condition is causal for the other. Rather, given the biological aetiologies described above for both syndromes, it is highly likely that diabetes impacts the development of frailty, and that frailty and its underlying biology contributes to the hyperglycaemia and/or diabetes frequently observed in frail, older adults. When attempting to answer the question of how might diabetes impact frailty, several potential pathophysiological pathways are possible (Figure 13.2). First and foremost, skeletal muscle appears to be negatively impacted by diabetes and glucose intolerance [18, 28, 29]. As skeletal muscle weakness is a key component of frailty, it is highly likely that skeletal muscle weakness drives much of the association between frailty and diabetes. The term 'sarcopenic obesity' was coined to help describe the phenomena of older, obese, insulin-resistant or diabetic individuals who have marked muscle weakness consistent with frailty [30]. The muscle decline in this subgroup of 'frail' older adults is likely profoundly influenced by both the fatty replacement of muscle tissue and by the insulin resistance, increased levels of cytokines, and increased levels of adiponectin observed in this population [30]. Additional pathophysiology related to diabetes may also influence frailty. Chronic fluxes in glucose levels related to diabetes appear to activate both the sympathetic nervous system (SNS) and the hypothalamic-pituitary-adrenal axis (HPA). The result of the chronic activation of stress pathways is the chronic elevation of cortisol in those with poorly

controlled diabetes, which in turn negatively impacts skeletal muscle. Furthermore, chronic inflammation is also known to negatively influence skeletal muscle strength in older adults, and is also known to be strongly related to incident frailty [15]. This association may be due to the accumulation of age-related glycosylated end products (AGE) which, when bound to specific receptors (RAGE, a signal transduction receptor), leads to the activation of nuclear factor-kappa B (NFκB)-related inflammatory pathways, which in turn leads to the chronic secretion of inflammatory cytokines such as IL-6; this causes a reinforcement of glucose intolerance as well as an acceleration of muscle mass decline [31]. Finally, it is also clear that a number of diabetes complications, such as renal failure and CVD, can also activate inflammatory pathways and influence multiple systems into decline [32].

13.4.2 How might frailty impact the development of diabetes?

Frailty is likely driven by multiple age-related molecular and physiological changes, many of which are known to impact impaired glucose intolerance and diabetes (Figure 13.3). At a molecular level, age-related declines in mitochondrial function are driven by damaged mitochondrial DNA. This cumulative change can result in lower levels of energy production, an impaired utilization of energy, and the increased production of free radicals of oxygen [23]. The lower levels of energy production result in glucose intolerance and lower metabolic rates in tissues such as skeletal muscle that normally have high energy requirements. The increased generation of free radicals associated with mitochondrial dysfunction leads directly to the activation of NFκB-related inflammatory pathways. Chronic activity of this pathway results in the chronic elevation of the pleotrophic cytokine IL-6, the elevation of which in turn has been shown to influence the development of glucose intolerance, which in susceptible individuals

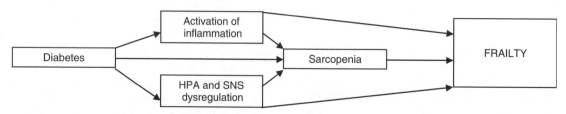

Figure 13.2 Schematic of key intermediate biology that connects diabetes to frailty. HPA = hypothalamic-pituitary-adrenal axis; SNS = sympathetic nervous system.

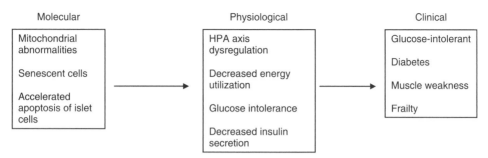

Figure 13.3 Modal pathway between age-related molecular changes, altered physiology and clinical outcomes. HPA axis = hypothalamic-pituitary-adrenal axis.

pushes towards the development of type 2 diabetes. In addition, there is considerable evidence that senescent cell types, including fibroblasts, endothelial cells and immune system cells, emerge with age. These cells appear to lose the ability to undergo apoptosis and develop inappropriate inflammatory characteristics. The resultant increase in inflammatory mediators may further reinforces the inflammatory milieu that influences late-life glucose intolerance. Finally, accelerated apoptosis – or programmed cell death – has also been hypothesized to be accelerated in frailty and in other aging-related conditions such as Parkinson's syndrome. Given the evidence that pancreatic beta-cell apoptosis is accelerated with ageing, it could be speculated that declines in insulin production, in parallel with increased insulin resistance, may push frail individuals towards the development of diabetes. On a more physiological level, circulating inflammatory mediators and increased cortisol secretion characterize frailty [5]. Chronic cortisol elevation has been demonstrated to influence impaired glucose intolerance. Furthermore, chronic elevations in inflammatory mediators such as IL-6 trigger glucose tolerance and hence may influence the development of diabetes in frail, older adults (Figure 13.3).

13.5 Geriatric syndromes and diabetes

In addition to the evidence for a strong relationship between diabetes and frailty, there is also evidence for the mutual interaction between diabetes and geriatric syndromes such as incontinence, immobility and cognitive or affective disorders [33]. Because of the strong relationship between diabetes and multiple geriatric syndromes, it will be increasingly important to

understand the biology that links the two, and to understand how best to treat older frail diabetics while maintaining a high quality of life. Many investigators have found that chronic disease, such as diabetes, poses a higher risk condition for the development of frailty (see Figure 13.3) or functional decline [34]. In fact, several studies have increasingly demonstrated the validity of the hypothesis that the elderly with diabetes have a higher prevalence of geriatric syndromes.

13.5.1 Mobility, falls and urinary incontinence

With increasing age, mobility begins to be affected in elderly individuals with diabetes. Park and coworkers identified an accelerated loss of leg muscle strength and quality in older adults with type 2 diabetes [18]. There is also a higher risk of hip fracture [35]. Activities in daily life are hindered, particularly those requiring mobility, and incontinence may be problematic [36]. Urinary incontinence is a common syndrome in the elderly with diabetes. In fact, its prevalence in women with impaired fasting glucose is almost double that in women with a normal fasting glucose [37]. A typical concomitant problem is the need to urinate arising suddenly ('urge'), with falls frequently occurring as the subject tries to reach the toilet 'in time'.

13.5.2 Malnutrition

Tooth loss and parodontitis are more prevalent in diabetes [38] and, together with problems in swallowing (e.g. after stroke), malnutrition and weight loss often occur; these are important components of frailty. In contrast to younger patients, in the elderly with diabetes undernutrition is more common; for this reason, restrictive diets are not advantageous for elderly patients with diabetes and should not be prescribed. Careful attention should be paid to patients with weight loss (indicator of frailty) or tooth loss, as functional pairs are very important for chewing.

13.5.3　Depression

Late-life depression is found commonly even in individuals without diabetes, reaching a prevalence of approximately 25%. Depression, reaching much higher rates in patients with diabetes, contributes to poor adherence to medication and dietary regimens. Depression is the most important determinant for reduced adherence to medications [47] and causes therefore poor glycaemic control. The depressed elderly have a reduced quality of life, and increased health care expenditures [39]. In younger adults, a history of depression increases the risk of diabetes [54]. Although depression is a risk factor for mortality in older patients with diabetes [55], the implementation of a depression management programme would have a decreased risk of mortality compared to depressed patients with diabetes in usual-care practices [56]. Before elderly patients take part in educational programmes for diabetes, depression should be screened for, and treated if indicated.

13.5.4　Cognition

Cognitive dysfunction and dementia are also more common in the diabetic older adult, and are in part correlated with diabetes control. This link was described by Reaven *et al.* in 1990 [57], but no explanation was provided at the time regarding the reasons. In the descriptive Rotterdam-Study [58] there was a double prevalence of vascular or degenerative dementia in patients suffering from diabetes. Only during the past few years have any studies provided any insight into the particular way in which diabetes might be linked to cognitive dysfunction. Type 2 diabetes is strongly associated with cognitive impairment, especially in semantic memory and perceptual speed, but not with episodic memory, working memory or visuospatial ability, nor with any measure of global cognition [59]. Importantly, *metabolic syndrome* is also significantly associated with declines in all cognitive measures. Among the single components of metabolic syndrome, hyperglycaemia was most strongly and significantly associated with cognitive function in a recent study [60]. The same study highlighted a significant interaction between metabolic syndrome and inflammation on cognition, indicating the close connection

of frailty, diabetes and cognitive impairment. In other studies, a correlation has been identified between cognitive dysfunction, as shown by a clock-drawing test or clock in a box and HbA_{1c} [40].

Cognitive dysfunction can be worsened by a concomitant depression or by other drugs such as benzodiazepines or pain medication [61]. Cognitive dysfunction may also render difficult all types of self-management skills of the elderly. Hyperglycaemia is associated with declines in cognitive function, and the extent of cognitive dysfunction in turn influences the ability to attain any quality of diabetes control. Thus, at times the goals of tight glucose control may need to be lowered.

13.5.5　Interaction between geriatric syndromes and diabetes

The mutually influencing effects of coexisting diabetes and geriatric syndromes are a very important field of future research. Treatment goals and strategies depend heavily on functional resources and deficits [36]. Examples of this interdependence are listed in Table 13.2, and the respective chapters in this book provide a deeper insight into the pathophysiological basis of depression or dementia and their connections to diabetes. As most of these geriatric syndromes are either directly or indirectly components of the frailty syndrome, it is imperative that professionals in this field should carefully examine for the presence of functional problems in elderly patients with diabetes.

13.6　Approaches for improving care for frail, older diabetics

With knowledge of these interactions and the impact on quality of life, new strategies for the comprehensive care of the geriatric patient with diabetes are needed.

13.6.1　Comprehensive geriatric assessment

Before frailty develops, the resources and deficits of the geriatric patient should be assessed and quantified by performing a comprehensive geriatric assessment. The effectiveness in reducing short-term mortality, the increased ability to live at home for at least one year, and improvement of physical and cognitive function, has been proven for those living in the community [41] as well as for hospitalized patients [42]. Some recommendations for the selection of elderly patients

Table 13.2 Interdependence of diabetes and geriatric syndromes [43].

Syndrome	Effect on diabetes	Diabetes causes
Dementia	• Worsens HbA_{1c} • Diabetes education and self-management rendered difficult • Controls obfuscated (retinopathy, blood-glucose and -pressure, foot, feeding and drinking)	• Prevalence of dementia higher • Worse metabolic control causes more severe cognitive impairment
Depression	• Worsens HbA_{1c} • Reduced compliance • 'Pseudodementia'	• Prevalence of depression higher • Depressive feeling augmented by fear of sequelae • Feeling guilty about 'diet errors'
Incontinence	• Voluntary reduced drinking amount causing dehydration and hyperglycaemia • Urinary tract infections causing worse metabolic control	• With hyperglycaemia, a large amount of urinary flow • High prevalence of urge incontinence • End-stage, often overflow, incontinence
Immobility	• Physical activity more difficult • Self-care difficult or impossible (foot-care, blood glucose self-control, insulin injection)	• Dizziness or fatigue hinders activity • Polyneuropathies cause afferent ataxia • Falls and hip fractures more often in diabetes

with diabetes who should undergo comprehensive geriatric assessment are listed in Table 13.3, together with some clues regarding the use of assessment tools.

13.6.2 Educational programmes

It has been perceived that conventional education programmes for diabetes patients are not as effective for the elderly; consequently, new approaches have been designed for application in elderly patients [43]. Apart from a particular didactic approach, age-specific subjects are also required. The general recommendations include individualized approaches, risk–benefit considerations, and the involvement of multiple disciplines and care partners [44]. Moreover. special educational programmes for care-givers in an out-patient setting or nursing home are needed.

13.6.3 Physical training

The classic approach of encouraging more physical activity for the younger patient with diabetes is most likely not workable for the elderly diabetic. Instead, low-threshold, slower approaches are encouraged which motivate the patient, combine the positive effects of physical activity on metabolism with the benefits on muscular strength, reduced risk of

falls and fractures, enhanced cognitive function, and generally the prevention of disease and frailty [45].

13.6.4 Nutrition

It is common practice today to advise the diabetic patient on diet; however, given the prevalence of undernutrition in the geriatric age group, therapeutic regimens calling for restrictive diets should clearly be stopped for these patients. Nutritional recommendations to geriatric patients should be realistic, individualized, and acceptable to the patient. Not only does food play an important role in the quality of life, but their body weight is also crucial when considering morbidity and mortality. A loss of body weight past the age of 75 years can be dangerous; a body mass index (BMI) $<22.7\,kg\,m^{-2}$ in old age is associated with above-average mortality rates, even in the apparently healthy [46].

13.7 Drug therapy in the frail elderly

The effects, side effects and particularities of drug therapy in the elderly with diabetes in general are described elsewhere; here, attention is focused on the

Table 13.3 Recommendations for selection of elderly patients with diabetes that should undergo comprehensive geriatric assessment [52] and recommended assessment tools [53].

Presence of a geriatric syndrome		Presence of several coexisting morbidities, apart from diabetes		Presence of disabilities resulting from lower-limb vascular disease or neuropathy requiring a rehabilitation programme	
Confused state	MMSE CDT CAM	Complex drug regimens	More than five different drugs	Diabetic foot syndrome	
Depression Falls	GDS TuG 5-Chair-Rise Modified Romberg test (Standing positions)	More than two drugs for the same condition More than once-daily administration of a drug		PNP	Peripheral neuropathy (Semmes–Weinstein-monofilament 10 g)
Immobility Pressure sores Incontinence Malnutrition	TCS Braden-Scale MNA NRS			PAD	Ankle-brachial index (Doppler)
In the absence of a terminal illness or severe dementia syndrome					

MMSE = Mini-Mental-State-Examination; CDT = clock-drawing test; CAM = Confusion Assessment Method; GDS = Geriatric Depression Scale; TuG = Timed Up & Go-Test; TCS = Trunk Control Scale; MNA = Mini-Nutritional Assessment; NRS = Nutritional Risk Score; PNP = peripheral neuropathy; PAD = peripheral arterial disease

administration of the medication. Adherence to therapy (either insulin or oral drugs) is generally low, ranging from 61 to 85% in a 6-month period of observation for oral medication to approximately 63% with insulin therapy [47]. Nikolaus *et al.* showed that, in a group of elderly patients, 10% failed to open at least one container of medication given in different dosage forms. This inability was associated with poor vision, impaired cognitive function and low manual dexterity. Compliance with prescribed medication correlated to cognitive function, ability to handle medication containers, number of prescribed drugs, and recent changes in drug prescriptions [48].

13.7.1 What about insulin?

Insulin therapy poses a major challenge in the treatment of geriatric patients. Insulin is not only a potent agent to normalize blood sugar, but it also acts as an anabolic drug, allowing 'doping' of the frail elderly [49]. Unfortunately, the administration of insulin is problematic for the elderly (see Table 13.4), as well as achieving the appropriate dosage – which if not correct will lead to hypo- or hyperglycaemia [50]. In order to determine the individual's ability to self-administer insulin correctly, the cognitive, visual and fine motor capacities of the patient should be examined. Here, for example, the timed money-counting test could be used [51]. Before the patient is provided with an insulin pen, the visus, cognitive capacity, ability to correctly self-dose and the obstacles to insulin self-application should be examined. It is necessary to carefully assess the benefits of self-management ('I can eat whenever I want') versus dependency ('I have to wait until the nurse has time for me'). It should also be determined if the elderly patient requires professional support for insulin therapy. As of yet, no insulin-injecting device specifically aimed for the elderly has been developed, but this would be helpful.

13.7.2 Assistive devices

There is a substantial demand for innovative assistive devices for the elderly with diabetes. This begins with age-appropriate devices for self-control of the blood sugar level. The obstacles when using existing devices are multiple: too small; non-user friendly; a need for calibration; digital numbers that could be

Table 13.4 Difficulties in self-administration of insulin in the elderly.

Forgetting injection (no dosage)
Forgetting that already injected (double dosage)
Wrong dosage ('U for 0' – 50 Units given, prescription 5U)
No mixing before injection of biphasic or NPH-Insulin
No change of needle – obstruction
Not waiting the appropriate time interval after injecting insulin
Waiting too long after self-administered medication (taking a nap)

misinterpreted if read upside-down, and so on. Intelligent blood glucose-monitoring systems for the elderly should be much easier to use. An advanced but simple system capable of providing advice that is easy to understand would be an example. For instance, similar to a traffic light where green indicates 'everything is fine', orange might mean 'take care', and red 'call for medical help'. Modern electronic and wireless technology could be included, quietly transmitting data, for example, to a nursing centre.

Devices used for insulin injection today are not optimal for the elderly. These should be constructed so that aspects such as limited motor ability or tremor, reduced visual function and diminished strength of the thumb (when using a pen) are considered. State-of-the-art technology could also be used in a device to enable the insulin-delivery system to provide the desirable dose for the moment automatically (an expert system might be connected to the glucose-monitoring system). Clearly, adaptations to the design of insulin devices would be one means of enabling the elderly to begin insulin therapy with more ease, comfort and acceptance, but further innovative studies are required to help facilitate the delivery of insulin and increase safety in this process.

When treating frail elderly with diabetes it is important to understand other basic assistive devices and their limitations. It is useful to test visual and hearing capacities by screening to identify a need for glasses or hearing aids, particularly before starting an educational programme. The prevention of falls and hip-fracture is also part of the care of the diabetic elderly. Canes, walkers or rolling-walkers are not only useful for individuals at high risk for falling (e.g. because of neuropathy and afferent ataxia), but can also be temporarily of help, for example when wearing a cast for a diabetic foot. Wearing hip-protectors can reduce

the incidence of hip-fracture after a fall. The prevention of falling is a priority and is achievable; as many falls occur in the bathroom, handles or grab-bars are advisable, installing a movement-sensor to turn on the light or putting a toilet-chair next the bed are simple to do. These basic procedures can facilitate remaining at home versus an unwanted move into a nursing home. For hospitalized patients with diabetes, socks with small rubber buttons to prevent slipping could be worn at night to avoid the need for putting on shoes. Sensor-mats that signal an alarm when the patient leaves the bed at night are useful for hospitalized patients, especially when at risk for disorientation or delirium. The aims of achieving a more comfortable, safe and acceptable existence for the elderly patient with diabetes, as well as extending the length of time living without dependence on others, can be attained by prudent operation of assistive devices.

13.8 Summary

In summary, it is increasingly clear that there are important interactions between diabetes, frailty and other geriatric syndromes in older adults. These interactions appear to have a deeply biological basis that impact profoundly upon skeletal muscle and are, in part, driven by neuroendocrine and inflammatory changes. Most importantly, as frail, older adults are more vulnerable to adverse health outcomes, it is critical to be able to identify the frailest subset of diabetic patients and to formulate a clear and coherent treatment plan that focuses on the quality of life and reduction of symptoms in these most vulnerable patients. The interaction of geriatric syndromes – mainly depression, dementia, malnutrition and diabetes – should, on the other hand, always be considered in the treatment plan. Multidisciplinary approaches targeting increased functionality and independent living can be effective in this regard, considering also the particularities and possibilities in drug therapy and the use of assistive devices.

References

1. Blaum C. (2008) Descriptive epidemiology of diabetes. In: M. Munshi and L. Lipsitz (eds). *Geriatric Diabetes Book*. Taylor and Francis Group, LLC, New York, pp. 1–10.
2. Fried LP, Tangen C, Walston J, Newman A, Hirsch CH, Gottdiener JS, Seeman T, Tracy R, Kop WJ, Burke G

and McBurnie MA. Frailty in older adults: evidence for a phenotype. Journal of Gerontology 2001; 56A (3): M1–11.

3. Rockwood K and Mitnitski A. Frailty in relation to the accumulation of deficits. J Gerontol A Biol Sci Med Sci 2007; 62 (7): 722–7.

4. Studenski S, Hayes RP, Leibowitz RQ, Bode R, Lavery L, Walston J, Duncan P and Perera S. Clinical Global Impression of Change in Physical Frailty: development of a measure based on clinical judgment. J Am Geriatr Soc 2004; 52 (9): 1560–6.

5. Walston J, Hadley EC, Ferrucci L, Guralnik JM, Newman AB, Studenski SA, Ershler WB, Harris T and Fried LP. Research agenda for frailty in older adults: toward a better understanding of physiology and etiology: summary from the American Geriatrics Society/National Institute on Aging Research Conference on Frailty in Older Adults. J Am Geriatr Soc 2006; 54 (6): 991–1001.

6. Chin APM, Dekker JM, Feskens EJ, Schouten EG and Kromhout D. How to select a frail elderly population? A comparison of three working definitions. J Clin Epidemiol 1999; 52 (11): 1015–21.

7. Studenski S, Perera S, Wallace D, Chandler JM, Duncan PW, Rooney E, Fox M and Guralnik JM. Physical performance measures in the clinical setting. J Am Geriatr Soc 2003; 51 (3): 314–22.

8. Leng S, Chaves P, Koenig K and Walston J. Serum interleukin-6 and hemoglobin as physiological correlates in the geriatric syndrome of frailty: a pilot study. J Am Geriatr Soc 2002; 50 (7): 1268–71.

9. Leng SX, Cappola AR, Andersen RE, Blackman MR, Koenig K, Blair M and Walston JD. Serum levels of insulin-like growth factor-I (IGF-I) and dehydroepiandrosterone sulfate (DHEA-S), and their relationships with serum interleukin-6, in the geriatric syndrome of frailty. Aging Clin Exp Res 2004; 16 (2): 153–7.

10. Varadhan R, Walston J, Cappola AR, Carlson MC, Wand GS and Fried LP. Higher levels and blunted diurnal variation of cortisol in frail older women. Journal of Gerontology: Medical Science 2008, 63 (2), 190–5.

11. Leng SX, Xue QL, Tian J, Walston J and Fried LP. Inflammation and frailty in older women. Journal of the American Geriatrics Society 2007; 55 (6): 864–71.

12. Puts MT, Visser M, Twisk JW, Deeg DJ and Lips P. Endocrine and inflammatory markers as predictors of frailty. Clin Endocrinol (Oxf) 2005; 63 (4): 403–11.

13. Chaves PH, Semba RD, Leng SX, Woodman RC, Ferrucci L, Guralnik JM and Fried LP. Impact of anemia and cardiovascular disease on frailty status of community-dwelling older women: the Women's Health and Aging Studies I and II. J Gerontol A Biol Sci Med Sci 2005; 60 (6): 729–35.

14. Walston J, McBurnie MA, Newman A, Tracy R, Kop WJ, Hirsch CH, Gottdiener JS and Fried LP. Frailty and activation of the inflammation and coagulation systems with and without clinical morbidities: Results from the Cardiovascular Health Study. Arch Intern Med 2002; 162: 2333–41.

15. Barzilay JI, Blaum C, Moore T, Xue QL, Hirsch CH, Walston JD and Fried LP. Insulin resistance and inflammation as precursors of frailty: the Cardiovascular Health Study. Arch Intern Med 2007; 167 (7): 635–41.

16. Walston J. Frailty – the search for underlying causes. Sci Aging Knowledge Environ 2004; (4): e4.

17. Fried LP, Hadley EC, Walston JD, Newman A, Guralnik JM, Studenski S, Harris TB, Ershler WB and Ferrucci L. From bedside to bench: research agenda for frailty. Sci Aging Knowledge Environ 2005; (31): e24.

18. Park SW, Goodpaster BH, Strotmeyer ES, Kuller LH, Broudeau R, Kammerer C, de RN, Harris TB, Schwartz AV, Tylavsky FA, Cho YW and Newman AB. Accelerated loss of skeletal muscle strength in older adults with type 2 diabetes: the health, aging, and body composition study. Diabetes Care 2007; 30 (6): 1507–12.

19. Meneilly GS and Elahi D. Metabolic alterations in middle-aged and elderly lean patients with type 2 diabetes. Diabetes Care 2005; 28 (6): 1498–9.

20. Meneilly GS, Veldhuis JD and Elahi D. Deconvolution analysis of rapid insulin pulses before and after six weeks of continuous subcutaneous administration of glucagon-like peptide-1 in elderly patients with type 2 diabetes. J Clin Endocrinol Metab 2005; 90 (11): 6251–6.

21. Fridlyand LE and Philipson LH. Reactive species, cellular repair and risk factors in the onset of type 2 diabetes mellitus: review and hypothesis. Curr Diabetes Rev 2006; 2 (2): 241–59.

22. Hughes VA, Roubenoff R, Wood M, Frontera WR, Evans WJ and Fiatarone Singh MA. Anthropometric assessment of 10-y changes in body composition in the elderly. Am J Clin Nutr 2004; 80 (2): 475–82.

23. Figueiredo PA, Mota MP, Appell HJ and Duarte JA. The role of mitochondria in aging of skeletal muscle. Biogerontology 2008, 9(2), 67–84.

24. Guerre-Millo M. Adiponectin: An update. Diabetes Metab 2008, 34 (1), 12–18.

25. Tilg H and Moschen AR. Role of adiponectin and PBEF/visfatin as regulators of inflammation: involvement in obesity-associated diseases. Clin Sci (Lond) 2008; 114 (4): 275–88.

26. Walston J and Silver K. (2008) The genetics of diabetes and its complications in older adults. In: M. Munshi and L. Lipsitz (eds). Geriatric Diabetes Book. Taylor and Francis Group, LLC, New York, pp. 11–28.

27. Libby P. Inflammatory mechanisms: the molecular basis of inflammation and disease. Nutr Rev 2007; 65 (12Pt 2): S140–6.

28. Goodpaster BH, Carlson CL, Visser M, Kelley DE, Scherzinger A, Harris TB, Stamm E and Newman AB. Attenuation of skeletal muscle and strength in the elderly: The Health ABC Study. J Appl Physiol 2001; 90 (6): 2157–65.

29. Park SW, Goodpaster BH, Strotmeyer ES, de RN, Harris TB, Schwartz AV, Tylavsky FA and Newman AB. Decreased muscle strength and quality in older adults with type 2 diabetes: the health, aging, and body composition study. Diabetes 2006; 55 (6): 1813–18.

30. Roubenoff R. Sarcopenic obesity: does muscle loss cause fat gain? Lessons from rheumatoid arthritis and osteoarthritis. Ann N Y Acad Sci 2000; 904: 553–7.

31. Ershler WB and Keller ET. Age-associated increased interleukin-6 gene expression, late-life diseases, and frailty. Annu Rev Med 2000; 51: 245–70.

32. Cesari M, Leeuwenburgh C, Lauretani F, Onder G, Bandinelli S, Maraldi C, Guralnik JM, Pahor M and Ferrucci L. Frailty syndrome and skeletal muscle: results from the Invecchiare in Chianti study. Am J Clin Nutr 2006; 83 (5): 1142–8.

33. Hader C, Beischer W, Braun A, Dreyer M, Friedl A, Fusgen I, Gastes U, Grunklee D, Hauner H, Kobberling J, Kolb G, von Laue N, Muller UA and Zeyfang A. Diagnosis treatment and follow up of diabetes mellitus in elderly. European Journal of Geriatrics 2006; 8: 1–57.

34. Gregg EW, Mangione CM, Cauley JA, Thompson TJ, Schwartz AV, Ensrud KE and Nevitt MC. Diabetes and incidence of functional disability in older women. Diabetes Care 2002; 25 (1): 61–7.

35. Lipscombe LL, Jamal SA, Booth GL and Hawker GA. The risk of hip fractures in older individuals with diabetes: a population-based study. Diabetes Care 2007; 30 (4): 835–41.

36. Zeyfang A. [Treating diabetes in the very old]. MMW Fortschr Med 2007; 149 (19): 29-3.

37. Brown JS, Vittinghoff E, Lin F, Nyberg LM, Kusek JW and Kanaya AM. Prevalence and risk factors for urinary incontinence in women with type 2 diabetes and impaired fasting glucose: findings from the National Health and Nutrition Examination Survey (NHANES) 2001-2002. Diabetes Care 2006; 29 (6): 1307–12.

38. Presson SM, Niendorff WJ and Martin RF. Tooth loss and need for extractions in American Indian and Alaska Native dental patients. J Public Health Dent 2000; 60 (Suppl. 1): 267–72.

39. Lustman PJ and Clouse RE. Depression in diabetic patients: the relationship between mood and glycemic control. J Diabetes Complications 2005; 19 (2): 113–22.

40. Munshi M, Grande L, Hayes M, Ayres D, Suhl E, Capelson R, Lin S, Milberg W and Weinger K. Cognitive dysfunction is associated with poor diabetes control in older adults. Diabetes Care 2006; 29 (8): 1794–9.

41. Stuck AE, Egger M, Hammer A, Minder CE and Beck JC. Home visits to prevent nursing home admission and functional decline in elderly people: systematic review and meta-regression analysis. JAMA 2002; 287 (8): 1022–8.

42. Gordon JN, Trebble TM, Ellis RD, Duncan HD, Johns T and Goggin PM. Thalidomide in the treatment of cancer cachexia: a randomised placebo controlled trial. Gut 2005; 54 (4): 540–5.

43. Zeyfang A. [Structured educational programs for geriatric patients with diabetes mellitus]. MMW Fortschr Med 2005; 147 (26): 43, 45-3, 46.

44. Suhl E and Bonsignore P. Diabetes self-management education for older adults: general principles and practical application. Diabetes Spectrum 2006; 19: 234–40.

45. Warburton DE, Nicol CW and Bredin SS. Health benefits of physical activity: the evidence. Canadian Medical Association Journal 2006; 174 (6): 801–9.

46. Breeze E, Clarke R, Shipley MJ, Marmot MG and Fletcher AE. Cause-specific mortality in old age in relation to body mass index in middle age and in old age: follow-up of the Whitehall cohort of male civil servants. Int J Epidemiol 2006; 35 (1): 169–78.

47. Cramer JA. A systematic review of adherence with medications for diabetes. Diabetes Care 2004; 27 (5): 1218–24.

48. Nikolaus T, Kruse W, Bach M, Specht-Leible N, Oster P and Schlierf G. Elderly patients' problems with medication. An in-hospital and follow-up study. Eur J Clin Pharmacol 1996; 49 (4): 255–9.

49. Sonksen PH. Insulin, growth hormone and sport. J Endocrinol 2001; 170 (1): 13–25.

50. Grissinger M. Top 10 adverse drug reactions and medication errors. Program and abstracts of the American Pharmacists Association Annual Meeting, 16 March 2007.

51. Nikolaus T, Bach M, Oster P and Schlierf G. The Timed Test of Money Counting: a simple method of recognizing geriatric patients at risk for increased health care. Aging (Milano) 1995; 7 (3): 179–83.

52. Sinclair AJ. Special Considerations in older adults with diabetes: meeting the challenge. Diabetes Spectrum 2006; 19 (4): 229–33.

53. Zeyfang A. (2006) In: *Diabetologie kompakt*, 4th edition. H. Schatz (ed.). Thieme, Stuttgart, Ch. 3.6, pp. 135–9.

54. Brown LC, Majumdar SR, Newman SC and Johnson JA. History of depression increases risk of type 2 diabetes in younger adults. Diabetes Care 2005; 28: 1063–7.

55. Katon WJ, Rutter C, Simon G, Lin EH, Ludman E, Ciechanowski P, Kinder L, Young B and Von Korff M. The association of comorbid depression with mortality

in patients with type 2 diabetes. Diabetes Care 2005; 28: 2668–72.

56. Bogner HR, Morales KH, Post EP and Bruce ML. Diabetes, depression, and death. A randomized controlled trial of a depression treatment program for older adults based in primary care (PROSPECT). Diabetes Care 2007; 30: 3005–10.

57. Reaven GM, LW Thompson, D Nahum and E Haskins. Relationship between hyperglycemia and cognitive function in older NIDDM patients. Diabetes Care 1990; 13: 16–21.

58. Ott A, Stolk RP, van Harskamp F, Pols HAP, Hofman A and Breteler MMB. Diabetes mellitus and the risk of

dementia: The Rotterdam Study. Neurology 1999; 53 (9): 1937–42.

59. Arvanitakis Z, Wilson RS, Li Y, Aggarwal NT and Bennett DA. Diabetes and function in different cognitive systems in older individuals without dementia. Diabetes Care 2006; 29 (3): 560–5.

60. Dik MG, Jonker C, Comijs HC, Deeg DJ, Kok A, Yaffe K and Penninx BW. Contribution of metabolic syndrome components to cognition in older individuals. Diabetes Care 2007; 30 (10): 2655–60

61. Nikolaus T and Zeyfang A. Pharmacological treatments for persistent non-malignant pain in older persons. Drugs Aging 2004; 21 (1): 19–41

14

Metabolic Decompensation in the Elderly

Giuseppe Paolisso and Michelangela Barbieri

Department of Geriatric Medicine and Metabolic Diseases, Second University of Naples (SUN), Piazza Miraglia, Napoli, Italy

Key messages

- Both, diabetic ketoacidosis and hyperosmolar hyperglycaemic state may be the presenting features in older people without a previous diagnosis of diabetes.
- Early detection and prompt treatment of both metabolic disturbances can minimize the excess mortality seen in ageing patients.

14.1 Introduction

Impaired glucose homeostasis plays an important role in aged individuals, its manifestations varying from light – often unrecognized – hyperglycaemia up to acute hyperglycaemic crises that frequently lead to hospital admission.

Hyperglycaemic complications include dehydration, mental status changes, increased risk of infection and, in severe cases, the possibility of ketoacidosis and hyperosmolar coma, a condition which is more often fatal in the elderly. In the elderly, whereas the mortality rate for diabetic emergencies associated with ketoacidosis has remained low, that for diabetic emergencies associated with a hyperosmolar state has, by contrast, remained considerably higher.

The attainment of glycaemic control in order to reduce acute complications associated with diabetes is a priority for all elderly patients. Although flexibility may be allowed in setting glycaemic parameters for individual treatment goals, the clinician also must take into account the need to prevent associated acute complications.

Not only higher glycaemic values, but also even more dangerous hypoglycaemic episodes, can disturb the frail equilibrium of older patients. Hence, achieving target glycaemic goals while avoiding hypoglycaemia represents a major challenge in the management of elderly patients with diabetes mellitus. Repeated episodes of hypoglycaemia may cause extreme emotional distress in such patients, even when the episodes are relatively mild.

14.2 Hypoglycaemia

Hypoglycaemia accounts for a relatively high number of emergencies requiring hospital admission. The condition occurs far more frequently as a consequence of an inadequate therapy in diabetes management, as demonstrated in the Diabetes Control and Complications Trial (DCCT) and the United Kingdom Prospective Diabetes Study (UKPDS) [1, 2]. The frequency of hypoglycaemic episodes increases with in-

Diabetes in Old Age. Third Edition. Edited by Alan J. Sinclair
© 2009 John Wiley & Sons, Ltd

creasing quality of glycaemic control assessed with HbA$_{1c}$. It is generally accepted that hypoglycaemia occurs when the capillary blood glucose level is below $0.6\,g\,l^{-1}$. Symptomatic hypoglycaemia can be distinguished from 'silent' hypoglycaemia, which is frequently associated with the occurrence of severe hypoglycaemia [1].

In older patients, susceptibility to hypoglycaemia is pronounced, and is exacerbated by older people having little knowledge about the symptoms and signs of the condition [3, 4]. While hypoglycaemic events are usually of minor importance, in some instances death or severe sequelae – including myocardial infarction and stroke – may occur. Hypoglycaemia in the elderly subject can have serious, sometimes life-threatening, consequences for the heart or brain, both in terms of morbidity and quality of life. In some cases the outcome may be permanent neurological damage, presumably because of an already compromised cerebral circulation [4].

Consequently, in older subjects the risk of hypoglycaemia must be evaluated as clearly as possible and balanced, on an individual basis, against the potential benefit of a near-normal glucose level.

The symptoms differ somewhat from those observed in younger subjects (notably blurred vision and instability), and are often blunted by an autonomous neuropathy or impaired cognitive function ('silent' hypoglycaemia). Hypoglycaemic symptoms in the elderly tend to present predominantly as neuroglycopenic symptoms, including impaired concentration, personality changes, focal neurological deficits, seizure or syncope. *Nocturnal hypoglycaemia* may present as morning headaches or disturbed sleep. Adrenergic symptoms (tremulousness, anxiety, diaphoresis, palpitation and hunger) are diminished, in part due to a loss of autonomic nerve function [5].

Glucose counter-regulatory hormones such as glucagon, epinephrine (adrenaline) and growth hormone (GH) are the most important hormones secreted in response to hypoglycaemia. When glucagon is deficient, epinephrine becomes critical, while GH and cortisol are important if the hypoglycaemia is prolonged [6]. The elderly exhibit an impaired response of glucose counter-regulatory hormones in the presence of decreased glucose. Furthermore, the rate of insulin clearance from the circulation declines with age, which may lead to an enhancement of the risk of hypoglycaemia in elderly people [7–9].

Changes in the release of counter-regulatory hormones may increase the susceptibility of the elderly to hypoglycaemia. Early studies of the effect of age on counter-regulatory hormone responses to hypoglycaemia produced inconsistent results [10, 11], although these studies were seen to be flawed because many of the elderly subjects included also suffered from underlying diseases. Recent investigations, in which older subjects free from disease have been carefully selected, have shown that healthy elderly subjects have impaired glucagon responses to hypoglycaemia [12, 13]. Epinephrine responses have been reported to be either impaired [12] or increased [13] in healthy elderly; cortisol responses have been found to be either normal [12] or increased [13], and GH responses may be impaired [12], although this has not been demonstrated conclusively.

A reduced epinephrine response to hypoglycaemia and a decreased responsiveness to β-adrenergic receptor stimulation may explain the reduced awareness of the autonomic symptoms of hypoglycaemia found in the healthy elderly when compared to young subjects [14].

In young adults, symptomatic responses to hypoglycaemia are generated at a blood glucose level that is higher than that at which cognitive function becomes impaired. This allows sufficient time to take corrective action before severe neuroglycopenia supervenes [15]. The difference between these glycaemic thresholds is $\sim$1.0 mmol l^{-1} (18 mg dl^{-1}). Indeed, in older persons the difference between the glycaemic threshold for subjective awareness of hypoglycaemia and that for the onset of cognitive dysfunction may be absent [16]. Thus, elderly patients who became hypoglycaemic are less likely to experience prior warning symptoms if their blood glucose level falls, and are at greater risk for injury or falls with fracture – all factors which have a disruptive effect on the frail subject.

However, two recent studies have described less serious consequences in elderly subjects provided with adequate care. For example, mortality was zero in a study conducted in Germany [5], while morbidity was only 4% in a study from Singapore [3]. An additional point was that elderly diabetics were less exposed to motor vehicle accidents [5], which is a serious complication of hypoglycaemia observed in the young population of the DCCT [1].

Hypoglycaemia is usually observed during the late morning and afternoon in insulin-treated patients. The favouring factors, other than age, include multiple comorbid conditions (psychiatric conditions and depression leading to variable food intake), renal impairment (sulphonylureas cause a ninefold increase in the risk of severe hypoglycaemia, especially if food intake is irregular), multiple medications (high-risk association with antibacterial sulfamides) and, more frequently, a poorly adapted behavior response. To this list should be added the rare use of self-monitoring and the absence of patient and caregiver education regarding the symptoms of hypoglycaemia. Furthermore, the direct cause of hypoglycaemia is generally related to a dietary error (53% of hypoglycaemic episodes follow a missed meal) and/or recent hospitalization (change in therapy poorly adapted to home life) [4], African-American race, and the use of five or more concomitant medications [17, 18]. The frequency of severe hypoglycaemia remains moderate among patients with type 2 diabetes (0.4 episode per 100 patient-years), irrespective of treatment, compared with insulin-treated patients (1.5 episodes per 100 patient-years).

Hypoglycaemia is a complication of insulin or any drug that increases pancreatic insulin secretion or release (sulphonylureas and glinides). Antidiabetic monotherapies that do not normally cause hypoglycaemia include metformin, the alpha-glucosidase inhibitors and the thiazolidinediones. However, if these therapies are added to insulin or drugs that promote insulin release, then the incidence of hypoglycaemia may increase.

Hypoglycaemia is threefold more frequent when insulin is used alone compared to antidiabetic drugs, with the combined treatments exposing the patient to an intermediary risk. Recent advances in molecular genetic engineering have made possible the development of insulin analogues with pharmacokinetics that more closely mimic the needs of patients with type 2 diabetes, thus reducing the risk of hypoglycaemia. Lys.Pro insulin and insulin aspart (both rapid-acting insulin analogues) administered immediately prior to the meal have demonstrated improved postprandial glucose control in comparison with regular insulin. Injection just before a meal, or even during a meal, represents a good way of adapting the dose to real food intake. However, in practice multiple injections are not always easy to implement in the elderly subject [19–22].

For oral antidiabetic drugs, α-glucosidases and metformin do not normally cause hypoglycaemia. The pharmacokinetic properties of sulfamides would favour the use of second-generation, short-acting drugs. The risk of severe hypoglycaemia is lower with glipizide

and tolbutamide than with glibenclamide or chlorpropamide, while hypoglycaemia is fourfold more frequent with glibenclamide than with gliclazide [17]. Prolonged-release glipizide is associated with severe hypoglycaemia in elderly subjects and/or in subjects with renal impairment. Unlike conventional sulphonylureas, glinides taken before a meal induce a rapid postprandial insulin response. The short half-life of these drugs ensures that insulin concentrations peak at 1–2 h, but by 6 h have returned to fasting concentrations with minimal risk of hypoglycaemia if the patient misses a meal; this, on the other hand, is a severe problem with the older sulphonylureas. Support for such clinical evidence is derived from studies which showed the risk of severe hypoglycaemia to be less than half that seen with traditional sulphonylureas [23].The short half-life and biliary elimination of glinides are interesting properties; however, as with glitazones, specific large-scale studies in elderly persons are lacking.

In the future, it would be useful to evaluate the effects of rapid insulin analogues and glinides on the hypoglycaemic risk in an elderly population aged over 70 years.

In conclusion, elderly type 2 diabetics suffer a higher frequency of hypoglycaemic episodes, with the highest frequency and most severe hypoglycaemia being observed in insulin-treated patients. Particular at-risk situations include chronic renal failure and polymedication, both of which are frequently present in this population. The prescription of long-acting sulphonylureas, especially glibenclamide, is not recommended in elderly patients. Targeting 'perfect' glycemic control, which is associated with a significant hypoglycaemic risk, is not justified in many elderly patients. In patients aged over 65 years, the recommended therapeutic targets for glycaemic control should be fixed at a higher level than for younger patients. In order to prevent severe – if not fatal – hypoglycaemia in old patients, a careful insulin scheduling (when necessary) should include preparations characterized by a shorter half-life and with minimal risk for nocturnal episodes. The short half-life sulfamides, and agents tolerated in cases of impaired renal and hepatic function, should be the first choice for geriatric care. Finally, due to the fact that elderly patients are often incapable of treating hypoglycaemia themselves, educational programmes should include advice and information relating to the detection and treatment of hypoglycaemia, including the criteria for hospital admission in cases of unresponsive hypoglycaemia [24].

14.3 Diabetic ketoacidosis and hyperosmolar hyperglycaemic state in the elderly

Diabetic ketoacidosis (DKA) and hyperosmolar non-ketotic coma (HONK) are two of the most serious acute complications in the spectrum of marked decompensated diabetes [25–28].

These hyperglycaemic emergencies persist as important causes of morbidity and mortality among diabetic patients, despite major advances in the understanding of their pathogenesis and more uniform agreement about their diagnosis and treatment. In contrast to DKA mortality, the mortality rate of hyperosmolar hyperglycaemic state (HHS) has remained high at ∼15%, compared to <5% in patients with DKA [27, 29–31]. Severe dehydration, older age and the presence of co-morbid conditions in patients with HHS account for the higher mortality in these patients [31].

DKA consists of the biochemical triad of hyperglycaemia, ketonaemia and metabolic high anion gap acidosis [29].

The terms 'hyperglycaemic hyperosmolar non-ketotic coma' and 'hyperglycaemic hyperosmolar non-ketotic state' have been replaced with the term 'hyperglycaemic hyperosmolar state' in order to reflect the facts that: (i) alterations of the sensoria may often be present without coma; and (ii) the hyperosmolar hyperglycaemic state may consist of moderate to variable degrees of clinical ketosis [26].

Although DKA most often occurs in patients with type 1 diabetes mellitus (T1DM), it may also occur in type 2 diabetes under conditions of extreme stress such as serious infection, trauma, cardiovascular or other emergencies. Less often, it will present as a manifestation of type 2 diabetes, a disorder known as 'ketosis-prone type 2 diabetes' [30]. Similarly, whereas HHS occurs most commonly in T2DM, it can be seen in T1DM in conjunction with DKA [32, 33].

Both, DKA and HHS are characterized by absolute or relative insulinopenia. Clinically, they differ only by the severity of dehydration, ketosis and metabolic acidosis [34, 35]. While both DKA and HHS can be seen in the elderly [36], DKA is rare and its features and management do not differ from those in younger diabetics. However, its mortality is greatest in old age, particularly because of associated cardiovascular disease (CVD) [36, 37] (Table 14.1). Older patients are less likely to be receiving insulin before they develop DKA, are less likely to have had a previous episode of

Table 14.1 The main features of diabetic ketoacidosis (DKA) and hyperosmolar hyperglycaemic state (HHS) in older people.

DKA

- Rare in the elderly
- Patients less likely to be receiving insulin before developing DKA
- Patients less likely to have had a previous episode of DKA
- More insulin required to treat the DKA
- A longer length of hospital stay
- Higher mortality rate
- No specific treatment guidelines available

HHS

- Occurs frequently in the elderly
- In ∼50% of cases diabetes mellitus has not been previously diagnosed or treated
- Frequent predisposing factors are:
  - impaired maintenance of serum osmolality;
  - decreased thirst perception (especially in elderly with dementia);
  - decreased access to water, especially in the bed-ridden and use of diuretics;
  - acute infection (pneumonia being the most common infection).
- Symptoms, signs, diagnosis, and treatment are otherwise similar to those in younger adults.

DKA, typically require more insulin to treat the DKA, have a longer length of hospital stay, and have a higher mortality rate (22% for those aged ≥ 65 years versus 2% for those aged <65) [36]. Causes of death include infection, thromboembolism and myocardial infarction [36]. Although concomitant diseases and high rates of morbidity must be considered when caring for older patients with DKA, no specific treatment guidelines are currently available.

HHS almost always occurs in older people, and in about half of the cases diabetes mellitus has not been previously diagnosed or treated [38]. The predisposition of the elderly to develop HHS can be explained by a combination of impaired maintenance of serum osmolality, a decreased thirst perception (especially in elderly with dementia), a decreased access to water (especially in the bed-ridden) and the use of diuretics. A reduced thirst perception renders the polydipsia less dramatic, thereby lessening recognition by self or others, leading to dehydration and ending up in hyperosmolar coma [39]. An acute infection is the most frequent predisposing factor (40–60%), with pneumonia being the most common infection. Other illnesses such as stroke, acute myocardial infarction, renal insufficiency and medications such as glucocorticoids can also be predisposing factors.

The symptoms, signs, diagnosis and treatment are otherwise similar to those in younger adults.

14.4 Pathogenesis of DKA and HHS

In both DKA and HHS, the underlying metabolic abnormality results from the combination of absolute or relative insulin deficiency and increased amounts of counter-regulatory hormones. Inadequate levels of circulating insulin lead to hyperglycaemia, which in turn can lead to progressive dehydration and hyperosmolarity and ultimately to HHS. If the insulin deficiency is severe enough, ketosis and ultimately acidosis will develop. A relative insulin deficiency – not an absolute insulin deficiency – is necessary for the development of both DKA and HHS. Even patients with T2DM and 'normal insulin levels' may develop DKA if the level of insulin resistance causes a sufficiently large increase in insulin requirement.

When insulin is deficient, the elevated levels of glucagon, catecholamines and cortisol will stimulate hepatic glucose production through increased glycogenolysis and enhanced gluconeogenesis [29]. Hypercortisolaemia will result in increased proteolysis, thus providing amino acid precursors for gluconeogenesis.

Low insulin and high catecholamine concentrations will reduce glucose uptake by the peripheral tissues. The combination of an elevated hepatic glucose production and a decreased peripheral glucose utilization is the main pathogenic disorder responsible for hyperglycaemia in DKA and HHS. The hyperglycaemia will lead to glycosuria, osmotic diuresis and dehydration. Initially, glycosuria causes an increase in the glomerular filtration rate (GFR), but when the hypovolaemia becomes significant the GFR is decreased and renal glucose losses may also decrease. As glucose clearance by the kidney declines, the hyperglycaemia and hyperosmolarity worsen.

In DKA, the low insulin levels, combined with increased levels of catecholamines, cortisol and GH will activate hormone-sensitive lipase; this causes the breakdown of triglycerides and the release of free fatty acids (FFAs). The FFAs are taken up by the liver and converted to ketone bodies that are released into the circulation. This process of *ketogenesis* is stimulated by the increase in glucagon levels [40]. Glucagon will activate carnitine palmitoyltransferase I, an enzyme that allows FFAs in the form of coenzyme A to cross the mitochondrial membrane following their esterification into carnitine. On the other hand, esterification is reversed by carnitine palmitoyltransferase II to form fatty acyl coenzyme A, which enters the β-oxidative pathway to produce acetyl coenzyme A. Most of the latter is utilized in the synthesis of β-hydroxybutyric acid and acetoacetic acid – two relatively strong acids that are responsible for the acidosis in DKA.

Normally, ketone bodies increase insulin release from the pancreas, and the insulin in turn suppresses ketogenesis. In the insulin-deficient state, however, the pancreatic β cells are unable to respond and the ketogenesis will proceed unchecked.

The reason for the absence of ketosis in the presence of insulin deficiency in HHS remains unknown [26]. The current hypothesis is that the absence may be due to the lower levels of FFAs or the higher portal vein insulin levels, or both [25, 41, 42]. It appears that in hyperglycaemic coma, most subjects with T2DM have just enough residual insulin secretion to suppress lipolysis and ketogenesis, thus avoiding DKA and developing a HONK coma instead. However, in one study similar insulin levels were found in subjects with DKA or HONK, whereas those with HONK had lower levels of counter-regulatory hormones, leading to less lipid breakdown and less hepatic ketogenesis [43]. It also appears that hyperosmolality not only worsens insulin resistance but also inhibits lipolysis [44].

14.4.1 Acid–base balance, fluids and electrolytes

Acidosis in DKA is due to the overproduction of β-hydroxybutyric acid and acetoacetic acid. At physiological pH, these two ketoacids dissociate completely, and the excess hydrogen ions bind the bicarbonate, resulting in decreased serum bicarbonate levels. Ketone bodies thus circulate in the anionic form, which leads to the development of anion gap acidosis that characterizes DKA. Despite substantial losses of ketoacids in the urine, the decrease in serum bicarbonate concentration and increase in the anion gap observed in DKA are almost equal [45]. Metabolic acidosis will induce hyperventilation through a stimulation of peripheral chemoreceptors and the respiratory centre in the brainstem, which will elicit a decrease in the partial pressure of carbon dioxide. This will partially compensate for the metabolic acidosis.

Hyperglycemia-induced osmotic diuresis results in severe fluid loss. The total body deficit of water is usually about 5–7 l in DKA and 7–12 l in HHS, which represents a loss of about 10–15% of body weight. The osmotic diuresis is associated with large losses of electrolytes in the urine. The sodium chloride deficit in DKA and HHS is usually 5–13 mmol kg^{-1} body weight for sodium, and 3–7 mmol kg^{-1} for chloride [26, 29, 41]. Initially, the increased glucose concentration is restricted to the extracellular space, which forces water from the intracellular to the extracellular compartment and induces a dilution of the plasma sodium concentration. Subsequently, further increases in the plasma glucose concentration will lead to osmotic diuresis, with losses of water and sodium chloride in the urine; the water loss usually exceeds that of the sodium chloride [29, 45].

Because of the osmotic shift of water, plasma sodium concentrations are usually low or normal in DKA, but may be slightly increased in HHS, despite extensive water loss [45, 46]. In this context, the plasma sodium concentration should be corrected for hyperglycaemia by adding 1.6 mmol to the reported sodium level for every 5.6 mmol l^{-1} increase in glucose above 5.6 mmol l^{-1} [29]. The plasma sodium concentration may also be artificially lowered by the presence of severe hyperlipidaemia.

Both, DKA and HHS are also associated with profound total body potassium depletion, ranging from 3 to 15 mmol kg^{-1} of body weight [27, 41, 47]. However, plasma potassium concentrations are typically normal or elevated at the time of presentation. As with sodium, the presence of hyperglycaemia leads to a shift of water and potassium from the intracellular to the extracellular space. The shift of potassium is further enhanced in the presence of acidosis, intracellular proteolysis and insulinopenia [48]. Potassium depletion is due to excessive urinary potassium loss secondary to osmotic diuresis, and leads to an increased delivery of fluid and sodium to the potassium secretory sites in the distal nephron [29]. This can be further exacerbated by a poor oral intake of potassium, vomiting and secondary hyperaldosteronism [29].

Phosphate, magnesium and calcium are other elements excreted in excess in urine during the development of DKA and HHS owing to osmotic diuresis, for a deficit of 1–2 mmol kg^{-1} on average [27, 41].

14.4.2 Precipitating factors

Infection remains the most important precipitating factor in the development of DKA and HHS. In 20–25% of cases, infections are the first manifestations of previously undiagnosed diabetes mellitus [48]. Omissions or inadequate insulin doses are frequent precipitating factors, particularly for DKA [41].

Other precipitating factors, especially for HHS, are silent myocardial infarction, cerebrovascular accident, mesenteric ischaemia, acute pancreatitis and the use of medications such as steroids, thiazide diuretics, calcium-channel blockers, propranolol and phenytoin [26]. In 2–10% of cases of DKA, no obvious precipitating factor can be identified [48].

14.5 Diagnosis of DKA and HHS

14.5.1 Clinical presentation

If a physical examination reveals dehydration along with a high capillary blood glucose level, with or without urine or increased plasma ketone bodies, then acute diabetic decompensation should be strongly suspected. A definitive diagnosis of DKA or HHS must be confirmed through laboratory investigations; however, the clinical presentation can provide helpful information for the preliminary bedside diagnosis [49].

DKA usually occurs in younger, lean patients with T1DM and develops within a day or so, whereas HHS is more likely to occur in elderly, obese diabetic patients, often those with decreased renal function who do not have access to water; in these cases the HHS may take days or weeks to fully develop [50].

The pathophysiological consequences of hyperglycaemia, hyperketonaemia and insulin deficiency account for many of the classic symptoms and physical findings seen in DKA and HHS. High glucose levels lead to an osmotic diuresis, dehydration and ultimately hypotension. The high ketone concentrations are responsible for the metabolic acidosis and also cause an osmotic diuresis.

Both, DKA and HHS often present with polyuria and polydypsia, although polydypsia may be absent in elderly patients with HHS. In both conditions, abdominal pain with nausea and vomiting can develop owing to acidosis *per se* or to decreased mesenteric perfusion, and can be mistaken for an acute surgical abdomen. Kussmaul–Kien respiration (rapid and deep respiration) with acetone on the breath is typical of DKA but is absent in HHS. Although dehydration occurs in both conditions, it is often more pronounced in HHS. Because DKA and HHS are usually accompanied by hypothermia, a normal or elevated temperature may indicate an underlying infection.

Although patients may be alert at the time of presentation, changes in their mental status are common and vary from confusion or disorientation to coma, usually as a result of extreme dehydration with or without prerenal azotaemia, hyperglycaemia and hyperosmolarity. In contrast to DKA, focal or generalized seizures and transient hemiplegia may occur.

14.5.2 Laboratory findings

Most patients presenting with DKA have a plasma glucose level of $14 \, \mathrm{mmol \, l^{-1}}$, or greater. However, most patients with T1DM who have such a plasma glucose level do not have ketoacidosis. On the other hand, ketoacidosis may develop in patients with a plasma glucose level below $14 \, \mathrm{mmol \, l^{-1}}$. In HHS, hyperglycaemia is usually more severe than in DKA, and a plasma glucose level $\geq 34 \, \mathrm{mmol \, l^{-1}}$ is arbitrarily one of the diagnostic criteria. Glucose is the main osmole responsible for the hyperosmolar syndrome. The increased serum osmolality can be calculated as follows: $[(2 \times \text{serum Na}) + \text{serum glucose}]$, with normal values being $290 \pm 5 \, \text{(SD)} \, \mathrm{mmol \, kg^{-1}}$ water. Blood urea nitrogen is not included in the calculation of effective osmolality because it is freely permeable in and out of the intracellular compartment [26, 51]. By definition, the osmolality must exceed $320 \, \mathrm{mmol \, kg^{-1}}$ to be diagnostic of HHS. However, it is not uncommon in DKA to have increased osmolality. In DKA the blood pH will be ≤ 7.3, and in HHS in isolation it will be >7.3. Venous blood can be used to measure pH and bicarbonate levels, unless information on oxygen transport is required. It must be remembered that venous blood, without arterial blood gas values, does not permit the identification of mixed acid–base disorders [52]. In DKA, a lower pH will usually be associated with a decrease in bicarbonate to $\leq 15 \, \mathrm{mmol \, l^{-1}}$, although a milder form of DKA may present with a bicarbonate level of $15–18 \, \mathrm{mmol \, l^{-1}}$. Less severe DKA is always accompanied by moderate to large amounts of ketones in the blood and urine, while trace amounts may also be found in cases of HHS [53]. Today, it is possible to measure blood β-hydroxybutyric acid levels at the bedside, using a reagent strip and a reflectance meter [54].

The majority of patients presenting with DKA and HHS have an elevated leukocyte count, usually in the range of $10.0–15.0 \times 10^9 \, \mathrm{l^{-1}}$, even in the absence of infection [25], this being attributed to stress and dehydration [48]. Amylase levels are often elevated in patients with DKA, but represent enzyme activity from non-pancreatic tissues such as the parotid gland. Lipase levels will usually be normal. Additional laboratory tests should include blood culture, urinalysis and urine culture, chest radiography and electrocardiography, as well as measurement of the lactate level, if indicated. Because a high fetal mortality rate is associated with ketoacidosis, it is important to eliminate the possibility of pregnancy in women of reproductive age.

14.6 Treatment of DKA and HHS

The therapeutic goals for the treatment of hyperglycaemic crises in diabetes consist of:

- Improving the circulatory volume and tissue perfusion.

- Decreasing the serum glucose and plasma osmolality towards normal levels.

- Clearing the serum and urine of ketones at a steady rate.

- Correcting electrolyte imbalances.

- Identifying and treating any precipitating events [55].

The successful treatment of DKA and HHS depends on the adequate correction of dehydration, hyperglycaemia, ketoacidosis and electrolyte deficits [56].

Any comorbid precipitating event should be identified and treated appropriately. Both, DKA and HHS are medical emergencies, and patients with these conditions must be admitted to hospital.

The treatment of HHS involves frequent and careful monitoring (Figure 14.1). Although $4–6 \, \mathrm{l}$ of fluid may be needed during the first $12 \, \mathrm{h}$, such rapid replacement may not be feasible in older persons, who often exhibit a poor cardiac reserve [57]. In most cases, insulin and intravenous fluids can be safely started simultaneously, the exceptions being patients with hypokalaemia or hypotension. In such cases, intravenous fluids should be given before insulin to prevent any worsening of hypokalaemia or hypotension that may occur in

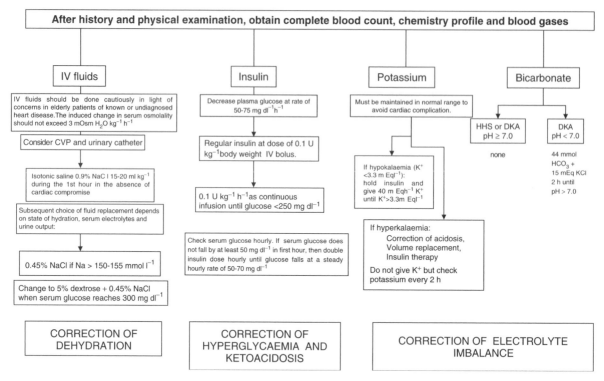

Figure 14.1   Management of patients with DKA and HHS.

response to insulin, and the resulting intracellular shift of glucose, potassium and water [58].

14.6.1   Fluid therapy

The objective of an initial fluid therapy is to expand the extracellular volume (intravascular and extravascular) and restore renal perfusion. In the absence of any major heart problems, it is suggested that treatment be started with an infusion of isotonic saline (0.9% NaCl) at a rate of 15–20 ml kg^{-1} h^{-1} during the first hour (1–1.5 l in an average adult) so as to rapidly expand the extracellular space. The subsequent choice of fluid replacement depends on the state of hydration, the electrolyte levels and urinary output. In general, this may be an infusion of 0.45% NaCl at a rate of 4–14 ml kg^{-1} h^{-1} if the serum sodium level is normal or elevated. The administration of hypotonic saline leads to a gradual replacement of the intracellular and extracellular compartments. As soon as the renal function is assured, potassium must be added to every litre of fluid. When the plasma glucose level reaches 12–14 mmol l^{-1}, each litre of fluid should contain 5% dextrose. Fluid replacement should correct the estimated water deficit over the

first 24 h. It is important that the change in osmolality does not exceed 3 mmol kg^{-1} h^{-1} [26, 27, 46, 59, 60].

In patients with kidney and heart problems, their cardiac, renal and mental statuses must be assessed frequently, with regular serum osmolality monitoring during rehydration to avoid iatrogenic water overload [26, 27, 46, 59, 60].

Caution is indicated in elderly patients with heart failure or renal insufficiency in order to avoid fluid overload. Along with frequent clinical and laboratory assessment, bladder catheterization and the monitoring of central venous pressure or pulmonary capillary wedge pressure may be warranted in order to assess fluid status more accurately.

14.6.2   Insulin therapy

There is general consensus that, in cases of DKA and HHS, regular insulin should be administered by means of continuous intravenous infusion in small doses through an infusion pump [29, 40, 59, 61].

Such low-dose insulin therapy provides insulin concentrations that are more physiological and produce a more gradual and steady fall in plasma glucose levels [62, 63]; the risk of hypoglycaemia and hypokalaemia is also decreased [29]. The available data do not support the subcutaneous or intramuscular route for insulin administration [29]. Although most proposed protocols suggest that a loading dose of insulin should be given at the initiation of insulin therapy, there are no data to support any advantage for such a recommendation [29, 63].

As soon as hypokalaemia (potassium concentration <3.3 mmol l^{-1}) has been excluded, a continuous infusion of regular insulin can be started at a dose of 0.1 U kg^{-1} h^{-1}, which should produce a gradual decrease in the plasma glucose level of 3–4 mmol l^{-1} h^{-1} [62]. When the plasma glucose level reaches 12–14 mmol l^{-1}, the insulin infusion rate may be decreased by 50% as the 5% dextrose is added. Thereafter, the insulin infusion dose must be adjusted to maintain the plasma glucose values until the acidosis in DKA or the clouded consciousness and hyperosmolality in HHS have been resolved.

When the ketoacidosis in DKA has been corrected (plasma glucose level <11.0 mmol l^{-1}, serum bicarbonate level ≥ 18 mmol l^{-1}, venous pH >7.3 and anion gap <12 mmol l^{-1}), the clouded consciousness and hyperosmolality in HHS have resolved, and patients are able to take fluids orally, then a multidose insulin regimen may be initiated based on the patient's treatment before the DKA or HHS developed.

Recent clinical studies have demonstrated the potency and cost-effectiveness of subcutaneous rapid-acting insulin analogues (lispro or aspart) in the management of patients with uncomplicated mild to moderate DKA [64, 65]. The patients received subcutaneous rapid-acting insulin doses of 0.2 U kg^{-1} initially, followed by 0.1 U kg^{-1} every hour, or an initial dose of 0.3 U kg^{-1} followed by 0.2 U kg^{-1} every 2 h until the blood glucose level was <250 mg dl^{-1} (13.7 mmol l^{-1}). The insulin dose was then decreased by half to 0.05 or 0.1 U kg^{-1}, respectively, and administered every 1 or 2 h until resolution of the DKA. No differences in the duration of hospital stay, total amount of insulin needed for the resolution of hyperglycaemia or ketoacidosis, or in the incidence of hypoglycaemia among treatment groups, were found [64, 65]. The use of insulin analogues allowed the treatment of DKA in general wards or the emergency department, and so reduced the cost of hospitalization by 30%, without any significant changes in hypoglycaemic events [65]. It is important to note here that the use of fast-acting insulin analogues is not recommended for patients with severe DKA or HHS, as there no studies have been conducted to support their use. Again, these agents may not be effective in patients with severe fluid depletion as they are given subcutaneously.

14.6.3 Potassium therapy

The treatment of DKA and HHS with rehydration and insulin is typically associated with a rapid decline in the plasma potassium concentration, particularly during the first few hours of therapy [45, 48]. This rapid decrease is due to several factors, the most significant being the insulin-mediated re-entry of potassium into the intracellular compartment. Other factors are extracellular fluid volume expansion, correction of acidosis, and continued potassium loss owing to osmotic diuresis and ketonuria. Despite major potassium depletion in the whole body, mild to moderate hyperkalaemia is not uncommon in patients in hyperglycaemic decompensation. Because treatment will rapidly induce decreased serum potassium concentrations, potassium replacement must be initiated as soon as levels fall below 5.0 mmol l^{-1}, assuming that the urine output is adequate. It is recommended that 20–30 mmol of potassium be added to each litre of infusion fluid to maintain the serum potassium concentration at 4–5 mmol l^{-1} [56]. If the serum potassium level is less than 3.3 mmol l^{-1}, then potassium replacement therapy should be started immediately with fluid therapy, and the initiation of insulin therapy should be delayed until the potassium concentration is restored to above 3.3 mmol l^{-1}, in order to avoid arrhythmia, cardiac arrest and respiratory muscle weakness [56].

Initially, the serum potassium level should be measured every 1–2 h because the most rapid change occurs during the first 5 h of treatment. Subsequently, it should be measured every 4–6 h, as indicated clinically.

14.6.4 Bicarbonate and phosphate therapy

Bicarbonate therapy

The use of bicarbonate in the treatment of DKA remains controversial [66]. Most current reviews do not recommend the routine use of alkali therapy in DKA, because the condition tends to correct with insulin therapy. Insulin administration inhibits ongoing lipolysis and ketoacid production and promotes ketoanion metabolism. Because protons are consumed during ketoanion metabolism, bicarbonate is regenerated, leading to a partial correction of any metabolic acidosis. The rationale for bicarbonate therapy is the (theoretical) assumption that severe acidosis could contribute to organ malfunction, such as of the liver, heart and brain.

However, few prospective, randomized studies of the use of bicarbonate in DKA have been conducted.

Studies of patients with a blood pH of 6.9 or higher have found no evidence that bicarbonate is beneficial [34], and some studies have even suggested that bicarbonate therapy might be harmful for these patients [35–37]. Because no studies have been conducted in patients with a blood pH below 6.9, the administration of bicarbonate as an isotonic solution is still recommended. However, it should be noted that, as bicarbonate therapy lowers the potassium levels, these will need to be monitored very carefully [67].

Phosphate therapy

The beneficial effect of phosphate therapy is purely theoretical. It would be expected to prevent potential complications associated with hypophosphataemia, such as respiratory depression, skeletal muscle weakness, haemolytic anaemia and cardiac dysfunction. Furthermore, the majority of controlled, randomized trials have been unable to demonstrate any clinical benefit of routine phosphate therapy [29], but still recommend that one-third of potassium replacement be given as potassium phosphate. No studies have been conducted on the use of phosphate therapy for HHS.

14.6.5 Clinical and laboratory follow-up

Vital signs should be monitored at 30-min intervals for the first hour, hourly for the next 4 h, and then every 2–4 h until resolution of the condition. An accurate record of hourly urine output is necessary to monitor kidney function. On admission, a comprehensive profile will include at least arterial or venous blood gas values, levels of plasma glucose, electrolytes, blood urea nitrogen and creatinine, ketone levels in the serum or urine (or both), and serum osmolality. Capillary blood glucose levels should be monitored hourly to allow any adjustment of the insulin infusion dose. Electrolyte levels should be measured every 1–2 h initially, and every 4 h thereafter. The measurement of venous pH can replace that of arterial pH, and should be undertaken every 4 h until the DKA has been corrected.

14.7 Treatment-related complications

Common complications of DKA include hypoglycaemia, hypokalaemia and recurrent hyperglycaemia, all of which may be minimized by careful monitoring. Hyperchloraemia is a common, but transient, finding that usually requires no special treatment.

Cerebral oedema is a rare but important complication of DKA. Although it can affect adults, it is more common in young patients. The early signs of cerebral oedema include headache, confusion and lethargy, but papilloedema, hypertension, hyperpyrexia and diabetes insipidus may also occur. Patients typically improve mentally with an initial treatment of DKA, but then suddenly worsen. Multiple factors in the treatment of DKA and HHS may contribute to the cerebral oedema, including: (i) the idiogenic osmoles, which cannot be dissipated rapidly during rehydration, thus creating a gradient and a shift of water into the cells [29]; (ii) insulin therapy *per se*, which may promote the entry of osmotically active particles into the intracellular space; and (iii) the rapid replacement of sodium deficits [27, 47].

In order to reduce the risk of cerebral oedema, it is recommended that physicians correct sodium and water deficits gradually, and avoid any rapid decline in plasma glucose concentration [25, 56].

14.7.1 Adult respiratory distress syndrome

Adult respiratory distress syndrome, or noncardiogenic pulmonary oedema, is a potentially fatal complication of DKA that fortunately occurs rarely [29]. The partial pressure of oxygen, which is normal on admission, decreases progressively during treatment to unexpectedly low levels. This change is believed to be due to increased water in the lungs and reduced lung compliance. These changes may be similar to those occurring in brain cells leading to cerebral oedema, which suggests that it is a common biological phenomenon in tissues [29].

14.7.2 Hypochloraemic metabolic acidosis

This phenomenon is not uncommon during the treatment of DKA [43]. A major mechanism is the loss of substrates (ketoanions) in the urine that are necessary for bicarbonate regeneration [43, 68]. Other mechanisms include: (i) intravenous fluids containing chloride concentrations exceeding that of plasma [68, 69]; (ii) volume expansion with bicarbonate-free fluids [68, 69]; and (iii) an intracellular shift of sodium bicarbonate during the correction of DKA [70]. This acidosis usually has no adverse effect and is corrected spontaneously in the subsequent 24–48 h through enhanced renal acid excretion [68–71].

14.7.3   Vascular thrombosis

Many features of DKA and HHS predispose the patient to thrombosis, including dehydration and contracted vascular volume, a low cardiac output, an increased blood viscosity and the frequent presence of underlying atherosclerosis [40, 51]. In addition, a number of haemostatic changes favour thrombosis [72]. This complication is more likely to occur when the osmolality is very high. Low-dose or low-molecular-weight heparin therapy should be considered for prophylaxis in patients at high risk of thrombosis, although no data are yet available demonstrating the safety or efficacy of this approach.

14.7.4   Hypoglycaemia and hypokalaemia

These complications are less common with current low-dose insulin therapy [29, 61, 62]. The potassium deficit should be adequately corrected and 5% dextrose added to infusion fluids as soon as the plasma glucose level falls below $12–14\,\mathrm{mmol}\,l^{-1}$.

14.8   Conclusions

Today, much remains to be done to reduce the incidence of DKA and HHS, and to improve the outcome of patients with these conditions. Although it has been suggested that the mortality rate associated with these complications is decreasing, it is still considered excessive [73]. The various factors that can precipitate hyperglycaemic decompensation in patients with diabetes should alert the physician to an early diagnosis and prompt therapy.

References

1. The Diabetes Control and Complications Trial Research Group. The effect of intensive treatment of diabetes on the development and progression of long-term complications in insulin-dependent diabetes mellitus. N Engl J Med 1993; 329: 977–86.
2. UK Prospective Diabetes Study (UKPDS) Group. Intensive blood-glucose control with sulphonylureas or insulin compared with conventional treatment and risk of complications in patients with type 2 diabetes (UKPDS 33). Lancet 1998; 352: 837–53.
3. Teo SK and Ee CH. Hypoglycaemia in the elderly. Singapore Med J 1997; 38: 432–4.
4. Lassmann-Vague V. Hypoglycaemia in elderly diabetic patients. Diabetes Metab 2005; 31: 5S51–5S55.
5. Holstein A, Plaschke A and Egberts EH. Clinical characterisation of severe hypoglycaemia: a prospective population-based study. Exp Clin Endocrinol Diabetes 2003; 111: 364–9.
6. Cryer PE. Glucose counterregulation in man. Diabetes 1981; 30: 261–4.
7. Reaven GN, Greenfield MS, Mondon CE, Rosenthal M Wright D and Reaven EP. Does insulin removal rate from plasma decline with age? Diabetes 1982; 31: 670–3.
8. Minaker KL, Rowe JW, Torino R and Pallotta JA. Influence of age on clearance of insulin in man. Diabetes 1982; 31: 851–5.
9. Fink RI, Revers RR, Kolterman OG and Olefsky JM. The metabolic clearance of insulin and the feedback inhibition of insulin secretion are altered with ageing. Diabetes 1985; 34 (3): 275–80.
10. Schramm VA, Push HJ Franke H and Haubitz I. Hormonal adaptive capacity in old age: behaviour of hormonal parameters after insulin hypoglycaemia in young and old patients. Fortsch. Med. 1981; 99: 1255–60.
11. Kalk WJ, Virik AI, Pimstone BL, Jackson WPU, Marker JC, Cryer PE and Clutter WE. Growth hormone response to insulin hypoglycaemia in the elderly. J Gerontol 1973; 28: 431–3.
12. Marker JC, Cryer PE and Clutter WE. Attenuated glucose recovery from hypoglycaemia in the elderly. Diabetes 1992; 41: 671–8.
13. Lenters KM, Ortiz RJ, Herman WH, Zobel D and Halter JB. (1990) Impaired glucose counterregulation in response to insulin-induced hypoglycaemia in the elderly. Clin Res. 38: 27OA.
14. Meneilly GS, Cheung E and Tuokko H. Altered responses to hypoglycaemia of healthy elderly people. J Clin Endocrinol Metab 1994; 78: 1341–8.
15. Mitraku A, Ryan C, Veneman T, Mokan M, Jenssen T, Kiss I, Durrant J, Cryer P and Gerich J. Hierarchy of glycemic thresholds for counterregulatory hormone secretion, symptoms and cerebral dysfunction. Am J Physiol 1991; 266: E67–74.
16. Matyka K, Evans M, Lomas J, Cranston I, Macdonald I and Amiel SA. Altered hierarchy of protective responses against severe hypoglycemia in normal aging in healthy men. Diabetes Care 1997; 20 (2): 135–41.
17. Shorr RI, Ray WA, Daugherty JR and Griffin MR. Incidence and risk factors for serious hypoglycemia in older persons using insulin or sulfonylureas. Arch Intern Med 1997; 157: 1681–6.
18. Saudek CD and Golden SH. Feasibility and outcomes of insulin therapy in elderly patients with diabetes mellitus. Drugs Aging 1999; 14: 375–85.
19. Madsbad S. Insulin analogues: have they changed insulin treatment and improved glycaemic control? Diabetes Metab Res Rev 2002; 18 (1): S21–8.

20. Hermansen K, Colombo M, Storgaard H, O Stergaard A, Kolendorf K and Madsbad S. Improved postprandial glycemic control with biphasic insulin aspart relative to biphasic insulin lispro and biphasic human insulin in patients with type 2 diabetes. Diabetes Care 2002; 25: 883–8.

21. Garber AJ, Clauson P, Pedersen CB and Kølendorf K. Lower risk of hypoglycemia with insulin detemir than with neutral protamine hagedorn insulin in older persons with type 2 diabetes: a pooled analysis of Phase III trials. J Am Geriatr Soc 2007; 55 (11): 1735–40.

22. Motta M, Bennati E, Ferlito L, Passamonte M, Cardillo E and Malaguarnera M. A review on the actual trends of insulin treatment in elderly with diabetes. Arch Gerontol Geriatr. 2008, 47 (1), 151–61.

23. Moses R. A review of clinical experience with prandial glucose regulator, repaglinde in the treatment of type 2 diabetes. Exp Opin Pharmacother 2001; 67: 1455–67.

24. Lecomte P. Diabetes in the elderly: consideration for clinical practice. Diabetes Metab 2005; 31: 5S51–5S55.

25. Kitabchi AE, Umpierrez GE, Murphy MB, Barrett EJ, Kreisberg, RA Malone JI and Wall BM. Management of hyperglycemic crises in patients with diabetes. Diabetes Care 2001; 24: 131–53.

26. Ennis ED, Stahl E and Kreisberg RA. The hyperosmolar hyperglycemic syndrome. Diabetes Rev 1994; 2: 115–26.

27. Kitabchi AE, Fisher JN, Murphy MB, *et al.* (1993) Diabetic ketoacidosis and hyperglycemic, hyperosmolar nonketotic state. In: CR Kahn and GC Weir (eds). Joslin's Diabetes Mellitus Textbook. Lea & Febiger, Philadelphia, pp. 753–60.

28. Fishbein H and Palumbo PJ. (1995) Acute metabolic complications in diabetes. In: National Diabetes Data Group. Diabetes in America. National Institutes of Health, National Institute of Diabetes and Digestive and Kidney Diseases, Bethesda, MD, pp. 283–91.

29. Kitabchi AE and Wall BM. Diabetic ketoacidosis. Med Clin North Am 1995; 79: 9–37.

30. Kitabchi AE and Nyenwe EA. Hyperglycemic crises in diabetes mellitus: diabetic ketoacidosis and hyperglycemic hyperosmolar state. Endocrinol Metab Clin N Am 2006; 35: 725–51.

31. Kitabchi AE, Umpierrez GE, Murphy MB and Kreisberg RA. Hyperglycemic crises in adult patients with diabetes. A consensus statement from the American Diabetes Association. Diabetes Care 2006; 29: 2739–48.

32. Kitabchi AE and Fisher JN. (1981) Insulin therapy of diabetic ketoacidosis: Physiologic versus pharmacologic doses of insulin and their routes of administration. In Handbook of Diabetes Mellitus, M. Brownlee (ed.). Vol. 5. Garland ATPM Press, New York, pp. 95–149.

33. Glaser N. Pediatric diabetic ketoacidosis and hyperglycemic hyperosmolar state. Pediatr Clin North Am. 2005; 52 (6): 1611–35.

34. Alberti KGMM. (2001) Diabetic acidosis, hyperosmolar coma, and lactic acidosis. In KL Becker (ed.). Principles and Practice of Endocrinology and Metabolism. 3rd ed. Lippincott Williams & Wilkins, Philadelphia, pp. 1438–50.

35. Kitabchi AE and Murphy MB. (2002) Hyperglycemic crises in adult patients with diabetes mellitus. In: Oxford Textbook of Endocrinology. JA Wass, SM Shalet and SA Amiel (eds). Oxford University Press, Oxford, pp. 1734–47.

36. Meneilly GS and Tessier D. Diabetes in the elderly. Diabet Med 1995; 12: 949–60.

37. MacIsaac RJ, Lee LY, McNeil KJ, Tsalamandris C and Jerums G. Influence of age on the presentation and outcome of acidotic and hyperosmolar diabetic emergencies. Intern Med J. 2002; 32 (8): 379–85.

38. Greene DA. Acute and chronic complications of diabetes mellitus in older patients. Am J Med 1986; 80: 39–53.

39. Singh I and Marshall MC Jr. Diabetes mellitus in the elderly. Endocrin Metab Clin N Am 1995; 24: 255–72.

40. Foster DW and McGarry JD. The metabolic derangements and treatment of diabetic ketoacidosis. N Engl J Med 1983; 309: 159–69.

41. Ennis ED and Kreisberg RA. (2000) Diabetic ketoacidosis and the hyperglycemic hyperosmolar syndrome. In: D. LeRoith, SI Taylor and JM Olefsky (eds). Diabetes mellitus. A fundamental and clinical text.: Lippincott Williams & Wilkins, Philadelphia, pp. 336–47.

42. Halperin ML, Marsden PA, Singer GG and West ML. Can marked hyperglycemia occur without ketosis? Clin Invest Med 1985; 8: 253–6.

43. Gerich JE, Martin MM and Recant L. Clinical and metabolic characteristics of hyperosmolar non-ketotic coma. Diabetes 1971: 20: 228–38.

44. Berger W and Keller U. Treatment of diabetic ketoacidosis and non-ketotic hyperosmolar diabetic coma. Balliere's Clin Endocrinol Metab 1992; 6: 1–22.

45. Adrogue HJ, Wilson H, Boyd AE, III, Suki WN and Eknoyan G. Plasma acid-base patterns in diabetic ketoacidosis. N Engl J Med 1982; 307: 1603–10.

46. Hillman K. Fluid resuscitation in diabetic emergencies – a reappraisal. Intensive Care Med 1987; 13: 4–8.

47. Kreisberg RA. (1990) Diabetic ketoacidosis. In: M Rifkin and D Porte (eds). Diabetes mellitus: theory and practice. Elsevier Science, New York, pp. 591–603.

48. Umpierrez GE, Khajavi M and Kitabchi AE. Review: diabetic ketoacidosis and hyperglycemic hyperosmolar nonketotic syndrome. Am J Med Sci 1996; 311: 225–33.

49. Gonzalez-Campoy JM and Robertson RP. Diabetic ketoacidosis and hyperosmolar nonketotic state: gaining control over extreme hyperglycemic complications. Postgrad Med 1996; 99: 143–52.

50. Braaten JT. Hyperosmolar nonketotic diabetic coma: diagnosis and management. Geriatrics 1987; 42: 83–92.

51. Lorber D. Nonketotic hypertonicity in diabetes mellitus. Med Clin North Am 1995; 79: 39–52.

52. Brandenburg MA and Dire DJ. Comparison of arterial and venous blood gas values in the initial emergency department evaluation of patients with diabetic ketoacidosis. Ann Emerg Med 1998; 31: 459–65.

53. Wachtel TJ, Tetu-Mouradjian LM, Goldman DL, Ellis SE and O'Sullivan PS. Hyperosmolarity and acidosis in diabetes mellitus: a three-year experience in Rhode Island. J Gen Intern Med 1991; 6: 495–502.

54. Wiggam MI, O'Kane MJ, Harper R, Atkinson AB, Hadden DR, Trimble ER, et al. Treatment of diabetic ketoacidosis using normalization of blood 3-hydroxybutyrate concentration as the endpoint of emergency management. Diabetes Care 1997; 20: 1347–52.

55. Tallis RC and Fillit HM. (2003) Geriatric Medicine and Gerontology, 6th edition. Churchill Livingstone, London.

56. American Diabetes Association. Hyperglycemic crises in patients with diabetes mellitus. Diabetes Care 2003; 26 (Suppl. 1): S109–17.

57. Lee M, Gardin JM, Lynch JC, et al. Diabetes mellitus and echocardiographic ventricular function in elderly men and women. The Cardiovascular Health Study. Am Heart J 1997; 133: 36–43.

58. Samos LF and Roos BA. Diabetes mellitus in older persons. Med Clin N Am 1998; 82 (4): 791–803.

59. Marshall SM, Walker M and Alberti KGM. (1997) Diabetic ketoacidosis and hyperglycemic non-ketotic coma. In: KGM Alberti, P Zimmet and RA DeFronzo (eds). International Textbook of Diabetes Mellitus. John Wiley & Sons, New York, pp. 1215–29.

60. Ennis ED, Stahl EJ and Kreisberg RA. (1997) Diabetic ketoacidosis. In: D Porte Jr and RS Sherwin (eds). Diabetes Mellitus: Theory and Practice. Elsevier, Amsterdam, pp. 827–44.

61. Fleckman AM. Diabetic ketoacidosis. Endocrinol Metab Clin North Am 1993; 22: 181–207.

62. Kitabchi AE. Low-dose insulin therapy in diabetic ketoacidosis: Fact or fiction? Diabetes Metab Rev 1989; 5: 337–63.

63. Burghen GA, Etteldorf JN, Fisher JN and Kitabchi AQ. Comparison of high-dose and low-dose insulin by continuous intravenous infusion in the treatment of diabetic ketoacidosis in children. Diabetes Care 1980; 3: 15–20.

64. Umpierrez GE, Latif K, Stoever J, et al. Efficacy of subcutaneous insulin lispro versus continuous intravenous regular insulin for the treatment of patients with diabetic ketoacidosis. Am J Med. 2004; 117: 291–6.

65. Umpierrez GE, Cuervo R, Karabell A, et al. Treatment of diabetic ketoacidosis with subcutaneous insulin aspart. Diabetes Care 2004; 27: 1873–8.

66. Barnes HV, Cohen RD, Kitabchi AE and Murphy MB. (1990) When is bicarbonate appropriate in treating metabolic acidosis including diabetic ketoacidosis? In: G Gitnick, HV Barnes, TP Duffy et al. (eds). Debates in Medicine. Yearbook, Chicago, p. 172.

67. Okuda Y, Adrogue HJ, Field JB, Nohara H and Yamashita K. Counterproductive effects of sodium bicarbonate in diabetic ketoacidosis. J Clin Endocrinol Metab 1996; 81: 314–20.

68. Oh MS, Carroll HJ and Uribarri J. Mechanism of normochloremic and hyperchloremic acidosis in diabetic ketoacidosis. Nephron 1990; 54: 1–6.

69. Adrogue HJ, Eknoyan G and Suki WK. Diabetic ketoacidosis: role of the kidney in the acid-base homeostasis re-evaluated. Kidney Int 1984; 25: 591–8.

70. Madias NE, Homer SM, Johns CA and Cohen JJ. Hypochloremia as a consequence of anion gap metabolic acidosis. J Lab Clin Med 1984; 104: 15–23.

71. Oh MS, Banerji MA and Carroll HJ. The mechanism of hyperchloremic acidosis during the recovery phase of diabetic ketoacidosis. Diabetes 1981; 30: 310–13.

72. Paton RC. Haemostatic changes in diabetic coma. Diabetologia 1981; 21: 172–7.

73. American Diabetes Association (1996) Acute complications. In: Diabetes 1996 Vital Statistics. American Diabetes Association, Alexandria, VA, pp. 29–44.

15

Nutritional Perspectives: Diabetes in Older People

Begoña Molina[1] and Alan J. Sinclair[2]

[1]*Servicio de Endocrinología y Nutrición, Hospital Infanta Cristina, Avda 9 de Junio, Parla, Madrid, Spain*
[2]*Bedfordshire and Hertfordshire Postgraduate Medical School, Putteridge Bury Campus, Luton, UK*

Key messages

- Although many older people with diabetes are obese, a proportion is recognized to have malnutrition or lesser degrees of nutritional impairment.
- The use of oral supplements to increase energy and nutrient intake should be considered at an early stage in nutritional planning, and may lessen several serious adverse outcomes.
- Nutritional recommendations for older people should particularly take into consideration food preferences, cultural background, socioeconomic factors and the support structure that is available to underpin management.
- Nutritional interventions in older people must become routine following a proper assessment; the presence of other comorbidities and chronic disease make this of paramount importance.

15.1 Introduction

In adults aged over 60 years, diabetes mellitus (DM) has reached almost epidemic proportions, affecting 8.6 million (18.3% of the population in the USA). When impaired fasting glucose (IFG) is also considered, the prevalence of both conditions in this population rises to 33.6%. Commencing at age 60, the lifetime risk of subsequently developing diabetes is also high – 22.4% for women and 18.9% for men [1].

To facilitate successful ageing in patients with diabetes, it is important to recognize the heterogeneity in the spectrum of health among older patients, so that an appropriate focusing of health interventions can take place. This must coincide with an assessment of functional status and the presence of geriatric syndromes. As a person's life expectancy may be shorter than the time needed to benefit from an intervention, it is important to prioritize treatment strategies. A realistic and individualized approach is mandatory, as any one of the comorbidities may take precedence over the actual management of the diabetes [2].

Several physiological changes associated with ageing predispose to the development of diabetes; moreover, once diabetes has been diagnosed, insulin resistance is invariably present and may be associated with obesity [3]. In contrast, it has also been shown that there is a high prevalence of malnutrition in the elderly, especially with regards to long-term care and hospital settings [4]. The impact of malnutrition could be more deleterious in elderly patients with diabetes if nutritional counselling is poor.

Diabetes in Old Age. Third Edition. Edited by Alan J. Sinclair
© 2009 John Wiley & Sons, Ltd

15.2　Basis of nutritional support

According to Peake [5], the following are the basic questions to bear in mind when designing nutrition programmes for patients with hyperglycaemia or diabetes:

- What is the nutritional status of the patient?
- Is artificial nutritional support indicated?
- Can the patient's requirements be met by oral nutritional support?
- Are there any disorders of gastrointestinal motility?
- Should enteral or parenteral feeding be used?
- What will be the best formula?
- What is an acceptable blood glucose range?
- What insulin regimen will be most effective?

15.2.1　Normal ageing and nutritional status

Changes in appetite and food intake with increasing age

A recognized correlation exists between an impaired sense of smell and a reduced interest in (and intake of) food. Hence, as the senses of taste and smell deteriorate with age – by 60–80% in some cases – people will tend to become less hungry and eat less as they grow older. Healthy older persons are less hungry, consume smaller meals more slowly, eat fewer snacks between meals, and become satiated more rapidly after eating a standard meal than do younger persons [6]. However, as the decrease in energy intake is greater than the decrease in energy expenditure, there is a tendency for the elderly to lose body weight. This physiological, age-related reduction in appetite and energy intake has been termed 'the anorexia of aging'.

Contributing to this are age-related changes with regards to gut motility (oesophagus, stomach and large intestine), while gastric emptying is slowed down in aged persons, but without causing the problems of neuropathy as seen in diabetic subjects. Together with a diminished distensibility of the stomach, this may induce an earlier satiety and therefore a minimization of food intake. Compared to the many other reasons for malnutrition in the elderly, these changes play only a minor role; however, in elderly patients with diabetes, gastroparesis might represent an important issue in nutritional terms.

Changes in body weight with increasing age

The results of large cross-sectional studies have shown that both body weight and body mass index (BMI) increase throughout adult life until the age of about 50–60 years, after which they decline. A substantial minority of older people undergoes a marked weight change over time. In one study [7], 17% of home-dwelling people in the USA aged >65 years lost ≥5% of their initial bodyweight over 3 years, whereas 13% gained 5% or more. A BMI range of 24–29 kg m^{-2} has been suggested as appropriate for the elderly population [8], especially for individuals aged over 70 years, as this higher than conventional BMI range has been associated with lower mortality rates. Morley suggested that weight reduction be considered only in those patients who were 20% above their desirable body weight, at which time a BMI of 29 kg m^{-2} may be a safer target for older people to achieve [9]. A weight loss of 5–10% from initial body weight is known to benefit blood pressure, glycaemic control and lipid profiles.

Changes in body composition with increasing age

With ageing, there is a progressive increase in fat and decrease in fat-free mass, which is due to a loss of skeletal muscle; such loss may be up to 3 kg of lean body mass per decade after the age of 50 years. Consequently, at any given weight, older people not only have more body fat than do young adults but it is also located in different places. The increase in body fat with ageing is multifactorial in origin; a decreased physical activity is a major cause, with contributions from reduced growth hormone secretion, declining sex hormone action, and reduced resting metabolic rate and thermic effects of food. In older people a greater proportion of body fat is intrahepatic, intramuscular and intra-abdominal (versus subcutaneous); these changes are associated with increased insulin resistance and, therefore, are likely to be associated with adverse metabolic outcomes [10].

The anorexia–sarcopenia–sachexia triad in the elderly

Malnutrition in the elderly seems to be caused by a diminished food intake leading to anorexia and, through inflammatory processes, inducing cachexia. Although anorexia, sarcopenia and cachexia partly have common backgrounds, anorexia mainly means a deficient caloric intake first leading to a loss of body fat mass.

This is distinct from sarcopenia, where primarily lean body mass (muscles) are lost, leading to loss of functionality (Table 15.1). Cachexia, on the other hand, leads to both a loss of fat and muscle mass, as seen in patients where cancer is at an advanced stage [11]. The resultant weight loss and associated undernutrition can contribute further to adverse outcomes, because a loss of body weight beyond the age of 60 years is disproportionately of lean body tissue, predominantly skeletal muscle. When excessive, this may lead to sarcopenia (defined as muscle mass more than two standard deviations below the sex-specific young-normal mean), which is present in 6–15% of people aged >65 years [12]. Unlike the loss of fat tissue, a loss of skeletal muscle is associated with metabolic, physiological and functional impairments; with disability, including increased falls; and with an increased risk of protein-energy malnutrition. In the National Health And Nutrition Examination Survey (NHANES) III study, older people who had marked sarcopenia were between 3.3-fold (women) and 4.7-fold (men) more likely to have a physical disability than were those with low-risk skeletal muscle mass [12].

Ageing *per se* seems to be partly triggered by inflammatory processes, increasing the oxidative stress, and accumulating over the whole life-span. Malnutrition in the elderly can be present in lean and obese patients. Both situations are caused by an inflammatory process described before. The first ones are malnourished because a diminished food intake leading to anorexia, and posterior cachexia. The second ones are malnourished because obesity can be associated to an increased fat body mass, and high BMI, but to a low lean body mass and sarcopenia. This lean mass has a very low metabolic rate and a poor response to low calorie diets that can lead to higher malnutrition. So both, malnourished elderly patients with diabetes and obese elderly patients with diabetes, reflect two types of inflammatory status and are completely different from a metabolic point of view, but require different nutritional approaches.

15.2.2 Undernutrition in older people

Prevalence

Protein-energy malnutrition is common in the elderly. Studies conducted in developed countries have shown that up to 15% of community-dwelling and home-bound elderly, between 23% and 62% of hospitalized patients, and up to 85% of nursing homes residents suffer from this condition [6]. Protein-energy malnutrition is associated with impaired muscle function, a decreased bone mass, immune dysfunction, anaemia, reduced cognitive function, poor wound healing, delayed recovery from surgery and, ultimately, increased morbidity and mortality. Epidemiological studies have shown that protein-energy malnutrition is a strong independent predictor of mortality in elderly people, regardless of whether they live in the community or in a nursing home, are patients in a hospital, or have been discharged from hospital during the past one to two years [13–15]. This mortality is even increased in the presence of other medical diseases (e.g. renal failure, cardiac failure, cerebrovascular disease), some of which are also increased in diabetes. Two of the most common markers of undernutrition and risk for morbidity and mortality are low body weight and loss of weight.

Estimation of the prevalence of malnutrition in elderly subjects depends on the tools used to evaluate the nutritional status, and on the setting of the studied population. In the past, methods used have included anthropometry, reports of recent weight loss, biochemical markers, and the Mini Nutritional Assessment or other composite nutritional evaluation tools. Various studies have reported an association between mortality and nutritional status, as assessed by BMI, weight loss, plasma levels of albumin or food intake. However – and especially in older people with

Table 15.1 Pathophysiology of malnutrition.

Triad of malnutrition	
Anorexia/ undernutrition	Deficient caloric intake (loss of fat mass)
Sarcopenia	Protein-deficient diet and lack of physical exercise (loss of muscle mass)
Cachexia	Catabolic state. Inflammatory parameters increased (TNF-α, IL-1, IL-6) (loss of both fat and muscle stores)

diabetes – it is important to take into account other potential predictors of adverse outcomes, such as illness severity, comorbidity and functional status.

In hospital, both age and albumin have significant effects on mortality. In one study of hospitalized patients, the lower the albumin levels on admission and the older the patient, the higher was the risk of death [16]. With regards to food intake, a total of 102 patients (21%) among a total of 497 aged $\geq$65 years had an average daily in-hospital nutrient intake of less than 50% of their calculated maintenance energy requirements, while the low nutrient intake group had a higher rate of in-hospital mortality (RR = 8.0; 95% CI 2.8–22.6) and 90-day mortality (RR = 2.9; 95% CI 1.4–6.1) [17]. The question is then, why should protein-energy malnutrition be important in old people with diabetes? It is not unusual to prescribe a low-energy, low-fat diet for patients with diabetes in a hospital setting, but restrictive diets can induce a marked reduction in the average daily nutrient intake of maintenance energy requirements, leading to a worse nutritional status. In older diabetic subjects, weight loss and malnutrition have also been associated with other adverse outcomes, such as length of stay in the hospital, hospital discharge location or time to readmission, infections, gait disorders, falls and fractures and poor wound healing.

Low body weight in older people

Body weight tends to decrease after the age of 60 years, and a loss of $\geq$5% of body weight is not uncommon in older people. The relationship between mortality and body weight is a J-shaped curve, with increased mortality at low and high BMI-values. For young adults, the BMIs associated with the greatest life expectancy are in the range of 20–25 kg m^{-2}. The BMI that is associated with maximum life expectancy increases with age. The lower end of the range increases to about 22–23 kg m^{-2}, while the upper end increases to 27–28 kg m^{-2} for people aged >65 years. Below a BMI of 22–23 kg m^{-2} there is a steady increase in risk of death, mainly at BMI values <18.5 kg m^{-2} in women and 20.5 kg m^{-2} in men [18].

Mortality was studied as a function of BMI in 8428 hospitalized patients. In those aged 20–40 years, mortality doubled in the most underweight (BMI <18 kg m^{-2}) compared to groups with BMIs between 20 and 40 kg m^{-2}; in patients aged 70–79 years there was a tripling in mortality for BMI <18 kg m^{-2} compared to that in groups with BMIs between 32 and 40 kg m^{-2} [19] (Figure 15.1). The conclusion is that being very underweight becomes increasingly lethal as patients age.

Causes of undernutrition in older people

Healthy aging is associated with a decline in energy (food) intake, the physiological 'anorexia of aging', and a reduction in function of homeostatic mechanisms that function in younger people to restore food intake in response to anorectic insults. Roberts and colleagues [20] proved this fact by underfeeding young and old men by approximately 750 kcal per day for 21 days, during which time both groups of men lost weight.

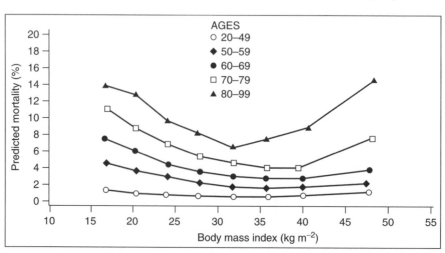

Figure 15.1 Association between BMI and mortality as a function of age in 8428 hospitalized patients. Reproduced from Ref. [19]

Following the underfeeding period, when the men were allowed to eat *ad libitum*, the young men ate more than at baseline and quickly returned to normal weight. In contrast, the old men did not compensate, returned only to their baseline intake, and did not regain the weight that they had lost.

Pathologic anorexia and undernutrition in older people

Protein-energy malnutrition is particularly likely to develop in the presence of other 'pathological' factors, many of which become more common with increased age. As most are responsive to treatment, recognition is important. Older people are more likely to live alone than are young adults, and social isolation and loneliness have been associated with decreased appetite and energy intake in the elderly. Moreover, they tend to consume substantially more food during a meal when eating in the company of friends than when eating alone [21].

Depression is a common problem in older people, it being present in 2–10% of community-dwelling older people and in a much greater proportion of those in institutions. Depression is more likely to manifest as a reduced appetite and weight loss in the elderly, and is an important cause of weight loss and undernutrition in this group. Depression is the cause in 30–36% of medical outpatients and nursing home residents who lose weight. Undernutrition – particularly if it produces folate deficiency – may worsen depression. The treatment of depression is effective in producing weight gain and improving other nutritional indices [22].

Another relevant factor is that poor dentition and ill-fitting dentures, both common in the elderly, may limit the type and quantity of food eaten. Complaints of problems with chewing, biting and swallowing are usual among nursing home residents, and those with dentures are more likely to have a poor protein intake [23]. The elderly often also take multiple medications, which increases the risk for drug interactions that can cause anorexia.

15.2.3 Overnutrition and obesity in older people

Prevalence

A substantial number of older people in westernized countries are overweight by standard BMI criteria, and the trend is increasing. In 2000, 58% of Americans aged ≥ 65 years had a BMI of $\geq 25\,kg\,m^{-2}$ or more, and the prevalence of obesity (BMI >30) in people in the USA who were aged >70 years increased by over one-third between 1991 and 2000, from 11.4% to 15.5% [24]. The increase in the relative risk of death associated with being obese is not as great in older adults as it is in young adults. In an assessment of 13 studies, in which non-hospitalized people aged >65 years were followed for at least 3 years [25], an association was found between mortality and high BMI in only a few cases, and then at BMIs only above $27–28.5\,kg\,m^{-2}$, with little or no increase in mortality at any BMI for people aged >75 years. Where an optimum BMI could be identified, it usually was in the range of $27–30\,kg\,m^{-2}$. The causes of increased mortality are essentially diabetes, hypertension, sleep apnoea, cardiovascular disease (CVD), and an increased risk with obesity for developing certain cancers, including breast, uterus, colon and prostate. Functional capacity and mobility are reduced significantly in the obese elderly, who have a lower quality of life, greater limitations of physical function, and are more likely to be homebound [26]. Obesity is predictive of a greater rate of future disability, declines in functional status, and an increased admission rate to nursing homes.

The most characteristic abnormality in glucose metabolism seen in ageing is a progressive rise in fasting and postprandial plasma insulin concentration, which suggests that ageing is an insulin-resistant state. The liver maintains normal glucose levels postprandially and during fasting; with ageing, more insulin is required to appropriately regulate hepatic glucose production and to avoid hyperglycaemia [27]. Failure of the beta cell to adequately secrete insulin in the face of hepatic and peripheral (muscle and fat) insulin resistance leads to the development of diabetes mellitus. Moreover, hyperglycaemia itself causes a further deterioration in muscle and liver sensitivity to insulin, and a continued impairment in beta-cell function (a phenomenon known as 'glucose toxicity'), which leads to a worsening of glucose tolerance in the patient with diabetes.

Insulin resistance and hyperinsulinaemia are associated with increases in total and visceral fat mass, which are typical of ageing. Insulin resistance is considered to be an independent risk factor for the development of coronary artery disease (CAD), and has been associated with hypertension, dyslipidaemia and dysfibrinolysis (the insulin resistance syndrome, or syndrome X), which is considered to be a major risk factor for atherosclerotic CVD, cancer and all-cause mortality, and is therefore related to a decreased life expectancy. A strong correlation between obesity and insulin resistance has been demonstrated in a variety of epidemiological studies; the fact that insulin sensitivity improves with weight loss in obese patients suggests a causality relationship between obesity and insulin resistance. It is speculated that the changes in body composition in the process of ageing are responsible for the development of insulin resistance, and consequently for the increased prevalence of type 2 diabetes with ageing.

All of these physiopathological considerations should be borne in mind when treating the insulin-resistant elderly patient with diabetes. Most therapeutic strategies are designed to induce an improvement in carbohydrate homeostasis by weight reduction (decreased fat), directly improving insulin sensitivity, and finally decreasing the deleterious effects of glucose toxicity.

Should overweight older people be advised to lose weight?

The adverse effects of obesity, reduced life expectancy at high BMIs up to the age of at least 70 years, and improvements in function that are associated with weight loss, must each be balanced against the detrimental effects of weight loss on muscle mass and bone density, and the proven association between all-cause weight loss and increased mortality in older people, even those who are overweight initially. It could be that an older person overweight to a degree that reduces life expectancy might be likely to die sooner if attempting to lose weight and succeeding than remaining weight-stable. Studies involving younger adults have found that intentional weight loss can reduce mortality in those who have obesity-related health problems (type 2 diabetes, ischaemic heart disease, hypertension) [28]. Available evidence suggests that it is safe to recommend weight loss to overweight older people who have obesity-related morbidities, particularly reduced mobility and function. Indeed, this group seems to have the most to gain.

15.3 Nutritional assessment

Before nutritional support is initiated, the indications, aims/objectives and ideal route of nutritional support must be determined, based on both the nutritional assessment of the patient and the clinical features of the condition being treated. Patients with hyperglycaemia form a heterogeneous group. It is vital to identify the aetiology of the hyperglycaemia in order to tailor appropriate clinical care with clear medical and nutritional management objectives. The stress response to trauma/illness commonly exacerbates hyperglycaemia in patients with pre-existing diabetes, and not infrequently produces significant hyperglycaemia in previously euglycaemic patients due to the increase in circulating counter-regulatory hormones (glucagon, cortisol, growth hormone, adrenaline), resulting in an increase in hepatic glucose production, a decrease in peripheral glucose uptake and an increase in insulin resistance. However, when assessing a patient with diabetes for nutritional support, their recent glycaemic control and treatment are highly relevant, as poor glycaemic control can compromise the patient's overall nutritional status.

A detailed discussion of methods that are used to diagnose undernutrition in older people with diabetes is beyond the scope of this chapter; there is no 'gold standard', and multiple methods have been used. The most important thing is to be aware of the diagnosis and to use effective tools for screening. An assessment is a more detailed and longer examination carried out by specially trained staff (clinician, dietician, or nutrition nurse) in those patients screened as being at nutritional risk, according to the ESPEN guidelines [29]. In addition, an intervention plan should be based on the results of the screening tool.

All elderly people aged >65 years should be screened once a year and weighed at regular intervals, particularly those in nursing homes or other institutions, because a weight loss of more than 5% is usually a key indicator. A BMI $<22\,\mathrm{kg\,m^{-2}}$ suggests undernutrition, which is particularly likely if the BMI is $<18.5\,\mathrm{kg\,m^{-2}}$.

Reduced serum albumin, haematocrit, lymphocyte count and serum folate are among the factors found to be associated with the risk for undernutrition and poor outcome [30]. Among the most widely used outpatient screening tools for undernutrition risk are the Mini Nutritional Assessment [31]. The short form of the Mini Nutritional Assessment (MNA) fulfils some of these expectations, having been derived from the original version of the MNA by identifying six items that are strongly correlated with the conventional nutritional assessment of experienced physicians. If the score amounts to 11 or less, the patient is classified as at risk of malnutrition and the full MNA must be carried out. In a multitude of studies, the MNA has been shown to correlates well with nutritional intake, anthropometry, laboratory data, functionality, morbidity, length of stay and mortality [32]. In nursing homes and hospitals there will be more obstacles that may hinder the successful application of the MNA. Many of these patients are not capable of cooperating, and under these circumstances the Nutritional Risk Screening (NRS) may be used as an alternative. In comparison with the MNA, the NRS emphasizes more the severity of concomitant diseases in the screening for risk. The NRS has been recommended for the nutritional screening of all hospital patients without age restriction, and its application seems to be most appropriate in this setting [33, 34]. If the total score is ≥ 3, then some form of nutritional support should be started. In Table 15.2 are shown the main validated methods for nutritional screening.

For special subgroups within this population who show a high prevalence of malnutrition, it is advised to proceed directly with the assessment tool. Examples might be frail elderly living largely independently in the community but relying on social services, elderly

Table 15.2 Validated methods for nutritional screening.

Technique	Use	Parameters studied
Mini Nutritional Assessment (MNA) [31]	Evaluation of nutritional status, validated in the elderly; for use in outpatient setting, community and nursing homes if possible.	*Anthropometrics*: weight, height, arm and calf circumferences and weight loss. *General assessment*: mobility, lifestyle and medication. *Dietary assessment*: food and fluid intake, number of meals, and autonomy of feeding. *Subjective assessment*: the patient's perception of their own health and nutrition.
Nutrition Risk Index (NRI) [33]	Evaluation of nutritional status in the elderly for all hospital patients without age restriction.	A 16-item questionnaire including: mechanics of food intake, dietary restrictions, morbid conditions affecting food intake, discomfort associated with outcome of food intake and significant changes in dietary habits.
Malnutrition Universal Screening Tool (MUST) [37]	Identifies adults, who are malnourished, at risk of malnutrition, or obese; for use in hospitals, community and other care settings.	A five-step screening tool using: height and weight, percentage unplanned weight loss, acute disease effect together to obtain overall risk of malnutrition.
Subjective Global Assessment (SGA) [38]	Identifies risk of developing nutrition-related complications.	*Nutritional history*: previous 6 months' weight loss, pattern of dietary intake, presence of gastrointestinal symptoms, functional capacity. *Physical examination*: loss of subcutaneous fat, muscle wasting, loss of fluid.
Prognostic Nutritional Index (PNI) [39]	Identifies increased risk of post-surgical complications	Combines anthropometry, delayed-hypersensitivity skin test and plasma protein levels – expressed as a single value.

Adapted from [36] Reilly, H.M. (1996) Screening for nutritional risk. *Proceedings of the Nutrition Society*, **55**, 841–53.
[37] Malnutrition Advisory Group (MAG). MAG guidelines for detection and management of malnutrition. 2000, Redditch, UK: British association for Parenteral and Enteral Nutrition. Available at: http://www.bapen.org.uk/must_tool.html
[38] Detsky, A.S., McLaughlin, J.R., Baker, J.P., Johnston, N., Whittake, S., Mendlson, R.A. and Jeejeebhoy, K.N. (1987) What is subjective global assessment of nutritional status? *Journal of Parenteral and Enteral Nutrition*, **11**, 8–13.
[39] Buzby, G.P., et al. (1980) Prognostic nutritional index in gastrointestinal surgery. *American Journal of Surgery*, **139**, 160–7.

with extensive comorbidities as diabetes, nursing home residents, and elderly hospital patients [29].

Initially, it is essential to obtain an accurate medical history of the patient. The most important clinical aspect leading to the diagnosis of malnutrition certainly addresses the course of the patient's weight and here especially weight loss, which should be expressed either in kilograms or as a percentage of the patient's usual weight. The interval since the weight loss started should also be explored. The patient should be asked whether they have suffered a loss of appetite, and/or it may be helpful to question the patient about restrictive diets and the consumption of alcohol or tobacco. Extra attention should be paid to physical signs of over-malnutrition (muscle atrophy, loss of subcutaneous fat and peripheral oedema as a consequence of hypoprotidaemia).

Since functional status in the elderly is closely correlated with their nutritional status, it is usually advisable to determine their basic and instrumental activities of daily living (ADLs and IADLs). Some additional information about the living conditions and the social relationships of the patient must also be obtained.

John Morley's mnemonic MEALS ON WHEELS summarizes a variety of treatable pathological causes [35]. Chronic diseases and medications can also be risk factors for malnutrition in the elderly through their effects on appetite, food intake, gastrointestinal function and metabolism (Tables 15.3 and 15.4).

Anthropometric measurements are an essential part of the nutritional assessment of the elderly [40], and comprise the determination of body height, body weight, circumference of the upper arm and calf, and measurement of the triceps skin fold. Special conditions such as oedema, ascites, pleural effusion and loss of body parts must be taken into account. Serial weights over days and weeks are more valuable than single measurements, and provide important information in the short term concerning fluid balance, and in the long term concerning changes in nutritional status. The BMI is a poorer reflection of changes in body composition in the elderly than in a younger population. For adults aged <65 years, the cut-off point below which malnutrition is highly probable has been set at $18.5\,\mathrm{kg\,m^{-2}}$, while in the elderly, for prognostic reasons, the cut-off point is usually set at 20–$22\,\mathrm{kg\,m^{-2}}$ [8]. With regards to the anthropometric parameters, an individual patient should not be judged to be malnourished on the basis of only one pathological value, but

Table 15.3 Mnemonic 'Meals on Wheels'. Adapted from Ref. [35].

- Medications (e.g. digoxin, theophylline, fluoxetine)
- Emotional causes (depression)
- Alcoholism
- Late-life paranoia
- Swallowing problems (dysphagia)
- Oral problems
- Nosocomial infections (TB, *Clostridium difficile*, *Helicobacter pylori*)
- Wandering (dementia)
- Hyperthyroidism, hyperparathyroidism, hypoadrenalism
- Enteral problems (malabsorption)
- Eating problems (inability to self-feed)
- Low-salt, low-fat diet
- Shopping and social problems

should also be assessed using a combination of all the anthropometric data (Table 15.5).

The most widely used laboratory parameter to assess the nutritional status has been serum albumin, although such levels may be influenced by a wide variety of acute and chronic inflammatory and malignant conditions; that is, serum albumin is a marker of disease severity rather than of malnutrition. Ageing, as well as hepatic and renal dysfunction, can also cause a decrease in serum albumin levels. A further disadvantage is that serum albumin has a long half-life of 18 days. Although a diminished serum albumin is rarely the consequence of a poor nutritional status alone, it may serve as a marker of the severity of a disease which itself carries a risk of developing malnutrition. Alternative parameters are transferrin, transthyretin, retinol-binding protein and insulin growth factor-1, but these will clearly increase laboratory costs.

Laboratory examinations are not an essential component of the diagnosis of malnutrition in the elderly. In a recent study, it was noted that weight loss and anthropometric data showed a stronger correlation with life-threatening complications among geriatric hospital patients than did either albumin or transthyretin [17].

Bioelectrical impedance analysis (BIA) and dual-energy X-ray analysis (DXA) measurements remain interesting fields of ongoing research in body

Table 15.4 Chronic diseases and drugs that may cause malnutrition in the elderly.

Chronic diseases	Drugs
• Chronic cardiac failure	• ACE-inhibitors
• Chronic pulmonary diseases	• Analgesics
• Cancer	• Antacids
• Chronic infectious diseases	• Anti-arrhythmic drugs
• Gastrointestinal diseases	• Antibiotics
• Diabetes	• Anti-epileptic drugs
• Severe osteoarthritis	• Antidepressants
• Hypothyroidism/hyperthyroidism	• β-blocking agents
• Cerebral ischaemia	• Calcium channel-blocking agents
• Intracerebral bleeding	• Digoxin/digitoxin
• Pressure ulcers	• H_2-receptor antagonists
• Parkinson's disease	• Laxatives
• Dementia	• NSAIDs
• Depression	• Oral antidiabetic substances
	• Potassium
	• Corticosteroids

Table 15.5 Essential parameters for the diagnosis of malnutrition in the elderly.

- Weight loss (expressed in kg or percentage of former/usual weight)
- Oral intake (simple documentation by e.g. the eye-ball method)
- Body mass index $<22\,\mathrm{kg\,m^{-2}}$ (showing an acceptable association with body fat stores)
- Calf circumference $<31\,\mathrm{cm}$ (showing a good correlation with muscle mass and functional status in the elderly)

composition, but neither is currently used in routine clinical practice.

15.3.1 Brief review of nutritional guidelines

A number of reviews of nutritional guidelines in people with diabetes (including older people) have been conducted, including ADA [41], IDF [42], ESPEN [66], ASPEN [69] and NICE [43].

Clinical advice has usually been based around the recommendations for all adults with diabetes. Clearly, these need to be individually modified with consideration of important factors, such as functional and mental ability and polypharmacy when prescribing diet or nutritional support to this age group. The ADA position statement concerning nutritional intervention for older adults with diabetes focuses only on weight management and physical activity, plus a multivitamin supplement recommendation for those older adults with reduced energy intake.

Current European recommendations are based on studies in younger age groups, which have then been extrapolated to the elderly, leading to a low quality of evidence for the specific effects in older age groups.

The most recent European recommendations for adults with diabetes emphasize energy balance and weight control, and recognize a wide variation in carbohydrate intake as being compatible with good diabetic control. The target is to help optimize glycaemic control and reduce the risk of CVD and nephropathy. The quality of life of the individual person must be considered when defining nutritional objectives, and health care providers must achieve a balance between the demands of metabolic control, risk factor management, patient well-being and safety.

15.3.2 Current dietary recommendations: applications to older people with diabetes

The National Diet and Nutrition Survey of people aged ≥65 years [44, 45] showed that two-thirds of free-living elderly were overweight or obese. While only 3% of men and 6% of women in the community were underweight, this figure rose to 17% for the elderly in institutions. Undernutrition in acutely ill hospitalized elderly patients has been estimated at 26% [46].

The following topics should be considered: body weight, physical activity and the specific micronutrient composition of the diet, including carbohydrates, protein, alcohol, sodium, vitamins and minerals. Undernutrition is as much a concern in older patients with diabetes as is obesity [47]. The first measure in the treatment of malnutrition may be dietary counselling. With previously malnourished patients a nutritional intervention should be started sooner. Phosphate, chromium and trace element deficiencies can cause hyperglycaemia by decreasing insulin sensitivity.

15.4 Energy intake: carbohydrates and fats

15.4.1 General recommendations

The optimal diet for diabetic patients remains unknown. Total dietary energy should be the same for elderly patients as for their younger counterparts, with no specific recommendation unless the person is overweight or gaining weight, when a reduction in total energy intake is advised. Carbohydrate should be in an acceptable range of 45–60% of the total energy [41]. A combined intake of 60–70% of total energy is recommended for carbohydrate and monounsaturated with cis-configuration fatty acids. The source of carbohydrate does not appear to affect glycaemic control if used with mixed meals, but carbohydrates rich in fibre or having a low glycaemic index are particularly recommended, while sucrose intake should not exceed 10% of the total energy. In addition, an increase in the proportion of carbohydrates from fruits, vegetables and legumes should be recommended.

With regards to fats, an acceptable range 25–35% of the total energy should be recommended, with saturated and trans-unsaturated fatty acids providing <7% of the total energy [41]. Polyunsaturated

fatty acids should not exceed 10% of the total energy. Mono-unsaturated fatty acids (MUFAs) with cis-configuration in combination with carbohydrate should provide 60–70% of the total energy, and one portion of oily fish per week plus other plant sources are recommended for n-3 fatty acids. However, dietary supplements of fish oils (or their derived preparations) and pharmacological doses of vitamins are not recommended. The daily cholesterol intake should not exceed 200 mg. Plant sterol and stanol esters block the intestinal absorption of dietary and biliary cholesterol. Among the general public, and in individuals with type 2 diabetes, a daily intake of 2 g of plant sterols and stanols has been shown to lower both plasma and LDL-cholesterol [41, 42]. If these products are used, they should displace – rather than be added to – the diet in order to avoid weight gain. Soft gel capsules containing plant sterols are also available.

Although guidelines exist that outline the appropriate use of food sources, these often change, reflecting the lack of clear evidence-based suggestions. However, it is important to note that, while a decreasing fat intake is warranted for weight loss, any oils used should consist of unsaturated fats (e.g. olive, corn, canola, and certain varieties of safflower and sunflower). Second, complex carbohydrates – long polymers of glucose found in starches, such as rice, potatoes and vegetables – should be the substitutes of simple sugars.

'Diabetic' foods are not recommended, and non-nutritive sweeteners afford an alternative means of providing sweetened foods and drinks that are palatable to the elderly. For hypertension control, the DASH diet (Dietary Approaches to Stop Hypertension) [48] suggested: (i) an emphasis on the use of fruits, vegetables and low-fat dairy products; (ii) the inclusion of whole grains, poultry and nuts; and (iii) a reduction in the intake of fats, red meat, sweets and sugar-containing beverages.

15.4.2 Malnourished diabetic patients

If a patient is eating very little, then the provision of palatable sugar-containing food may help to stimulate the appetite. The inclusion of high-fat food is valuable in helping the patient maximize their energy intake in smaller portions. Conversely, the inclusion of high-fibre diets (complex carbohydrates) may limit food intake by causing early satiety. The provision of extra high-protein and energy snacks may be sufficient to meet a patient's nutritional requirement [49]. These dietary modifications are likely to increase the intake of simple sugar and the glycaemic index of the diet, but these potentially adverse changes must be offset against the risks of malnutrition. Some foods with a high energy content have a low glycaemic index, and it may be advantageous to encourage the intake of foods such as ice-cream, custard, yoghurt, sponge cake and muffins to minimize the glycaemic response.

15.4.3 Obese diabetic patients

The typical patient with insulin-resistant type 2 diabetes is obese, and the control of diabetes mellitus will be improved after only a slight weight loss. Insulin sensitivity increases when obese patients are on a negative caloric balance. Thus, as the major goal in improving insulin sensitivity is weight loss, a decrease in caloric intake should be emphasized [50]. As fat contains more than twice as many calories as carbohydrate and protein per gram, it should be limited in the hypocaloric diets of overweight patients with type 2 diabetes. Rather, patients should switch to diet drinks or water to save a significant number of calories, in addition to decreasing their intake of simple sugars. Low-carbohydrate diets (which restrict the total carbohydrate to <130 g per day) are not recommended in the treatment of overweight/obesity, as the long-term effects of these diets are unknown. Although they produce short-term weight loss, the maintenance of weight loss is similar to that with low-fat diets, and the impact on the CVD risk profile is uncertain.

A trained dietician should instruct the patient with diabetes about appropriate dietary strategies. This approach, which often includes the spouse, may restructure the patient's eating habits – an action that is critical for the long-term successful dietary treatment of diabetes.

15.4.4 Exercise

The benefits of exercise for all diabetics have been well documented, and are irrespective of body weight or age. Exercise will lead to an improvement in metabolic and cardiovascular risk factors, as well as improving strength, flexibility, balance and function [51]. In an eight-year prospective study from the NHIS of 2896 adults with diabetes, walking for at least 2 h each week was associated with a 39% lower all-cause mortality rate and a 34% reduction in coronary heart disease (CHD) mortality. The magnitude of these benefits persisted after controlling for age, gender,

obesity, functional limitations, duration of diabetes, or the presence of other comorbid conditions [52]. Physical training also increases insulin sensitivity – that is, patients respond better to insulin injection or to endogenous insulin.

The current guidelines from the Centers for Disease Control and Prevention [53] recommend that a 30-min period of moderate activity on most days is achievable for many older people. Individuals should be encouraged to do what they can achieve, to do it regularly, and to gradually build up in intensity and frequency. Even very frail older people can manage certain activities and, over time, should be able gradually to improve their strength.

15.4.5 Protein

Protein intake should account for 10–20% of the total energy. The European Association for the Study of Diabetes [42] has recognized that recommendations for the dietary protein content is based on incomplete evidence. Overall, the incidence of nephropathy in the elderly population has increased over the past 20 years, one possible explanation being that the improved treatment of CHD and hypertension has resulted in more patients with type 2 diabetes living long enough to develop nephropathy and end-stage renal failure (ESRF).

In a recent review which examined protein ranges between 0.3 and 0.8 g kg^{-1} body weight per day, high protein intakes contributed to the development of nephropathy [54]. Reducing protein intake appears to slow the progression to renal failure, although the level of restriction that is both effective and acceptable to patients is unknown. Current guidelines are based mainly on individuals with type 1 diabetes, and often use proxy indicators such as creatinine clearance rather than hard clinical end-points such as time to dialysis or death from ESRF. The current European recommendations suggest that patients with diabetes, who exhibit evidence of microalbuminuria or established nephropathy, should have a protein intake at the lower end of the normal range (0.7–0.9 g kg^{-1} body weight per day).

Protein intakes below this level increase the risk of malnutrition during chronic illness or catabolic states. In some elderly patients with diabetes, the balance between the risk of malnutrition and the possible benefits of a reduced protein intake to delay nephropathy must be carefully assessed.

15.4.6 Fibre

Fibre is a particularly important component to encourage in an older person's diet. Soluble fibre such as oat bran, pectin and guar lowers the plasma glucose levels and may improve the plasma lipid profile. Soluble fibre does not appear to interfere with the absorption of minerals in elderly patients with diabetes. *Constipation* is common among diabetics, and increasing the fibre intake can reduce laxative use and improve bowel function. The ADA[41] recommendation is 14 g per 1000 kcal of intake mainly from food containing whole grains, this means mainly insoluble fibre. However, fibrous foods tend to have a greater satiating effect and should be advised with caution in those with a depressed appetite. An increased fibre intake, particularly in the oldest elders, may cause bowel impaction if the liquid intake is poor.

15.4.7 Sodium intake

Both, taste and smell decline with age, beginning around the age of 60 years but becoming more marked above 70 years. Salt and monosodium glutamate are commonly used as taste enhancers, and can improve dietary intake in elderly people. On the other hand, sodium intake is linked with the development or exacerbation of hypertension, and when salt intake is reduced the blood pressure may fall. A balance between using flavour enhancers to encourage dietary intake for underweight people, while not exacerbating hypertension, must be made. Sodium restriction requires a salt intake of <6 g per day [41, 48].

15.4.8 Alcohol

Older people are more susceptible to the effects of alcohol, and are likely to develop problems at relatively lower levels of consumption, due to the age-related body composition changes. Moderate intakes of alcohol appear to benefit blood pressure, glycaemic control and reduce the risk of thrombosis. Alcohol can also act as an appetite stimulant, which may be beneficial. A large intake of alcohol has been shown to increase the risk of stroke, hypertension, hypoglycaemia and both lactic and ketoacidosis [55]. The intake should be restricted to 1–2 units per day for women, or 2–3 units per day for men., though the lower end of these ranges is probably preferable. When using insulin or sulphonylureas it is advisable that alcohol is consumed together with carbohydrate-containing foods.

15.4.9 Vitamins and minerals

Elderly persons with diabetes are at risk of micronutrient deficiency, whether due to a low food intake, to the presence of chronic disease, or to drugs. The second evaluation of the Euronut-SENECA study population [4] was made in 1993, when subjects were aged 74–79 years ($n = 1005$). Among this population, 23.9% of the men and 46.8% of the women had low dietary intakes for at least one of the following micronutrients: calcium, iron, retinol, β-carotene, thiamine, pyridoxine or vitamin C. Vitamin D plasma levels were low in 36% of the men and 47% of the women. A cobalamin deficiency was described in 23.8% of the subjects. In both institutionalized and hospitalized elderly persons, the prevalence of micronutrient deficiency appeared to be higher, especially for thiamine, pyridoxine, cobalamin, folates, vitamin C, vitamin E and selenium. Among the survey population, between 10 and 40% were shown to have multiple vitamin deficiencies, while 10% were anaemic. Notably, the levels of deficiencies were higher when an individual was receiving institutionalized care.

The micronutrient status of elderly individuals with diabetes is controversial, with limited information available and the recommendation that any intervention should be carried out with caution until further research is completed [56]. The authors concluded that micronutrient supplementations for people with diabetes should be individualized and based on clinical findings, dietary history and laboratory results. The most important of these are discussed in the following sections.

Specific mineral and vitamin deficiencies

Vitamin D Vitamin D deficiency causes osteomalacia, rickets and myopathy, and is associated with reduced bone density, impaired mobility and an increased rate of falls and fractures. In ambulatory older people, mobility was seen to decline markedly when serum 25-hydroxyvitamin D levels were $<40 \, \text{pmol} \, l^{-1}$, although vitamin D supplementation reduced the rate of falls in nursing home residents (even those not deficient in vitamin D). Treatment with vitamin D at dosages of 700–800 IU per day, with or without calcium, reduced the relative risk for hip and other non-vertebral fractures by 23–26% compared to calcium or placebo in ambulatory or institutionalized older persons [57, 58].

A plasma 25-hydroxyvitamin D level <40 nmol/L (or <16 µg/L) is widely considered to represent vitamin D deficiency that is in need of treatment. If the more generous definition of this condition is used (serum 25-hydroxyvitamin D <80 nmol/L), a much larger proportion of the population has the problem. Most circulating 25-hydroxyvitamin D derives from exposure of the skin to UV-B radiation in sunlight; the remainder is obtained via the dietary intake of foods rich in vitamin D (predominantly oily fish), supplements and vitamin D-fortified food. Dietary requirements are greater in older people due to a reduced production in the skin, decreased sun exposure, an age-related thinning of the skin, and other skin changes. For that reason the recommended dietary reference intakes are higher for older adults; in the USA, it is 10 mg (400 IU) for people 51 to 70 years of age. The USA and Canada have mandatory vitamin D fortification of milk, and Canada also requires it in margarine, whereas other countries have variable levels of non-mandatory fortification [58].

Vitamin D therapy is safe, inexpensive and easy to administer. The prevalence of vitamin D deficiency is so high among the institutionalized elderly that routine supplementation with doses of 800–1000 IU per day, without testing, is being recommended and increasingly adopted. The most effective form of replacement is oral cholecalciferol, which can be given in intermittent boluses at intervals of one to six months, in doses not usually totalling more than 50 000 IU per month or as 500–2000 IU per day [59].

Calcium Guidelines for daily dietary intakes of calcium, developed with the aim of optimizing bone health, usually recommend higher intakes for older adults. Few older people achieved an adequate daily calcium intake (1200 mg) without taking a calcium supplement; the median daily dietary intake for American men and women aged ≥ 60 years is approximately 600 mg [60]. One tablet per day of a supplement containing 500–700 mg of elemental calcium is usually sufficient to achieve an adequate intake, but people with a low dietary intake should take two tablets. An adequate vitamin D status is essential for calcium uptake by the gut and bone formation and remodelling; hence, any vitamin D deficiency should be identified and corrected in older people who take calcium. Alternatively, vitamin D should be added routinely to the calcium treatment [61].

The risk of fractures due to falls and osteoporosis when diabetes is present may be further increased by peripheral neuropathy, autonomic neuropathy, hypoglycaemic episodes and poor eyesight. Sunlight on the skin should be sufficient for vitamin D synthesis for most adults, with the face and arms being exposed for 30 min each day. Further studies are required to clarify the assessment of vitamin and mineral status in elderly patients with diabetes.

Vitamin B_{12} (Cobalamin) Vitamin B_{12} deficiency is more common in older people than in young adults. In the Framingham study, 11.3% of elderly subjects had a serum vitamin B_{12} concentration <258 pmol l^{-1}, together with elevated plasma homocysteine and methylmalonic acid levels, compared to 5.3% of younger adults. In elderly people living in institutions, the prevalence of deficiency may reach 30–40%. Because the signs and symptoms of vitamin B_{12} deficiency often are subtle (macrocytic anaemia, subacute combined degeneration of the spinal cord, neuropathies, ataxia, glossitis, and possibly dementia), there should be a low threshold for testing older people, in particular those who are malnourished, those who have a neurologic or neuropsychiatric presentation that is consistent with vitamin B_{12} deficiency, and those who are in institutions, including psychiatric hospitals [62].

There is evidence that homocysteine damages blood vessel walls, and that there is a significant association between increased plasma homocysteine levels and an increased risk for CVD. The increased prevalence of deficiency in the elderly is due mainly to an increased rate of food cobalamin malabsorption and pernicious anaemia, which account for approximately 60–70% and 15–20% of cases, respectively [63].

Both, vitamin B_{12} and folate deficiencies coexist frequently in older people. The most common predisposing factor is gastric atrophy, which is present in more than 40% of people aged >80 years. Numerous factors predispose to the development of gastric atrophy, including *Helicobacter pylori* infection, chronic alcoholism, bacterial overgrowth, the long-term ingestion of metformin and antacids, and gastric bypass surgery for obesity.

Clinically apparent causes should be treated when possible, but a reversible cause of vitamin B_{12} deficiency often is not found, and so treatment with vitamin B_{12} usually is needed for life. The recommended daily intake of vitamin B_{12} is 2–5 mg in older adults. A vitamin B_{12} deficiency (<150 pmol l^{-1}) that is due to dietary inadequacy is best treated initially with intramuscular (i.m.) vitamin B_{12}, or at least with 100 mg per day of oral vitamin B_{12}. Food malabsorption is treated best with i.m. vitamin B_{12} or possibly high-dose oral vitamin B_{12} (e.g. 500 mg per day), whereas pernicious anaemia requires lifelong i.m. therapy [62]. When folate deficiency coexists, vitamin B_{12} should be given with appropriate folate doses; in any case, it is reasonable to coadminister a multivitamin that contains folate.

Folate Foods that are rich in folate include orange juice, dark green leafy vegetables, peanuts, strawberries, dried beans and peas, and asparagus. The synthetic folic acid found in vitamin supplements and fortified foods does not require intestinal cleavage and is absorbed more readily. The recommended daily intake of folate and folic acid is 400 mg, with an upper limit of 1000 mg of synthetic folic acid which, in high doses, may mask the features of coexistent vitamin B_{12} deficiency in older people. Folate deficiency causes macrocytic anaemia and increased homocysteine concentrations, and is associated with increased rates of colorectal cancer and, possibly, also cervical cancer, cognitive impairment, depression and dementia. The prevalence of folate deficiency among older people varies from 4% to 50%, depending on the population studied, and is particularly common among persons in institutions. Most folate deficiency is due to an inadequate dietary intake; an impaired use due to drug intake (e.g. methotrexate, anticonvulsants, sulfasalazine) or alcohol consumption is much less common. When folate deficiency is due to dietary insufficiency, attempts should be made to improve the diet by increasing the intake of fruit and vegetables. Folic acid supplements are also indicated to ensure treatment success, and are essential when the cause is not dietary, but should be excluded before starting treatment with folic acid (0.5–5 mg per day) [64].

Other vitamins and minerals [65]

- Zinc: zinc deficiency is associated with abnormalities in a wide variety of biological functions, including anorexia, T-cell abnormalities, wound healing, impotence and, possibly, macular degeneration. There is currently no definitive evidence that zinc deficiency causes diabetes or exacerbates glucose homeostasis. The recommended daily allowance (RDA) for zinc for men aged >50 years remains at 15 mg per day and 12 mg per day for women. For patients with leg ulcers, impotence or poor wound healing, a 3-month course of zinc supplementation (70 mg elemental zinc daily) is recommended. Overall, there is a consensus that nutrition is important for wound healing.

- Chromium (Cr): chromium has an important role in the regulation of glucose and lipid metabolism, and

symptoms of deficiency include weight loss, neuropathy and impaired glucose tolerance. The prevalence of Cr deficiency in diabetes is uncertain, but Cr supplementation enhances glucose tolerance in patients with diabetes; however, the significance of this finding in elderly diabetic subjects remains to be tested.

- Copper: the clinical relevance of elevated copper levels in the elderly patient with diabetes is still unknown. The recommended range of copper consumption has recently been extended to 1.5–3.0 mg per day.

- Iron: currently, there appears to be no evidence of any major alteration in iron status in diabetic patients who do not have renal failure or neuropathy with delayed absorption, but the uptake and utilization of iron is delayed. Although the iron status in elderly diabetic patients has not been studied, the elderly diabetic patient is most likely not at an increased risk of iron deficiency in the absence of other causes of iron loss.

- Magnesium (Mg): magnesium plays an important role in glucose homeostasis, and diabetes is associated with an increased urinary losses of this ion, especially when hyperglycaemia is present, and more so in elderly patients. The intake recommended for healthy adult males is 420 mg/d and for women is 320 mg/d. Open and double blind studies on the effects of the treatments of magnesium deficiency and of magnesium depletions in geriatic populations are too scarce. Magnesium supplementation (3 g per day) resulted in a significant improvement in response to glucose and arginine in a clinical trial in the elderly, but more studies are required to confirm this.

- B and A vitamins: these are used in a variety of metabolic functions, their primary source being green leafy vegetables (that occasionally are lacking in the diet of many elderly patients). For patients with neuropathy, a 2-month trial of vitamin B_1 or B_6 has been suggested, but the efficacy of such a regimen has not been proven. No deficiency has been found in most studies of serum vitamin A in the aged.

- Vitamin C: serum deficiency states of vitamin C are commonly noted in both elderly and younger patients with diabetes. The tissues stores of vitamin C are also depleted in the presence of chronic hypergly-caemia, but are associated with impaired leukocyte function and microangiopathy. The UK Department of Health currently recommends a reference nutrient daily intake of 40 mg of vitamin C, but not routine supplementation. These vitamin C requirements are based on the prevention of scurvy, and further research into the benefits of higher intakes is required. However, ADA does not recommend routine supplementation with antioxidants, such as vitamins E and C and carotene due to a lack of evidence and concern relating to long-term safety, unless for older adults with a reduced energy intake in whom a daily multivitamin supplement might be appropriate.

15.5   Nutritional oral supplements

If dietary counselling alone proves insufficient, the next step may be to increase the energy and protein concentration of the food. According to ESPEN guidelines for enteral nutrition in geriatric patients, oral supplementation increases both energy and nutrient intake [66]. Oral supplements should be given at an early stage, when there is evidence of insufficient intake, of weight loss exceeding 5% in a 3-month period or >10% in 6 months, or when the BMI is <22 kg m^{-2}.

Oral supplements are available in a wide range of savoury and sweet flavours. There is also a wide variety of presentations, including powders, pre-made carton sip feeds, glucose polymers (powders and syrups) and protein powders. These products may be nutritionally complete. A recent meta-analysis [67] showed a reduced mortality and fewer complications among undernourished hospital patients treated with supplements. The best results in terms of mortality were obtained in those aged >75 years, in those taking >400 kcal of supplement daily, those in a poor general condition, and those who were initially undernourished. In long-stay patients (>4 weeks), however, there was a tendency for even the initially well-nourished patients to become malnourished. This may be prevented by using supplements. In the above meta-analysis, there also was a trend towards a reduced length of stay in hospital for the intervention group.

For most patients, supplements should be prescribed for a limited period of time, and continued only after a positive effect has been documented. The compliance and acceptance of supplementation by patients may become problematic. Supplements should be given between meals and occasionally before bedtime, in order to avoid a reduced intake at meal times. The consumption of each supplement should take no longer than 30 min, and it should ideally be controlled and documented by the nursing staff (even better, on the drug rounds, when the consumption can be supervised). For most supplements, 1 ml is equal to 1 kcal, but hyper-caloric drinks (1.5–2 kcal ml^{-1}) are available and may be useful under certain circumstances. High-protein supplements may be indicated in cases of severe protein depletion. A realistic goal for energy intake from nutritional supplements is 400 kcal per day, although in some cases this may need to be increased to 600 kcal per day.

The sugar content of the supplement is often offset by the patient's reduced dietary carbohydrate intake, and can be invaluable in preventing hypoglycaemia during periods of poor oral intake. Spicy snacks may sometimes be helpful and induce old people with impaired taste to eat more [49]. In particular, among those ambulant, demented patients in residential homes, who tend to forget meal times and wander off, a finger-food buffet to which patients help themselves as they wish has proved superior in terms of total intake, to fixed mealtimes and sit-down meals.

15.6   Artificial nutrition

The nutritional management of hospitalized adult patients with diabetes covers the aetiology of hypergly-caemia, the effects of diabetes on nutritional status, the metabolic consequences of stress and specific nutrient mixes. Artificial nutritional support can also exaggerate the hyperglycaemic response to stress caused by injury or illness, unmasking glucose intolerance in the previously glucose-tolerant. Enteral and parenteral nutrition are valid options in the malnourished elderly, both in the hospital and at home. Elderly patients share most indications and complications with adult patients, though perhaps a greater focus should be placed on function and quality of life than on mortality.

Out of hospital, the focus for good glycaemic control is to minimize any long-term diabetic complications. In hospital, the rationale for good glycaemic control is to ensure a metabolic environment that promotes the best possible immune activity and wound healing. Hyperglycaemia has a detrimental effect on the immune system, adversely affecting chemotaxis, granulocyte adhesion, phagocytosis, intracellular killing and complement function [68]. The optimal blood glucose level for ill patients receiving nutritional support is unclear, but various reports have provided many different blood glucose targets and approaches to avoid both hyper- and hypoglycaemia. The specific targets for glycaemic control for each patient must take into consideration some of the following variables: age, prognosis, aetiology of the hyperglycaemia, level of consciousness, severity of any infection, degree of metabolic stress and immune status.

Although the metabolic consequences of diabetes are known to involve fat metabolism and to result in a significant dyslipidaemia, there are few defined management targets for serum lipids when giving nutritional support to diabetic patients. The degree of dyslipidaemia is frequently disproportional to the degree of hyperglycaemia, and requires monitoring and control which is separate from the diabetes. Some of the clinical consequences of hyperlipidaemia include: impairment of the immune response, endothelial dysfunction, an increased tendency to develop a coagulopathy and an exacerbation of insulin resistance.

Each hospital should have clearly stated monitoring protocols for nutritional support [66, 67]. The frequency of monitoring depends on the clinical situation, and must be individualized. Patients with hyperglycaemia, and those who are severely malnourished, should be monitored closely to prevent metabolic complications, including the potential life-threatening re-feeding syndrome associated with profound electrolyte disturbances and fluid overload. During refeeding there is a switch from fat to carbohydrate metabolism with an increase in insulin release. During carbohydrate repletion, insulin- stimulated glucose uptake is accompanied by an increased cellular uptake of potassium, phosphorus and water, and magnesium requirements will increase as a consequence of stimulation the sodium-potassium adenosine triphosphatase (ATPase) pump [5].

Medical management must be employed in the elderly patient with diabetes on nutritional support to achieve the objectives of glycaemic control. Oral hypoglycaemic agents (OHAs) are relatively contraindicated during critical illness. Metformin is not usually suitable for ill patients because there is a formal contraindication for its use in patients undergoing any form of imaging that requires contrast media. The OHAs most suited to hospital use are the short-acting insulin secretagogues, such as repaglinide or nateglinide. Long-acting sulphonylureas should be avoided as these are a potent cause of hypoglycaemia, particularly in the elderly. If necessary, OHAs may be uses in clinically stable patients receiving enteral (gastric administration)

feeds, but this is really only suitable when the enteral tube is pre-pyloric.

Insulin is required for all patients with type 1 diabetes and for those with type 2 diabetes with significant hyperglycaemia or critical illness. The type of insulin regimen used will be tailored to the particular circumstances of the patient, ranging from a continuous infusion to the use of subcutaneous, intermittent, quick-acting insulin on a background of once- or twice-daily long-acting insulin. It should be noted that if insulin is added to a parenteral nutrition bag, some will be adsorbed onto the plastic of the bag and cannulas.

15.6.1 Is artificial nutritional support necessary?

Artificial nutritional support is indicated for those patients who are malnourished, or who would become malnourished if not treated in this way. In order to benefit, patients must be fed for seven days or more [70]. The goals of nutritional support for patients with diabetes are to maintain or improve nutritional status, to promote wound healing, to optimize glycaemic control and optimal lipid control, and to avoid either hyperglycaemia or hypoglycaemia.

15.6.2 Route of artificial support [5, 66, 67]

When a decision has been made that nutritional support is required, the optimal route must be determined. Enteral nutrition should be used whenever possible, as it enjoys many advantages over parenteral nutrition, including economic considerations, the avoidance of infections associated with parenteral nutrition, and a more physiological impact on the intestinal bacterial milieu.

Enteral nutrition is suited to patients with diabetes due to the more physiological delivery of nutrients. The first line of nutritional support is an oral diet, and only if the patient is at risk of aspiration or cannot meet their nutritional requirements orally should other routes be considered. The decision requires a consensus from the clinical team and, if possible, the agreement of the patient and/or caregivers. The options are: oral diet; nutritional oral supplements; and tube feeding, whether pre-pyloric or post-pyloric.

When enteral nutrition is prolonged due to persistent anorexia or dysphagia, then percutaneous endoscopic gastrostomy (PEG) will often be the route of choice for artificial nutrition in the elderly. For this, three groups of patients can be identified:

(i) diabetes patients who will need prolonged home enteral nutrition, probably due to persistent dysphagia after a resolute disease; (ii) those who will obtain a short-term benefit before resuming oral nutrition, such as with secondary anorexia after stress; and (iii) those who will die while on home enteral nutrition, due to their primary disease. In these patients enteral nutrition can be considered as palliative.

As might be expected, both life expectancy and the health-related quality of life under nutritional support are poorer in elderly patients compared to younger patients. This is true for survival in home enteral nutrition patients [5], and after procedures such as PEG [71]. For obvious ethical reasons, no study has been designed to demonstrate any benefit of artificial nutrition versus an absence of nutritional support in comparable groups. Rather, the only studies performed not only provided conflicting results but were also either observational or had non-comparable groups.

15.7   Enteral tube feeding [43, 69]

Enteral tube feeding (ETF) may be continuous, intermittent or overnight. When the regimen to be applied has been decided, the type of enteral tube feed must be selected, based on the nutritional and fluid requirements. The approximate composition of generic feeds are as follows:

- Standard enteral tube feeds (1 kcal ml^{-1}; osmolarity 201–250 mOs l^{-1}): these contain 15–16% of energy as whole protein (milk protein-casein), 30–35% of energy as a mixture of long- and medium-chain fats [40% MUFA, 30% short-chain fatty acid (SFA) and poly-unsaturated fatty acids (PUFA)], such as linseed, sunflower, safflower or rapeseed oil, and may also contain fish oil. Carbohydrates provide 50–56% of the energy content of the feed (mainly present as maltodextrins), but may also contain sucrose, oligosaccharides, polysaccharides, corn syrups and starches.

- High-energy feeds (1.5 kcal ml^{-1}; osmolarity 300 mOs l^{-1}): these have the same percentage energy from macronutrients as the standard formula. The osmolarity of these products is increased to 300 mOs l^{-1} due to the reduced volume of the product.

- Fibre feeds: the amount of fibre per 100 ml is usually between 1–2 g. The type of fibre ranges from soy, inulin wheat fibre, fructo-oligosaccharides, oat fibre and gums, from a mixed or single source. The ratio of soluble to insoluble fibre in the mixed fibre source feeds varies, with some products having 50%/50% proportions while others contain 75% insoluble and 25% soluble fibre.

- Specialist feeds: for the management of patients with special needs, additional feeds are also available. Typical patients will have renal failure, malabsorption, electrolyte restrictions, milk protein intolerance and inflammatory bowel disease. As a general rule, elemental or semi-elemental feeds have an osmolarity between 300 and 500 mOs l^{-1}.

15.7.1   Composition of specialist feeds for the management of hyperglycaemia

Most of the evidence used to support the use of specialized enteral feeds in diabetic management has been extrapolated from the general diabetic literature, and is aimed at avoiding hyperglycaemia. Specialist feeds for people with diabetes are available, and aim to reduce the usual high liquid carbohydrate content of standard feeds (>50% of calories as carbohydrate). A high liquid carbohydrate content tends to exacerbate hyperglycaemia, and often necessitates insulin therapy. Tube feeding is associated with a more rapid increase in postprandial glucose than solid diets of similar nutritional composition. High postprandial glucose levels predispose to hypertriglyceridaemia [72].

Compared with standard formulas, diabetes-specific formulas are typically higher in fat (40–50% of energy, with a large contribution from MUFAs, e.g., >60% of fat), with a lower carbohydrate content (35–40% of energy) and up to 15% of energy from fructose. These nutrients could facilitate glycaemic management by delaying gastric emptying (fat and fibre), delaying the intestinal absorption of carbohydrate (fibre), and producing smaller glycaemic responses (fructose). A high proportion of MUFAs may also have beneficial effects on lipid profiles.

Only short-term studies have been fulfilled using specialized oral diets in which the carbohydrate content is reduced by increasing the MUFA content. These have been undertaken either as single test meals or over short periods of time, and have involved relatively few subjects.

Many of the nutrients included in tube feeds must be chemically modified to enable delivery from a tube. As the glycaemic response of a food is dependent on its physical properties, changing nutrients from a solid phase to a liquid phase can radically alter the glycaemic properties. With respect to glycaemic control, while there is good evidence of the beneficial effect of fibre in a solid diet, the addition of fibre to a liquid diet has not been shown to be of benefit [73]. In addition, fibre supplementation to tube feeding can be problematic, as optimal fibre blends increase the feed viscosity, which makes the formula flow through fine-bore feeding tubes extremely difficult. Indeed, the biophysical properties of a fibre in a liquid may be the reason why there has been a lack of improvement in glycaemic control with tube feeds containing fibre. For tube feeds, the postprandial insulin and glucose responses are related to the carbohydrate load, and not to its fibre content.

The meta-analyses of Pohl and colleagues, based on studies of patients of medium age (70 years), with insulin-treated type 2 diabetes, HbA$_{1C}$ <7.0% and an indication for tube feeding due to dysphagia caused by neurological disorders, have shown that the use of diabetes-specific oral and tube formulas (containing high proportions of MUFAs, fructose and fibre) are associated with improved glycaemic control compared to standard formulas. This shows that the use of diabetes-specific formulas, given either as oral nutritional supports (ONSs) or enteral tube feeding (ETF), results in a significantly lower postprandial rise in blood glucose, peak blood glucose concentrations and the glucose-versus-time area under the curve (AUC) in patients with diabetes. This was achieved without any evidence of hypoglycaemia, and suggests that glycaemic control may be facilitated by the use of diabetes-specific enteral formulas compared to standard formulas in patients with diabetes.

The current meta-analyses found that the postprandial rise in glucose concentration was lower, and the peak glucose concentration reduced, following diabetes-specific compared to standard formulas. Recent studies have also demonstrated a strong correlation between postprandial glucose regulation and cardiovascular complications in patients with diabetes, impaired glucose tolerance, and all-cause mortality, whereas no such correlation was demonstrated for fasting glucose control [74]. This implies that, by improving glycaemic control, the long-term use of diabetes-specific versus standard enteral formulas may reduce cardiovascular complications in patients with diabetes, although this proposal was not assessed by the studies reviewed.

In some studies, diabetes-specific formulas reduced the quantity of hypoglycaemic medication, and in some cases also prevented the need for insulin injections.

Very few long-term studies have been reported examining clinical outcome. One study of ETF [73] showed the diabetes-specific formula to be associated with a trend towards a reduced incidence of pneumonia, fever and urinary tract infection relative to the standard formula. This may have clinical relevance for those hyperglycaemic patients who are at increased risk of infections. Further common comorbidities in patients with diabetes include CVD and hyperlipidaemia. Although diabetes-specific feeds had a higher fat content than standard feeds, it was suggested that diabetes-specific formulas had no detrimental effect on total cholesterol, HDL-cholesterol or triglycerides. For ETF studies, it was impossible to evaluate how far the administration of the feeds might have influenced the metabolic effects. A further consideration was the amount of feed administered, as patients receiving ONSs may obtain only 25% of their daily energy from this source, compared with up to 100% for tube-fed patients.

National organizations [41, 42] generally recommend low-fat (25–35% of energy) and high-carbohydrate diets (45–60%), rich in complex carbohydrates, for those with diabetes. The situation for MUFAs is less clear, with the American Diabetes Association reporting that there is a lack of evidence that MUFAs exert any long-term effects on glucose control or other metabolic parameters [41]. Formulas that have a particularly high proportion of fructose should probably be administered with some caution to critically ill patients, who are at risk of lactic acidosis.

Dietary therapy or enteral tube feeding, when given under medical supervision, can be individualized to include a more liberal use of fat (e.g. MUFAs), which is particularly important in the treatment of malnourished patients to increase their dietary energy intake [75]. There is clearly a need for further research to determine the role of enteral nutritional support and diabetes-specific formulas on the management, clinical outcome and quality of life of malnourished patients with diabetes.

15.7.2 Complications of enteral nutritional support

Gastrointestinal symptoms are the most frequent byproducts of tube feeding, with gastroparesis and diarrhoea being the most common complications.

Gastroparesis is extremely common among patients with diabetes and affects 30–75% of all patients undergoing nutritional enteral feeding [5]. Gastroparesis reduces the tolerance to enteral nutritional support, as well as causing bloating, satiety, nausea and vomiting. The irregular and unpredictable rate of gastric emptying associated with gastroparesis can result in poor glycaemic control, and also can cause an exacerbation of gastroparesis. In addition to changing the enteral formula, a number of prokinetic drugs are available that can improve gastric emptying. If these strategies are unsuccessful, then a change to jejunal feeding may be helpful.

Chronic *diarrhoea* occurs in 20–85% of people with diabetes receiving enteral feeding, and can be a difficult management problem because it demands a systematic approach, including an awareness of the patient's bowel history and any altered bowel habits prior to tube feeding. It is important to consider all possible contributory factors for the diarrhoea, to take note of all prescribed and non-prescribed medications being taken (notably broad-spectrum antibiotics), and to consider any bacterial overgrowth and specific infections (e.g. *Clostridium difficile*) or other bowel pathology. It must also be borne in mind that enteral feeding itself may be a cause of diarrhoea, due to the use of hyperosmolar feeds or feeds with an inadequate sodium content, as well as rapid administration (e.g. bolus feeding).

15.8   Parenteral nutrition [43, 69]

Parenteral nutrition (PN) provides no added value over enteral feeding in patients with a functioning gastrointestinal tract, and is related to an increased risk of complications and health costs [76]. Parenteral nutrition is only indicated when enteral nutrition is contraindicated, which usually occurs when the gastrointestinal tract is either non-functioning or not accessible.

Parenteral nutrition, for example, can result in approximately 30% of patients developing transient diabetes, and at least 15% developing hyperglycaemia [77]. Intravenous catheter-related infections are fivefold more prevalent in patients receiving central PN, a figure which is higher still in the presence of hyperglycaemia.

Parenteral nutrition is hyperosmolar and requires access via a large central vein. Central access can be achieved either by a peripherally inserted central catheter (PICC) threaded up into a larger central vein (which is more suitable for short-term PN), or by direct access to a central vein (PICC <15 cm; Hickman line or Portacath, as long-term lines).

The energy content in PN is provided by a mixed source of fat and carbohydrate (usually 50%

non-protein energy from carbohydrate and fat). The inclusion of fat improves substrate utilization, enables the delivery of fat-soluble vitamins, and also reduces the osmolarity of feeds which may be used for simultaneous peripheral feeding. The protein component in PN is made up of essential amino acids and soluble, non-essential amino acids.

Parenteral nutrition is usually applied in an all-in-one bag. A variety of PN pre-compounded bags are available, designed to meet the nutritional requirements for most patients but, if possible, some hospital pharmacies are able to compound PN bags for individual patients. Parenteral nutrition should preferably be administered continuously over a 24 h period, using a suitable infusion pump to minimize infusion errors, and prevent marked swings in blood glucose and electrolyte values or rapid changes in fluid balance.

Individuals with stress-induced glucose intolerance, and all diabetic patients, will require insulin during PN administration for glycaemic control, and all oral hypoglycaemic agents must be stopped. The glycaemic management during parenteral nutrition must be tailored and adapted to the nutritional support required, taking into consideration that blood glucose levels reflect the underlying illness rather than the route of nutritional support [77].

Parenteral nutrition support can be optimized to minimize both hyperglycaemia and hypoglycaemia by adhering to the following points:

1. Prevent overfeeding.

2. Ensure that the infusion rate of carbohydrate in the PN does not exceed the patient's glucose oxidation rate ($6–7\,\mathrm{mg\,kg^{-1}\,min^{-1}}$), because exceeding this value may increase the metabolic rate and worsen glucose tolerance [78]. Alternative sugars have been tried experimentally as potential carbohydrate substitutes, including fructose, sorbitol, xylitol and glycerol, but have not successfully prevented or improved the hyperglycaemia.

3. Optimize the fat to carbohydrate ratio. Some groups have advocated increasing the fat component to 60–70% of non-protein energy in PN in order to reduce the carbohydrate component to 30–40%. A high fat content in PN increases the possibility of hyperlipidaemia, and this has the potential in septic or critically ill patients to precipitate pancreatitis and renal failure. Reducing the carbohydrate component in patients with hyperglycaemia will reduce

the glucose load of the feed, but this may not be sufficient to allow the withdrawal of insulin.

4. Reduce the rate of the PN to prevent rebound hypoglycaemia before stopping PN.

15.9   A specific nutrition support formula for elderly patients?

There is no evidence in favour of a specific formula in EN or PN in the elderly. Recently, Rees *et al.* [79] have proved high-energy, high-protein EN diets capable of reaching a positive nitrogen balance very rapidly, which may be valuable in stressed elderly patients. However, sodium reabsorption is lower and the threshold for thirst higher in elderly subjects, which highlights the needs for water intake ($30 \, \mathrm{ml \, kg^{-1}}$ per day), and this should be considered in the prescription of EN/PN formulas. Semi-elemental EN formulas are not preferable to their polymeric counterparts. Finally, fibre supplementation is able to improve bowel function with a reduced stool frequency and a more solid stool consistency, without affecting the nutritional efficiency of enteral feeding in hospitalized geriatric patients [80].

15.10   Ethical issues

Ethical issues are crucial in deciding when to start an elderly patient on artificial nutrition, there having been much recent public controversy regarding life-sustaining technologies for elderly people. The patient's informed consent is essential, although a family member or a caregiver may act as possible surrogates. The decision must always be based on evidence, but if this is unavailable then the patient's wishes (or those of his/her family) must be taken into account. In a therapeutic project, even if artificial nutrition may be withheld, it best not to do so.

15.10.1   Geriatric syndromes and nutrition in the older diabetic patient

In contributing to their generally poorer quality of life, older persons with diabetes have higher rates of CHD, hypertension and stroke, and are also at greater risk for developing one of the common – but frequently overlooked – geriatric syndromes than their age-matched, non-diabetic counterparts. These syndromes include depression, cognitive impairment, injurious falls, polypharmacy, persistent pain and urinary

incontinence. Any one of these can adversely affect the quality of life and result in a vicious cycle of decline, deterioration in self-management, greater demands on caregivers, loss of independence and possible institutionalization.

An inadequate intake of energy and nutrients is a common problem in demented patients. Such undernutrition may be caused by several factors, including anorexia (commonly caused by polypharmacotherapy), insufficient oral intake (forgetting to eat), depression, apraxia of eating or, less often, an enhanced energy requirement due to hyperactivity (constant pacing). In the advanced stages of dementia, dysphagia may develop, and this might be an indication for EN in a few cases. Enteral nutrition may be recommended during the early stages of the disease, or after an acute weight loss in patients with Alzheimer's disease. For patients with terminal dementia, EN is not recommended however (grade of recommendation C) [66].

15.10.2   Neurological dysphagia

Nutritional therapy depends on the type and extent of the swallowing disorder. This may range from normal food, to mushy meals (modified consistency), thickened liquids of different consistencies or to total EN delivered via a nasogastric tube or PEG. In a Cochrane analysis of interventions for dysphagia in acute stroke, EN delivered via PEG was associated with a greater improvement of nutritional status compared to EN delivered via a nasogastric tube [81]. As dysphagia will rarely improve after two weeks, should severe dysphagia persist for longer than 14 days after the acute event, then a PEG should be placed immediately [66].

15.10.3   Pressure sores and diabetic foot

Malnutrition increases the risk for the occurrence of pressure sores, which are associated with an increased risk of morbidity and mortality. Pressure sores develop in 4–10% of newly hospitalized patients, increasing to 14% in long-term elderly care. Patients with diabetes are a vulnerable group with poor wound healing. To date, there is insufficient evidence to support the routine supplementation of micronutrients for wound or leg ulcer healing using either multivitamins or vitamin C, with or without zinc. An improved healing of leg ulcers and wounds has been reported following a 3-month period of zinc supplementation, given as 70 mg of zinc three times each day. A review on nutrition and wound healing concluded that, while the supplementation of hospitalized patients with zinc and vitamin C may be reasonable, the routine use of vitamin C supplementation alone was unlikely to be beneficial [56, 82].

Low protein and energy intake, BMI and albuminaemia are all risk factors for the development of pressure sores in elderly patients. Additionally, oral nutritional supplements could significantly reduce the incidence of pressure ulcer development in at-risk patients (Odds ratio 0.75, 95% CI: 0.62–0.89) [82, 83]. As with the effect of nutritional status on the healing of existing pressure ulcers, the scarce amount of available data suggests that malnutrition slows the healing process, and that an increase in protein and energy intake raises the rate of healing. A systematic review by Stratton et al. showed that enteral nutritional support may significantly reduce (by 25%) the risk of developing pressure ulcers. [84].

15.10.4 Oral health

Diabetes adversely affects oral health, increasing the risk of gingivitis and other oral infections. Gingivitis is a major cause of tooth loss and pain that can affect oral intake. Poor oral and dental health is linked with chewing difficulties that can cause malnutrition, poor general health and a reduced quality of life. There are dietary implications for those with no teeth or partial dentures, as difficulties in eating can lead to a reduction in the variety of food choices and an overall reduction in nutrient intake. Full dentures can cause a reduction in food consumption due to the mouth feeling full, to a greater time needed to eat, to causing embarrassment, and to changes in food flavours [85]. All patients should be encouraged to maintain good oral hygiene, with special attention given to those with dry mouths or who eat more frequently due to a small appetite or, in the case of a patient with type 1 diabetes, to a need for frequent snacks. Dental advice is required for patients with chewing difficulties, pain and other oral health problems.

15.11 Conclusions

The dietary treatment of diabetes has long been the cornerstone of management of this common disease, especially in the elderly diabetic, who may present a major challenge to the physician. Nutritional recommendations for these patients should be highly individualized,

taking into consideration their food preferences, their cultural background, financial resources and support systems. A series of simple recommendations, drafted with the help of the patient or their caregiver, would more likely be successful. The elderly are often at risk of nutritional deficiency and malnutrition, and the presence of a chronic disease such as diabetes profoundly affects their metabolism, placing them at still higher risk. Unfortunately, our present understanding of this problem is somewhat limited, and additional research in this area is clearly required, mainly in order to ameliorate the quality of life of the elderly diabetic.

References

1. Narayan KM, Boyle JP, Thompson J et al. Lifetime risk for diabetes mellitus in the United States. JAMA 2003; 290: 1884–90.
2. Gu K, Cowie CC and Harris MI. Mortality in adults with and without diabetes in a national cohort of the U.S. population, 1971–1993. Diabetes Care 1998; 21: 1138–45.
3. Meneilly GS and Tessier D. Diabetes in elderly adults. J Gerontol A: Biol Sci Med Sci 2001; 56: M5–13.
4. Euronut – SENECA. Nutrition and the elderly in Europe. 1st European Congress on Nutrition and Health in the Elderly. The Netherlands, December. 1991 Eur J Clin Nutr 1991; 45 (Suppl 3). 1–196.
5. Peake H. (2003) Inpatient nutritional support of sick patients with diabetes. In: G. Frost, A. Dornhorst and R. Moses (eds). *Nutritional Management of Diabetes Mellitus*. John Wiley & Sons, Ltd. England. 2003; chapter 14; pp 215–229.
6. Morley JE. Anorexia of aging: physiologic and pathologic. Am J Clin Nutr 1997; 66 (4): 760–73.
7. Newman AB, Arnold AM, Burke GL et al. Cardiovascular disease and mortality in older adults with small abdominal aortic aneurysms detected by ultrasonography: The Cardiovascular Health Study. Ann Intern Med 2001; 134 (3): 182–90.
8. Flodin L, Svensson S and Cederholm T. Body mass index as a predictor of 1 year mortality in geriatric patients. Clin Nutr 2000; 19: 121–5.
9. Morley JE and Perry HM, III. The management of diabetes mellitus in older individuals. Drugs 1991; 41: 548–65.
10. Beaufrere B and Morio B. Fat and protein redistribution with aging: metabolic considerations. Eur J Clin Nutr 2000; 54 (Suppl. 3): S48–53.
11. Morley JE, Thomas DR and Wilson MMG. Cachexia: pathophysiology and clinical relevance. Am J Clin Nutr 2006; 83: 735–43.

12. Janssen I, Baumgartner RN, Ross R *et al.* Skeletal muscle cutpoints associated with elevated physical disability risk in older men and women. Am J Epidemiol 2004; 159 (4): 413–21.

13. Campbell AJ, Spears GF, Brown JS *et al.* Anthropometric measurements as predictors of mortality in a community population aged 70 years and over. Age Ageing 1990; 19 (2): 131–5.

14. Morley JE and Silver AJ. Nutritional issues in nursing home care. Ann Intern Med 1995; 123 (11): 850–9.

15. Cederholm T, Jagren C and Hellstrom K. Outcome of protein-energy malnutrition in elderly medical patients. Am J Med 1995; 98 (1): 67–74.

16. Herrmann FR, Safran C, Levkoff SE and Minaker KL. Serum albumin level on admission as a predictor of death, length of stay, and readmission. Arch Intern Med 1992; 152: 125–30.

17. Sullivan DH, Sun S and Walls RC. Protein-energy undernutrition among elderly hospitalized patients: a prospective study. JAMA 1999; 281: 2013–19.

18. Calle EE, Thun MJ, Petrelli JM *et al.* Body-mass index and mortality in a prospective cohort of US adults. N Engl J Med 1999; 341 (15): 1097–105.

19. Potter JF, Schafer DF and Bohi RL. In-hospital mortality as a function of body mass index: an age-dependent variable. J Gerontol 1988; 43: M59–63.

20. Roberts SB, Fuss P, Heyman MB *et al.* Control of food intake in older men. JAMA 1994; 272 (20): 1601–6.

21. Walker D and Beauchene RE. The relationship of loneliness, social isolation, and physical health to dietary adequacy of independently living elderly. J Am Diet Assoc 1991; 91 (3): 300–4.

22. Thomas P, Hazif-Thomas C and Clement JP. Influence of antidepressant therapies on weight and appetite in the elderly. J Nutr Health Aging 2003; 7 (3): 166–70.

23. Wilson MM, Vaswani S, Liu D *et al.* Prevalence and causes of undernutrition in medical outpatients. Am J Med 1998; 104 (1): 56–63.

24. Flegal KM, Carroll MD, Ogden CL *et al.* Prevalence and trends in obesity among US adults, 1999–2000. JAMA 2002; 288 (14): 1723–7.

25. Heiat A, Vaccarino V and Krumholz HM. An evidence-based assessment of federal guidelines for overweight and obesity as they apply to elderly persons. Arch Intern Med 2001; 161 (9): 1194–203.

26. Villareal DT, Apovian CM, Kushner RF *et al.* Obesity in older adults: technical review and position statement of the American Society for Nutrition and NAASO, The Obesity Society. Am J Clin Nutr 2005; 82 (5): 923–34.

27. Meneilly GS. Diabetes in the elderly. Med Clin N Am 2006 (90): 909–23.

28. Fontaine KR and Allison DB. Does intentional weight loss affect mortality rate? Eat Behav 2001; 2 (2): 87–95.

29. Kondrup J, Allison SP, Elia M, Vellas B and Plauth M. ESPEN Guidelines for Nutrition Screening 2002. Clin Nutr 2003; 22: 415–21.

30. Fuhrman MP, Charney P and Mueller CM. Hepatic proteins and nutrition assessment. J Am Diet Assoc 2004; 104 (8): 1258–64.

31. Guigoz Y, Lauque S and Vellas BJ. Identifying the elderly at risk for malnutrition. The Mini Nutritional Assessment. Clin Geriatr Med 2002; 18 (4): 737–57. (Available at: http://mna-elderly.com)

32. Bauer JM, Vogl T, Wicklein S, Trögner J, Möhlberg W and Sieber CC. Comparison of Mini Nutritional Assessment, Subjective Global Assessment and Nutritional Risk Screening (NRS 2002) for Nutritional Screening and Assessment in Geriatric Hospital Patients. Z Gerontol Geriat 2005; 38: 322–7.

33. Kondrup J, Rasmussen HH, Hamberg O, Stanga Z, and the Ad Hoc ESPEN Working Group. (2003) Nutritional risk screening (NRS 2002): a new method based on an analysis of controlled clinical trials. Clin Nutr 2003; 22: 321–36.

34. Kondrup J, Allison SP, Elia M, Vellas B and Plauth M. (2003) ESPEN Guidelines for Nutrition Screening 2002. Clin Nutr 2003; 22: 415–21.

35. Morley JE. Pathophysiology of anorexia. Clin Geriatr Med 2002; 18: 661–3.

36. Reilly HM. Screening for nutritional risk. Proc Nutr Soc 1996; 55: 841–53.

37. Malnutrition Advisory Group (MAG). MAG guidelines for detection and management of malnutrition. 2000, Redditch, UK: British association for Parenteral and Enteral Nutrition. (Available at:www.bapen.org.uk/must _tool.html)

38. Detsky AS, McLaughlin JR, Baker JP, Johnston S, Whittake S, Mendlson RA and Jeejeebhoy KN. What is subjective global assessment of nutritional status? JPEN. 1987; 11: 8–13.

39. Buzby GP, *et al.* Prognostic nutritional index in gastrointestinal surgery. Am J Surg 1980; 139: 160–167.

40. Omran ML and Salem P. Diagnosing undernutrition. Clin Geriatr Med 2002; 18: 719–36.

41. American Diabetes Association. (2007) Nutrition Recommendations and Interventions for Diabetes. A position statement of the American Diabetes Association. Diabetes Care 2007; 30 (Suppl. 1): S48–65.

42. IDF (Europe). A desktop guide to Type 2 diabetes mellitus. European Diabetes Policy Group, *Diabet Med* 1999; 16 (9): 716–30.

43. NICE guidelines (2006). Nutrition support in adults: Oral nutrition support, enteral tube feeding and parenteral nutrition. Published by the National Collaborating Centre for Acute Care at The Royal College of Surgeons of England. (Available at: www.rcseng.ac.uk or www.nice.org.uk).

44. Milton JE, Briche B, Brown IJ, Hickson M, Robertson CE and Frost GS. Relationship of glycaemic index with cardiovascular risk factors: analysis of the National Diet and Nutrition Survey for people aged 65 and older. Public Health Nutr. 2007; 10 (11): 1321–35.

45. Finch S, Doyle W, Lowe C, Bates CJ, Prentice A, Smithers G and Clarke P. *National Diet and Nutrition Survey: people aged 65 years and over.* Vol. 1. Report of the Diet and Nutrition Survey. The Stationary Office, London, 1998.

46. Chapman IM. Nutritional disorders in the elderly. Med Clin N Am 2006; 90 (5): 887–907.

47. Hickson M. Malnutrition and ageing. Postgrad Med J 2006; 82: 2–8.

48. Nitzke S, Freeland-Graves J and the American Dietetic Association. (2007) Position of the American Dietetic Association: total diet approach to communicating food and nutrition information. J Am Diet Assoc. 2007; 107 (7): 1224–32.

49. Zizza CA, Tayie FA and Lino M. Benefits of snacking in older Americans. J Am Diet Assoc. 2007; 107 (5): 800–6.

50. Hickson M and Wright L. (2003) Nutritional management of the elderly person with diabetes. In: G. Frost, A. Dornhorst and R. Moses (eds). *Nutritional Management of Diabetes Mellitus.* John Wiley & Sons, Ltd. England. 2003; chapter 10; pp 147–168.

51. American College of Sports Medicine Position Stand. (1998) Exercise and physical activity for older adults. Med Sci Sports Ex 1998; 30: 992–1008.

52. Gregg EW, Gerzoff RB, Caspersen CJ *et al.* Relationship of walking to mortality among US adults with diabetes. Arch Intern Med 2003; 163: 1440–7.

53. Physical Activity Guidelines for Americans (2008). Chapter 5: Active older adults. Available at: www.health.gov/paguidelines/guidelines/chapter5.aspx. Available as pdf-document at: www.health.gov/paguidelines/pdf/paguide.pdf.

54. Waugh NR and Robertson AM. Protein restriction for diabetic renal disease. Cochrane Database Syst Rev 2000; 2: CD002181.

55. Swade TF and Emanuele NV. Alcohol and diabetes. Compr Ther 1997; 23: 135–40.

56. Mooradian A, Failla M, Hoogwerf BJ, Maryniuk M and Wylie-Rosett J. Selected vitamins and minerals in diabetes. Diabetes Care 1994; 17: 464–79.

57. Flicker L, MacInnis RJ, Stein MS *et al.* Should older people in residential care receive vitamin D to prevent falls? Results of a randomized trial. J Am Geriatr Soc 2005; 53 (11): 1881–8.

58. Hanley DA and Davison KS. Vitamin D insufficiency in North America. J Nutr 2005; 135 (2): 332–7.

59. Hollis BW. Circulating 25-hydroxyvitamin D levels indicative of vitamin D sufficiency: implications for establishing a new effective dietary intake recommendation for vitamin D. J Nutr. 2005; 135 (2): 317–22.

60. Ervin RB and Kennedy-Stephenson J. Mineral intakes of elderly adult supplement and non supplement users in the third National Health and Nutrition Examination Survey. J Nutr 2002; 132 (11): 3422–7.

61. Grant AM, Avenell A, Campbell MK *et al.* Oral vitamin D3 and calcium for secondary prevention of low-trauma fractures in elderly people (Randomised Evaluation of Calcium Or vitamin D, RECORD): a randomised placebo-controlled trial. Lancet 2005; 365 (9471): 1621–8.

62. Andres E, Loukili NH, Noel E *et al.* Vitamin B12 (cobalamin) deficiency in elderly patients. Can Med Assoc J 2004; 171 (3): 251–9.

63. Wald DS, Law M and Morris JK. Homocysteine and cardiovascular disease: evidence on causality from a meta-analysis. Br Med J 2002; 325 (7374): 1202.

64. Rampersaud GC, Kauwell GP and Bailey LB. Folate: a key to optimizing health and reducing disease risk in the elderly. J Am Coll Nutr 2003; 22 (1): 1–8.

65. Joshi S and Morley JE. Vitamins and minerals in the elderly. In: MSJ Pathy, AJ Sinclair and JE Morley (eds). *Principles and practice of geriatric medicine.* 4th ed. John Wiley & Sons Ltd. Chichester, England. 2006; Vol. 1, pp. 329–46.

66. Volkert D, Berner YN, Berry E, Cederholm T, Coti Bertrand P, Milne A, Palmblad J, Schneider S, Sobotka S, Stanga Z, DGEM (German Society for Nutritional Medicine), Lenzen-Grossimlinghaus R, Krys U, Pirlich M, Herbst B, Schütz T, Schröer W, Weinrebe W, Ockenga J, Lochs H. ESPEN Guidelines on Enteral Nutrition: Geriatrics. Clin Nutr 2006; 25(2): 330–60.

67. Milne AC, Avenell A and Potter J. Meta-analysis: Protein and energy supplementation in older people. Ann Intern Med 2006; 144: 37–48.

68. Pomposelli JJ, Baxter JK, Babineau TJ, Pomfret EA, Driscoll DF, Forse RA and Bistrain BR. Early post operative glucose control predicts nosocomial infection rate in diabetes patients. J Parenter Enteral Nutr 1998; 22: 77–81.

69. Task Force of A.S.P.E.N; American Dietetic Association Dietitians in Nutrition Support Dietetic Practice Group, Russell M, Stieber M, Brantley S, Freeman AM, Lefton J, Malone AM, Roberts S, Skates J, Young LS; A.S.P.E.N. Board of Directors; ADA Quality Management Committee. American Society for Parenteral and Enteral Nutrition (A.S.P.E.N.) and American Dietetic

Association (ADA): standards of practice and standards of professional performance for registered dietitians (generalist, specialty, and advanced) in nutrition support. Nutr Clin Pract. 2007; 22 (5): 558–86.

70. Sandstrom R, Drott C, Hyltander A, Arfvidsson B, Schersten T, Wickstrom I and Lundholm K. The effect of postoperative intravenous feeding (TPN) on outcome following major surgery evaluated in a randomized study. Ann Surg 1993; 217: 185–95.

71. Schneider SM, Raina C, Pugliese P, Pouget I, Rampal P and Hebuterne X. Outcome of patients treated with home enteral nutrition. J Parenter Enteral Nutr. 2001; 25: 203–9.

72. Schrezenmeir J. Rationale for specialized nutrition support for hyperglycaemic patients. Clin Nutr 1998; 17 (Suppl. 2): 26–34.

73. Craig LD, Nicholson S, Silverstone FA and Kennedy RD. Use of a reduced carbohydrate, modified-fat enteral formula for improving metabolic control and clinical outcomes in long-term care residents with type 2 diabetes: results of a pilot trial. Nutrition 1998; 14: 529–34.

74. Heine RJ, Balkau B, Ceriello A, Del Prato S, Horton ES and Taskinen MR. What does postprandial hyperglycaemia mean? Diabet Med 2004, 21: 208–13.

75. Elia M, Ceriello A, Laube H, Sinclair AJ, Engfer M and Stratton R. Enteral nutritional support and use of diabetes-specific formulas for patients with diabetes: A systematic review and meta-analysis. Diabetes Care 2005; 28: 2267–79.

76. Woodcock NP, Zeigler D, Palmer D, Buckley P, Mitchell CJ and MacFie J. Enteral versus parenteral nutrition: a pragmatic study. Nutrition 2001; 17: 1–12.

77. Pitts DM, Kilo KA and Pontious SL. Nutritional support for the patient with diabetes. Crit Care Nurs Clin North Am 1993; 5: 47–56.

78. Orr ME. Hyperglycemia during nutritional support. Crit Care Nurs 1992; 12: 64–70.

79. Rees RG, Cooper TM, Beetham R, Frost PG and Silk DB. Influence of energy and nitrogen contents of enteral diets on nitrogen balance: a double blind prospective controlled clinical trial. Gut. 1989; 30(1): 123–9.

80. Vandewoude MF, Paridaens KM, Suy RA, Boone MA and Strobbe H. Fibre-supplemented tube feeding in the hospitalised elderly. Age Ageing 2005; 34: 120–4.

81. Bath PM, Bath FJ and Smithard DG. Interventions for dysphagia in acute stroke. Database Syst Rev. 2000: CD000323.

82. Collins C. A practical guide to nutrition and pressure sores. Compl Nutr 2001; 1: 25–7.

83. Guérin O, Andrieu S, Schneider SM et al. Different modes of weight loss in Alzheimer disease: a prospective study of 395 patients. Am J Clin Nutr. 2005; 82: 435–41.

84. Stratton RJ, Ek AC, Engfer M, Moore Z, Rigby P, Wolfe R and Elia M. Enteral nutritional support in prevention and treatment of pressure ulcers: a systematic review and meta-analysis. Ageing Res Rev 2005; 4(3): 422–50.

85. Mojon P, Budtz-Jorgensen E and Rapin CH. Relationship between oral health and nutrition in very old people. Age Ageing 1999; 28: 463–8.

16

Early Management of Type 2 Diabetes

Alan Sinclair

Bedfordshire and Hertfordshire Postgraduate Medical School, University of Bedfordshire, Putteridge Bury Campus, Luton, UK

Key messages

- Many older people with diabetes have a set of unique characteristics which must be considered when planning initial management.
- High circulating glucose levels in the elderly can produce a varied symptom and sign profile which is distinct from the common osmotic profile.
- Achieving high-quality diabetes care can be realized by use of a five-step management protocol.

16.1   Introduction

Diabetes mellitus in ageing subjects is a chronic metabolic disorder associated with macrovascular disease, a spectrum of functional impairments and, in many cases, premature death [1]. Some evidence of improved care has emerged during the decade-and-a-half since the plight of elderly people with diabetes was first highlighted, when there was a call for interventional strategies to reduce early functional decline. The call was also made for an individual-based plan of care, giving details of realistic targets of glycaemia, regular screening for complications, and involving both patients and carers in educational programmes [2]. As with several other chronic disease states, care for people with diabetes is complex and often expensive, with 60% of total health care expenditure being related to hospitalizations [3]. In addition, informal carers (care-givers) may lose up to $20 000 per year in lost employment [4].

Although, type 2 diabetes is clearly not limited to older people, the disease's unique characteristics begin to surface in those subjects with this condition who are of advanced age (>75 years), may have additional major comorbidities and multiple medications, and who have personal and diabetes care issues that may not be coordinated in the community [5, 6]. These characteristics are listed in Table 16.1. It is also important to identify those patients who are 'frail' because their management will be modified, their aims of care

Table 16.1 Defining characteristics of older subjects with diabetes.

- High levels of medical comorbidities
- Age-related impairment of functional ability
- Increased vulnerability to hypoglycaemia
- Overlapping and often limited medical follow-up by primary-care physicians, and hospital-based specialists
- A management system which involves spouses and informal carers to a greater extent

Diabetes in Old Age. Third Edition. Edited by Alan J. Sinclair
© 2009 John Wiley & Sons, Ltd

adjusted, and their prognosis affected. Frailty is likely in the presence of significant physical or cognitive decline, care home residency, malnourishment, and when long-term vascular disease such as coronary artery disease (CAD) is present, which limits severely both quality of life and well-being. The adjustment of both glycaemic and blood pressure targets for the presence of frailty has been recommended [7, 8] although the evidence base to justify this is weak due to a lack of data.

16.2 Developing the case for high-quality diabetes care

The presentation of diabetes in the older patient is varied, and the symptoms and signs profiles of those with hyperglycaemia are often unexpected (Table 16.2). Many cases are detected by noting hyperglycaemia during hospital admissions for other morbidities or acute illnesses, although with detailed enquiry directly related symptoms of diabetes can be confirmed in a large number of cases. Some patients do not have the classic features of either diabetic ketoacidosis (DKA) or hyperosmolar non-ketotic (HONK) coma, but present with a 'mixed' disturbance of hyperglycaemia (blood glucose levels 15–25 mmol l^{-1}, an arterial blood pH of 7.2–7.3 (i.e. not particularly acidotic), and without marked dehydration or any change in their level of consciousness.

The insidious presentation may delay diagnosis and partially account for the high prevalence of diabetic complications at the time of diagnosis. A better screening for complications at the time of diagnosis is, therefore, part of the rationale for promoting quality diabetic care for older patients with diabetes (Table 16.3). Other recommendations relating to metabolic control, eye screening and specialist follow-up complement this

Table 16.2 The varying relationship between raised plasma glucose levels (>9 mmol l^{-1}) and patient symptom and sign profile.

Lethargy	Usually glucose >11 mmol l^{-1}
Increased micturition	Disturbed sleep patterns Increased fall rate Dehydration Incontinence
Visual impairment	Increased fall rate Poor mobility
Erectile impotence	Complicated by vascular disease
Pain	Limb pain and decreased threshold
Cognitive impairment	Memory disorder Psychomotor slowing
Depressive symptoms	Irritability and intolerance

Table 16.3 Rationale for high-quality diabetes care for older people.[a]

Screening and early diagnosis may prevent progression of undetected vascular complications	*Level of evidence 2++, Grade of recommendation (C)*
Improved metabolic control will reduce cardiovascular risk	*Level of evidence 2++, Grade of recommendation (B)*
Improved screening for maculopathy and cataracts will reduce visual impairment and blind registrations	*Level of evidence 2+, Grade of recommendation (C)*
An integrated approach to management of peripheral vascular disease and foot disorders will reduce amputation rate	*Level of evidence 2++, Grade of recommendation (B)*
Improved primary care and specialist follow-up will reduce hospital admission rate	*Level of evidence 3, Grade of recommendation (D)*

[a]Adapted from Ref. [8].

approach. Although few long-term studies have specifically involved older patients (e.g. aged >75 years) and none has attempted to assess the benefits of intervention in frail subjects, a number of potential benefits may accrue from enhancing metabolic control. These include the removal of fatigue, a reduced risk of metabolic decompensation and admission to hospital, a reduced carer support, and the avoidance of early functional decline.

16.3 Aims in the early management

The overall assessment schedule for an older patient with newly diagnosed diabetes should mimic that of a younger individual, and form part of an integrated plan of diabetes care. This will involve a comprehensive history, physical examination and laboratory work-up. The essential components of this are well described in the Standards of Medical Care document of the American Diabetes Association [9].

The essential aims of management are summarized in Table 16.4, and reflect the approach that aims are not fixed, vary with time, and have different perspectives. In situations where life expectancy is estimated to be at least 7 years, the aims of care should be tailored

Table 16.4 Aims in managing diabetes in the elderly.

Health professional-oriented

- To reduce fatigue due to raised glucose levels
- To assess the impact on management and patient outcome of coexisting disease (e.g. ischaemic heart disease, peripheral vascular disease)
- To prevent undesirable weight loss and maintain nutritional well-being
- Avoid hypoglycaemia and other adverse drug reactions
- To screen for and prevent complications
- To reduce the risk of functional impairment and disability
- To achieve a normal life expectancy for patients where possible

Patient (and family/carer)-oriented

- To maintain general social and health well-being and good quality of life
- To acquire skills and knowledge and understanding to adapt to changing requirements in their lifestyle
- Avoid dependency and institutionalization

to reducing vascular complications, maintaining functional status and ensuring the highest quality of life commensurate with effective care.

16.3.1 Acute presentation

Diabetes in elderly patients with type 2 diabetes may present acutely in several ways: in DKA or as HONK coma or, more commonly, as hyperglycaemia without significant ketosis or increased osmolality with or without coexisting acute illness; for example, an acute cerebrovascular accident (a mixed metabolic disturbance). Various precipitating factors for HONK coma have been identified (Table 16.5), and patients may present comatose due to the combined effects of marked hyperglycaemia (glucose levels >30 mmol l^{-1}) and dehydration (serum osmolality >650 mOsm). In all cases of presentation in a coma, other non-diabetes-related causes should be excluded, such as head injury, stroke, alcohol or drug overdose.

Seriously ill patients require insulin therapy (especially those with ketones), given either as an intravenous infusion or by regular subcutaneous injections of short-acting insulin, complemented by intravenous rehydration. In all severe cases, arterial blood gases should be measured to assess the acid–base balance.

16.3.2 Non-acute presentation

The majority of elderly type 2 diabetic patients are not severely unwell at presentation, and should ideally be managed in the community by an interested general practitioner or member of a primary care team with some additional competencies in diabetes care. At this stage there are four important objectives: (i) to satisfy yourself that the patient has diabetes; (ii) to screen for complications; (iii) to identify who will be responsible

Table 16.5 Hyperosmolar non-ketotic coma (HONK): precipitating factors.

- 50% Unknown
- Infection
- Operation (surgery)
- Myocardial infarction
- Stroke
- Drugs: propranolol, thiazides
- Steroids, dialysis, (glucose drinks)

for diabetic care (i.e. the patient or somebody else); and (iv) to initiate treatment.

Making the diagnosis

A detailed discussion of the criteria used to make a diagnosis of diabetes can be found in Chapter 3.

It should be appreciated, however, that many patients may not be able to provide an accurate history of symptoms. Moreover, the 'classic' symptoms of polyuria and polydipsia due to excessive glycosuria may be absent owing to the raised renal threshold found in elderly subjects. A true fasted blood sample is often difficult to obtain, and may be normal in any case [10], while an oral glucose tolerance test (OGTT) may be thought of as time-consuming and inconvenient. In addition, many patients have elevated plasma glucose levels which are secondary to acute illness, diabetogenic drug therapy, or other stress-inducing disorders. If the physician has any doubt about the diagnosis of diabetes, it is wise not to treat but to retest later and to use an OGTT if necessary.

Screening for complications at diagnosis

A detailed history may reveal symptoms of a distal sensory diabetic neuropathy, such as numbness, paraesthesiae, burning pains and hyperaesthesiae from bedclothes at night-time. Symptoms of postural hypotension (especially after treatment for coexisting hypertension with vasodilators has been started), diarrhoea or constipation and impotence should provide an alert to the possibility autonomic neuropathy. Symptoms of claudication should be inquired about. A physical examination requires the measurement of lying and standing blood pressures, and an assessment of the peripheral blood vessels.

Visual acuity (VA) can be checked using a 3 m Snellen chart; patients with a VA worse than 6/6 (US 20/20) in either eye should be examined using the pinhole test, which will partially correct for a refractive error. Alternatively, they may use their distance glasses (if worn). In patients with poor VA which remains unaltered or worsens in the pinhole test, the retina should be closely inspected for lesions, particularly those of maculopathy.

Direct ophthalmoscopy should start with the lens at zero and a red reflex obtained. When present, this indicates that there is no significant evidence of a cataract, vitreous haemorrhage or retinal detachment. By setting the lens at +10 D initially, and using a

succession of less powerful lenses, a direct inspection of the cornea, anterior chamber and lens is possible. *Diabetic retinopathy* should be looked for after pupillary dilation using 0.5–1.0% tropicamide eye-drops. Relative contraindications for this include those with previous eye surgery, lens implants or a history of narrow-angle glaucoma. The precipitation of previously undiagnosed acute glaucoma, although distressing at the time, may be a service to the patient in the long run as treatment may prevent further visual loss. Patients with scattered microaneurysms and blot haemorrhages require review at 6 months. This part of the examination may be aided by a red-free filter to improve blood vessel examination. Diabetic maculopathy can be sight-threatening and requires urgent referral to the ophthalmologist. Other reasons for referral include the presence of yellow, waxy hard exudates, proliferative retinopathy, severe cataract formation, or rapid decrease in VA, for example within the previous 3 months (noticed by the patient – subjective; or evidence of a two-line deterioration in VA using a Snellen chart – objective).

Examination of the *limbs* for sensory neuropathy should include an assessment of knee and ankle reflexes, sensation by testing with a nylon monofilament (e.g. 5.07 Semmes–Weinstein), pin-prick and cotton wool, vibration sense by 128 Hz tuning fork (bearing in mind the age-associated loss of vibration sense) and proprioception. Infection, foot ulceration, the presence of pressure areas and the presence of sharp, poorly cut nails requires referral to the podiatrist. Management may also include radiology, antibiotic therapy, rest, use of pressure-relieving devices, and even surgery. Effective education, including advice about suitable footwear, reduces the risk of new foot lesions [11] but a recent targeted approach to secondary prevention did not demonstrate benefit [12].

Other investigations include: serum creatinine, glycosylated haemoglobin (HbA_{1c}), lipid profile [triglycerides, total and high-density lipoprotein (HDL) cholesterol] in those aged less than 75 years, especially those with CAD. In patients who may have had undiagnosed diabetes for some time with marked hyperglycaemia, hyperlipidaemia may be present. In these cases, it is worth rechecking the patient's lipid profile after 6 months to determine whether the treatment has reversed the abnormality. An electrocardiogram seeking ischaemia, arrhythmias and ventricular hypertrophy is useful.

Urinalysis (in the absence of infection) may demonstrate proteinuria, although this is not particularly common at diagnosis in the elderly. Microalbuminuria is also common at diagnosis, but this may occur secondary to hypertension or congestive heart failure. It is routinely screened for in the author's diabetic clinic when the dipstick test is negative for protein. A Barthel scale and mini-mental state examination to assess both physical disability and mental function should be completed [13]. Brain failure may make the patient totally dependent on others (spouse, other relative or community nurse) for both treatment and monitoring.

Identifying responsibilities in diabetes management

In most situations, an individual care plan must be adopted and agreed by all concerned. This may be organized by the primary care physician (general practitioner), although diabetes specialist nurses can play an important role in this decision-making. This will consist of identifying the principal informal carer, setting realistic glycaemic goals, planning the timing and frequency of visits, and being aware of the indications for hospital referral to a specialist (Table 16.6) or admission. Ideally, the health care team should aim to provide written information about diabetes for each newly diagnosed patient (and informal carer where appropriate) and organize several educational tutorials over the next 6–12 months.

Wherever possible, a multidisciplinary approach and philosophy shared with the patient (or informal carer) is recommended, with the promotion of self-advocacy being an important goal. With diabetic elders from ethnic minority backgrounds, who may pose special problems of language and communication, access and availability of services, cultural and dietary differences, it is important to tailor the educational package to meet their needs and provide information about any regional or national societies/organizations involved in diabetes care.

16.4 Initial treatment

In patients whose glucose values lie between 8 and 17 mmol l^{-1}, and who are not troubled by symptoms, an initial 6- to 12-week course of dietary instruction only is warranted. The main elements of a suitable dietary plan include consuming 50–55% of total energy intake as carbohydrate (including a daily fibre intake of at least 30 g), 30–35% fat intake (<10% saturated fat) and 10–15% protein.

Dietetic treatment will depend on several factors, but must include the patient's ability to cooperate, physical and mental well-being, and their natural desire to be independent. This process is a form of negotiation, and some dieticians are today developing a 'Getting Started' diet sheet for initial management. There is a shift away from traditional 'food exchanges' towards a more generalized plan of healthy eating (provision of 'healthy eating messages'). In those patients who are overweight, a plan of fat restriction may be beneficial. Other practical advice, including alcohol consumption and the benefits of exercise, are often given at this time.

When dietary advice fails to reduce levels of glycaemia or improve patient well-being, or when initial random glucose levels are greater than 14 mmol l^{-1} and/or a patient feels unwell, then several treatment options are available (Table 16.7), although in most cases oral agents are then prescribed.

Table 16.6 Indications for referral to hospital specialist for elderly patients with diabetes.

- Patients with severe complications (e.g. maculopathy, foot ulceration, peripheral vascular disease)

- Patients whose metabolic symptom control is suboptimal irrespective of treatment (e.g. oral agents or insulin)

- Complex management problems in those with coexisting disease (e.g. patients with chronic pulmonary disease taking steroids)

- Patients with increasing dependency and immobility (e.g. post-stroke)

- Patients not adequately cared for in primary care

Table 16.7 Treatment options for diet failures.

- Further period of intense dietary therapy requiring inputs from both physician and dietician

- Specified and appropriate exercise programme

- Guar gum: little used in UK clinical practice

- Acarbose: an alpha-glucosidase inhibitor

- Oral hypoglycaemic agents: sulphonylureas, metformin, a meglitinide, thiazolidinediones

- Insulin therapy: usually considered on a temporary basis in well- defined circumstances only, such as acute illness

16.4.1 Physical activity and exercise

Structured physical activity (exercise) as part of a lifestyle intervention programme (as an adjunct to proper diet and weight control) protects against the development of type 2 diabetes [14]. Brisk walking for 30 min each day, or swimming for 45–60 min up to three times per week are appropriate for older people. Aerobic exercise of this nature has been associated with varying improvements in glycaemia, weight, lipid profile and blood pressure [15]. Combined training which also involves moderate intensity resistance training (two sets of 12–20 repetitions) on a regular basis can also lead to increases in muscle strength and increased glucose disposal rates [16]. Prolonged or unusual exercise may be harmful, however, especially in those with underlying cardiovascular disease, those receiving insulin therapy (because of delayed hypoglycaemia), and those with sensory loss in their feet, where tissue damage may be sustained.

In general, exercise has several beneficial actions: the lowering of hyperinsulinaemia and an improvement in glucose tolerance occurs probably secondary to a reduction in insulin resistance. The lipid profile becomes less atherogenic, with a reduction in total plasma cholesterol and triglycerides while increasing HDL-cholesterol. A fall in blood pressure may occur not only as a direct result of exercise but also as the effect of weight loss. Some patients (especially older patients) are unable to participate in exercise programmes because of decreased joint mobility due to diabetes-related joint stiffness and/or osteoarthritis, or because of a previous stroke. The age-related loss of muscle mass seen in adults aged ≥50 years can be pronounced in those in their 70s or 80s. Moreover, when this is combined with reduced energy expenditure and decreased exercise levels, it often leads to an increase in weight, skeletal muscle fat deposition, and reduced lower limb muscle power. Limited exercise only is possible in those with poor metabolic control and ketosis, or those with ischaemic heart disease, advanced retinal or renal disease.

The importance of promoting weight loss in overweight patients cannot be overemphasized, since obese patients with type 2 diabetes pose several unique problems in diabetic management. First, an increasing bodyweight makes the attainment of normoglycaemia by dietary manipulation exceedingly difficult. Second, both insulin resistance and hyperinsulinaemia will exacerbate type 2 diabetes, and may also promote the development of hypertension and dyslipidaemia, which

in turn increases the risk of cardiovascular disease. The term 'syndrome X' or metabolic syndrome encompasses these relationships, which also includes dyslipidaemia [17]. Third, treatment with sulphonylureas, a meglitinide or insulin is associated with hyperinsulinaemia, which may promote both weight gain and paradoxically increase insulin resistance. These factors are important and should be considered when antidiabetic therapy is instituted.

16.4.2 Oral agents

In choosing a specific antidiabetic drug, several factors must be considered, including renal and hepatic function, coexisting disease, possible drug interactions, and the likelihood of producing significant hypoglycaemia. There are no oral agents in routine practice which are not recommended in older people, but knowledge of their varying clinical pharmacology and the effect of ageing can be helpful in optimizing patient safety. For this reason, glibenclamide (glyburide) and chlorpropamide, both of which have prolonged durations of action, can accumulate in renal dysfunction, and have a high associated risk of hypoglycaemia, sometimes with fatal consequences [18]. Hence, they should not be prescribed for diabetic subjects aged ≥60 years. Patients should be warned of the possibility of hypoglycaemia developing, and educated with practical advice on how to both avoid and prevent this potentially serious situation developing. In relatively newly diagnosed patients, a failure to achieve acceptable glycaemic targets with diet and a single antidiabetic agent (e.g. a sulphonylurea) after 6 months should lead to a further review of treatment.

The International Diabetes Federation (European region) has published guidelines of diabetes care for type 2 diabetes [19], and a new updated version will be available in 2009. In the current guidance, no specific stepwise algorithm has been adopted for drug treatment, leaving the choice to the individual practitioner. One of the important messages from this document is that a regular review of treatment is essential, as a deterioration in glucose control over time should be expected and this will require an increase in therapy, with insulin likely to be needed in many patients after a variable period of time after diagnosis.

In 2004, evidence-based clinical guidelines for older people were made available [8]. Both levels of evidence and grades of recommendations were given based on the most up-to-date trial data, although the relative lack of major published trials in older people of

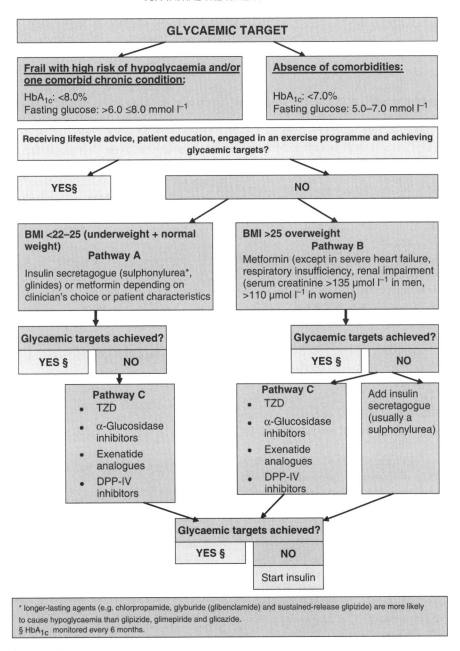

Figure 16.1 Glycaemic targets.

antiglycaemic therapies has limited the power of some of this guidance. A new up-to-date Executive Summary of the guidelines is being made available for 2009. A revised algorithm from the European guidelines has been included (Figure 16.1), based on treatment pathways determined by the body mass index (BMI).

Recent concern with the use of thiazolinediones (TZDs) in increasing the risk of myocardial infarction

and heart failure (predominantly attributed to rosiglitazone) [20] prompted a reappraisal of their use in diabetes treatment pathways. Whilst TZDs should not be given to patients with a history of serious cardiovascular disease or heart failure, they are still regarded as very effective glucose-lowering agents and considered safe when prescribers adhere to guidance. As other recent concerns have included an increased risk of fractures (mainly in women), the use of TZDs must be supervised by clinicians with significant diabetes care experience. These agents may be added to treatment with either metformin or a sulphonylurea (or both).

Newer agents such as exenatide (an incretin mimetic agent) requires subcutaneous injection, and functions by activating the glucagon-like peptide 1 (GLP-1) receptor. Amylin analogues such as pramlintide (a synthetic analogue) offer alternative approaches to glucose lowering in elderly patients, although there is limited trial evidence of long-term benefit, and they should not be used routinely at this stage. In patients whose BMI is very high (e.g. $>35\,kg\,m^{-2}$), or in those who are 'failing' on metformin and sulphonylurea therapy, exenatide may be considered. Inhibitors of the enzyme responsible for degrading GLP-1 (dipeptidyl peptidase IV inhibitors) are also now available (sitagliptin, vildagliptin), and these have consistent effects on lowering HbA_{1c} with relatively good tolerability and few adverse side effects. Their place in the overall treatment of older diabetes subjects needs to be determined, however.

A more recent consensus document on the treatment of type 2 diabetes by the American Diabetes Association and the European Association for the Study of Diabetes [21] provided an algorithm for insulin initiation and recommendations for these newer agents. These emphasize a practical goal of lowering the HbA_{1c} to $<7\%$, the effective incorporation of lifestyle modification as an adjunct to management, rapid titration with medications to achieve target glucose levels, and earlier use of insulin where necessary.

16.4.3   Insulin therapy

Few newly diagnosed elderly diabetic subjects require insulin therapy to sustain life and prevent DKA, although some patients may have a slowly developing form of type 1 diabetes and will inevitably require insulin in the future. In everyday clinical practice, the usual indications to start insulin are:

- persisting symptoms with poor patient well-being

- continued weight loss

- a failure to achieve satisfactory glycaemic control with diet and oral agents, usually failing to achieve a HbA_{1c} $<7.5\%$.

A common error in managing elderly type 2 diabetics is an undue reluctance to start insulin therapy – a view often shared by patients until they try insulin. The underlying reasons for the patient's attitudes include a horror of injections, awful stories of 'hypos', fear of further hospitalization, and the belief that taking insulin will change their lives for the worse [22]. It is imperative that the decision to start insulin be taken after full discussion with the patient (and carers, as appropriate). Although there are no time limits for when this decision should be taken, it is suggested that a maximum of 6 months' perseverance with diet and oral agents be undertaken before insulin is initiated. In practice, this decision may have been delayed already for several years. Able patients can begin insulin at home, much like their younger counterparts, with treatment organized by a diabetes specialist nurse (whose professional roles are increasing; see Table 16.8), in cooperation with the general practitioner. A structured education programme with frequent telephone support during the first 2–3 weeks is essential. Those patients who are unwell, or who have other severe medical problems, or where community support is absent, need to be considered for hospital admission although this should be avoided if possible.

Usually, treatment can start with about 8–14 units of insulin per day and adjusted thereafter. Although NPH insulin is often advised, the recommendation is to start with a longer-acting analogue such as glargine or determir, in combination with an existing oral agent (e.g. metformin). This basal insulin regimen can be

Table 16.8 Roles of a diabetes specialist nurse for older adults with diabetes.

- Teaching, advising and counselling patients and carers, both in the clinic and in the patient's home

- Educating patients to achieve self-care where possible

- Teaching self-monitoring of blood glucose: use of special techniques for patients with physical disability or visual loss

- Initiating insulin in the community and instructing patients and informal carers about insulin administration

- Commencement of insulin in the patient's home

- Liaising with other health professionals to ensure optimal treatment of the patient

- Advising residential care home staff about care of residents with diabetes

- Providing continuing support and advice to patients and carers tailored to the individual, and should avoid significant hypoglycaemia, especially at night. If mealtime glucose levels are a problem, then additional pre-meal insulin is also required. A number of insulin devices are available which are easy to use, although in certain cases – such as those patients with confusion, visual loss or arthritis – the technique of insulin administration should be taught to the spouse or to another relative or friend.

The success of insulin may be evaluated objectively by factors such as glycaemic control, patient well-being, episodes of hypoglycaemia or the frequency of hospital admissions due to diabetes.

16.5 Establishing an individual diabetes care plan

The elements of an initial care plan for diabetic elders are listed in Table 16.9. This is usually applicable during the first 3–6 months after diagnosis [13]. The care plan should state precisely what the roles of the involved individuals are, and where the boundaries of responsibility lie. The timing and components of the follow-up can be predetermined, as can the date and format of the annual review process, which is a mandatory requirement for all diabetic elders.

The effective self-monitoring of glycaemic control is a worthwhile objective for most patients with type 2 diabetes, especially for those receiving insulin or who have frequent acute illnesses or hypoglycaemic episodes. In some cases, with the appropriate level of education, patients learn the effects of dietary changes and exercise on blood glucose levels, by frequent use of self-monitoring.

Table 16.9 Components of an initial diabetes care plan.

1. Establish realistic glycaemic and blood pressure targets.

2. Ensure that all parties are agreed on the principal aspects of diabetes care: patient, spouse or family, GP, informal carer, community nurse or hospital specialist, where appropriate.

3. Offer instruction in diabetes self-care management

4. Define the frequency and nature of diabetes follow-up.

5. Organize glycaemic monitoring by patient or carer.

6. Refer to social or community services as necessary.

7. Provide advice on stopping smoking, exercise, and alcohol intake.

Urine testing for glucose remains a common practice but is inconvenient, messy, and often misleading because of the raised renal threshold of the elderly. Both, patients and physicians are also often uncertain about the significance of glycosuria, and the routine use of this parameter is no longer advised. Testing for the presence of ketones (when poor control is present – persistent values of blood glucose >17 mmol l^{-1}, or during severe acute illness) is worth carrying out if patients and informal carers have been suitably educated regarding its significance.

Blood glucose monitoring (e.g. using BM reagent strip measurements) should be encouraged in all those able to cooperate. Measurements can be taken twice weekly: pre-meal and before-bedtime estimations are ideal, but few patients are this compliant. In other cases, spouses, district nurses or diabetes specialist nurses may monitor control.

Guidelines for reasonable diabetic control in the elderly are as follows: a fasting glucose of 5–7 mmol l^{-1}, and a random level of 6–8 mmol l^{-1}. These limits should allow patients to remain well and be relatively free of symptoms of hyperglycaemia, and to avoid the risk of hypoglycaemia. It should be remembered that even glucose levels of 9 mmol l^{-1} can make some patients feel lethargic, and will need to be lowered. A HbA$_{1c}$ value $<7\%$ should be aimed for. Glycaemic targets for relatively frail patients with diabetes are provided in Figure 16.1.

16.5.1 Metabolic targeting

Whilst few clinicians would institute aggressive metabolic control in patients aged >80 years, there is increasing evidence of benefits from glucose lowering, blood pressure reduction and lipid lowering in older populations. Therapies for the latter two areas are covered elsewhere in this book. Metabolic targeting in geriatric diabetes (see Table 16.10) has a partial evidence base, and this has been extensively reviewed elsewhere [8]. Most guidelines of diabetes care assume a single-disease model when recommendations are offered, but for older people there is an increased risk of significant other comorbidities and/or frailty, and care must be interpreted on an individual basis. Patients in these latter categories may be care-home residents, have evidence of cognitive impairment, serious mood disturbance, or generally lack self-caring. Unfortunately, about one-third of patients fall into this latter category, according to the results of a large community-based sample of

Table 16.10 Metabolic targeting in geriatric diabetes.

1. Independent in self-care, mobile and mentally alert/single medical disorder:
   Aim Strict glycaemic, blood pressure and lipid control

2. Relatively independent with some evidence of functional decline and several comorbidities:
   Aim: Optimize glucose and blood pressure control; consider lowering lipids

3. High dependency and frailty; may be a resident of a nursing home and/or cognitively impaired; life expectancy <3 years:
   Aim: Symptom control; avoid fatigue; avoid hypoglycaemia and intrusive monitoring

people aged >65 years with diabetes, where objective measures of dependency were based on the Barthel ADL score, Extended ADL score and the Mini-Mental State Examination score [23].

16.5.2 Prioritizing diabetes care for diabetic elders

Diabetes care in older adults requires prioritization, and a five-step approach is recommended to provide a framework to develop an individual intervention programme (Table 16.11). These interventions may include, for example, the aggressive treatment of blood glucose and blood pressure, specific rehabilitation programmes for older people with diabetes, or fast-track vascular work-up and early surgical referral [24].

Charts such as those of Yudkin and Chaturvedi [25] permit an estimate of the overall level of vascular risk to be derived which can be used to inform the physician about which thresholds apply for therapeutic intervention. However, it is important to individualize these

Table 16.11 Prioritizing diabetes care in older adults: a five-step approach.

1. Functional assessment including cognitive testing and screening for depression.

2. Vascular risk assessment with advice on lifestyle modification and vascular prophylaxis.

3. Metabolic targeting (individualized): single-disease model versus frailty model.

4. Consider specific interventions for diabetes-related disabilities.

5. Assess suitability for self-care versus carer assistance.

estimates very carefully in diabetic elders, as it is likely that they will have several other comorbidities that may influence the decision to treat. In addition, applying the standard threshold for intervention based on a 10-year risk of coronary heart disease event of 20%, few of the older patients with diabetes encountered in every clinical practice would not require intervention.

16.6 Conclusions

The management of the older diabetic patient represents a major challenge to any physician, whether based in the community or in a hospital setting. Hospital physicians without specialist training in diabetes should seek the advice of a consultant diabetologist for patients whose glycaemic control is persistently unacceptable or those with severe diabetic complications; for example, extensive foot ulceration, autonomic neuropathy or painful neuropathy. Patients with significant diabetic eye disease, such as proliferative or preproliferative retinopathy or maculopathy, require prompt referral to a consultant ophthalmologist.

A detailed assessment of other cardiovascular risk factors is beyond the scope of this chapter, although the presence of hypertension, ischaemic heart disease or hyperlipidaemia may warrant further attention and interventions. The development of local specifications for diabetes care, providing an integrated approach to management and agreed by all health professionals involved, will help this process of referral to occur efficiently and to provide the most benefit for each patient.

References

1. Sinclair A.J. (ed./Guest ed.) Diabetes in Senior Citizens: a major threat to personal independence. *Br J Diab Vasc Dis* 2005; **5** (1): 3–5.

2. Sinclair AJ and Barnett AH (1993) Special needs of elderly diabetic patients. *British Medical Journal*, **306**, 1142–3.

3. Krop JS, Powe NR, Weller WE, Shaffer TJ, Saudek CD and Anderson GF. (1998) Patterns of expenditures and use of services among older adults with diabetes. Implications for the transition to capitated managed care. *Diabetes Care*, **21** (5), 747–52.

4. Holmes J, Gear E, Bottomley J, Gillam S, Murphy M and Williams R. (2003) Do people with type 2 diabetes and their carers lose income? (T2ARDIS-4). *Health Policy* **64** (3), 291–6.

5. Sinclair AJ (1999) Diabetes in the elderly: a perspective from the United Kingdom. *Clinics in Geriatric Medicine*, **15**, 225–37.

6. Hendra TJ and Sinclair AJ (1997) Improving the care of elderly diabetic patients: the final report of the St Vincent Joint Task Force for Diabetes. *Age and Ageing*, **26**, 3–6.

7. Brown AF, Mangione CM, Saliba D and Sarkisian CA. Guidelines for improving the care of the older person with diabetes. *J Am Geriatr Soc* 2003; **51** (5 Guidelines): S265–80.

8. The European Diabetes Working Party for Older People. Clinical Guidelines for Type 2 Diabetes Mellitus 2001–2004. (Available at: www.eugms.org.)

9. American Diabetes Association. Standards of Medical Care 2008. *Diabetes Care* 2008; **31**: S12–54.

10. DECODE Study (Diabetes Epidemiology: Collaborative Diagnostic Criteria in Europe) (1999) Consequences of the new diagnostic criteria for diabetes in older men and women. *Diabetes Care*, **22**, 1667–71.

11. Apelqvist J. The foot in perspective. *Diabetes Metab Res Rev* 2008; **24** (1): S110–15.

12. Lincoln NB, Radford KA, Game FL and Jeffcoate WJ. Evaluation for secondary prevention of foot ulcers in people with diabetes: a randomized controlled trial. *Diabetologia* 2008; **51** (11): 1954–61.

13. Sinclair AJ, Turnbull CJ and Croxson SCM (1996) Document of care for older people with diabetes. *Postgraduate Medical Journal*, **72**, 334–8.

14. Knowler WC, Barrett-Connor E, Fowler SE, Hamman RF, Lachin JM, Walker EA, Nathan DM and the Diabetes Prevention Program Research Group. Reduction in the incidence of type 2 diabetes with lifestyle intervention or metformin. *N Engl J Med* 2002; **346** (6): 393–403.

15. Gold-Haber Fiebert JD, Goldhaber-Fiebert SN, Tristan ML, *et al.* Randomised controlled community-based nutrition and exercise intervention improves glycaemia and cardiovascular risk factors in type 2 diabetic patients in rural Costa Rica. *Diabetes Care* 2003; **26** (1): 24–9.

16. Cuff DJ, Meneilly GS, Martin A, *et al.* Effective exercise modality to reduce insulin resistance in women with type diabetes. *Diabetes Care* 2003; **26** (11): 2977–82.

17. Reaven GM (1988) Role of insulin resistance in human disease. *Diabetes*, **37**, 1595–607.

18. Asplund K, Wilholm BE and Lithner F (1983) Glibenclamide-associated hypoglycaemia: a report of 57 cases. *Diabetologia*, **24**, 412–17.

19. European Diabetes Policy Group (1999) *A Desktop Guide to Type 2 Diabetes Mellitus*. International Diabetes Federation (European Region), Brussels, Belgium.

20. Singh S, Loke YK and Furberg CD. Long-term risks of cardiovascular events with rosiglitazone: a meta-analysis. *JAMA* 2007; **298** (10): 1189–95.

21. Nathan DM, Buse JB, Davidson MB, Heine RJ, Holman RR, Sherwin R and Zinman B. Medical management of hyperglycaemia in Type 2 diabetes: A consensus algorithm for the initiation and adjustment of therapy: A consensus statement of the American Diabetes Association and the European Association for the Study of Diabetes. *Diabetes Care* 2006; **29** (8): 1963–72.

22. Taylor R (1992) Use of insulin in non-insulin-dependent diabetes. *Diabetes Review*, **1**, 9–11.

23. Sinclair AJ and Bayer AJ (1998) *All Wales Research in Elderly (AWARE) Diabetes Study*. Department of Health Report (UK Government), 121/3040, London.

24. Sinclair AJ (2000) Diabetes in old age: changing concepts in the secondary care arena. *Journal of the Royal College of Physicians of London*, **34**, 240–4.

25. Yudkin JS and Chaturvedi N (1999) Developing risk stratification charts for diabetic and nondiabetic subjects. *Diabetic Medicine*, **16**, 219–27.

Drug Therapy: Current and Emerging Agents for Hyperglycaemia

Joe M. Chehade and Arshag D. Mooradian

*Division of Endocrinology Diabetes and Metabolism, University of Florida College of Medicine,
Jacksonville, FL, USA*

Key messages

- Type 2 diabetes is a heterogeneous disease.
- The goal for glycaemic control in the elderly diabetic is to achieve euglycaemia without the undue risk of hypoglycaemia.
- If possible, the management should be tailored to the individual's needs. Drug regimens may change over time as the disease progresses.
- Postprandial hyperglycaemia is becoming an important target of the management of diabetes.

17.1 Introduction

The Diabetes Control and Complications Trial (DCCT) [1] and the United Kingdom Prospective Diabetes Study (UKPDS) [2] have proven the benefit of improved glycaemic control beyond any reasonable doubt. Furthermore, in elderly people, diabetes control is an important quality of life issue. Type 2 diabetes is very common in old age, and the rate of development of some diabetic complications – including macroangiopathy, nephropathy and neuropathy – appear to be accelerated in this age group [3, 4].

With advanced disease, the achievement of glycaemic control can be challenging for both the physician and patient. Often, a combination of two or more oral anti-diabetic agents is needed [5, 6]. Another challenging aspect of treating type 2 diabetes is targeting postprandial hyperglycaemia (PPHG) which, in fact, may be a better predictor of diabetes complications than fasting hyperglycaemia. Today, this may be targeted with some newer agents [7].

During the past decade, the pharmacological options for treating diabetes have grown considerably such that, today, six classes of agent are available that target hyperglycaemia through different mechanisms (Figure 17.1):

Sulphonylureas and meglitinides increase insulin secretion from pancreatic β-cells.

Biguanides decrease hepatic gluconeogenesis and, to a lesser extent, enhance glucose uptake in skeletal muscles.

Thiazolidinediones enhance the insulin sensitivity in the liver, muscles and adipose tissue.

Alpha-glucosidase inhibitors delay carbohydrate absorption from the gut.

- Incretin mimetics and incretin enhancers stimulate insulin release from the β-cells and

Diabetes in Old Age. Third Edition. Edited by Alan J. Sinclair
© 2009 John Wiley & Sons, Ltd

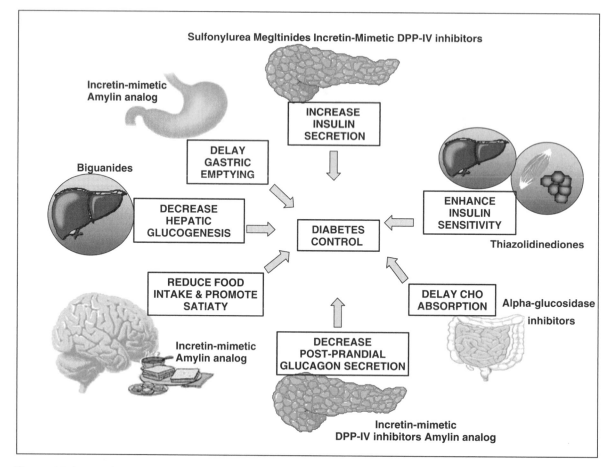

Figure 17.1   Mechanisms of action of the currently available oral agents for the treatment of type 2 diabetes. CHO = carbohydrate.

inhibit glucagon secretions from alpha cells in a glucose-dependent manner.

- Pramlintide, by modulating gastric emptying, can prevent the postprandial rise in glucagon and enhance satiety.

Although additional pharmacological agents are required to manage other risk factors such as hypertension and dyslipidaemia, in this chapter attention is focused only on those agents that control blood glucose.

17.2   Sulphonylureas

Sulphonylureas have been used extensively worldwide since the introduction of tolbutamide and carbutamide in 1956. Shortly thereafter, other compounds were developed, including acetohexamide, tolazamide

and chlorpropamide. These so-called 'first-generation' sulphonylureas were followed by the development of 'second-generation' sulphonylureas such as glyburide or glibenclamide, glipizide, gliclazide, gliquidone and glimeperide (Table 17.1).

The primary mechanism of action of sulphonylureas is through the depolarization of pancreatic β-cells by blocking ATP-dependent potassium channels, causing an influx of calcium and stimulating insulin release [8]. A decrease in plasma glucagon levels was also noted in some studies [9]. Although other extra-pancreatic effects have also been described, sulphonylureas are ineffective in patients with type 1 diabetes who lack islet β-cells [10]. The reported increased insulin sensitivity in peripheral tissues is thought to be mainly a consequence of the reduction of hyperglycaemia and an alleviation of glucotoxicity [11, 12]. A reduced hepatic insulin extraction was demonstrated with glipizide

Table 17.1 Comparative pharmacological profile of sulphonylurea agents.

Drug	Dose range (mg)	Duration of action (h)	Doses per day	Metabolism
First-generation				
Acetohexamide	250–1500	8–24	2	60% hepatic, active renal metabolism
Tolbutamide	500–3000	6–12	2–3	Hepatic with renal excretion
Tolazamide	100–1000	12–24	1–2	Hepatic with renal excretion
Chlorpropamide	100–500	24–72	1	30% renal excretion, some hepatic metabolism
Second-generation				
Glipizide	2.5–40	16–24	1–2	Hepatic, renal excretion of inactive metabolites
Glipizide XL (Glucotrol XL)	5–20	24	1	Hepatic, renal excretion of inactive metabolites
Glyburide	1.25–20	12–24	1–2	Hepatic with renal excretion of active metabolites
Glyburide Micronized (Glynase)	1.25–10	12–24	1	Hepatic with renal excretion of active metabolites
Glimepiride	1–8	12–24	1	Hepatic with renal excretion of active metabolites
Gliquidone	15–60	8–10	1–2	Hepatic with renal excretion of inactive metabolites
Gliclazide	40–320	10–15	1–2	Hepatic with renal excretion of inactive metabolites

[13] and glibenclamide [14]. However, this effect is probably secondary to increased insulin secretion.

The pharmacological characteristics of the sulphonylureas are summarized in Table 17.1. They are rapidly absorbed, and detectable levels can be found in the serum within an hour of ingestion. They are 90–99% bound to serum proteins, mainly albumin [15], and can be displaced by other drugs. On a milligram per milligram basis, second-generation sulphonylureas have 100-fold the potency of the first-generation agents [16] (Table 17.1). Moreover, since their binding to plasma proteins is mainly to non-ionic sites, drug–drug interactions are less likely than with first-generation agents. Even though there are some differences in the pharmacokinetic and pharmacodynamic properties of various sulphonylureas, to date no clinical evidence has been submitted of the superiority of any particular agent. Sulphonylureas are mainly converted by the liver to inactive, less active – or, in the case of acetohexamide, more active – metabolites. First-generation drugs and their metabolites are largely excreted by the kidney, while second-generation agents are excreted via both the kidney and bile in varying proportions (Table 17.1). Although differences in absorption, metabolism and elimination do not affect long-term efficacy, they are important in terms of the frequency and severity of adverse effects in elderly people. Of special concern is the prolonged half-life of chlorpropamide, along with its water-retaining properties. Of note is that the UKPDS showed that the incidence of hypoglycaemia with glyburide (glibenclamide) therapy was as high as with

chlorpropamide. While the long-acting preparation of glipizide (glipizide GITS) can be administered once daily, its longer duration of activity may result in a higher incidence of hypoglycaemia.

On average, sulphonylureas lower plasma glucose by 3.3–3.9 mmol l^{-1} (60–70 mg dl^{-1}), with a concomitant reduction in HbA$_{1c}$ of 1.5–2% [8,17]. Some 10–15% of subjects with type 2 diabetes fail to respond to this class of agent – a situation known as 'primary failure'. Annually, an additional 5–10% of initial responders have 'secondary failure' of response to sulphonylureas [18]. The most frequent side effect of sulphonylureas is hypoglycaemia [19]. UKPDS data showed that, over a six-year treatment period with sulphonylureas, 45% of patients experienced at least one hypoglycaemic episode, and 3% had severe hypoglycaemia [20]. It is noteworthy that continuous dextrose infusions for several days may be required to treat sulphonylurea-induced hypoglycaemia. A retrospective study conducted by the Swedish Board of Health and Welfare between 1975 and 1982 revealed that all serious causes of hypoglycaemia secondary to sulphonylureas were associated with advanced age, drug–drug interactions and acute energy deprivation due to gastroenteritis [21]. Due to the high prevalence of polypharmacy in elderly people, caution should be taken when sulphonylureas are combined with agents that potentiate their efficacy.

Tolazamide and *glyburide* have active metabolites that accumulate when creatinine clearance is reduced. Low-dose tolbutamide and glipizide may therefore be preferable for elderly patients with mild renal insufficiency. However, because of its short half-life, tolbutamide may need to be given three times a day, but compliance with such regimen is often difficult. None of the sulphonylureas should be used in patients in whom the creatinine clearance is less than 30 ml min^{-1} [22].

Other potential disadvantages of sulphonylureas are the associated hyperinsulinaemic state and weight gain. Over a nine-year period, subjects assigned to sulphonylureas in the UKPDS gained on average 4 kg compared to 2 kg for those treated with diet alone. In contrast, people in the metformin arm maintained a steady weight [2, 20]. This side effect of sulphonylureas is undesirable in obese subjects, bit in older subjects – where being underweight is common [23] – the weight gain-promoting properties of sulphonylureas may not be a serious deterrent to their use. However, obesity [body mass index (BMI) >30 g m^{-2}] continues to increase mortality risk at any age [24]. The potential advantages of sulphonylureas include their long track record, ease of use, and affordability. However, hypoglycaemia remains the main limiting factor in elderly people.

17.3 Biguanides

Metformin (dimethylbiguanide) and phenformin (phenethyl biguanide) were introduced for the treatment of type 2 diabetes in 1957, and buformin was introduced a year later [25]. During the 1970s, phenformin and buformin were withdrawn in many countries due to their association with lactic acidosis [26]. Metformin is now the biguanide of choice and is extensively used worldwide. The bioavailability of metformin after a standard dose of 500 mg is approximately 50–60%. The presence of food decreases the extent and slightly delays absorption of the drug. In contrast to sulphonylureas, metformin is not significantly bound to plasma proteins, and steady-state plasma concentrations are achieved within 24–48 h of dosing [27]. Metformin does not undergo any hepatic metabolism and is excreted unchanged in the urine [25]. Because the renal clearance of metformin is 3.5-fold greater than the creatinine clearance, tubular secretion appears to be the main route of elimination. In healthy elderly subjects, the total plasma clearance is decreased and thus the half-life of the drug is prolonged. These pharmacokinetic changes with ageing are the result of decreased renal function. No pharmacokinetic studies have been conducted in subjects with hepatic insufficiency.

Unlike sulphonylureas, metformin has no insulinotropic effect and does not cause hypoglycaemia when used as monotherapy [28]. As such, it is considered as an antihyperglycaemic agent rather than a hypoglycaemic agent. The antihyperglycaemic action of metformin is primarily due to a reduction in hepatic gluconeogenesis, thereby reducing basal glucose output. To a lesser extent, it enhances glucose uptake in the peripheral tissue, mainly muscle [25, 28]. The reduction of fatty acid oxidation in metformin-treated subjects may account for some of its antihyperglycaemic action [29].

A dose–response relationship of the antihyperglycaemic effect of metformin was demonstrated in a double-blind, placebo-controlled trial over 14-week period. At doses between 500 to 2000 mg daily, metformin reduced the adjusted mean fasting plasma glucose (FPG) from baseline by 1.04–4.62 mmol l^{-1} (19–84 mg dl^{-1}) and adjusted mean HbA$_{1C}$ by 0.6–2.0% [30]. The maximum efficacy is observed with a daily dose of 2000 mg [30].

Metformin has been used extensively both as monotherapy and in combination with sulphonylureas or insulin [31, 32]. It is noteworthy that individuals with primary or secondary failure of sulphonylureas are unlikely to respond to metformin alone. However, when metformin is combined with sulphonylureas in individuals who appear to have secondary failure, a substantial blood glucose lowering occurs [33].

Metformin has a favourable effect on plasma lipid levels and on blood pressure [34]. There is a moderate reduction in triglyceride levels due to decreased hepatic synthesis of very low-density lipoprotein (VLDL)-cholesterol and a slight increase in the high-density lipoprotein (HDL) level [35]. Perhaps the most attractive feature of this agent is that it is often associated with weight loss, and so counteracts the weight gain associated with sulphonylureas or insulin therapy [31]. However, obesity is much less of a problem in elderly people than in the middle-aged [24, 36]. In the UKPDS, metformin monotherapy in overweight subjects was the only arm of the study which showed a significant reduction in cardiovascular events and overall mortality [31]. The precise underlying mechanism of this favourable outcome is not known, however.

The most common and troublesome side effects of metformin include gastrointestinal discomfort, nausea, diarrhoea, anorexia, and rarely, a metallic taste. Starting therapy with 500 mg daily and increasing the dose gradually can attenuate these side effects. The biguanide-associated malabsorption of vitamin B_{12} (cyanocobalamin) and folate is usually not of a major clinical concern [37]. However, this should be borne in mind when prescribing for elderly subjects who have a relatively high incidence of atrophic gastritis and vitamin B_{12} deficiency. Although rare, the most dreaded side effect is *lactic acidosis*, the incidence of which is approximately 9 per 100 000 persons per year in metformin users [38], almost 10-fold lower than that associated with phenformin. Therefore, any clinical condition associated with, or predisposing, to lactate generation or a decreased ability to clear lactate is a contraindication to the use of metformin. These conditions include hepatic disease, alcoholism, congestive heart failure, peripheral vascular disease, obstructive airway disease and particularly renal impairment, all of which are relatively common in elderly people. Metformin is absolutely contraindicated when the serum creatinine level is >132 mmol l^{-1} (1.5 mg dl^{-1}) in men and >124 mmol l^{-1} (1.4 mg dl^{-1}) in women. Because the risk of lactic acidosis increases with the degree of renal impairment and the patient's age, metformin should not be initiated in patients aged over 80 years. Above the age of 70, careful monitoring of renal function and at least a baseline creatinine clearance is a requirement. Metformin should be promptly withdrawn with the acute onset of dehydration, hypoxaemia, sepsis or the use of contrast media. In this setting, metformin should not be reinstituted unless renal function is demonstrably normal.

Although the efficacy of metformin is comparable to that of sulphonylureas and its use is not limited by hypoglycaemia, for the above reasons it is not necessarily the agent of first choice for many older patients with type 2 diabetes.

17.4 Alpha-glucosidase inhibitors

More than 50% of type 2 diabetic patients receiving oral conventional therapy have persistent postprandial hyperglycaemia [39]. The alpha-glucosidase inhibitors (AGIs) are a class of agent that primarily target postprandial hyperglycaemia. *Acarbose* was the first such agent to be made available commercially, and both acarbose and miglitol are now available in many countries; a third agent, voglibose, is available in Japan.

Alpha-glucosidases are hydrolase enzymes within the brush border of the small bowel, and are responsible for cleavage of the non-absorbable oligo- and dissaccharides into monosaccharides, which are then rapidly absorbed from the gastrointestinal tract. The improvement of postprandial hyperglycaemia is through a reversible inhibition of the brush border glucosidases, resulting in a redistribution of carbohydrate absorption from the upper portion of the gut to a more extended surface area covering the whole length of the small intestine [40]. However, this may result in a higher level of fermentable carbohydrate reaching the large bowel where they are metabolized by colonic microflora to short-chain fatty acids and then absorbed [41]. There is no substantial caloric loss in the faeces. Due to the high specificity of these agents for α-glucosidases, β-glucosidases, like lactoses, are not inhibited and lactose intolerance is not a clinical problem. Based on its mode of action, several inferences can be made. One is that these agents should be effective in every individual who has postprandial hyperglycaemia and ingests sufficient amounts of carbohydrates. The second inference is that this agent will be effective only when given with meals. Being a competitive inhibitor of carbohydrate digestion, it will not be effective when given on an empty stomach. The third inference is that AGIs may cause gastrointestinal flatulence and loose stools in some individuals. Less than 2% of an oral dose of acarbose is absorbed as active drug. Acarbose is metabolized exclusively within the gastrointestinal tract, primarily by the intestinal microflora and to a lesser extent by digestive enzymes. A fraction of these metabolites (34% of the oral dose) is absorbed and subsequently excreted in the urine [42].

Other mechanisms of action of acarbose may include an enhancement of glucagon-like peptide-1 (GLP-1) response; however, this effect is probably a minor contributor (if any) to the antihyperglycaemic effects of these agents [43].

Miglitol absorption is saturable at high dose. When an oral dose of 25 mg is given, it is almost completely absorbed, whereas a dose of 100 mg is only 50–70% absorbed. Miglitol is not metabolized and is eliminated unchanged by renal excretion. The elimination half-life is 2 h. In renal failure, the miglitol plasma concentration increases but a dose adjustment is not recommended because the drug acts locally. Plasma concentrations of both acarbose and miglitol are increased in renal impairment, and no safety data are available when creatinine clearance is less than $25 \, ml \, min^{-1}$ [44].

Acarbose treatment reduced HbA_{1C} by 0.5–0.7% in monotherapy compared to 0.5–1.2% when combined with a sulphonylurea or biguanide [45, 46]. On average, the postprandial glucose surge was reduced by $2.7–3.3 \, mmol \, l^{-1}$ ($50–60 \, mg \, dl^{-1}$), but the effect on fasting glucose levels was more modest at $1.1–1.6 \, mmol \, l^{-1}$ ($20–30 \, mg \, dl^{-1}$) [45].

AGIs are best tolerated when started at a low dose (25 mg once daily with the beginning of the meal), and then increased gradually over a 6- to 8-week period to a maximum dose of 100 mg t.i.d. with meals. In subjects weighing <60 kg, the total daily dose should not exceed 150 mg. In older subjects, a dose–response study showed that the efficacy of acarbose is near-maximal at 25 mg when the meal size does not exceed 483 kcal and contains only 61 g of carbohydrates [47]. Similarly, in an elderly population with a median age of 70 years, miglitol achieved near-maximal metabolic benefits at a low dosage of 25 mg t.i.d. [48]. The Precose Resolution of Optimal Titration to Enhance Current Therapies (PROTECT) study showed that there was no difference in efficacy or safety of acarbose when subjects aged over 60 years were compared to younger subjects [49, 50]. In a study of patients with impaired glucose tolerance (IGT), acarbose treatment was associated with a significant reduction in the risk of cardiovascular disease and hypertension [51].

Like bigaunides, this class of agents is considered to be antihyperglycaemic, since when used as monotherapy, they do not result in hypoglycaemia. Another potential advantage of AGIs when used as monotherapy is that there is no associated hyperinsulinaemia or weight gain. However, if patients are treated with a combination of an AGI and a hypoglycaemic agent such as insulin or a sulphonylurea, glucose should be used to treat the hypoglycaemic reactions since sucrose or a complex carbohydrate will not be readily effective.

Hypoglycaemia is a major concern and a limiting factor in treating elderly patients with type 2 diabetes. Considering the favourable tolerability and safety profile of AGIs, some diabetologists therefore choose these agents as first-line therapy in elderly type 2 diabetic subjects with fasting blood glucose levels of $<11.0 \, mmol \, l^{-1}$ [52]. However, the relatively higher cost of these agents, the need for multiple daily dosing and the adverse gastrointestinal side effects have limited their widespread use.

17.5 Thiazolidinediones

Thiazolidinediones (TZDs) enhances insulin sensitivity in the liver, adipose tissue and muscle, without affecting insulin secretion. Their site of action is mediated through selective activation of peroxisome proliferator-activated receptor gamma (PPAR-γ), a nuclear receptor that plays an important role in adipogenesis [53]. So far, the precise mechanisms that lead to the transcriptional regulation of genes involved in insulin sensitization and lipid metabolism have not been elucidated.

Troglitazone, the first compound in this class to become available, was introduced in 1997 but withdrawn from the market shortly afterwards due to severe hepatotoxicity. Two other agents, rosiglitazone and pioglitazone, are still available. The TZDs are antihyperglycaemic agents, and do not cause hypoglycaemia when used as monotherapy. However, TZD monotherapy will also fail in patients without enough endogenous or exogenous insulin. The TZDs are 99% bound to plasma proteins, notably albumin, while the plasma elimination half-lives range between 3 and 7 h for rosiglitazone and pioglitazone. In the case of rosiglitazone, a twice-daily regimen (4 mg b.i.d.) was more efficacious than a once-daily dosing (8 mg q.d.), with reductions in HbA_{1c} from baseline of 0.7% and 0.3%, respectively [54].

All TZDs undergo major hepatic metabolism. Unlike troglitazone, rosiglitazone does not appear to induce cytochrome P_{450} (CYP)3A4-mediated metabolism and is, therefore, likely to experience fewer drug–drug interactions. The TZDs are mainly excreted in bile, either unchanged or as metabolites, and then eliminated via the faeces. Consequently, there is no need for dose adjustment in patients with renal impairment. On the other hand, the TZDs are contraindicated in patients with active liver disease or if serum aminotransferase (ALT) is more than 2.5-fold the normal level at baseline.

The efficacy of the TZDs has been demonstrated in multiple clinical trials [55, 53]. In monotherapy with troglitazone or rosiglitazone, the mean decline in HbA_{1C} from baseline ranged between 0.6 and 1% [55]. A more pronounced drop in HbA_{1C} of 1.0–1.4% was noted when combined with insulin, however. A head-to-head comparison study for pioglitazone and rosiglitazone has now been conducted [56] wherein the mean decline in HbA_{1C} from baseline at 24 weeks was

0.7% and 0.6% for pioglitazone and rosiglitazone, respectively. Both LDL- and HDL-cholesterol tend to increase with TZD therapy, while serum triglyceride levels may decrease with troglitazone and pioglitazone but not with rosiglitazone. Although rosiglitazone has a pure PPAR-γ agonist activity, pioglitazone and troglitazone have in addition some PPAR-α activity that may contribute to their triglyceride-lowering effect. Compared to baseline, the reduction in triglyceride level may be as high as 26% with troglitazone and pioglitazone therapy [53]. The effect of pioglitazone and rosiglitazone is different on plasma lipids, independent of glycaemic control or concomitant lipid-lowering or other antihyperglycaemic therapy. Pioglitazone, compared with rosiglitazone, is associated with significant improvements in triglycerides, HDL-cholesterol, LDL particle concentration and LDL particle size [56].

On average, 20–50% of individuals fail to respond to this class of agent [55]. It appears that obese and hyperinsulinaemic individuals are more likely to respond than those who have insufficient insulin. When combined with sulphonylureas, TZDs were as effective as the combination of metformin and sulphonylureas [57, 58]. A major disadvantage of the combination of TZDs and sulphonylureas is the associated weight gain, which may be as high as 6.5 kg after one year of therapy. A modest increase in body weight is also observed when TZDs are used as monotherapy.

The major concern of serious hepatotoxicity seen with troglitazone seems not to be a class-related issue. After eight years of post-marketing, the available data suggest that pioglitazone and rosiglitazone do not have an increased incidence of hepatotoxicity. During a 48-week study with rosiglitazone and pioglitazone, the improving insulin sensitivity resulted in improved histological markers of non-alcoholic steatohepatitis (NASH) [59, 60].

The controversy surrounding the increased risk of cardiovascular events with rosiglitazone has raised major safety concerns, and caused a major dilemma for practitioners. In a meta-analysis study, rosiglitazone was associated with a significant increase in the risk of myocardial infarction, with an odds ratio of 1.43 (95% CI: 1.03–1.98; P = 0.03) [61]. In a prospective randomized trial of 5238 patients with type 2 diabetes and macrovascular disease, pioglitazone did not increase the risk of myocardial ischaemia. Rather, there was a trend towards a benefit in regard to all-cause mortality, non-fatal myocardial infarction, stroke and acute coronary syndrome [62]. On 30th July 2007, the United States Food and Drug Administration (FDA)

acknowledged the increase risk of cardiac events associated with rosiglitazone, especially in a subgroup of patients, yet opted to keep the drug on the US market with the addition of a 'black box' warning.

The TZDs are usually well tolerated and, when used as monotherapy, there is no associated risk of hypoglycaemia. Peripheral oedema is occasionally seen in monotherapy, more so with the concomitant use of insulin, mainly as a result of the plasma volume expansion. Therefore, these agents are not recommended in patients with New York Heart Association (NYHA) Class III or IV congestive heart failure. A minor decrease in haematocrit and haemoglobin is another observation correlates with the dilutional effect of fluid retention.

The once-daily dosing regimen and lack of associated hypoglycaemia make the TZDs an attractive option in elderly subjects. On the other hand, recent concerns about cardiovascular safety, suboptimal efficacy in underweight subjects and costs may limit their usefulness, particularly as a first-line agent.

17.6 Meglitinides

Meglitinide belongs to a novel group of insulinotropic agents known as the non-sulphonylurea insulin secretagogues [63]. Both, repaglinide and mitiglinide are benzoic acid derivatives, while nateglinide is a phenylalanine derivative. As with the sulphonylureas, the insulinotropic effect is mediated through the ATP-regulated potassium channels but via different binding sites on the β cells [64]. After oral administration, meglitinides are rapidly absorbed from the gastrointestinal tract, with maximum plasma concentrations being reached within 0.8 h and the drug rapidly eliminated with an approximate half-life ($t_{1/2}$) of 1–1.7 h [65, 66]. However, the wide variability of $t_{1/2}$ of repaglinide elimination kinetics ranging between 0.5 and 8 h is of concern. The absorption of nateglinide is increased when the medication is taken 10 min before a meal, whereas the C_{max} is decreased by 34% and the T_{max} increased by 22% when the drug is given after the meal. The absorption is also reduced during fasting. The influence of food on the pharmacokinetics of repaglinide is of lesser importance.

The pharmacokinetic profile makes meglitinides a suitable agent for targeting postprandial hyperglycaemia [7]. Meglitinides are completely metabolized by the liver, with 90% of repeglinide being excreted via the biliary route and only 8% via the urine. In contrast, 90% of nateglinide is excreted via the urine and 10% via the bile [65, 66]. When comparing healthy young individuals with people aged ≥ 65 years, there was no difference in the pharmacokinetic parameters. However, elderly type 2 diabetic subjects had a significantly higher mean diurnal plasma concentration and a reduced clearance when compared to healthy controls [67]. Although the area under the plasma concentration–time curve (AUC) and C_{max} were significantly increased in subjects with various degrees of renal impairment, a dose adjustment was not necessary. However, the authors recommended a careful and gradual increase in the initial dose. Following a single dose of repaglinide, patients with moderate to severe liver disease had higher and more prolonged serum concentrations [68]. Although liver disease did not significantly increase the risk of hypoglycaemic episodes in this latter study, the safety of repaglinide remains questionable in this subgroup of patients.

A 1-year comparison study of repaglinide and glimepiride, with an 8-week titration period, showed similar reductions of HbA_{1c} (−1.2% versus − 1.1%) and FPG levels (−2.11 versus − 2.7 mmol l^{-1}), but repaglinide resulted in a greater reduction in FPG level than glimepiride (−2.56 versus -1.17 mmol l^{-1}) [69]. When the efficacy of repaglinide was compared to glyburide in a multicentre, randomized, double-blind study over one year, the reduction in HbA_{1C} was similar in both groups [70]. However, when added to metformin in suboptimally controlled diabetes ($HbA_{1C} = 8.5\%$), the HbA_{1C} fell by 1.4% [71]. A combination therapy achieved a better control than either drug alone. Repaglinide and nateglinide have been also tested in association with TZD [72, 73]. As with the sulphonylureas, weight gain and hypoglycaemia were the two most frequent adverse effects, although there was a reduced risk of hypoglycaemia when a meal was omitted and the repaglinide dose withheld. [74].

The potential for a reduced risk of hypoglycaemia is an interesting feature of this class of agent, especially in older individuals. However, additional studies are required to define the relative value of these agents. Of concern is the wide range of variability in drug elimination kinetics with repeglinide. In addition, a preprandial dosing regimen may be an obstacle to achieving long-term compliance in some individuals. Nateglinide pharmacokinetics are more favourable in terms of improving postprandial hyperglycaemia. Finally, the real advantage of these relatively costly agents compared

to a small dose of short-acting sulphonylurea is still not clear [75].

17.7 Incretin mimetics and enhancers: Glucagon-like peptide-1 and dipeptidyl peptidase IV inhibitors

Over 40 years ago, the observation that enteral glucose provided a more pronounced insulinotropic effect compared with an isoglycaemic intravenous challenge led to the development of the incretin concept [76]. Incretins are intestinal hormones which are released after meal ingestion and play an important role in normal glucose homeostasis. Glucose-dependent insulinotropic polypeptide (GIP) – the first incretin to be identified – is synthesized in duodenal and jejunal enteroendocrine K cells in the proximal small bowel. Glucagon-Like Peptide-1 (GLP-1) is a very potent insulinotropic peptide hormone secreted by the L-cells of the intestinal mucosa in the lower gut [77, 78]. The insulinotropic effect is mediated at the level of the L-cells through a stimulation of adenylate cyclase and protein kinase A activity [79]. Unlike sulphonylurea agents, GLP-1 has no hypoglycaemic effect in the absence of glucose [80]. Its secretion increases in response to unabsorbed nutrient within the intestinal lumen. In addition, it has an inhibitory effect on glucagon secretion and the gastric emptying rate [77]. Although fasting hyperglycaemia can be reduced with GLP-1, its primary target is postprandial hyperglycaemia [81, 82].

In clinical studies, the two shorter forms of GLP-1, the (7–37) and (7–36) amides, have been used. These peptides have a short duration of action (<1 min) and should be given parenterally. Although, both GLP-1 and GIP act as incretin hormones in healthy subjects, more attention has been focused on GLP-1 because of the observation that in type 2 diabetes the GLP-1 level is reduced yet the response to GLP-1 is preserved, whereas GIP secretion is normal but the response to GIP is blunted or absent. Circulating levels of both GLP-1 and GIP decrease rapidly due to enzymatic degradation, mainly by the action of dipeptidyl peptidase IV (DPP-IV) and renal clearance.

Exenatide is the synthetic version of exendin-4, an incretin hormone originally found in the saliva of the Gila monster, *Heloderma suspectum*. Exenatide has a greater potency and a longer duration of action than the native GLP-1 when administered subcutaneously [83].

Exenatide shares with the native GLP-1 its biological actions and is resistant to DPP-IV degradation. Following subcutaneous (sc) administration, it reaches median peak plasma concentrations in 2.1 h, and is eliminated predominantly by glomerular filtration. No dose adjustment is required in mild to moderate renal impairment. Exenatide is administered sc within a 60-min period before the two main meals of the day, 6 h or more apart, at a starting dose of 5 µg twice daily (b.i.d.) and then titrated to 10 µg b.i.d. after 4 weeks [84]. The main adverse events are nausea, vomiting, diarrhoea, headache and dizziness. The risk of hypoglycaemia is increased when exenatide is used in combination with sulphonylureas. The drug was approved by the FDA in April 2005 as an adjunct therapy for type 2 diabetes in conjunction with sulphonylureas, biguanides and TZDs. At 30 weeks, the HbA_{1c} reduction from baseline was between -0.8% and -0.9% in the metformin, sulphonylurea and metformin-sulphonylurea combination subgroup, with weight reductions of 1.6 kg in the sulphonylurea and metformin-sulphonylurea arms, and 2.8 kg in the metformin-alone arm [85, 86, 87]. The reductions in HbA_{1c} and body weight were sustained at 2.5 years at -1% and 5 kg, respectively [88]. In combination with TZD, the HbA_{1c} reduction was -0.8% at 16 weeks with a 1.5 kg weight loss [88]. The efficacy of a long-acting release (LAR) exenatide is currently undergoing Phase III studies at a weekly dose of 0.8 to 2 mg.

Due to the rapid degradation of GLP-1 by DPP-IV, attempts have been made to develop specific inhibitors. DPP-IV is a ubiquitous membrane-spanning, cell-surface aminopeptidase that is expressed in many tissues, such as liver, lung, kidney, lymphocytes, endothelial cells and intestinal brush border [89]. DPP-IV catalyzes the cleavage of GIP and GLP-1 to bioinactive GIP_{3-42} and $GLP-1_{9-37}$ or $GLP-1_{9-36}$ amide, respectively [90]. Two DPP-IV inhibitors, vildagliptin and sitagliptin, have completed Phase III clinical trials, and their efficacy in both monotherapy and combination therapy regimens was examined. Both, vildagliptin and sitagliptin significantly lowered HbA_{1c} when used either as an initial monotherapy, or in combination with other oral anti-diabetic agents such as biguanides, thiazolidinediones or sulphonylureas. The average fall in HbA_{1c} in most reports was between 0.5 and 0.8% from baseline, with no associated weight gain. DPP-IV inhibitors had an increased risk of infection [risk ratio 1.2 (95% CI: 1.0–1.4) for nasopharyngitis and 1.5 (95% CI: 1.0–2.2) for urinary tract infection] and headache [risk ratio 1.4 (95% CI: 1.1–1.7)]. Gastrointestinal (GI) side effects were infrequent and hypoglycaemic episodes very rare and insignificant [91, 92]. The first DPP-IV inhibitor (sitagliptin) was approved for the treatment of type 2 diabetes in the United States in October 2006.

Further clinical experience is required before the incretin approach can be accepted as an alternative to the currently available hypoglycaemic agents to treat the elderly population with type 2 diabetes. Although the risk of hypoglycaemia with GLP-1 analogues is less compared to sulphonylureas and it has a favourable weight change profile, the sc route of administration and the frequent GI side effects may be problematic. For DPP-IV inhibitors, the once-daily regimen, the lack of weight gain and almost no hypoglycaemia may make this class of agents an excellent first-line therapy, especially in those patients with mild glucose elevation. However, cost reduction, careful post-marketing surveillance for adverse effects and continued evaluation in longer-term studies are required to determine the role of this new class among current pharmacotherapies. The recommended dose of sitagliptin is 100 mg once daily, with or without food, as monotherapy or as combination therapy with metformin or a TZD. A dosage adjustment is recommended in patients with moderate or severe renal insufficiency or with end-stage renal disease (ESRD) requiring dialysis. In these patients, the initial dose should be 50 mg once daily if the creatinine clearance (CrCl) is $\geq 30-<50$ ml min^{-1}, and 25 mg once daily if <30 ml min^{-1}. No dosage adjustment is required based on age; however, because sitagliptin is excreted substantially by the kidney it may be useful to assess renal function in elderly patients prior to initiation, and periodically thereafter.

17.8 Amylin analogues

Amylin was identified in 1987 [93] as a 37-amino acid hormone secreted in conjunction with insulin by the pancreatic β-cells in response to a glucose load or other insulin secretagogues [94]. In type 1 diabetes, the reduction in amylin concentration parallels the decline in insulin secretion [95]. When compared to a population of lean, healthy subjects, basal and stimulated amylin secretion were significantly higher in obese patients with or without impaired glucose tolerance [96]. However, in long-standing type 2 diabetes, the amylin concentration decreases in conjunction with β-cell failure [97]. The effect of amylin on glucose metabolism

Table 17.2 Comparative profile of available oral agents for treatment of type 2 diabetes (in monotherapy).

	Sulphonylureas	Meglitinides	Biguanides	TZD	AGI	GLP-1	DPP-IV inhibitors
Mode of action	Stimulate insulin release from β-cells	Stimulate insulin release from β-cells	Decrease hepatic gluconeogenesis	Enhance insulin sensitivity in muscles and liver	Reversible inhibition of the intestinal brush border glucosidase	Stimulate insulin release from β-cells, Decrease post-prandial glucagon secretion from α-cells Inhibits gastric emptying Reduces food intake	Stimulate insulin release from β-cells, Decrease post-prandial glucagon secretion from α-cells
Potency ↓ in HbA$_{1c}$	1.5–1.8	1.0–1.5	1.0–1.5	0.7–1.5	0.5–0.7	0.8–0.9	0.6–0.7
Body weight change	↑↑	↑↑	↓ or neutral	↑↑	↓ or neutral	neutral to ↓↓	neutral
Hypoglycaemia	+++	++	0	0	0	+	0
Side effects	Prolonged hypoglycaemia	Hypoglycaemia	Gastrointestinal	Oedema, slight increase risk of CHF, may increase risk of CAD (Rosiglitazone)	Gastrointestinal Flatulence	Gastrointestinal (nausea, vomiting and diarrhoea)	Nasopharyngitis, headaches and upper respiratory infections
Contraindications	Renal failure (risk of prolonged hypoglycaemia)	Renal failure (risk of hypoglycaemia)	Renal impairment Liver failure Hypoxaemic states (risk of lactic acidosis)	NYHA III-IV Liver failure	Diarrhoea	Gastroparesis Creatinine clearance <30 ml min^{-1}	Need dose adjustment with renal impairment
Cost	+	++	+	+++	++	+++	+++

CHF: Chronic heart failure; NYHA: New York Heart Association; CAD: Coronary artery disease; TZD: thiazolidiones; AGI: Alpha-glucosidase inhibitors; GLP-1: Glucagon-like-peptide-1; DPP-IV: Dipeptidyl peptidase IV.

involves several mechanisms. By slowing the rate of gastric emptying, it limits the proportion of nutrients delivered to the gut, thus preventing the postprandial hyperglycaemic surge [98]. Amylin also suppresses postprandial glucagon secretion, helps replenish glycogen stores [7, 99], promotes satiety, and reduces caloric intake. However, due to its short half-life and its tendency to aggregation, amylin is not suitable for clinical use.

The amylin analogue 'pramlintide' is an injectable synthetic analogue that is structurally identical to human amylin, but with the exception of a proline substitution at positions 25, 28 and 29 [100]. Clinical studies have demonstrated a substantial decrease in postprandial hyperglycaemia in healthy individuals, as well as in patients with type 1 or type 2 diabetes after sc or intravenous administration [101]. Pramlintide was approved in the US market in 2005 for the treatment of type 1 and 2 diabetes in conjunction with insulin. The half-life of pramlintide in healthy subjects is 48 min, and the drug is metabolized and excreted primarily via the kidneys. Patients with moderate or severe renal impairment (creatinine clearance >20 to $<50\,\text{ml}\,\text{min}^{-1}$) did not show an increase in pramlintide exposure, or reduced clearance. The pramlintide starting dose is 15 µg prior to the major meals, and this must be titrated every 3–7 days to a maximum of 60 µg before meals in type 1 diabetes, and up to 120 µg in type 2 diabetes. The most common adverse side effects include nausea, headache, anorexia, vomiting and abdominal pain. Pramlintide alone does not cause hypoglycaemia, although coadministration of the drug with insulin can aggravate the risk of insulin-induced hypoglycaemia, especially in type 1 diabetes. With the initiation of pramlintide therapy, the insulin dose will need to be reduced in order to prevent severe hypoglycaemic episodes.

In a 52-week, double-blind, placebo-controlled study of 656 patients with type 2 diabetes, treatment with pramlintide 120 µg b.i.d. led to a sustained reduction from baseline in HbA_{1c} of -0.62%, and this was accompanied by a mean body weight loss of $-1.4\,\text{kg}$ compared to $+0.7\,\text{kg}$ with placebo [102]. In a similar 1-year study of 651 type 1 diabetic patients, the addition of pramlintide 60 µg t.i.d or q.i.d. to insulin led to significant reductions in HbA_{1c} from a baseline of 0.29% ($P < 0.011$) and 0.34% ($P < 0.001$), respectively, compared to a 0.04% reduction in the placebo group. This HbA_{1c} reduction occurred without any increase in concomitant insulin use, and was accompanied by a significant reduction in body weight from baseline to week 52 of 0.4 kg in the 60 µg t.i.d.

($P < 0.027$) or q.i.d. ($P < 0.040$) treatment groups, compared to a 0.8 kg weight gain in the placebo group [103].

The frequency and the route of administration of pramlintide have raised major concerns regarding the suitability of such agents in the elderly population.

17.9 Insulin and insulin analogues

As insulin therapy in diabetes is discussed extensively in Chapter 18, this section will deal mainly with the role of some of the newer insulin preparations. Multiple clinical trials have proven that intensive glycaemic control can be achieved with insulin therapy in both type 1 [1] and type 2 diabetes [2, 31].

The most commonly used human insulin preparations, all of which differ in their pharmacokinetics, are summarized in Table 17.3. Hypoglycaemia remains the most frequently encountered side effect of insulin therapy, and is the major limiting factor in intensive glycaemic control [1, 2]. Hypoglycaemia is commonly precipitated by erratic meal timing, excessive insulin dosage and unplanned exercise. The failure to administer regular insulin in a timely manner (30–45 min before a meal) also increases the risk. In addition to the increased risk of hypoglycaemia, the recommended timing of the injection of short-acting insulin prior to meals can be inconvenient and may disrupt the patient's lifestyle.

Recombinant DNA technology has been used to design insulin molecules that overcome the limitations of short-acting regular insulin. Yet, safety issues are a concern with these alternatives, as the alteration of the three-dimensional structure may modify the interaction with the insulin and/or IGF-I receptors and, as a result, lead to the activation of alternative metabolic and mitogenic signalling pathways. It is, then, essential to apply cautious study to the acute and long-term effects in a preclinical state, as insulin therapy is meant to be a lifelong treatment.

Ultra-short-acting insulin analogues were originally developed with the hope of overcoming these limitations. Lispro insulin is identical to human regular insulin, but with a minor transposition of a lysine and proline in the beta chain. This transposition results in an acceleration of the dissociation rate of the insulin hexamers, such that lispro insulin acts quickly within 10–20 min, peaks on average at 1–2 h, and is essentially cleared from the system within 4–5 h [104]. Thus, lispro provides a greater flexibility in insulin

Table 17.3   Some of the most commonly used insulin preparations.

Insulin preparations	Action profile (h)		
	Onset	Peak	Duration
Ultra-Rapid acting analogues (Human)			
Lispro	0.25–0.5	0.5–2	3–4
Aspart	0.25–0.5	0.5–2	3–4
Glulisine	0.25–0.5	0.5–2	3–4
Short-acting insulin (Human)			
Regular	0.5–1	2–3	6–8
U-500	1–3	6–12	12–18
Short-acting inhaled insulin Exubera	0.16–0.3	2	5–6
Intermediate-acting (Human)			
NPH	1.5	4–10	16–24
Intermediate-acting analogues			
Detemir	1–2	6–8	14–24
Long-acting analogues			
Glargine	1–1.5	No peak	20–24
Mixtures*			
Humulin 70/30 NPH 70%, regular 30%	0.5–1	3–12	16–24
Humulin 50/50 NPH 50%, regular 50%	0.5–1	2–12	16–24
Mixtures analogues*			
Humalog 75/25 NPL 75%, Lispro 25%	0.3–0.5	1–6.5	Up to 24
Humalog 50/50 NPL 50%, Lispro 50%	0.3–0.5	0.8–4.8	Up to 24
Novolog 70/30 NPL 70%, Aspart 30%	0.3–0.5	1.6–3.2	Up to 24

*Mixtures with different proportions of NPH and regular, and more recently a mixture of lispro insulin and its protamine derivative, are also available but less commonly used.

administration, and can be given 5–10 min before a meal. Another modest advantage of lispro insulin has been the improvement in postprandial hyperglycaemia in both type 1 and type 2 diabetic subjects, and a reduction in the number of hypoglycaemic episodes in type 1 subjects [104, 105]. However, this latter advantage over regular insulin has not been consistently demonstrated in type 2 subjects [104]. Overall, glycaemic control as reflected by HbA$_{1C}$ levels does not differ between lispro insulin and human regular insulin-treated groups [106].

Two other short-acting insulin analogues are available currently. 'Insulin aspart' (B28 Asp) has a proline at position B28 replaced with a negatively charged aspartic acid [107, 108]. Insulin glulisine has an asparagine replaced with lysine at position B2 and lysine with glutamic acid at B29 [108, 109]. In addition to their rapid onset of action, insulin aspart and glulisine also have a favourable effect on postprandial hyperglycaemia in both type 1 and type 2 diabetic subjects, while their pharmacokinetics resemble that of lispro insulin.

The clinical utility of these short-acting insulin analogues and their advantages over the regular insulin in the elderly population has yet to be established.

Many attempts have been made to identify an alternate method of insulin delivery, through nasal, oral, buccal, transdermal or inhaled routes. *Inhaled insulin* is a theoretically attractive approach, mainly because of the large absorptive surface of the lung alveoli with relatively little proteolytic activity to cause insulin degradation. One such product, Exubera (Pfizer), has already been granted approval for clinical use in the United States and the European Union, and other products [AERx (Novo Nordisk) and AIR (Eli Lilly)] are currently in the advanced stages of clinical trials. In clinical studies in patients with type 1 and type 2 diabetes, following the inhalation of Exubera, serum insulin reached a peak concentration more quickly than after sc injection of regular human insulin, namely 49 min (range 30–90 min) compared to 105 min (range 60–240 min). With inhaled insulin, the onset of glucose-lowering activity in healthy volunteers occurred within 10–20 min, with the maximum effect on glucose lowering being exerted approximately 2 h after inhalation. The duration of the glucose-lowering activity was approximately 6 h. There were no apparent differences in the pharmacokinetic properties of Exubera when comparing patients aged >65 years with younger, adult patients [110]. There is little doubt that treatment with inhaled insulin is associated with a small (ca. 5%) decline in lung function, when measured by parameters such as the diffusion capacity of the lung, and forced expiratory volume in 1 s. The results of a recent study indicated that treatment group differences in lung function between inhaled and sc insulin in adult patients with type 1 diabetes were small, developed early, and were non-progressive for up to 2 years of therapy [111]. There is a theoretical concern for an increased risk of cancer with the long-term use of inhaled insulin, since it is a potent growth factor. It might, therefore, be prudent to monitor for this potential serious side effect that may take many years to emerge.

Longer-acting insulin preparations are prepared with different chemical modifications of insulin. A protamine derivative of lispro insulin (NPL) is currently available that has an intermediate duration of action. When NPL was premixed with lispro in a ratio of 75:25%, it was shown to improve postprandial glycaemic control compared to premixed human NPH and regular insulin in a 30:70% ratio [112].

Other intermediate- and long-acting insulin analogues include glargine and detemir. *Insulin glargine* differs from human insulin in that the amino acid asparagine at position A21 is replaced by glycine, and two arginines are added to the C-terminus of the B-chain. Insulin glargine is a human insulin analogue that has been designed to have low aqueous solubility at neutral pH. After injection into the subcutaneous tissue, the acidic solution is neutralized, leading to the formation of microprecipitates from which small amounts of insulin glargine are slowly released; this results in a relatively constant concentration–time profile over 24 h, with no pronounced peak. This pharmacokinetic profile of glargine allows once-daily dosing as the patient's basal insulin [113]. Compared to bedtime NPH insulin, insulin glargine is associated with less nocturnal hypoglycaemia in patients with type 2 diabetes (28.8% versus 12.6%, P = 0.011) [114].

Insulin detemir differs from human insulin in that the amino acid threonine in position B30 has been omitted, and a C_{14} fatty acid chain has been attached to the amino acid B29. Insulin detemir is a soluble, long-acting basal human insulin analogue with a relatively flat action profile. The mean duration of action of insulin detemir ranged from 5.7 h at the lowest dose to 23.2 h at the highest dose, and the serum C_{max} was reached at 6–8 h after administration [115]. *Note:* Glargine and detemir should not be diluted or mixed with any other insulin preparations.

There is currently no strong rationale favouring glargine, neutral protamine of Hagedorn insulin, insulin detemir or fixed-ratio insulin preparations as the preferred agent for initiating insulin therapy. Rather, an insulin regimen should be tailored to each patient's needs [114].

17.10 The choice of an anti-diabetic agent in elderly people

In general, the management of type 2 diabetes should be individualized and tailored to the clinical status of the individual, coexisting diseases, body weight, goals of therapy, expectations, involvement in care, functional impairment, ease of administration, side effect profile, cost of therapy, baseline blood sugar and the urgency of blood sugar normalization. Although difficult to generalize when considering all these parameters, some guidelines can be suggested based on blood sugar levels and the known clinical efficacy and tolerability of the various classes of anti-diabetic agents. (Table 17.2)

As in middle-aged individuals, lifestyle modification, including diet-control and exercise, remain the cornerstone of every treatment plan for type 2 diabetes. However, under-nutrition is common in elderly patients with type 2 diabetes, especially in those who live in nursing homes [23, 116]. In this subgroup, the patient's nutritional status should be carefully evaluate and an appropriate caloric consumption recommended. Elderly subjects also have more difficulties with the acquisition, preparation and sometimes ingestion of food, and this can affect their nutritional status and increase the risk of hypoglycaemic episodes [117]. Here, a support system that can provide the appropriate meals in a timely manner is helpful. When there is no major physical limitation, physical activity and exercise should be encouraged within reason. On the other hand, a careful medical evaluation – and sometimes also a limited stress test – should be undertaken before starting any exercise programme, due to the high incidence of subclinical coronary artery disease in this population.

Although it should be individualized, the trigger point to start pharmacological intervention in the elderly is not generally different from that in middle-aged diabetic people [118]. The goal for glycaemic control in the elderly diabetic is to achieve euglycaemia without the undue risk of hypoglycaemia. Ideally, the following blood glucose values should be sought: A FBG of 4.4–6.6 mmol l^{-1} (80–120 mg dl^{-1}); a 1-h postprandial glucose $<8.8\,\mathrm{mmol\,l^{-1}}$ $(160\,\mathrm{mg\,dl^{-1}})$; and $\mathrm{HbA_{1C}} <7\%$. Additional action is suggested if the FBG is $>7.8\,\mathrm{mmol\,l^{-1}}$ $(140\,\mathrm{mg\,dl^{-1}})$, the postprandial glucose is $>10\,\mathrm{mmol\,l^{-1}}$ $(180\,\mathrm{mg\,dl^{-1}})$, or the $\mathrm{HbA_{1C}}$ is $>7\%$. In order to avoid the deleterious effect of hypoglycaemia in the frail elderly diabetic patient, no attempt should be made to lower the FBG or bedtime blood glucose below $5.5\,\mathrm{mmol\,l^{-1}}$ $(100\,\mathrm{mg\,dl^{-1}})$.

Although many physicians have traditionally relied only on the FBG and the $\mathrm{HbA_{1C}}$ measurement to guide pharmacological therapy, postprandial hyperglycaemia is becoming an important target of the management [7, 36]. The rationale behind this approach is that self-monitoring FBG and postprandial glucose are readily available for patients and clinicians, and can be used to expedite the titration and changes in drug therapy. In addition, it appears that individuals with isolated postprandial hyperglycaemia are at

increased risk of atherosclerotic heart disease. Postprandial hyperglycaemia is probably one of the reasons why some individuals with a FBG within the target range $(4.4–6.6\,\mathrm{mmol\,l^{-1}})$ have already established microvascular and macrovascular complications.

Despite the fact that non-pharmacological interventions alone may be sufficient at early stages of the disease, these measures will fail in most patients as the disease progresses [2, 31]. An initial approach to drug therapy of type 2 diabetes in elderly people is illustrated in Figure 17.2. When the FBG levels are consistently over $16.7\,\mathrm{mmol\,l^{-1}}$ $(300\,\mathrm{mg\,dl^{-1}})$, it is most likely that the patient has either a profound insulin deficiency or severe insulin resistance, or both. Insulin treatment – at least initially – is the preferred choice for these individuals. Insulin therapy should be initiated in a hospital setting if the patient is symptomatic

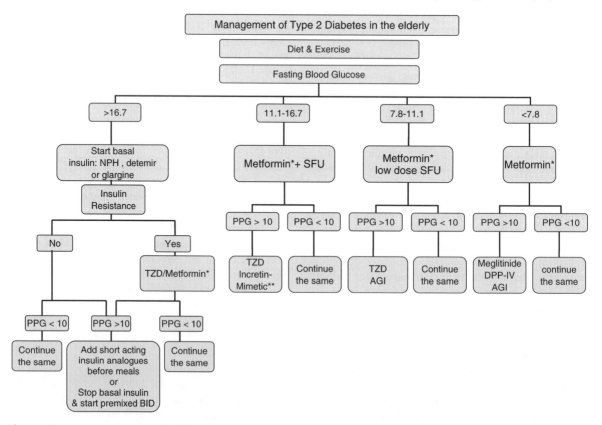

Figure 17.2 A suggested algorithm for the initial choice of therapeutic agents based on fasting blood glucose (in $\mathrm{mmol\,l^{-1}}$). The initial choice might be only for a brief period of time. PPG is 1 h postprandial blood glucose (in $\mathrm{mmol\,l^{-1}}$). SFU = sulphonylurea; AGI = alpha-glucosidase inhibitor; TZD = thiazolidinediones; DPP-IV = dipeptidyl-peptidase IV inhibitors; BID = twice daily. *If metformin is contraindicated, consider low-dose SFU, AGI, DPP-IV or TZD. **Adding insulin at this stage might be more cost-effective.

with mental status changes or severe dehydration; otherwise, it can be started in the doctor's surgery. The dose will be titrated during follow-up visits, and if there is any evidence of significant insulin resistance then insulin sensitizers, such as thiazolidinediones or metformin, can be added if there are no contraindications. It is noteworthy, however, that some individuals (and especially obese subjects) who present with a FBG >16.7 mmol l^{-1} may only require insulin for a short period until the glucose toxicity resolves and glycaemic goals can then be achieved by switching to oral agents.

When attending to with lean patients with an average FBG of 11.1–16.7 mmol l^{-1} (200–300 mg dl^{-1}), the initial drug of choice can be either a sulphonylurea or insulin. For obese subjects (i.e. BMI $\geq$30 kg m^{-2}), metformin would be added, although due to a high prevalence of contraindications to biguanides in the elderly, TZD – particularly pioglitazone – might be an alternative to metformin. It is important that the potential for cardiovascular events associated with these agents is thoroughly discussed with the patients. If the FBG is within target, but postprandial hyperglycaemia remains a problem, then consideration should be given to adding a GLP-1 mimetic or initiating insulin therapy.

For individuals with a FBG of 7.8–11.1 mmol l^{-1} (140–200 mg dl^{-1}), metformin should be the initial drug and subsequently a low dose of sulphonylurea can be added. Alternatively, a TZD might be added or started, if metformin were contraindicated.

The cost of a triple oral therapy is of concern (as are drug–drug interactions), and this should probably be reserved for those individuals who refuse insulin therapy. When the FBG is <7.8 mmol l^{-1} (140 mg dl^{-1}), a trial of an exercise programme with a weight-reducing diet for a 2-month period is initially appropriate. Subsequently, if the glycaemic goals are not within target, then metformin should be the initial drug and an AGI, DPP-IV inhibitor or meglitinide added as appropriate. The addition of a sulphonylurea is definitely more cost-effective, but the risk of hypoglycaemia will be increased. Alternatively, consideration could be given to adding or starting with a thiazolidinedione, especially when metformin is contraindicated

One common problem in clinical practice is that monotherapy with oral agents either fails initially, or fails over time. This important clinical observation was confirmed in the UKPDS. In order to achieve an optimal outcome, multiple drug therapy or a combination of oral agents and insulin is often needed. An important question that must be explored here is whether triple oral therapy, when used to avoid insulin use in the elderly, has any potential advantages over insulin therapy alone. When using such a regimen, it is important to consider the high cost of therapy and the possible increased adverse events as a result of drug–drug interactions. This latter concern is very legitimate when dealing with a frail population with multiple coexisting medical conditions, and where polypharmacy is common. Further studies are required to evaluate the advantages and disadvantages of triple or quadruple oral therapy in the elderly diabetic people and its impact on the quality of life when compared to insulin monotherapy.

Until more data are available, the primary approach is to tailor the management to individual needs. Different individuals require different drug regimens, and this may change over time as the disease progresses. It should be borne in mind that type 2 diabetes is a heterogeneous disease. Now that multiple pharmacological agents are available, with distinct mechanisms of action, it should be more possible than ever to individualize management by matching the appropriate agent to the underlying pathophysiology of type 2 diabetes.

References

1. The Diabetes Control and Complications Trial Research Group (1993) The effect of intensive treatment of diabetes on the development and progression of long-term complications in insulin-dependent diabetes mellitus. N Engl J Med, 329, 977–86.
2. UK Prospective Diabetes Study Group 33 (1998) Intensive blood-glucose control with sulfonylureas or insulin compared with conventional treatment and risk of complications in patients with type 2 diabetes (UKPDS 33). Lancet, 352, 837–53.
3. Morley JE, Mooradian AD, Rosenthal MJ and Kaiser FE (1987) Diabetes mellitus in elderly patients: is it different? Am J Med, 83, 533–44.
4. Rosenthal MJ and Morley JE (1992) Diabetes and its complications in older people. In: Endocrinology and Metabolism in the Elderly, JE Morley and SG Korenman (eds), Blackwell Scientific Publications, Boston, pp. 373–87.
5. Oiknine R and Mooradian AD. (2003) Drug therapy of diabetes in the elderly. Biomed Pharmacother. 57, 231–9.
6. Mooradian AD. (2004) Towards single-tablet therapy for type 2 diabetes mellitus: rationale and recent developments. Treat Endocrinol. 3, 279–87.
7. Mooradian AD and Thurman J (1999) Drug therapy of postprandial hyperglycemia. Drugs, 97 (1), 19–29.

8. Groop LC (1992) Sulfonylureas in NIDDM. Diabetes Care, 19, 737–54.

9. Pfeiffer MA, Beard JC, Halter JB, Judzewitsch R, Best JD and Porte D Jr. (1983) Suppression of glucagon secretion during a tolbutamide infusion in normal and noninsulin-dependent diabetic subjects. J Clin Endocrinol Metab, 56, 586–91.

10. Keller U, Muller R and Berger W (1986) Sulfonylurea therapy fails to diminish insulin resistance in type 1 diabetic subjects. Horm Metab Res, 18, 599–603.

11. Kolterman OG and Olefsky JM (1984) The impact of sulfonylurea treatment upon the mechanisms responsible for the insulin resistance in type II diabetes. Diabetes Care, 7 (Suppl. 1), 81–8.

12. Mooradian AD (1987) The effect of sulfonylureas on the in vivo tissue uptake of glucose in normal rats. Diabetologia, 30, 120–1.

13. Groop L, Groop PH, Stenman S, Saloranta C, Tötterman KJ, Fyhrquist F and Melander A (1988) Do sulfonylureas influence hepatic insulin clearance? Diabetes Care, 11, 689–90.

14. Beck-Nielsen H, Hother Nielsen O, Andersen PH, Pederson O and Schmitz O (1986) In vivo action of glibenclamide. Diabetologia, 29 (Abstract No. 26), 515A.

15. Kahn CR and Schecte Y (1993) Oral hypoglycemic agents. In: The Pharmacologic Basis of Therapeutics, AG Gilman, TW Rall, AS Nies, P Taylor (eds), McGraw-Hill, New York, p. 1485.

16. Melander A, Bitzén PO, Faber O and Groop L (1989) Sulphonylurea antidiabetic drugs: an update of their clinical pharmacology and rational therapeutic use. Drugs, 37, 58–72.

17. Scheen AJ (1997) Drug treatment on non-insulin-dependent diabetes mellitus in the 1990s. Achievements and future developments. Drugs, 54 (3), 355–68.

18. Groop L, Schalin C, Franssila-Kallunki A, Widén E, Ekstrand A, Eriksson J. Characteristics of non-insulin-dependent diabetic patients with secondary failure to oral antidiabetic therapy. Am J Med. 1989; 87 (2): 183–90.

19. Jennings AM, Wilson RM and Ward JD (1989) Symptomatic hypoglycemia in NIDDM patients treated with oral hypoglycemic agents. Diabetes Care, 12, 203–8.

20. UK Prospective Diabetes Study Group 16 (1995) U.K. Prospective Diabetes Study. Overview of 6years' therapy of Type II diabetes: a progressive disease. Diabetes, 44, 1249–58.

21. Asplund K, Wiholm BE and Lithner F (1983) Glibenclamide-associated hypoglycemia: a report of 57 cases. Diabetologia, 24, 412–17.

22. Rosenkranz B, Profozic V, Metelko Z, Mrzljak V, Lange C and Malerczyk V (1996) Pharmacokinetics and safety of glimepiride at clinically effective doses in diabetic patients with renal impairment. Diabetologia, 39, 1617–24.

23. Mooradian AD, Osterweil D, Petrasek D and Morley JE (1988) Diabetes mellitus in elderly nursing home patients: a survey of clinical characteristics and management. J Am Geriatr Soc, 36, 391–6.

24. Horani MH and Mooradian AD. (2002) Management of obesity in the elderly. Special considerations. Treatments in Endocrinology, 1, 387–98.

25. Bailey CJ (1992) Biguanides and NIDDM. Diabetes Care, 15, 755–72.

26. Williams RH and Palmer JP (1975) Farewell to phenformin for treating diabetes mellitus. Ann Intern Med, 83, 567–8.

27. Bristol-Myers Squibb (1995) Glucophage® (metformin hydrochloride tablets) 500 mg and 850 mg. Prescribing information. Princeton, New Jersey: Bristol-Myers Squibb Company.

28. Bailey CJ and Turner RC (1996) Metformin. New Engl J Med, 334, 574–9.

29. Perriello G, Misericordia P, Volpi E, Santucci A, Santucci C, Ferrannini E, Ventura MM, Santeusanio F, Brunetti P and Bolli GB (1994) Acute antihyperglycemic mechanisms of metformin in NIDDM: evidence for suppression of lipid oxidation and hepatic glucose production. Diabetes, 43, 920–8.

30. Garber AJ, Duncan TG, Goodman AM, Mills DJ and Rohlf JL (1997) Efficacy of metformin in type II diabetes: Results of a double-blind, placebo-controlled, dose response trial. Am J Med, 102, 491–7.

31. UK Prospective Diabetes Study Group 34 (1998) Effect of intensive blood-glucose control with metformin on complications in overweight patients with Type 2 diabetes (UKPDS 34). Lancet, 352, 854–65.

32. Yki-Jarvinen H, Ryysy L, Nikkilä K, Tulokas T, Vanamo R and Heikkila M (1999) Comparison of bedtime insulin regimens in patients with Type 2 diabetes mellitus. A randomized controlled trial. Ann Intern Med, 130, 389–96.

33. Defronzo RA and Goodman AM, (1995) Multicenter Metformin Study Group. (1995) Efficacy of metformin in patients with non-insulin diabetes mellitus. N Engl J Med, 333, 541–9.

34. Stumvoll M, Nurjhan N, Perriello G, Dailey G and Gerich JE (1995) Metabolic effects of metformin in non-insulin-dependent diabetes mellitus. N Eng J Med, 333, 550–4.

35. Grosskopf I, Ringel Y, Charach G, Maharshak N, Mor R, Iaina A and Weintraub M (1997) Metformin enhances clearance of chylomicrons and chylomicron remnants in nondiabetic mildly

overweight glucose-intolerant subjects. Diabetes Care, 20, 1598–602.

36. Mooradian AD (1996) Drug therapy of non-insulin-dependent diabetes mellitus in the elderly. Drugs, 6, 931–41.

37. Bergman U, Boman G and Wilholm BE (1978) Epidemiology of adverse drug reactions to phenformin and metformin. Br Med J, 2 (6135), 464–6.

38. Stang M, Wysowski DK and Butler- Jones D (1999) Incidence of lactic acidosis in metformin users. Diabetes Care, 22, 925–7.

39. Rabasa-Lhoret R and Chiasson JL (1998) Potential of α-glucosidase inhibitors in elderly patients with diabetes mellitus and impaired glucose tolerance. Drugs and Aging, 13 (2), 131–43.

40. Clissold SP and Edwards C (1988) Acarbose. A preliminary review of its pharmacodynamic and pharmacokinetic properties, and therapeutic potential. Drugs, 35, 214–43.

41. Santeusanio F and Compagnucci P (1994) A risk-benefit appraisal of acarbose in the management of non-insulin-dependent diabetes mellitus. Drug Safety, 11, 432–44.

42. Bayer Corporation (1998) Precose® (acarbose). Prescribing information. Bayer Corporation, West Haven, CT, USA.

43. Deleon MJ, Chandurkar V, Albert SG and Mooradian AD. (2002) Glucagon-like peptide-1 (GLP-1) response to acarbose in elderly type 2 diabetic subjects. Diabetes Research and Clinical Practice, 56, 101–6.

44. Pharmacia and Upjohn 1998. Glyset® (miglitol). Prescribing information. Pharmacia & Upjohn Company, Kalamazoo, MI, USA.

45. Chiasson JL, Josse RG, Hunt JA, Palmason C, Rodger NW, Ross SA, Ryan EA, Tan MH and Wolever TM (1994) The efficacy of acarbose in the treatment of patients with non-insulin dependent diabetes mellitus. A multicenter controlled clinical trial. Ann Intern Med, 121, 928–35.

46. Holman RR, Cull CA and Turner RC (1999) A randomized double-blind trial of acarbose in type 2 diabetes shows improved glycemic control over 3years. (U.K. Prospective Diabetes Study 44). Diabetes Care, 22, 960–4.

47. Mooradian AD, Albert SG, Wittry S, Chehade J, Kim J and Bellrichard B. (2000) Dose-response profile of acarbose in older subjects with Type 2 diabetes. Am. J. Med. Sci., 319, 334–7.

48. Johnston PS, Lebovitz HE and Coniff R (1997) Advantages of monotherapy with alpha-glucosidase inhibitors in elderly NIDDM patients (abstract). Diabetes, 46 (Suppl. 1), 158A.

49. Baron A and Neumann C (1997) PROTECT interim results: A large multicenter study of patients with type II diabetes. Clin Ther, 19, 282–95.

50. Baron A and Neumann C. PROTECT interim results: a large multicenter study of patients with type II diabetes. Precose Resolution of Optimal Titration to Enhance Current Therapies. Clin Ther. 1997; 19 (2): 282–95.

51. Chiasson JL, Josse RJ, Gomis R, Hanefeld M, Karasik A, Laakso M and the STOP-NIDDM TRIAL research group (2003) Acarbose treatment and the risk of cardiovascular disease and hypertension in patients with impaired glucose tolerance: the STOP-NIDDM trial. JAMA, 290(4), 486–94.

52. Johnston PS, Lebovitz HE, Coniff RF, Simonson DC, Raskin P and Munera CL (1998) Advantages of alpha glucosidase inhibition as monotherapy in elderly type 2 diabetic patients. J Clin Endocrinol Metab, 83, 1515–22.

53. Mooradian AD, Thurman JE and Chehade JM (2002) The role of thiazolidinediones in the treatment of patients with type 2 diabetes mellitus. Treat Endocrinol. 1, 13–20.

54. SmithKline Beecham (1999) Avandia (Rosiglitazone) tablets. Prescribing information. Philadelphia, Pennsylvania, USA.

55. Maggs DG, Buchanan TA, Burant CF, Cline G, Gumbiner B, Hsueh WA, Inzucchi S, Kelley D, Nolan J, Olefsky JM, Polonsky KS, Silver D, Valiquett TR and Shulman GI (1998) Metabolic effects of troglitazone monotherapy in Type 2 diabetes mellitus. A randomized double blind placebo controlled trial. Ann Intern Med, 128, 176–85.

56. Godlberg RB, Kendall DM, Deeg MA, Buse JB, Zagar AJ, Pinaire JA, Tan MH, Khan MA, Perez AT, Jacober SJ and the GLAI Study investigators (2005). A comparison of lipid and glycemic effects of pioglitazone and rosiglitazone in patients with type 2 diabetes and dyslipidemia. Diabetes Care, 28 (7), 1547–54.

57. Schnieder R, Egan J and Houser V (1999) Pioglitazone 101 Study Group. Combination therapy with pioglitazone and sulfonylurea in patients with type 2 diabetes. Diabetes, 48 (Suppl. 1), Abstract 458 A106.

58. Gomis R, Jones NP, Vallance SE and Ratwardhan R (1999) Low dose rosiglitazone provides additional glycemic control when combined with sulfonylureas in type 2 diabetes. Diabetes, 48 (Suppl. 1), Poster 266 A63.

59. Promrat K, Lutchman G, Uwaifo GI, Freedman RJ, Soza A, Heller T, Doo E, Ghany M, Premkumar A,

Park Y, Liang TJ, Yanovski JA, Kleiner DE and Hoofnagle JH (2004) A pilot study of pioglitazone treatment for nonalcoholic steatohepatitis. Hepatology, 39 (1), 188–96.

60. Neuschwander-Tetri BA, Brunt EM, Wehmeier KR, Oliver D and Bacon BR (2003) Improved nonalcoholic steatohepatitis after 48 weeks of treatment with the PPAR-gamma ligand rosiglitazone. Hepatology, 38 (4), 1008–17.

61. Nissen SE and Wolski K (2007) Effect of rosiglitazone on the risk of myocardial infarction and death from cardiovascular causes. N Engl J Med, 356, 2457–71.

62. Dormandy JA et al. and the PROactive investigators. Secondary prevention of macrovascular events in patients with type 2 diabetes in the PROactive Study (PROspective pioglitAzone Clinical Trial In macroVascular Events): a randomised controlled trial. Lancet, 2005; 366 (9493): 1279–89.

63. Malaisse WJ. Stimulation of insulin release by non-sulfonylurea hypoglycemic agents: the meglitinide family. Horm Metab Res. 1995; 27 (6): 263–6.

64. Balfour JA and Faulds D (1998) Repaglinide. Drugs and Aging, 13, 173–80.

65. Novo Nordisk (1997) Prandin® (repaglinide). Prescribing information. Novo Nordisk Pharmaceuticals, Princeton, NJ, U.S.A.

66. McLeod JF. Clinical pharmacokinetics of Nateglinide (2004) A rapidly-absorbed, short-acting insulinotropic agent. Clin Pharmacokinet, 43, 97–120.

67. Hatorp V (2002) Clinical pharmacokinetics and pharmacodynamics of repaglinide. Clin Pharmacokinet., 41 (7), 471–83.

68. Marbury TC, Ruckle JL, Hatorp V, Andersen MP, Nielsen KK, Huang WC and Strange P (2000) Pharmacokinetics of repaglinide in subjects with renal impairment. Clin Pharmacol Ther., 67(1), 7–15.

69. Derosa G, Mugellini A, Ciccarelli L, et al. (2003) Comparison between repaglinide and Glimepiride in patients with type 2 diabetes mellitus: a one-year, randomized, double-blind assessment of metabolic parameters and cardiovascular risk factors. Clin Therapeutics, 25, 472–84.

70. Marbury T, Huang WC, Strange P, Lebovitz H (1999) Repaglinide versus glyburide: a one-year comparison trial. Diabetes Res Clin Pract., 43 (3), 155–66.

71. Moses R, Slobodniuk R, Boyages S, Colagiuri S, Kidson W, Carter J, Donnelly T, Moffitt P and Hopkin H (1999) Effect of repaglinide addition to metformin monotherapy on glycemic control in patients with type 2 diabetes. Diabetes Care, 22 (1), 119–24.

72. Fonseca V, Grunberger G, Gupta S, et al. (2003) Addition of Nateglinide to Rosiglitazone monotherapy suppresses mealtime hyperglycemia and improves overall glycemic control. Diabetes Care, 26, 1685–90.

73. Jovanovic L, Hassman DR, Gooch B, et al. (2004) Treatment of type 2 diabetes with a combination regimen of repaglinide plus pioglitazone. Diab Res Clin Pract, 63, 127–34.

74. Tornier B, Marbury TC, Dambso P and Windfield K (1995) A new oral hypoglycemic agent, Repaglinide, minimizes risk of hypoglycemia in well controlled Type 2 diabetic patients. Diabetes, 44 (Suppl. 1), 70A, Abstract.

75. Mooradian AD (1998) Repaglinide: A viewpoint. Drugs and Aging, 13 (2), 181.

76. Elrick H, Stimmler L, Hlad CJ and Arai Y (1964) Plasma insulin response to oral and intravenous glucose administration. J Clin Endocrinol Metab, 24, 1076–82.

77. Holst JJ (1994) Glucagon-like peptide-1 (GLP-1) - a newly discovered gastrointestinal hormone. Gastroenterology, 107, 1848–55.

78. Ørskov C (1992) Glucagon-like peptide-1, a new hormone of the enteroinsular axis. Diabetologia, 35, 701–11.

79. Drucker DJ, Philippe J, Mozsov S, Chick W and Habener JF (1987) Glucagon-like peptide I stimulates insulin gene expression and increases cyclic AMP levels in a rat islet cell line. Proc Natl Acad Sci USA, 84, 3434–8.

80. Göke R, Wagner B, Fehmann HC and Göke B (1993) Glucose-dependency of the insulin stimulatory effect of glucagon-like peptide-1 (7-36) amide on the rat pancreas. Res Exp Med, 193, 97–103.

81. Willms B, Werner J, Holst JJ, Orskov C, Creutzfeldt W and Nauck MA. Gastric emptying, glucose responses, and insulin secretion after a liquid test meal: effects of exogenous glucagon-like peptide-1 (GLP-1)-(7-36) amide in type 2 (noninsulin-dependent) diabetic patients. J Clin Endocrinol Metab. 1996; 81 (1): 327–32.

82. Gutniak MK, Larsson H, Sanders SW, Juneskans O, Holst JJ and Ahrén B (1997) GLP-1 tablet in type 2 diabetes in fasting and postprandial conditions. Diabetes Care, 20 (12), 1874–9.

83. Parkes DG, Pittner R, Jodka C, Smith P and Young A (2001) Insulinotropic actions of exendin-4 and glucagon-like peptide-1 in vivo and in vitro. Metabolism, 50 (5), 583–9.

84. Amylin Pharmaceuticals 2005. Byetta (package insert). Amylin, San Diego, CA.

85. DeFronzo RA, Ratner RE, Han J, Kim DD, Fineman MS and Baron AD (2005) Effects of exenatide (exendin-4) on glycemic control and weight over 30

weeks in metformin-treated patients with type 2 diabetes. Diabetes Care, 28 (5), 1092–100.

86. Buse JB, Henry RR, Han J, Kim DD, Fineman MS, Baron AD and the Exenatide 113 Clinical Study Group (2004) Effects of exenatide (exendin-4) on glycemic control over 30 weeks in sulfonylurea-treated patients with type 2 diabetes. Diabetes Care, 27 (11), 2628–35.

87. Kendall DM, Riddle MC, Rosenstock J, Zhuang D, Kim DD, Fineman MS and Baron AD (2005) Effects of exenatide (exendin-4) on glycemic control over 30 weeks in patients with type 2 diabetes treated with metformin and a sulfonylurea. Diabetes Care, 28 (5), 1083–91.

88. Klonoff DC, Buse JB, Nielsen LL, Guan X, Bowlus CL, Holcombe JH, Wintle ME and Maggs DG. Exenatide effects on diabetes, obesity, cardiovascular risk factors and hepatic biomarkers in patients with type 2 diabetes treated for at least 3years. Curr Med Res Opin. 2008; 24 (1): 275–86.

89. Mentlein R (1999) Dipeptidyl-peptidase IV (CD-26)-role in the inactivation of regulatory peptides. Regul Pept, 85, 9–24.

90. Drucker DJ and Nauck MA (2006) The incretin system: glucagon-like peptide-1 receptor agonists and dipeptidyl peptidase-4 inhibitors in type 2 diabetes. Lancet, 368 (9548), 1696–705.

91. Nauck MA, Meininger G, Sheng D, Teranella L, Stein P for the Sitagliptin Study Group (2007) Efficacy and safety of the dipeptidyl peptidase-4 inhibitor, sitagliptin, compared with the sulfonylurea, glipizide, in patients with type 2 diabetes inadequately controlled on metformin alone: a randomized, double-blind, non-inferiority trial. Diabetes Obes Metab. 2, 194–205.

92. Amori RE, Lau J and Pittas AG (2007) Efficacy and safety of incretin therapy in type 2 diabetes: systematic review and meta-analysis. Lancet, 298 (2), 194–206.

93. Cooper GJS, Willis AC, Clark A, Turner RC, Sim RB and Reid KB (1987) Purification and characterization of a peptide from amyloid-rich pancreas of type 2 diabetic patients. Proc Natl Acad Sci USA, 84, 8628–32.

94. Inoue K, Hisatomi A, Umeda F and Nawata H (1991) Release of amylin from perfused rat pancreas in response to glucose, arginine, beta-hydroxybutyrate, and gliclazide. Diabetes, 40, 1005–9.

95. Koda JE, Fineman M, Rink TJ, Dailey GE, Muchmore DB and Linarelli LG (1992) Amylin concentrations and glucose control. Lancet, 339 (8802), 1179–80.

96. Ludvik B, Lell B, Hartter E, Schnack C and Prager R (1991) Decrease of stimulated amylin release precedes

impairment of insulin secretion in Type II diabetes. Diabetes, 40, 1615–19.

97. Fineman MS, Giotta MP, Thompson RG, Kolterman OG and Koda JE (1996) Amylin response following Sustacal ingestion is diminished in type II diabetic patients treated with insulin. Diabetologia, 39 (Suppl. 1), A149, Abstract.

98. Kolterman OG, Gottlieb A, Moyses C, Colburn W. Reduction of postprandial hyperglycemia in subjects with IDDM by intravenous infusion of AC137, a human amylin analogue. Diabetes Care 1995; 18 (8): 1179–82.

99. Gedulin BR, Rink TJ and Young AA (1997) Dose-response for glucagonostatic effect of amylin in rats. Metabolism, 46, 67–70.

100. Thompson RG, Gottlieb A, Organ K, Koda J, Kisicki J, Kolterman OG. Pramlintide: a human amylin analogue reduced postprandial plasma glucose, insulin, and C-peptide concentrations in patients with type 2 diabetes. Diabet Med. 1997; 14 (7): 547–55.

101. Thompson RG, Pearson L, Schoenfeld S and Kolterman OG (1998) The Pramlintide in Type 2 Diabetes Group. Pramlintide, a synthetic analog of human amylin, improves the metabolic profile of patients with type 2 diabetes using insulin. Diabetes Care, 21 (6), 987–93.

102. Hollander PA, Levy P, Fineman MS, Maggs DG, Shen LZ, Strobel SA, Weyer C and Kolterman OG (2003) Pramlintide as an adjunct to insulin therapy improves long-term glycemic and weight control in patients with type 2 diabetes: a 1-year randomized controlled trial. Diabetes Care, 26 (3), 784–90.

103. Ratner RE, Dickey R, Fineman MS, Maggs DG, Shen LZ, Strobel SA, Weyer C and Kolterman OG (2004) Amylin replacement with pramlintide as an adjunct to insulin therapy improves long-term glycaemic and weight control in Type 1 diabetes mellitus: a 1-year, randomized controlled trial. Diabet Med., 21 (11), 1204–12.

104. Holleman F and Hoekstra JB (1997) Insulin Lispro. N. Engl. J. Med., 337, 176–83.

105. Anderson JH, Jr, Brunelle RL, Keohane P, Koivisto VA, Trautmann ME, Vignati L and DiMarchi R (1997) Mealtime treatment with insulin analog improves postprandial hyperglycemia and hypoglycemia in patients with non-insulin-dependent diabetes mellitus. Arch Intern Med, 157, 1249–55.

106. Anderson JH, Jr, Brunelle RL, Koivisto VA, Pfutzner A, Trautmann ME, Vignati L and Dimarchi R (1997) Reduction of postprandial hyperglycemia and frequency of hypoglycemia in IDDM patients on insulin-analog treatment. Diabetes, 46, 265–70.

107. Simpson KL and Spencer CM (1999) Insulin Aspart. Drugs, 57 (5), 759–65.

108. Oiknine R, Bernbaum M and Mooradian AD. (2005) A critical appraisal of the role of insulin analogues in the management of diabetes. Drugs, 65 (3), 325–40.

109. Becker RH (2007) Insulin glulisine complementing basal insulins: a review of structure and activity. Diabetes Technol Ther, 9 (1), 109–21.

110. Pfizer (2006) EXUBERA® (insulin human [rDNA origin]). Inhalation Powder US Package Insert.

111. Skyler JS, Jovanovic L, Sol Klioze S, Reis J, Duggan W, for the Inhaled Human Insulin Type 1 Diabetes Study Group (2007) Two-year safety and efficacy of inhaled human insulin (Exubera) in adult patients with type 1 diabetes. Diabetes Care, 30, 579–85.

112. Roach P, Yue L and Arora V (1999) Improved postprandial glycemic control during treatment with Humalog M; a novel protamine-based insulin lispro formulation. Humalog Mix25 Study. Diabetes Care, 22, 1258–61.

113. Sanofi-Aventis (2000) Lantus® (insulin glargine [rDNA origin] injection). Prescribing information. Sanofi-Aventis, Bridgewater, NJ, USA

114. Mooradian AD, Bernbaum M and Albert SG (2006) A narrative review: a rational approach to starting insulin therapy. Annal Intern Med, 145 (2), 125–34.

115. Novo Nordisk (2005) Levemir (insulin detemir [rDNA origin] injection). Package insert, Novo Nordisk, Princeton, NJ.

116. Mooradian AD, Kalis J and Nugent CA (1990) The nutritional status of ambulatory elderly type II diabetic patients. Age, 13, 87–9.

117. Reed RL and Mooradian AD (1990) Nutritional status and dietary management of elderly diabetic patients. Clin Geriatr Med, 6, 883–901.

118. Chehade JM and Mooradian AD (2000) A rational approach to drug therapy of type 2 diabetes mellitus. Drugs, 60, 95–113.

18

Insulin Therapy

Dennis Yue and Marg McGill

Diabetes Centre, Royal Prince Alfred Hospital, Camperdown, NSW, Australia

Key messages

- Insulin therapy may be required at some stage in up to 30% of older people, and is usually prescribed to optimize metabolic control.
- Insulin regimens used in younger patients are equally applicable to the elderly, although in rather frail or highly dependent patients, the regimen is usually once-daily insulin plus or minus tablet therapy.
- Starting insulin therapy in older people requires the consideration of several patient-related factors, the likelihood of carer involvement, and the agreed goals of treatment.

18.1   Introduction

Diabetes is a condition that becomes more prevalent with age and, indeed, is one of the most common chronic diseases of elderly people [1]. It is inevitable therefore that, as the population ages, the number of older people with diabetes will increase. Most people with diabetes have the type 2 condition, and almost half of all persons known to have type 2 diabetes are aged >65 years [2]. Occasionally, type 1 diabetes can appear for the first time in the elderly and, with better general medical care, many patients with type 1 diabetes survive more than 50–60 years with the condition [3]. However, these scenarios are rare, and in the context of starting insulin therapy, type 2 diabetes comprises the majority of patients encountered. Such patients will usually provide a history of having diabetes for more than a few years and then gradually losing their responsiveness to oral hypoglycaemic agents, which is now known to be a consequence of the inevitable decline in pancreatic beta-cell function. This profile is so characteristic that, from a clinical perspective, if an elderly patient has a short duration of diabetes and then rapidly becomes insulin requiring, one should consider the presence of an underlying pancreatic carcinoma causing insulin deficiency.

There is a general consensus worldwide that insulin therapy is not used early or often enough in the treatment of diabetes. Many young patients languish for years on supra-maximal dosages of oral hypoglycaemic agents whilst hyperglycaemia insidiously but unrelentingly causes tissue damage and complications. The failure to introduce insulin therapy sufficiently early is, in many countries, due to lack of resources, but in others it is due to inappropriate and entrenched attitudes of health professionals and people with diabetes, alike. Obviously, such factors affecting the use of insulin in a particular country would also impact on the use of insulin therapy in the elderly in the community. However, some other factors may also play a role, in that the use of insulin in the elderly can vary considerably in many developed countries of similar health care standards [4]. For example, in the United States insulin therapy is used in up to 25% of elderly people with diabetes, whereas in a population-based cohort of persons aged ≥65 years in France, insulin was found to be used by only 6.5% of such patients [5]. In contrast,

Diabetes in Old Age. Third Edition. Edited by Alan J. Sinclair
© 2009 John Wiley & Sons, Ltd

in United Kingdom nursing homes insulin was found to be used in 25–47% of elderly people with type 2 diabetes [6].

In younger diabetic individuals whose glycaemic control is not adequately achieved after an appropriate period of treatment with dietary measures and oral medications, the introduction of insulin therapy is almost always indicated and correct. This has the proven benefit of reducing the development and severity of chronic diabetic complications, this being a matter of great importance not only to the individuals but also to the nation from a health economics point of view. In the elderly, however, the same is not always true. Elderly patients can be unnecessarily commenced on insulin therapy, causing inconvenience to the person and his/her family, with little possibility of improving health outcomes. Furthermore, as tight glycaemic control is often associated with an increased risk of severe hypoglycaemia in the elderly, this can have serious consequences such as precipitating a fall with fractures, or exacerbating ischaemic heart disease. It is noteworthy that the median age of patients with severe hypoglycaemia in Sweden was 75 years, and 21% of these were aged >85 years, with an overall fatality rate of 20% [7]. On the other hand, elderly patients, even more than their younger counterparts, are often denied insulin therapy because of their age alone [6]. Thus, when – and how – to start elderly patients on insulin therapy is an important issue for which there is relatively little evidence-based data to guide the clinicians. Rather, they must instead rely on their commonsense and clinical skills, not only as a health care provider but often also as a psychologist and a social worker. In the following section, we provide a perspective on what are becoming increasingly common issues in the practical care of the elderly person with diabetes.

18.2 What glycaemic threshold should trigger insulin therapy in the elderly?

The American Geriatric Society has published guidelines regarding glucose control for older ambulatory adults with diabetes [8]. These guidelines acknowledged the possible risks associated with tight glycaemic control, and therefore suggested a modified HbA_{1c} goal of <8%. Conceptually, this needs to be modified according to the status of microvascular complications and life expectancy. On this basis, the

US Veterans Health Administration guidelines suggest aiming for a HbA_{1c} of:

- <7% if the person's predicted lifespan is ≥15 years, and there are no microvascular complications; or ≥10 years if early to moderate microvascular complications are present.
- <8% if the life span is 5–15 years if no microvascular complications are present, or 5–10 years if early to moderate microvascular complications are present.
- <9% if the lifespan is thought to be <5 years, with or without microvascular complications.

Implicit in these guidelines is the fact that glycaemic goals should be individualized to the specific circumstances of the elderly, balancing the need to prevent microvascular complications against life expectancy, largely governed by comorbidities such as stroke, cancer and severe heart failure [9], all of which are less amenable to the benefits of tight glycaemic control. In this regard, the duration of diabetes should also be taken into consideration in making this decision. It is true that many patients have hyperglycaemia well before being discovered to have diabetes, and thus may have microvascular complications soon after presentation. However, by and large the development of microvascular complications is still a function of known duration of diabetes. Therefore, the risk of developing severe microvascular complications in a patient diagnosed in their 70s or 80s is not high, provided that they do not already have evidence of complications at presentation. These individuals can afford to have glycaemic targets that are less tight compared to a person who has been diagnosed for many years and is now in their 70s, or older.

18.3 Other indications for insulin therapy in the elderly

It is important to recognize that the application of the above guidelines should be completely over-ridden by any need to use insulin therapy to control hyperglycaemic symptoms and infection. If an elderly person is experiencing distressing thirst, nocturia and either skin, vaginal or penile monilial infection, then insulin therapy is indicated irrespective of the patient's age or life expectancy [10]. Elderly patients often do not volunteer these symptoms. Questions such as "Do you have to get up at night to go to the toilet?", "Is it worse than last year?" and "Do you have any itch in your front passage?" are simple tools which cannot be readily replaced by investigations, and the response would greatly influence our decision to implement insulin therapy. Other clinical parameters that can be added to this list include tiredness, poorer general health and weight loss. Whilst the first two are harder to quantify, a well-documented weight loss of several kilograms is an important sign indicative of insulin deficiency and the need to commence insulin therapy, provided that other causes seem unlikely.

In assessing elderly people's symptoms and well-being with regards to insulin therapy, it is worth bearing in mind the findings of Berger *et al.* [11]. In this study, 15 elderly people with type 2 diabetes and a fasting blood glucose (FBG) level of >9 mmol l^{-1} all claimed to feel well and to be asymptomatic, but agreed to start insulin therapy. Over the 8 months of the study period there was a significant fall in HbA$_{1c}$, and at the end of the study only two people wished to return to tablet therapy. The authors concluded that 'asymptomatic' hyperglycaemia in elderly people is often associated with a reduced well being which can only be unmasked by a trial of insulin.

The elderly are more likely to have medical comorbidities, such as renal disease and heart failure, which may preclude the use of other glucose-lowering medications. Metformin is contraindicated in persons with compromised renal function [12], and it is generally recommended that the administration of this agent is ceased in those individuals with an estimated glomerular filtration rate (GFR) of <40 ml min^{-1}. A study by Beebe and Patel [13] showed that the glitazones functioned well in the elderly, although significant fluid retention with a worsening of previously compensated or unrecognized heart failure is a well-known problem in this age group. Moreover, as a general principle, considering the recent information regarding the use of glitazones in those with ischaemic heart disease, the glitazones probably should be used with caution, and not as first line agents in the elderly. The glitazones have also been shown to increase peripheral fractures and to reduce bone density, and for this reason are also not preferred agents in the elderly. In elderly patients the potent long-acting sulphonylurea glibenclamide has the potential to cause hypoglycaemia which is severe, persistent, resistant to treatment, and not infrequently results in death or permanent disability. Among this group of susceptible elderly patients, insulin represents a safer therapeutic alternative than glibenclamide.

A variety of data, albeit limited, has demonstrated that those being cared for in nursing homes often do not receive care of an adequate standard. As a consequence, many people unnecessarily live with elevated blood glucose levels that interfere with their quality of life and make them more susceptible to infection and coma. One of the reasons for this may be the lack of nursing staff in some institutions, which makes the delivery of insulin injections problematic when the majority of staff are care assistants. A further contributor to the situation is the staff's fear of hypoglycaemia due to the unreliable eating pattern of some elderly people. However, the nursing home person is more likely to suffer from episodes of non-ketotic hyperosmolar coma, often triggered by an infection such as a foot infection or urinary tract infection. Thus, the judicious use of insulin therapy in elderly persons at risk of these complications is warranted. As a consequence of this situation, individuals living in nursing homes and residential care require a structured care plan with regular reviews of both the goals of treatment and the educational needs of the formal carers.

18.4 Some of special considerations of elderly people and insulin therapy

Cognitive dysfunction is common in the elderly, and individuals with diabetes are not exempt from this. Whilst some studies have demonstrated the level of dysfunction correlates with degree of hyperglycaemia [14] the correction of hyperglycaemia generally only has, at most, marginal effects on improving the situation. So, the assessment of mental capacity is not so much to determine if insulin is indicated but rather to evaluate to what extent a person can cope with insulin therapy without assistance.

Elderly people are often more frail, and an assessment of their physical function is also essential. Whilst most current insulin delivery devices appear simple to use, they still require a certain level of manual dexterity. Nevertheless, studies have generally found that prefilled insulin pens are well accepted and used effectively by elderly patients [15]. An assessment of vision is also required to ensure that an elderly person can administer the correct insulin dosage. About one-third of elderly people with diabetes have some degree of visual disability, often due to cataract, glaucoma or macular degeneration rather than to retinopathy [16]. Hence, the use of a device that 'clicks', so that the number of units of insulin dialled up for delivery can be heard and counted, would be necessary in some cases.

Before commencing an older person on insulin therapy, apart from a mental and physical assessment (as described above), a thorough history of their social situation should also be taken. Typical questions asked would include "Who lives at home with you?"; "Do you cook for yourself?"; and "Does someone visit you regularly?". The replies will help to provide important information about the particular individual, such as how great is the risk of hypoglycaemia, what is the best time for the insulin to be administered and, indeed, if insulin is needed at all.

Often, it is the clinician who feels that the elderly person may have a fear of injections, and so is reluctant to broach the subject. However this is rarely the case if the situation is handled sensitively and not used as a threat. All people with type 2 diabetes should be advised early during the course of their disease that the natural history of diabetes is such that approximately 50% will require insulin after about 5 years [17, 18]. In this way, they will realize that the need to receive insulin therapy is often inevitable, and is not their 'fault'. It is often also helpful to ask the patient if they know anyone else who takes insulin therapy, as this can influence their acceptance or, not, of such treatment. It is also a good opportunity to dispel the myths and misconceptions related to insulin therapy; an example is that "...my father had an amputation after he went onto insulin".

One practical tip used in the authors' Diabetes Centre is that, whenever the subject of insulin therapy is first raised, the person is assisted in giving themselves a practice injection. In this way they realize the needle does not hurt, the insulin is simple to administer, and they leave the consultation feeling that they are capable of commencing such therapy. Having their anxieties allayed also means that a patient will be more likely to accept insulin therapy!

18.5   Glucose-lowering medications and the introduction of insulin therapy

Today, it is standard practice – not only in the elderly but virtually for all patients – to start insulin therapy but to maintain the same oral glucose-lowering medications, at least for the first year of insulin therapy.

The question of whether combined oral drug and insulin treatment provides a better glycaemic control than insulin alone has been examined extensively. Yet, this is in a sense a meaningless question, because the answer would depend on how much insulin was used. Although the oral agents have 'failed' in the situation of 'secondary failure', they are still exerting considerable effects in lowering glucose levels. Clinical studies have shown that if either sulphonylurea or metformin is stopped, then each would need to be replaced by an extra 20–30 units of insulin per day. In other words, if sulphonylurea and metformin at maximum dosage are stopped, the insulin dosage would generally need to exceed about 40–60 units per day before any significant improvement in glycaemic control would occur. All too commonly, a deterioration in glycaemic control has been witnessed when both oral drugs were stopped and not replaced with sufficient insulin. An insulin-only therapy would require a more complicated regimen and a more rapid titration schedule, making the process of beginning insulin treatment much more difficult, as it would involve more clinic visits and a higher risk of hypoglycaemia. Whilst applicable to all age groups, this would create particular difficulties for the elderly.

It is, however, quite common to modify the oral agent regimen in the following situations:

• If the person is taking a supra-maximal dosage of any oral drugs, it is reduced to what is recommended in the product information.

• If the person is suffering from the gastrointestinal adverse effects of metformin, it is reduced to a dosage which is tolerated.

• If the person is taking a third glucose-lowering medication, such as acarbose or a glitazone, this would be stopped. In the case of acarbose, this would be because of the drug's relatively weak action and inconvenient side effect of flatulence. In the case of a glitazone, it would be because of potentially serious side effects in the face of a presumed lack of great efficacy (otherwise, insulin therapy would not be required).

• If the person chooses to have more insulin injections and at a higher dosage (which, in our experience, is a rare situation).

Generally, it is easier to persuade patients to undertake combined oral drugs and insulin treatment. They are often comforted by the knowledge that this allows them to take insulin only once a day, in the privacy of their own home, and without a great deal of disturbance to their daytime routine. It is also a gentle way of easing them into insulin therapy. When they are familiar with insulin injections they will be more accepting if a second injection were to be required.

Occasionally, patients develop frequent daytime hypoglycaemia on combined treatment. When this happens, the sulphonylurea dosage should be reduced or ceased if necessary. Apart from this, and in the absence of any contraindications (e.g. renal failure or allergy), there is no good evidence to indicate that glucose-lowering medications must be stopped at any stage. In fact, the current policy is to continue them while the glycaemic control remains satisfactory, albeit at a reduced dosage if the patient has renal or cardiac comorbidities. Some patients may wish to reduce the number of tablets they take each day, especially if they are receiving multiple medications for blood pressure and lipid control. There is no problem in reducing one or more of the oral hypoglycaemic drugs when the patient has been established on insulin therapy, but it is essential that the insulin dose is titrated.

18.6 Which insulin regimen should be used in the elderly?

Bearing in mind the above considerations, the most commonly used insulin regimen is to introduce a long-acting insulin before bedtime, while maintaining oral agent treatment. The starting dose should be low; 10 units would normally be a reasonable starting point. As insulin is an 'additional' treatment, the patient's condition will not deteriorate and usually will start to improve from that point onward. If the patient is very nervous or reluctant, and it is imperative to minimize the risk of hypoglycaemia – however small – then an even lower insulin dosage can be used to start the process and to gain the patient's confidence.

With regards to the choice of insulin, until recently an isophane type of insulin has normally been used. The availability of long-acting insulin analogues such as Lantus and Levemir has today made them quite popular choices [19], mainly because they have the advantage of longer and flatter actions. Consequently, they are less likely to cause hypoglycaemia and more likely to require only one injection a day. Their pharmacokinetic properties also make less important the timing of their injection and relationship to meal times. For example, if an elderly person needs to have insulin administered by a relative or a nurse who can only visit at mid-morning tea, it is perfectly safe for the patient to maintain their existing meal schedule and to have the insulin injected before or after morning tea. Provided that the injections are given at about the same time each day, the precise relationship to meals is not of great concern. On this basis, if cost is not a consideration, the use of a long-acting insulin analogue would be recommended over a conventional isophane insulin. It is important that the premixed insulins should not be administered just before bed time, as their short-acting component would most likely cause nocturnal hypoglycaemia. On the other hand, the main food intake of some patients – including some elderly people – is a major meal in the evening. This may be a lifetime habit which is difficult to break, or it may be necessary because this is the only time that family members can gather for a meal. In this situation, there is often a large postprandial hyperglycaemic peak in the evening. Under such circumstances, a premixed insulin given before dinner is a good alternative of providing both post-prandial and basal insulin supplies [20]. For this, the type of premixed insulin which contains a short-acting insulin analogue is favoured, because its rapid onset and shorter action profile is best for controlling post-prandial hyperglycaemia, with less risk of causing nocturnal hypoglycaemia.

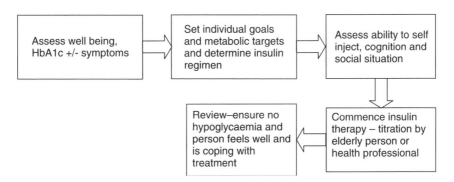

18.7 Titrating the insulin dosage and monitoring progress

A major feature of combination therapy is that insulin is added to an existing treatment. Glycaemic control should therefore improve immediately and, for practical purposes, should not deteriorate. This means that the dose of insulin can be increased slowly, minimizing the risk of hypoglycaemia. A titration regimen previously described suggests increasing the insulin dosage by 4 units per day if the FBG exceeded $8 \, \text{mmol} \, l^{-1}$ on three consecutive days, and by 2 units per day if it exceeded $6 \, \text{mmol} \, l^{-1}$. Depending on the patients, this can sometimes be implemented directly by the patients or assisted by health professionals after discussing the blood glucose-monitoring results by telephone. In the elderly, such a titration can be made slightly more slowly, such as every 1–2 weeks. This slower pace will help to gain the person's confidence and reduce the risk of hypoglycaemia. In accordance with the philosophy that, in elderly people, it is not always necessary – or indeed desirable – to aim for excellent glycaemic control, a less ambitious FBG target is sometimes used. For patients in their seventh decade of life, the aim is to achieve a FBG of $7 \, \text{mmol} \, l^{-1}$, while for those in their eighth decade the target is $8 \, \text{mmol} \, l^{-1}$, and so forth.

After 2–3 months, the patient is likely to be receiving about 20–30 units of insulin each day, together with maximum oral drug therapy. Measurement of the HbA_{1c} concentration after this interval helps to quantify the overall level of glycaemic control, such that further increases in insulin dosage can be made accordingly. There is often a reduction in HbA_{1c} of up to 2% and an increase in body weight of several kilograms. If these changes are not evident, then the possibility should be considered that the patient has not been taking the insulin regularly, or that somebody unfamiliar with the regimen has either reduced or stopped one or more of the oral hypoglycaemic drugs. At any time, if a patient is noticing significant hypoglycaemia, the sulphonylurea and then the insulin dosage should be reduced.

18.8 What should patients be told on the day they start insulin?

Although everyone has different educational needs and capacities to learn, the comprehensive information provided when starting insulin may confuse elderly patients – and, for that matter, many young patients! If the patients are overloaded with information on a stressful day such as this, they may not remember the more important messages, and indeed some may even be scared away from insulin treatment altogether. The best practice is to concentrate on teaching the patient or carer how, and when, to inject the insulin subcutaneously into the abdomen, using injection devices which are extremely user-friendly, such that the technique can be taught in a matter of minutes. The day of starting insulin therapy is also not an ideal time for detailed dietary advice. The current practice is to emphasize only the need to have regular meals and snacks (including one before bed) containing carbohydrates. In fact, the patients are often told that "nothing else needs to change", and experience suggests that both patients and relatives derive considerable comfort and reassurance from this approach.

At this stage of diabetes, most patients would be familiar with glucose monitoring and should be asked to perform the task [21]. As the adjustment of insulin dosage in this regimen is primarily dependent on the morning FBG concentrations, testing at this time point is the first priority and should be included every day. For some elderly patients who cannot test their blood glucose, it may be necessary to commence insulin without such monitoring, and to rely on blood glucose monitoring at the doctor's surgery, at the same time measuring HbA_{1c} concentrations and assessing symptoms to make dose adjustments.

Hypoglycaemia is the only risk in starting insulin therapy, and however much such a risk is minimized, it cannot be completely eliminated [22]. How much information should be provided to patients – especially the elderly ones – is a difficult question. Too much detail would incur the risk of scaring a reluctant patient away from the correct treatment, but not enough information would open the door to negligence. This dilemma is, of course, not unique to commencing insulin, and each doctor must make a decision with an individual patient. It is reassuring that, in patients with type 2 diabetes, hypoglycaemia due to insulin is usually less severe.

When possible, the patient should also be seen a few days after starting insulin therapy in order to review their injection technique. If this is satisfactory, then the stabilization of glycaemic control can be achieved by telephone or e-mail communication every few days, until the target blood glucose levels are achieved. In

Table 18.1 Clinical data acquired from patients with type 2 diabetes (n = 493) who attended the authors' Diabetes Centre, and were commenced on insulin therapy.

Parameter	Age of patients	
	<60 years (n = 218)	≥60 years (n = 275)
Duration of diabetes at start of insulin therapy (years)	8.1 (6.3–11.4)	12.0 (8.2–16.2)
Insulin dosage on once-daily injection (units)	23 (20–33)	20 (14–25)
Change in HbA$_{1c}$ (%) from start of insulin therapy to first review	−0.3 (−1.4−0.6)	−0.4 (−1.0−0.3)
Time between once- and twice- daily injections (years)	2.0 (1.2–3.8)	2.2 (1.3–3.7)
No. of injections (%)		
1	61	59
2	31	36
≥3	8	5
Hypoglycaemia reported at last visit (%)	1.8	2.9

this situation a family member or friend is invaluable in assisting with communication, and it is normally suggested that such a companion attend at least the first visit, if at all possible.

18.9 When should more complex insulin regimens be introduced?

After a couple of years on a single insulin injection, a second injection – usually given in the morning before breakfast – may need to be introduced, depending on the subject's age and well-being. In this situation, a small starting dose of medium-acting insulin or a premixed insulin in the order of 6–12 units would be reasonable [23]. Based on experience, patients normally accept additional insulin injections much more readily than the first one, having realized that the injection is not a major difficulty. Occasionally, elderly individuals may adapt quite well to use of a basal bolus regimen, and in some cases also to insulin pump therapy [24].

18.10 Favourable outcomes

According to a computerized database, elderly people respond to insulin therapy in a similar manner to their younger counterparts. Between 2003 and 2006, a total of 493 individuals with type 2 diabetes attending

the present authors' Diabetes Centre were commenced on insulin therapy (see Table 18.1). Of these, 275 individuals were aged >60 years.

The goal of treatment in elderly patients is to optimize glycaemic control to an extent consistent with the avoidance of hypoglycaemia and the prevention of acute complications. Age-related physiological changes, life expectancy and comorbidities will influence the type of treatment implemented. Consequently, the management plan should be individualized so as to ensure that the elderly person enjoys a balance between quality of life and the diabetes regimen. In this, the 'art' of medicine will prevail, even more than the 'science' of medicine.

References

1. DeFronzo, R.A. (1988) Pathogenesis of type 2 diabetes mellitus. *Medical Clinics of North America*, 88, 787–835.
2. Gossain, V.V., Carella, M.J. and Rovner, D.R. (1994) Management of diabetes in the elderly: a clinical perspective. *Journal of the Association for Academic Minority Physicians*, 5, 22–31.
3. Gambert, S.R. (1990) Atypical presentation of diabetes mellitus in the elderly. *Clinics in Geriatric Medicine*, 6, 721–9.
4. Rosenstock, J. (2001a) Insulin therapy: optimizing control in type 1 and type 2 diabetes. *Clinical Cornerstone*, 4, 50–64.

5. Bourdel-Marchasson, I., Dubroca, B., Manciet, G., De-camps, A., Emeriau, J. P. and Dartigues, J.F. (1997) Prevalence of diabetes and effect on quality of life in older French living in the community: the PAQUID Epidemiological Survey. *Journal of the American Geriatrics Society*, 45, 295–301.

6. Hendra, T.J. (2002) Starting insulin therapy in elderly patients. *Journal of the Royal Society of Medicine*, 95, 453–5.

7. Gale, E.A., Dornan, T.L. and Tattersall, R.B. (1981) Severely uncontrolled diabetes in the over-fifties. *Diabetologia*, 21, 25–8.

8. Brown, A.F., Mangione, C.M., Saliba, D., Sarkisian, C.A. and the California Healthcare Foundation/American Geriatrics Society Panel on Improving Care for Elders with diabetes. (2003) Guidelines for improving the care of the older person with diabetes mellitus. *Journal of the American Geriatrics Society*, 51, S265–80.

9. Meneilly, G.S. and Tessier, D. (2001) Diabetes in elderly adults. [see comment]. *Journals of Gerontology Series A – Biological Sciences and Medical Sciences*, 56, M5–13.

10. Singh, I. and Marshall, M.C., Jr (1995) Diabetes mellitus in the elderly. *Endocrinology and Metabolism Clinics of North America*, 24, 255–72.

11. Berger W. (1988) Insulin therapy in the elderly type 2 diabetic patient. *Diabetes Res Clin Pract* 4 (Suppl), 124–8.

12. Cusi, K., Consoli, A. and Defronzo, R. A. (1996) Metabolic effects of metformin on glucose and lactate metabolism in noninsulin-dependent diabetes mellitus. *Journal of Clinical Endocrinology and Metabolism*, 81, 4059–67.

13. Beebe, K. and Patel, J. (2003) Rosiglitazone is effective and well tolerated in patients >65 years with type 2 diabetes [abstract]. *Diabetes* 99; 42 (Suppl. 1), A111.

14. Reaven GM, Thompson LW, Nahum D and Haskins E. (1990) Relationship between hyperglycemia and cognitive function in older NIDDM patients. *Diabetes Care*, 13(1), 16–21.

15. Coscelli, C., Lostia, S., Lunetta, M., Nosari, I. and Coronel, G. A. (1995) Safety, efficacy, acceptability of a pre-filled insulin pen in diabetic patients over 60 years old. *Diabetes Research & Clinical Practice*, 28, 173–7.

16. Klein, R. (1991) Age-related eye disease, visual impairment, and driving in the elderly. *Human Factors*, 33, 521–5.

17. Matthews, D.R., Cull, C.A., Stratton, I.M., Holman, R.R. and Turner, R.C. (1998) UKPDS 26: Sulphonylurea failure in non-insulin-dependent diabetic patients over six years. UK Prospective Diabetes Study (UKPDS) Group. *Diabetic Medicine*, 15, 297–303.

18. Sinclair, A.J. and Meneilly, G.S. (2000) Re-thinking metabolic strategies for older people with type 2 diabetes mellitus: implications of the UK Prospective Diabetes Study and other recent studies. *Age & Ageing*, 29, 393–7.

19. Rosenstock, J., Schwartz, S.L., Clark, C.M., Jr, Park, G.D., Donley, D.W. and Edwards, M.B. (2001) Basal insulin therapy in type 2 diabetes: 28-week comparison of insulin glargine (HOE 901) and NPH insulin. *Diabetes Care*, 24, 631–6.

20. Coscelli, C., Calabrese, G., Fedele, D., Pisu, E., Calderini, C., Bistoni, S., Lapolla, A., Mauri, M.G., Rossi, A. and Zappella, A. (1992) Use of premixed insulin among the elderly. Reduction of errors in patient preparation of mixtures. *Diabetes Care*, 15, 1628–30.

21. Skyler, J.S. (1997) Glucose control in type 2 diabetes mellitus. *Annals of Internal Medicine*, 127, 837–9.

22. Rosenstock, J. (2001) Management of type 2 diabetes mellitus in the elderly: special considerations. *Drugs & Aging*, 18, 31–44.

23. Turner, H.E. and Matthews, D.R. (2000) The use of fixed-mixture insulins in clinical practice. *European Journal of Clinical Pharmacology*, 56, 19–25.

24. Rizvi AA. (2002) Benefits of insulin pump therapy in the elderly. *Geriatric Times* 3 (4), 23–30.

19

Treatment of Hypertension

Peter Fasching

5th Medical Department, Wilhelminenspital, Vienna, Austria

Key Messages

- Hypertension is the commonest complication associated with diabetes mellitus. A large proportion of older patients may have unsatisfactory blood pressure levels, despite treatment.
- Treatment of hypertension can be effective in substantially reducing cardiovascular risk, stroke rate and death.
- A general blood pressure target is 140/80 mmHg or less in patients with diabetes, but much lower levels should be aimed for in those able to tolerate therapy.
- Treatment of hypertension in patients with diabetes should include an ACE inhibitor or angiotensin-receptor blocker.

19.1   Introduction

According to the results of recently published studies, hypertension (with a prevalence of 66%) is the most frequent comorbidity in type-2 diabetic patients aged >65 years [1]. Adequate diabetic management and prevention of cardiovascular complications are regarded as crucial for controlling health care costs in this group of patients. On the other hand, a recent survey showed that 73% of male diabetic patients with a mean age of 66 years had a blood pressure >140/90 mmHg and received less intensive antihypertensive medication therapy than patients without diabetes [2].

19.2   Risk assessment from observational studies

In a meta-analysis of 61 prospective observational studies of blood pressure and mortality which included 9 58 074 participants and an analysis of 12.7 million person-years at risk, it was shown that within each decade of age a proportional benefit of a low blood pressure down to 115 mmHg systolic blood pressure (SBP) and 75 mmHg diastolic blood pressure (DBP), was evident [3]. At the age of 40–69 years, each reduction of 20 mmHg SBP (or, approximately equivalently, of 10 mmHg usual DBP) is associated with more than a twofold lowering of the death rate from stroke, and with a twofold lowering of death rates from ischaemic heart disease and other vascular causes. Whilst all of these proportional reductions in vascular mortality are only about a half in persons aged 80–89 years when compared with subjects aged 40–49 years, the annual absolute difference in risk is greater in old age. For predicting vascular mortality from a single blood pressure measurement, the average of SBP and DBP is slightly more informative than either alone, and pulse pressure is much less informative. Yet, the number of included diabetic patients is not specified in the report. In contrast, smaller epidemiological studies have shown that in men aged ≥85 years, a higher systolic blood pressure is associated with a better survival [4, 5].

Diabetes in Old Age. Third Edition. Edited by Alan J. Sinclair
© 2009 John Wiley & Sons, Ltd

Table 19.1 Indications for initial treatment and goals for adult hypertensive diabetic patients, according to ADA (2008).

	Systolic BP (mmHg)	Diastolic BP (mmHg)
Goal (mmHg)	<130	<80
Lifestyle therapy alone (max. 3 months), then add pharmacological treatment	130–139	80–89
Lifestyle therapy + pharmacologic treatment	>140	>90

19.3 Target values for hypertension treatment in patients with diabetes

Several authorities have issued guidelines for treatment of blood pressure within diabetic populations. The American Diabetes Association recommendations are listed in Table 19.1, whilst other published recommendations are listed in Tables 19.2–19.4, for comparison.

In the American JNC 7 Report [6], a SBP of 120–139 mmHg or a DBP of 80–89 mmHg is defined as 'Pre-hypertension', and lifestyle modification is advised to prevent cardiovascular complications.

Table 19.2 Blood pressure control assessment level according to diabetes type 2 Desktop Guidelines 1998–1999. European Diabetes Policy Group (IDF-European Region) [8].

- Low risk (mmHg) <140/85

- Life-style management of raised blood pressure should be given a good trial before beginning antihypertensive drugs

- If antihypertensive drugs are necessary use:
  - single-agent therapy at rising doses until target achieved (or intolerance)
  - multiple therapy if targets not reached on maximum doses of single agents
  - once-daily drug administration regimes

In the recent European guidelines [7], Grade 1 hypertension (mild) is defined as SBP 140–159 mmHg and/or DBP 90–99 mmHg. An isolated systolic hypertension (ISH) is present if the SBP is >140 mmHg and DBP is <90 mmHg. In patients aged over 50 years, a SBP >140 mmHg represents a markedly more important risk factor for cardiovascular disease (CVD) than does the DBP.

As a therapeutic aim, a reduction in SBP and DBP below 140/90 mmHg is recommended in all patients who tolerate this, and in diabetic patients below 130/80 mmHg. Yet, it must be recognized that in ISH in older patients it is difficult to reach systolic Riva-Rocchi (RR)-values below 140 mmHg.

All recommendations have in common that they do not differentiate with regards to the age of the patients. The recommendation by the ADA [9] sets a goal of <130/<80 mmHg systolic/diastolic, which is most ambitious compared to the older IDF or recent German guidelines [10] (where the common goal is <140/<85 mmHg). A European-wide primary care approach to the treatment of hypertension in diabetes is provided in Table 19.4.

None of the previous guidelines has included specific and detailed sections on managing the older patient, or those with frailty. Evidenced-based clinical guidelines for type 2 diabetes in older patients were presented in 2004 [12], and recommendations were made in these areas. A more recent update is planned

Table 19.3 Therapeutic target values for antihypertensive therapy for adult patients with diabetes mellitus type 2, according to the clinical guidelines of the German Diabetes Association (Praxis-Leitlinien der Deutschen Diabetes Gesellschaft (DDG).

Clinical scenario	Therapeutic target for blood pressure	
	Systolic BP (mmHg)	Diastolic BP (mmHg)
Diabetes with essential hypertension	<140	<85
Good tolerance of BP <140/85 mmHg	<130	<80
Diabetes with microalbuminuria	<130	<80
With/or manifest nephropathy	better <120	–

Table 19.4 Recommendations according to the SVDPCDG Guidelines Working Group. St Vincent Declaration Primary Care Diabetes Group. Approved Guidelines for Type 2 Diabetes 2002 [11].

- The general practitioner (GP) determines body mass index (BMI) based on height and weight and blood pressure. A patient with DBP >85 mmHg or SBP >150 mmHg is a candidate for follow-up measurements.

- Determination of the urine albumin concentration or the albumin:creatinine ratio in patients aged >50 years is not recommended. From a cardiovascular point of view, this group should already be receiving optimal treatment by a tight regulation of dyslipidaemia and reduction of blood pressure to <150/85 mmHg. It is not known whether the treatment of microalbuminuria in patients aged >50 years, without hypertension, is worthwhile in the prevention of nephropathy.

- There is evidence that, in patients with type 2 diabetes mellitus, maintaining the DBP <90 mmHg and SBP <160 mmHg reduces the risk of microvascular and macrovascular complications. It is, therefore, recommended that the target blood pressure should be <150/85 mm Hg. Whether the reduction of blood pressure is achieved using thiazide diuretics, ACE-inhibitors or β-blockers leads to virtually the same reduction in microvascular and macrovascular complications.

- The following steps are recommended:
  - Step 1: a low dose of thiazide diuretic, hydrochlorothiazide or chlorthalidone 12.5 mg
  - Step 2: add an ACE-inhibitor or a β-blocker.
  - Step 3: a combination of the three aforementioned drugs.

- Any initial kidney function deterioration must be monitored when prescribing an ACE-inhibitor in older patients.

for the IDF Conference in Montreal, 2009, when the threshold for treatment is expected to recommended as 140/80 mmHg or higher present for 3 months, and measured on at least three separate occasions. A lower value is recommended for those patients who are able to tolerate the therapy and to self-manage, and/or those with concomitant renal disease. For frail subjects (dependent; multisystem disease; care home residency, including those with dementia), an acceptable blood pressure is recommended to be <150/90 mmHg. Although this is supported in part by others, a lower DBP is suggested for the oldest of elderly subjects (aged >80 years), namely <150/80 mmHg [13].

19.4 Available evidence from randomized controlled trials

19.4.1 Meta-analysis: old versus new drugs

The first meta-analysis (which included nine randomized trials comparing treatment in 62 605 hypertensive patients) investigated whether antihypertensive drugs offered cardiovascular protection beyond blood pressure lowering. Compared with 'old' drugs (e.g. diuretics and β-blockers), calcium-channel blockers and angiotensin-converting enzyme (ACE) inhibitors offered a similar overall cardiovascular protection, but the calcium-channel blockers provided more reduction against the risk of stroke but less reduction

against the risk of myocardial infarction (MI) [14]. A meta-regression across 27 trials (1 36 124 patients) showed that the odds ratio could be explained by the achieved differences in systolic pressure. Thus, these findings emphasize that blood pressure control is important. Although all antihypertensive drugs have similar long-term efficacy and safety, calcium channel blockers might be especially effective in stroke prevention. It was not found that ACE inhibitors or alpha-receptor blockers affected cardiovascular prognosis beyond their antihypertensive effects [14].

Similar conclusions have also been reached following an overview of placebo-controlled trials of ACE inhibitors, calcium channel blockers and other blood pressure-lowering drugs (15 studies; 74 696 individuals; mean age 62 years; no specification as to age or presence of diabetes, although studies as ABCD, HOPE and Syst-Eur have been included) [15].

Recently, it was questioned whether beta-blocker therapy should remain first choice in the treatment of primary hypertension, since in a meta-analysis in comparison with other antihypertensive drugs the effect appeared to be less than optimum with a raised risk of stroke [16]. A Cochrane analysis also concluded that the available evidence does not support the use of beta-blockers as first-line drugs in the treatment of hypertension. This conclusion was based on the relatively weak effect of beta-blockers to reduce stroke and the absence of an effect on coronary heart disease when compared to placebo or no treatment.

More importantly, it was based on the trend towards worse outcomes in comparison with calcium-channel blockers, renin–angiotensin system (RAS) inhibitors and thiazide diuretics. Most of the evidence of these conclusions was derived from trials where atenolol was used as the beta-blocker (75% of beta-blocker participants in this review). However, it is not known at present whether beta-blockers have differential effects on younger and elderly patients, or whether there are differences between the different subtypes of beta-blocker [17].

With regards to the age-dependent effect, another meta-analysis advised that beta-blockers should not be considered first-line therapy for older hypertensive patients without another indication for these agents. However, in younger patients beta-blockers were associated with a significant reduction in cardiovascular morbidity and mortality [18]. In comparison to other agents, a systematic review by Bradley *et al.* found beta-blockers to be inferior to calcium channel blockers and also to inhibitors of the RAS for reducing several important hard endpoints. Compared to diuretics, they had similar outcomes, but were less well tolerated [19].

19.4.2 Prospective studies: old versus new drugs

The Antihypertensive and Lipid-Lowering Treatment to Prevent Heart Attack Trial (ALLHAT) was a placebo-controlled trial conducted to determine whether treatment with a calcium-channel blocker or an ACE inhibitor would lower the incidence of coronary heart disease (CHD) or other CVD events in comparison to treatment with a diuretic [20]. After a mean follow-up of 4.9 years in a group of 33 357 participants aged ≥55 years (mean age 66.9 years) who had at least one other CHD risk factor, thiazide-type diuretics (chlorthalidone, 12.5–25 mg daily) were seen to be equal in preventing one or more major forms of CVD, and to be less expensive. Approximately 36% of the participants were known diabetics at the start of the study. The results, even when comparing individual therapy arms, were also consistent for subgroups of participants – that is, older and younger, male and female, diabetic and non-diabetic. Thus, for the important diabetic population, lisinopril appeared to have no special advantage, while amlodipine had no particular detrimental effect for most CVD and renal outcomes when compared to chlorthalidone.

In fact, chlorthalidone was superior to lisinopril for several CVD outcomes, and superior to amlodipine for heart failure in both the diabetic and non-diabetic participants. The study arm with doxazosin was stopped at an early stage because of a large excess of heart failure with a need for hospitalization. Doxazosin should therefore be avoided as a first-line antihypertensive drug, and particularly so in patients with heart failure [21].

One detrimental effect of diuretic therapy in the ALLHAT study was a slightly elevated fasting blood glucose in non-diabetic patients compared to the other treatment options.

Especially, high-dose diuretic therapy and β-blockers can cause a significant increase in the prospective diabetic risk [22]. Of interest also was a recent post-hoc analysis of the Systolic Hypertension in the Elderly Program (SHEP), which showed that the participants who had hypokalaemia after one year of treatment with a low-dose diuretic did not experience the reduction in cardiovascular events achieved among those without hypokalaemia [23].

The HOPE study, where the active treatment ACE-inhibitor ramipril (10 mg) was compared to placebo, showed cardiovascular protection in a large group of individuals with high cardiovascular risk, including also diabetic persons [24]. In the OnTarget study, the angiotensin-receptor blocker (ARB) telmisartan (80 mg per day) was compared to the 'gold standard' ramipril (10 mg per day), and to a combination of both drugs, in over 25 000 persons with high cardiovascular risk. After a mean follow-up of 56 months, telmisartan was equivalent to ramipril in patients with vascular disease or high-risk diabetes, and associated with less angioedema. The combination of the two drugs was associated with a greater number of adverse events, but without any increase in benefit [25]. At baseline, the mean age of patients was 66 years, and 38% had diabetes. In a subgroup analysis, age (also for those aged >75 years) and the presence of diabetes showed no influence on the study results.

19.4.3 Prospective studies in old people

A subgroup meta-analysis of randomized, controlled trials of antihypertensive drugs in very old people (aged >80 years; n = 1670) suggested that treatment prevented 34% of strokes. The rates of major cardiovascular events and heart failure were significantly decreased, by 22% and 39%, respectively. However, there was no treatment benefit for cardiovascular death, and a significant 6% (range from − 5% to 18%) relative excess of death from all causes. These inconclusive findings for mortality contrasted with the benefit of treatment for non-fatal events. The percentage of diabetic patients was reported as 14% of the total number. No separate analysis was carried out, however, most likely due to the small absolute number [26].

In the STOP-Hypertension-2 trial, a total of 6614 patients aged 70–84 years with hypertension ($RR_{systolic}$ >180 mmHg; $RR_{diastolic}$ >105 mmHg, or both) were randomly assigned to conventional antihypertensive drugs (β-blockers, diuretics) or newer drugs (ACE-inhibitors, calcium-channel blockers) [27]. The blood pressure was seen to decrease to a similar degree in all treatment groups, and the 'old' and 'new' antihypertensive agents were similar in terms of their prevention of cardiovascular mortality or major events. A decrease in blood pressure was of major importance for the prevention of cardiovascular events. Among the total patient cohort, 10.9% (n = 719; 433 females, 286 males, mean age 75.8 years) had diabetes at baseline, but the treatment effects did not differ significantly in terms of the primary endpoint (treatment duration 4–5 years).

In a subgroup analysis of the Syst-Eur Study [28], diabetic patients aged >70 years showed a greater clinical benefit of the blood pressure-lowering afforded by the calcium channel-blocker nitrendipine than their age-matched, non-diabetic counterparts.

In the very recently reported HYVET study [13], a total of 3845 patients aged >80 years (mean age 83.6 years) with a sustained SBP ≥160 mmHg received (at random) either active treatment with the diuretic indapamide, or a matching placebo, The ACE-inhibitor perindopril or placebo was added if necessary to achieve a target blood pressure of 150/80 mmHg. After 2 years the mean blood pressure was 15.0/6.1 mmHg lower in the indapamide-treated group than in the placebo group. This in turn led to a 30% reduction in the rate of fatal and non-fatal stroke (borderline significance, p = 0.06) and to a significant (21%) reduction in mortality rate from any cause (p = 0.02). Overall, there was a 39% reduction in death from stroke, and a 23% reduction in death from cardiovascular causes, after a median follow-up of 1.8 years. Unfortunately, such a very small proportion (<7%) of diabetic patients at baseline was remarkable in that age group,

and hinted at a degree of selection bias towards very healthy old individuals.

19.4.4 Prospective studies in type 2 diabetic patients

A total of 11 140 type 2 diabetic patients (mean age 66 years) was enrolled in the ADVANCE trial, conducted by the Advance Collaborative Group [29]. The patients were randomized to a fixed combination of the ACE-inhibitor perindopril and indapamide or placebo, in addition to current therapy. After a mean of 4.3 years of follow-up, those assigned active therapy had a mean reduction in SBP of 5.6 mmHg and in DBP of 2.2 mmHg. The relative risk of a major macrovascular or microvascular event was reduced by 9% (p = 0.04), of death from CVD by 18% (p = 0.03), and of death from any cause by 14% (p = 0.03). Hence, in this study, over a period of 5 years, the number of patients required to be treated in order to prevent one death was 79 for the blood pressure arm.

Major benefits of blood pressure-lowering in type 2 diabetic patients by treatment with either an ACE-inhibitor or β-blocker versus placebo were demonstrated by the hypertension arm of the UKPDS some 10 years earlier [30, 31], albeit with a higher median blood pressure in each group. The ADVANCE blood pressure values at baseline were similar to those in the tightly controlled groups of the UKPDS.

The long-term follow-up data acquired for the tight control of type 2 diabetes was published some 10 years after that of the UKPDS, in 1998 [32]. The differences in blood pressure between treatment groups had disappeared within 2 years following termination of the trial. Neither was any risk reduction seen during the long-term follow-up for MI, nor death from any cause. The suggestion was, therefore, that good blood pressure control must be continued if the benefits are to be maintained. Yet, this finding was in contrast to the 10-year follow-up of intensive glucose control arm of the UKPDS, which had been published simultaneously [33]. Despite an early loss of the glycaemic differences between groups, a continued reduction in microvascular risk and emergency risk reduction for MI and death from any cause were observed during a 10-year post-trial follow-up. A continued benefit after metformin therapy was evident among overweight patients, however.

19.5   Antihypertensive therapy as part of a multifactorial intervention

The combined effects of glycaemic control and blood pressure control in the UKPDS were reported in an epidemiological manner, highlighting the additive effects of both intervention to reduce microvascular and macrovascular complications and the risk of death [34].

The recently reported details of the glucose-lowering arm of the ADVANCE study demonstrated a significant reduction in a combined primary end-point (sum of macro- and microvascular complications). The additive efficacy of a tight control of blood glucose and blood pressure in elderly type 2 diabetic patients was demonstrated at the EASD meeting in Rome, in September 2008. Among patients included in the group, with both optimal control of blood pressure and blood glucose, an 18% reduction in all-cause mortality was observed ($p = 0.04$), as well as a 24% reduction in cardiovascular mortality ($p = 0.035$) and a 33% reduction in new or worsening nephropathy ($p = 0.005$). These effects were greater than were observed in each separate treatment arm, while the effects of both interventions were independent from each other and fully additive.

Thus, antihypertensive therapy in older patients with diabetes must be seen as one part of the multifactorial intervention necessary in diabetes management to prevent and/or delay cardiovascular complications, as shown in the Steno-2 Study [35]. In an observational follow-up of this cohort (n = 160) over another 5.5 years following the intervention (i.e. a total follow-up 13.3 years), it appeared that intensive multifactorial therapy was associated with a lower risk of death from cardiovascular causes (-57%, $p < 0.04$), of cardiovascular events (-59%, $p < 0.001$), of end-stage renal disease ($p = 0.04$), and also of the need for retinal photocoagulation (-55%, $p = 0.02$) [36].

The prevention or delay of visual and sensory loss, of coronary, cerebrovascular and peripheral vascular events in diabetic patients is of crucial importance in order to preserve self-competence and independence in further life.

19.6   Pharmacological therapy of hypertension in diabetes

According to the recommendations of the American Diabetes Association [9], any pharmacological therapy for patients with diabetes and hypertension should include either an ACE inhibitor or an ARB. If one class of drug is not tolerated, then the other should be substituted. If needed to achieve blood pressure targets, a thiazide diuretic should be added to the therapy of those patients with an estimated glomerular filtration rate (eGFR) $>50 \, \text{ml min}^{-1}$ per $1.73 \, \text{m}^{-2}$, and a loop diuretic for those with an eGFR $<50 \, \text{ml min}^{-1}$ per $1.73 \, \text{m}^{-2}$.

Multiple drug therapy (two or more agents at maximal doses) is generally required to achieve blood pressure targets. If ACE inhibitors, ARBs or diuretics are used, then kidney function and serum potassium levels should be closely monitored [9].

In older individuals, kidney function is a critical factor in clinical practice. Severe disturbances of electrolyte concentrations (high and low potassium/hyponatraemia and hypernatraemia are common in patients, especially when receiving multiple medications (i.e. ACE-inhibitors, ARBs, aldosterone-antagonists, diuretics, antidepressants and antipsychotics inducing the inappropriate secretion of antidiuretic hormone). Long-acting calcium-channel blockers are associated with good evidence of stroke prevention, and are neutral with regards to metabolism, electrolytes and kidney function [28]. Beta-blockers should be considered if there is an additive indication besides primary hypertension, as is often the situation in older diabetic patients (i.e. status post-MI, heart failure, tachycardia, coronary heart disease). Any contraindications for beta-blocker therapy must be ruled out before prescribing this class (i.e. severe chronic obstructive pulmonary disease, acute myocardial insufficiency, critical peripheral disease, bradycardia consequent to sick-sinus syndrome). Diabetes mellitus *per se* in NOT a contraindication for beta-blocker therapy.

References

1. Niefeld MR, Braunstein JB, Wu AW, Saudek CD, Weller WE and Anderson GF. Preventable hospitalization among elderly Medicare beneficiaries with Type 2 diabetes. Diabetes Care 26: 1344–49, 2003.
2. Berlowitz DR, Ash AS, Hickey EC *et al.* (2003) Hypertension management in patients with diabetes: the need for more aggressive therapy. Diabetes Care 26: 355–9.
3. Prospective Studies Collaboration. (2002) Age-specific relevance of usual blood pressure to vascular mortality: a meta-analysis of individual data for one

million adults in 61 prospective studies. Lancet, 360, 1903–13.

4. Satish S, Freeman DH, Ray L and Goodwin JS. The relationship between blood pressure and mortality in the oldest old. J Am Geriatr Soc 49: 367–374, 2001.

5. Van Bemmel T, Gussekloo J, Westemdorp RGJ, Blauw GJ. In a population-based prospective study, no association between high blood pressure and mortality after age 85years. J Hypertension 24: 287–292, 2006.

6. Chobanian AV, Bakris GL, Black HR et al. and the National High Blood Pressure Education Program Coordinating Committee. The seventh report of the Joint National Committee on prevention, detection, evaluation, and treatment of high blood pressure. The JNC 7 Report. JAMA 289: 2560–2572, 2003.

7. Guidelines Committee ESH/ESC: 2003 European Society of Hypertension – European Society of Cardiology guidelines for the management of arterial hypertension. J Hypertension 21: 1011–1053, 2003.

8. Alberti G., for the European Diabetes Policy Group 1998-1999. (1999) Guidelines for Diabetes Care. A Desktop Guide to Type 2 Diabetes Mellitus. International Diabetes Federation, IDF (European Region). Diabetic Medicine, 16, 716–30.

9. American Diabetes Association ADA: Standards of Medical Care in Diabetes - 2008. Hypertension/blood pressure control – Recommendations. Diabetes Care 31 (Suppl. 1): S24–6, 2008.

10. Scherbaum WA, Landgraf für die Leitlinienkommission der DDG. Praxis-Leitlinien der Deutschen Diabetes-Gesellschaft (DDG). Diabetes & Stoffwechsel, 11 (Suppl. 2): 20, 2002.

11. Rutten GEHM, Verhoeven S, Heine RJ, De Grauw WJC, Cromme PVM, Reenders K, Van Ballegooie, Wiersma TJ and torgnamhe St Vincent Declaration Primary Care Diabetes Group. (1999) Approved Guidelines for Type 2 Diabetes 2002. Huisarts en Wetenschap 42(2): 67–84.

12. The European Diabetes Working Party for Older People, 2001-2004. Clinical Guidelines on Type 2 Diabetes Mellitus. Available at www.eugms.org.

13. Beckett NS, Peters R, Fletcher AE et al. for the HYVET Study Group. Treatment of hypertension in patients 80years of age or older. N Engl J Med 358: 1887–1898, 2008.

14. Staessen JA, Wang J-G and Thijs L. Cardiovascular protection and blood pressure reduction: a meta-analysis. Lancet 358: 1305–15, 2001.

15. Blood Pressure Lowering Treatment Trialists' Collaboration. Effects of ACE inhibitors, calcium antagonists, and other blood-pressure-lowering drugs: results of prospectively designed overviews of randomised trials. Lancet 355: 1955–64, 2000.

16. Lindholm LH, Carlberg B and Samuelsson O. Should beta blockers remain first choice in the treatment of primary hypertension. A meta-analysis. Lancet 366: 1545–53, 2005.

17. Wiysonge CS, Bradley H, Mayosi BM, Maroney R, Mbewu A, Opie LH, Volmink J. Beta-blockers for hypertension. Cochrane Database Syst Rev Jan 24 (1): CD002003, 2007.

18. Khan N and McAllister FA. Re-examining the efficacy of beta-blockers for the treatment of hypertension: a meta-analysis. Canadian Medical Association Journal 174: 1737–42, 2006.

19. Bradley HA, Wiysonge CS, Volmink JA, Mayosi BM and Opie LH. How strong is the evidence for use of beta-blockers as first-line therapy for hypertension? Systematic review and meta-analysis. J Hypertens 24: 2131–41, 2006.

20. The ALLHAT Officers and Coordinators for the ALLHAT Collaborative Research Group. Major outcomes in high-risk hypertensive patients randomised to angiotensin-converting enzyme inhibitor or calcium channel blocker vs. diuretic: the Antihypertensive and Lipid-Lowering Treatment to Prevent Heart Attack Trial (ALLHAT). JAMA 288: 2981–97, 2002.

21. The ALLHAT Officers and Coordinators for the ALLHAT Collaborative Research Group. Major cardiovascular events in hypertensive patients randomised to doxazosin vs. chlorthalidon: the Antihypertensive and Lipid-Lowering Treatment to Prevent Heart Attack Trial (ALLHAT). JAMA 283: 1967–75, 2000.

22. Gress TW, Nieto J, Shahar E, Wofford MR, Brancati FL for the Atherosclerosis Risk in Communities Study. Hypertension and antihypertensive therapy as risk factors for type 2 diabetes mellitus. N Engl J Med 342: 905–12, 2000.

23. Franse LV, Pahor M, Di Bari M, Somes GW, Cushman WC and Apllegate WB. Hypokalemia associated with diuretic use and cardiovascular events in the Systolic Hypertension in the Elderly Program. Hypertension 35: 1025–30, 2000.

24. Heart Outcomes Prevention Evaluation (HOPE) Study Investigators. Effects of ramipril on cardiovascular outcomes in people with diabetes mellitus: results of the HOPE study and MICRO-HOPE substudy. Lancet 355: 253–9, 2000.

25. The ON TARGET Investigators. Telmisartan, ramipril, or both in patients at high risk for vascular events. N Engl J Med 358: 1547–59, 2008.

26. Gueyffier F, Bulpitt C, Boissel J-P, Schron E, Ekbom T, Fagard R, Casiglia E, Kerlikowske K, Coope J, for the INDANA Group. Antihypertensive drugs in very old people: a subgroup meta-analysis of randomised controlled trials. Lancet 353: 793–6, 1999.

27. Hansson L, Lindholm LH, Ekbom T, Dahlöf B, Lanke J, Schersten B, Wester P-O, Hedner T, de Faire U, for the STOP-Hypertension-2 Study Group. Randomised trial of old and new antihypertensive drugs in elderly patients: cardiovascular mortality and morbidity the Swedish Trial in Old Patients with Hypertension-2 study. Lancet 354: 1751–61, 1999.

28. Tuomilehto J, Rastenyte D, Birkenäger WH *et al.* for the Systolic Hypertension in Europe Trial Investigators. Effects of calcium-channel blockade in older patients with diabetes and systolic hypertension. N Engl J Med 340: 677–84, 1999.

29. Advance Collaborative Group. Effects of a fixed combination of perindopril and indapamide on macrovascular and microvascular outcomes in patients with type diabetes mellitus (the ADVANCE trial): a randomised controlled trial. Lancet 370: 829–40, 2007.

30. UK Prospective Diabetes Study Group. Tight blood pressure control and risk of macrovascular and microvascular complications in type 2 diabetes: UKPDS 38. Br Med J 317: 703–13, 1998.

31. UK Prospective Diabetes Study Group. Efficacy of atenolol and captopril in reducing risk of macrovascular and microvascular complications in type 2 diabetes UKPDS 39. Br Med J 317: 713–20, 1998.

32. Holman RR, Paul SK, Bethel MA, Neil HAW, Matthews DR. Long-term follow-up after tight control of blood pressure in type 2 diabetes. N Engl J Med 359: 1565–76, 2008.

33. Holman RR, Paul SK, Bethel MA, Matthews DR and Neil HAW. 10-year follow-up of intensive glucose control in type 2 diabetes. N Engl J Med 359: 1577–89, 2008.

34. Adler AI, Stratton IM, Neil HAW, Yudkin JS, Matthews DR, Cull CA, Wright AD, Turner RC, Holman RR, on behalf of the UK Prospective Diabetes Study Group. Association of systolic blood pressure with macrovascular and microvascular complications of type 2 diabetes (UKPDS 36): prospective observational study. Br Med J 321: 412–419, 2000.

35. Gaede P, Vedel P, Larsen N, Jensen GVH, Parving HH and Pedersen O. Multifactorial intervention and cardiovascular disease in patients with type 2 diabetes. N Engl J Med 348: 383–93, 2003.

36. Gaede P, Lund-Andersen H, Parving HH and Pedersen O. Effect of a multifactorial intervention on mortality in type 2 diabetes. N Engl J Med 358: 580–91, 2008.

20

Treatment of Dyslipidaemia

Peter Fasching

5th Medical Department, Wilhelminenspital, Vienna, Austria

Key messages:

- Older patients with diabetes are often under-treated in terms of lipid-lowering, and may be at risk of preventable cardiovascular disease.
- Standard assessments of cardiovascular risk in older patients may be misleading and underestimate this risk; under these circumstances the threshold for lipid lowering may need to be adjusted.
- Statins are effective in significantly reducing cardiovascular risk in older patients aged up to 80 years with type 2 diabetes, but the effect on mortality is inconsistent.

20.1   Introduction

Elderly and old patients with diabetes mellitus suffer from increased cardiovascular risk [1–3]. Coronary heart disease is a major cause of physical disability, particularly in the rapidly growing population of elderly persons [4]. Cross-sectional data concerning lipid management, however, show that patients with diabetes – and especially those of advanced age – are strikingly undertreated for reasons apparently not related to LDL-cholesterol levels [5]. Thus, special attention to cardiovascular risk factor management is obligatory, as the prevention of subsequent coronary events and the maintenance of physical functioning in such

patients are major challenges in preventive care [6].

20.2   Risk assessment and treatment targets

Categories of risk based on lipoprotein levels in adults with diabetes mellitus according to most international recommendations are given without modification concerning age and duration of diabetes [7, 8] (Table 20.1). Since general cardiovascular risk is increasing with both variables – and especially age – the cardiovascular risk in elderly diabetic and non-diabetic patients is generally underestimated according to non-age-specific risk assessment [9]. A more specific approach is calculating individual risk by risk tables on the basis of epidemiological data [10].

Principally, target values for treatment decisions based on LDL-cholesterol level in adults should be adopted without age limitation, especially in otherwise healthy and independent individuals ('single disease model') and yet, particular considerations for old (>75 years) and very old (>85 years) patients are advisable in case of multimorbidity, dependency and end-stage dementia ('multi-disease model') due to limited life expectancy [11]. This may also involve the consequences of competing non-cardiovascular causes for death such as cancer and infections [12, 13]. In these cases, lipid-lowering therapy should be initiated only on the basis of special individual causes.

Diabetes in Old Age. Third Edition. Edited by Alan J. Sinclair
© 2009 John Wiley & Sons, Ltd

Table 20.1 Treatment decisions based on LDL-cholesterol level in adult with diabetes according to the American Diabetes Association.

- Lifestyle modification focusing on the reduction of saturated fat, trans fat and cholesterol intake; weight loss; increased physical activity should be recommended to improve the lipid profile in patients with diabetes.
- Statin therapy should be added to life-style therapy, regardless of baseline lipid levels, for diabetic patients:
  - with overt cardiovascular disease (CVD); or
  - without CVD who are aged >40 years and have one or more other CVD risk factors.
- For patients at lower risk than those mentioned above (e.g. without overt CVD and aged <40 years), statin therapy should be considered in addition to lifestyle therapy if LDL-cholesterol remains >100 mg dl^{-1}, or in those with multiple CVD risk factors.
- In individuals without overt CVD, the primary goal is an LDL-cholesterol <2.6 mmol l^{-1} (100 mg dl^{-1}).
- In individuals with overt CVD, a lower LDL-cholesterol goal of <1.8 mmol/l (70 mg dl^{-1}), using a high dose of a statin, is an option.
- If drug-treated patients do not reach the above targets on maximal tolerated statin therapy, a reduction in LDL-cholesterol of ∼40% from baseline is an alternative therapeutic goal.
- Triglyceride levels <1.7 mmol l^{-1} (150 mg dl^{-1}) and HDL-cholesterol levels >1.0 mmol l^{-1} (40 mg dl^{-1}) in men and >1.3 mmol l^{-1} (50 mg dl^{-1}) in women are desirable. However, LDL-cholesterol-targeted statin therapy remains the preferred strategy.
- Combination therapy using statins and other lipid-lowering agents may be considered to achieve lipid targets, but this has not been evaluated in outcome studies for either CVD outcomes or safety.

20.3 Available evidence from randomized controlled trials

High cholesterol levels in older subjects are associated with increased cardiovascular events and mortality, and indeed, there is a positive relationship between the serum cholesterol level and cardiovascular risk. *Statins* are effective in lowering serum cholesterol levels, and reducing the risk of cardiovascular events. There is no evidence of a threshold below which lower cholesterol levels are not associated with a lower risk, which suggests that cholesterol reduction is useful for all individuals at high cardiovascular risk, regardless of their baseline cholesterol level.

The evidence for cholesterol lowering is evident for individuals up to the age of 80 years. For those aged >80 years, there is some evidence of benefit from observational studies (e.g. [14]). No mortality benefit was found for those aged >80 years who received a statin, whereas those aged 65–79 years showed a significant 11% reduction in mortality. There was evidence, however, of a trend towards benefit in those aged 80–85 years compared to those aged >85 years [15]. Although the positive association between total and LDL-cholesterol and cardiovascular risk becomes attenuated with advancing age – and more so in

men than in women [16] in the Cholesterol Treatment Trialists Collaborators (CTTC) (a systematic prospective meta-analysis which reported data from 14 randomized trials) – those aged >65 years (n = 6446) had a 19% reduction in the risk of major cardiovascular events, a benefit similar to the 22% reduction in risk experienced by those aged <65 years (n = 7902) [17].

Statins reduce the proportional risk as effectively in older as in younger people, although only limited data are available for elderly patients with type 2 diabetes. In the CTTC meta-analysis, which included 18 686 patients with diabetes among a total of 90 056 participants, there was a 21% reduction (95% CI: 19–23%) in major vascular events per 1 mmol l^{-1} reduction in serum LDL-cholesterol level, and no difference in treatment effect between patients with and without diabetes [17].

Scientific evidence for the clinical effects of lipid lowering in elderly diabetic and non-diabetic patients on the basis of large randomized controlled trials (RCTs) is therefore scarce. In the meantime, the details of two statin trials – the HPS [18] and PROSPER [19] trials – have been reported which have included increased numbers of older patients with diabetes.

Statin therapy based on once-daily simvastatin or pravastatin (40 mg) has been shown to significantly reduce the relative risk (RR) of combined cardiovascular endpoints and coronary events to a similar extent (ca. 20%; range 15–25%) in older (>70 years) and diabetic subcohorts in both the HPS and PROSPER studies. In contrast to a reduction of all-cause-mortality by 12.9% in the HPS study, the PROSPER trial found no effect on total mortality. In the HPS study, however, the therapeutic effects could be discriminated at the earliest after one year of treatment.

In the CARDS trial, the efficacy of atorvastatin (10 mg daily) versus placebo was examined in 2838 type 2 diabetic patients aged 40–75 years. Unfortunately, however, the study was terminated 2 years earlier than expected after a median follow-up of 3.9 years, because the prespecified early stopping rule for efficacy had been met. Here, a 10 mg daily dose of atorvastatin reduced all major cardiovascular events by 37% (p = 0.001), acute coronary heart disease events by 36%, coronary revascularizations by 31%, the rate of stroke by 49%, and mortality rate by 27% (p = 0.059) [20].

A review of several large-scale clinical trials assessing the efficacy of atorvastatin in the primary and secondary prevention of cardiovascular events in patients with diabetes mellitus and/or metabolic syndrome, underlined the integrative place of atorvastatin in this indication [21]. However, no differentiation with regards to patients of different ages was presented.

The effect of statin therapy on the prevention of strokes is heterogeneous, and consequently no general recommendation can yet be provided for the primary prevention of stroke besides the secondary prevention of coronary disease.

20.3.1 Statin therapy and adverse side effects

Statin therapy with simvastatin and pravastatin (40 mg, once daily) is well tolerated in older and diabetic people (partly on multiple drug therapy) (HPS, PROSPER). In the CARDS study, no excess of adverse events was noted in the atorvastatin group when compared to the placebo group [20].

20.3.2 Statin therapy and special clinical scenarios

A number of smaller RCTs have suggested particular beneficial effects of statin therapy in special clinical scenarios, which might have implications for the treatment of older patients with diabetes mellitus (e.g. unstable angina and non-Q-wave infarction [22];

status post-percutaneous coronary intervention [23]; multivessel coronary disease [24]).

20.3.3 Fibrate therapy

Because of the limited number of older diabetic subjects included in RCTs with gemfibrozil or fibrates, it is not possible to draw definite conclusions concerning hard clinical endpoints for this special group of patients [25, 26].

In the FIELD study, which included 9795 participants aged 50–75 years with type 2 diabetes mellitus who were not receiving statin therapy at study entry, micronized fenofibrate (200 mg daily) caused no significant reduction in the risk of primary outcome of coronary events compared to placebo after the 5-year study duration [27]. Yet, fenofibrate was shown to reduce total cardiovascular events (–11%, p = 0.05), due mainly to fewer non-fatal myocardial infarctions (−24%, p = 0.010) and revascularization (−21%, p = 0.003). Mortality due to coronary heart disease was increased by 19%, albeit non-significantly. In conclusion, at present no firm recommendation can be provided for the use of fibrate as first-line therapy in diabetic patients.

Evidence-based clinical guidelines focusing on elderly people [28] have presented recommendations for lipid lowering in older patients with type 2 diabetes. Their emphasis is, quite rightly, on good glycaemic control, statin therapy for all those with abnormal lipid profiles, fibrate therapy for those with persistent raised triglycerides (≥ 2.3 mmol l^{-1}), and referral to a specialist lipid or diabetes clinic for those with triglyceride levels >10 mmol l^{-1}.

20.3.4 Other pharmacological therapies

Until now, only one intervention study with hard clinical end points has been reported with the cholesterol-resorption inhibitor, ezetimibe. Since hyperlipidaemia is suggested as a risk factor for stenosis of the aortic valve, 1873 patients (mean age 67.5 years) with mild-to-moderate asymptomatic aortic stenosis were included in the SEAS trial, and randomized to daily treatment with either 40 mg simvastatin plus 10 mg ezetimibe, or placebo [29]. After a mean follow-up period of 52.2 months, the primary endpoint (a composite of major cardiovascular events) was similar in both groups. Although there was no change in the need for aortic valve replacement, fewer patients in the simvastatin-ezetimibe group had ischaemic cardiovascular events (−22%, p = 0.02), due mainly to the smaller number of patients who underwent coronary artery bypass grafting.

A large-scale, randomized double-blind study involving 15 067 patients at high cardiovascular risk was conducted to evaluate the effect of a combination of atorvastatin and the cholesteryl ester transfer protein (CETP) inhibitor torcetrapib, compared to atorvastatin alone [30]. While, in the torcetrapib group, the HDL-cholesterol was increased by 72% and LDL-cholesterol decreased by 25% compared to baseline, after a 12-month treatment period there was a significantly increased risk of cardiovascular events ($+25\%$, p = 0.001) and death from any cause ($+58\%$, p = 0.006), albeit of unknown mechanism.

20.4   Eligibility for lipid-lowering therapy

Lipid lowering in older patients with diabetes must be seen as one part of the multifactorial intervention process necessary in diabetes management to prevent and/or delay cardiovascular complications [31, 32].

Lipid-lowering therapy in patients with type 2 diabetes seems the case for early intervention. Yet, in view of the divergent study results and outstanding data, an assessment of the risk of the individual with type 2 diabetes is mandatory to assist clinical decision-making when initiating lipid therapy [33].

The denial of an otherwise recommended lipid-lowering therapy in older patients with diabetes mellitus is not justified on the basis of present knowledge, if the patient is principally eligible for invasive procedures such as coronary angiography, percutaneous transluminal coronary angiography and stenting for coronary heart disease or surgery (i.e. coronary bypass or heart valve surgery, or carotid endarterectomy).

Finally, in very frail individuals, great caution must be exercised before embarking on lipid lowering with a statin, largely because of the likely increased risk of muscle disease-related side effects. Patient safety and balancing the risks and benefits are important priorities when managing older patients, and are hallmarks of the careful clinician.

References

1. Sinclair AJ, Robert IE and Croxon SCM. Mortality in older people with diabetes mellitus. Diabetic Med 14: 639–47, 1997.

2. Brun E, Nelson RG, Benett PH, Imperatore G, Zoppini G, Verlato G and Muggeo M. Diabetes duration and cause-specific mortality in the Verona Diabetes Study. Diabetes Care 23: 1119–23, 2000.

3. Bertoni AG, Krop JS, Anderson GF and Brancati FL. Diabetes-related morbidity and mortality in a national sample of U.S. elders. Diabetes Care 25: 471–5, 2002.

4. Pinsky JL, Jette AM, Branch LG, Kannel WB and Feinleib M. The Framingham Disability Study: relationship of various coronary heart disease manifestations to disability in older persons living in the community. Am J Public Health 80: 1363–7, 1990.

5. Massing MW, Sueta CA, Chowdhury M, Biggs DP and Simpson RJ. Lipid management among coronary artery disease patients with diabetes mellitus or advanced age. Am J Cardiol 87: 646–9, 2001.

6. Ades PA. Cardiac rehabilitation and secondary prevention of coronary disease. N Engl J Med 345: 892–902, 2001.

7. American Diabetes Association ADA: Standards of Medical Care - 2008. Dyslipdemia/lipid management: Recommendations. Diabetes Care 31 (Suppl. 1): S26–7, 2008.

8. Executive Summary of the Third Report of the National Cholesterol Education Program NCEP Expert Panel on Detection, Evaluation and Treatment of High Blood Cholesterol in Adults (Adult Treatment Panel III). JAMA 285: 2486–97, 2001.

9. D'Agostino RB, Russell MW, Huse DM, et al. (2000) Primary and subsequent coronary risk appraisal∼: new results from the Framingham study. Am Heart J 139: 272.

10. Rutten GEHM, Verhoeven S, Heine RJ, De Grauw WJC, Cromme PVM, Reenders K, Van Ballegooie, Wiersma TJ and the St Vincent Declaration Primary Care Diabetes Group. (1999) Approved Guidelines for Type 2 Diabetes 2002. Huisarts en Wetenschap 42 (2): 67–84.

11. Sinclair AJ. Diabetes in old age: changing concepts in the secondary care arena. J Roy Coll Phys 2000; 34: 240–4.

12. Weverling-Rijnsburger AW, Blauw GJ, Lagaay AM, Knook DL, Meinders AE and Westendorp RG. Total cholesterol and risk of mortality in the oldest old. Lancet 350: 119–23, 1997.

13. Schatz IJ, Masaki K, Yano K, Chen R, Rodriguez BL and Curb JD. Cholesterol and all-cause mortality in elderly people from the Honolulu Heart Program: a cohort study. Lancet 358: 351–5, 2001.

14. Aronow WS and Ahn C. Incidence of new coronary events in older persons with prior myocardial infarction and serum low-density lipoprotein cholesterol ≥125 mg/dl treated with statins versus no lipid-lowering drug. Am J Cardiol. 2002; 89: 67–9.

15. Foody JM, Rathore SS, Galusha D, *et al.*. Hydroxy-methylglutaryl-CoA reductase inhibitors in older persons with acute myocardial infarction: evidence for an age statin interaction. J Am Geriatr Soc. 2006; 54: 421–30.

16. Anum EA and Adera T. Hypercholesterolemia and coronary heart disease in the elderly: a meta-analysis. Ann Epidemiol. 2004; 14: 705–21.

17. Baigent C, Keech A, Kearney PM, *et al.* The Cholesterol Treatment Trialists' (CTT) Collaborators: Efficacy and safety of cholesterol-lowering treatment: prospective meta-analysis of data from 90,056 participants in 14 randomised trials of statins. Lancet 2005; 366: 1267–78.

18. Heart Protection Study Collaborative Group. MRC/BHF Heart Protection Study of cholesterol lowering with simvastatin in 20 536 high-risk individuals: a randomised placebo-controlled trial. Lancet, 360, 7–22, 2002.

19. Shepherd J, Blauw GJ, Murphy MB, *et al.* On behalf of the PROSPER study group. Pravastatin in elderly individuals at risk of vascular disease (PROSPER): a randomised controlled trial. Lancet 360: 1623–30, 2002.

20. Colhoun HM, Betteridge DJ, Durrington PN, Hitman GA, Neil HA, Livingstone SJ, Thomason MJ, Mackness MI, Charlton-Menys V, Fuller JH and the CARDS investigators. Primary prevention of cardiovascular disease with atorvastatin in type 2 diabetes in the Collaborative Atorvastatin Diabetes Study (CARDS): multicentre randomised placebo-controlled trial. Lancet 364: 685–96, 2004.

21. Arca M. Atorvastatin efficacy in the prevention of cardiovascular events in patients with diabetes mellitus and/or metabolic syndrome. Drugs 67 (Suppl. 1): 43–54, 2007.

22. Waters DD, Schwartz GG, Olsson AG, *et al.* for the MIRACLE Study Investigators. Effects of atorvastatin on stroke in patients with unstable angina or non-Q-wave myocardial infarction. A myocardial ischemia reduction with aggressive cholesterol lowering (MIRACLE) substudy. Circulation 106: 1690–5, 2002.

23. Serruys PWC, de Feyter P, Macaya C, *et al.* for the Lescol Intervention Prevention Study (LIPS) Investigators. Fluvastatin for prevention of cardiac events following successful first percutaneous coronary intervention. A randomised controlled trial. JAMA 287: 3215–22, 2002.

24. Pitt B, Waters D, Brown WV, *et al.* for the Atorvastatin versus Revascularization Treatment Investigators. Aggressive lipid-lowering therapy compared with angioplasty in stable coronary artery disease. N Engl J Med 341: 70–6, 1999.

25. Rubins HB, Robins SJ, Collins D, Fye CL, Andersen JW, Elam MB, Faas FH, Linares E, Schaefer EJ, Schectman G, Wilt TJ, Wittes J. Gemfibrozil for the secondary prevention of coronary heart disease in men with low levels of high-density lipoprotein cholesterol: Veterans Affairs High-Density Lipoprotein Cholesterol Intervention Trial Study Group. N Engl J Med 341: 410–18, 1999.

26. Diabetes Atherosclerosis Intervention Study Investigators. Effect of fenofibrate on progression of coronary-artery disease in type 2 diabetes: the Diabetes Atherosclerosis Intervention Study, a randomised study. Lancet 357: 905–10, 2001.

27. Keech A, Simes RJ, Barter P, Best J, Scott R, Taskinen MR, Forder P, Pillai A, Davis T, Glasziou P, Drury P, Kesäniemi YA, Sullivan D, Hunt D, Colman P, d'Emden M, Whiting M, Ehnholm C, Laakso M and the FIELD study investigators. Effects of long-term fenofibrate therapy on cardiovascular events in 9795 people with type 2 diabetes mellitus (the FIELD study): randomised controlled trial. Lancet 366: 1849–61, 2005.

28. The European Diabetes Working Party for Older People, 2001-2004. Clinical Guidelines for Type 2 Diabetes Mellitus. (available on www.eugms.org).

29. Rossebo AB, Pedersen TR, Boman K, *et al.* for the SEAS Investigators. Intensive lipid lowering with simvastatin and ezetimibe in aortic stenosis. N Engl J Med 359: 1343–56, 2008.

30. Barter PJ, Caulfield M, Eriksson M, *et al.* for the ILLUMINATE Investigators. Effects of torcetrapib in patients at high risk for coronary events. N Engl J Med 357: 2109–22, 2007.

31. Gaede P, Vedel P, Larsen N, Jensen GVH, Parving HH and Pedersen O. Multifactorial intervention and cardiovascular disease in patients with type 2 diabetes. N Engl J Med 348: 383–93, 2003.

32. Gaede P, Lund-Andersen H, Parving HH and Pedersen O. Effects of a multifactorial intervention on mortality in type 2 diabetes. N Engl J Med 358: 580–91, 2008.

33. Steinmetz A. Lipid-lowering therapy in patients with type 2 diabetes: the case for early intervention. Diabetes Metab Res Rev 24: 286–93, 2008.

21

Hypoglycaemia

Vincent McAulay[1] **and Brian M. Frier**[2]
[1]*Department of Diabetes, Crosshouse Hospital, Kilmarnock, UK*
[2]*Department of Diabetes, Royal Infirmary, Edinburgh, UK*

Key Messages

- The frequency and severity of hypoglycaemia in the elderly is commonly underestimated, and often mis-attributed to other conditions.
- The symptoms of hypoglycaemia are different in the elderly compared to younger people, partly as a function of ageing.
- The increasingly stringent glycaemic targets inherent in modern diabetes care demands that patients, and their relatives and carers, are fully informed about the symptoms and effects of hypoglycaemia and its emergency management.

21.1 Introduction

Hypoglycaemia is the most serious and disruptive side effect of the treatment of diabetes in the elderly. While it is a recognized clinical consequence of the use of insulin and sulphonylureas in all age groups requiring such therapy, the frequency of hypoglycaemia is underestimated in elderly people with diabetes. This may be because its clinical manifestations are unrecognized or are wrongly attributed to other pathological conditions such as cerebral ischaemia or degenerative disorders. The effects of hypoglycaemia can be severe in elderly patients, many of whom are physically frail and have coexisting macrovascular disease. They may therefore be at increased risk of suffering a major vascular event such as myocardial infarction and stroke as a consequence of hypoglycaemia. In addition, frequent and unpredictable hypoglycaemia in an old person, causing problems such as dizziness, disturbed balance, weakness, transient loss of consciousness and falls, can undermine their self-confidence and have a destabilizing effect on their independence and ability to live alone. The imposition of the burden of prevention and treatment of hypoglycaemia on relatives and carers, many of whom may also be elderly, may provoke further domestic difficulties, threatening the independence of the affected individual, and possibly precipitating their transfer to residential care. The emergence of hypoglycaemia as a prominent problem in an elderly person with diabetes may influence their management by encouraging health attendants to avoid the risk of exposure to a low blood glucose and to accept poor or suboptimal glycaemic control.

Most people who develop diabetes later in life have type 2 diabetes, the prevalence of which is rising in association with increasing longevity, and treatment with insulin is increasing in elderly people as a consequence of the decline in pancreatic beta-cell function that occurs as diabetes progresses in severity. In addition, some older people have an insulin-deficient form of diabetes, and require insulin from the time of diagnosis, while many more people with type 1 diabetes now survive into old age. Although hypoglycaemia was considered to be a relatively uncommon side effect of oral antidiabetic agents [1], many sulphonylureas promote hypoglycaemia of varying frequency

Diabetes in Old Age. Third Edition. Edited by Alan J. Sinclair
© 2009 John Wiley & Sons, Ltd

and severity. The increasing popularity of combining oral antidiabetic agents with insulin in the treatment of type 2 diabetes may possibly augment the magnitude of this problem, particularly in the elderly patient. The risk of exposure to insulin-induced hypoglycaemia is, therefore, rising steadily in older people with diabetes.

Before examining the epidemiology and morbidity of hypoglycaemia in the elderly population with diabetes, it is important to ascertain whether age *per se* affects the symptomatic awareness of – and counter-regulatory hormonal response to – acute hypoglycaemia, and how these fundamental responses to a low blood glucose may be modified by the presence of type 2 diabetes in an ageing population.

21.2 Physiological responses to hypoglycaemia

21.2.1 Counter-regulation

The human brain is dependent upon glucose as its principal source of fuel, and requires a continuous supply of glucose via the cerebral circulation. Depriving the brain of glucose rapidly causes neuroglycopenia which has various effects, including impairment of cognitive function.

In humans, several mechanisms have evolved to maintain glucose homeostasis and so protect the integrity and function of the brain [2]. A decline in blood glucose concentration activates a characteristic hierarchy of responses, commencing with the suppression of endogenous insulin secretion, the release of several counter-regulatory hormones, and the subsequent development of characteristic symptoms (Figure 21.1). These alert the informed individual to the development of hypoglycaemia, so allowing them to take early and appropriate action (the ingestion of carbohydrate) to assist recovery. Such protective responses are usually effective in maintaining the arterial blood glucose concentration within a normoglycaemic range (which can be arbitrarily defined as a blood glucose above 3.8 mmol l^{-1}), which protects the brain from exposure to neuroglycopenia caused by protracted glucose deprivation. Glucose counter-regulation is controlled from centres within the brain (mainly the ventromedial hypothalamus), assisted by activation of hypothalamic autonomic nervous centres with stimulation of the peripheral sympathoadrenal system. This contributes to glucose counter-regulation through the peripheral actions of catecholamines, and

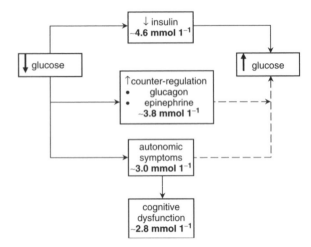

Figure 21.1 Hierarchy of responses to hypoglycaemia in non-diabetic humans.

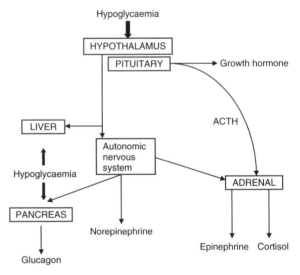

Figure 21.2 Principal components of glucose counter-regulation in humans.

also by the generation of characteristic autonomic warning symptoms (Figure 21.2). Although glucagon is the most potent counter-regulatory hormone, the role of epinephrine (adrenaline) becomes paramount if the secretory response of glucagon is deficient [3]. Other counter-regulatory hormones, such as cortisol and growth hormone, have greater importance in promoting recovery from prolonged hypoglycaemia.

Both, glucagon and epinephrine stimulate hepatic glycogenolysis, releasing glucose from glycogen stored in the liver, and also promote gluconeogenesis from three-carbon precursors such as alanine, lactate and glycerol. The energy for this process is provided by the hepatic oxidation of free fatty acids that are released by lipolysis. Catecholamines inhibit insulin secretion, diminish the peripheral uptake of glucose, stimulate lipolysis and proteolysis and promote glycogenolysis in peripheral muscle to provide lactate, which is utilized for gluconeogenesis in the liver and kidney.

21.2.2 Symptoms

Both the sympathetic and parasympathetic divisions of the autonomic nervous system are activated during hypoglycaemia, leading to the direct neural stimulation of end-organs via peripheral autonomic nerves, and the physiological effects are augmented by the secretion of epinephrine from the adrenal medulla [4] (Figure 21.3). Studies in young adults using physiological and pharmacological methods to assess the symptoms of hypoglycaemia, have confirmed that the symptoms of pounding heart, tremulousness and feeling nervous or anxious are adrenergic in nature [5]. The sweating response to hypoglycaemia is mediated primarily via sympathetic cholinergic stimulation [5, 6], with circulating catecholamines possibly contributing through the activation of α-adrenoceptors [7]. When the brain is deprived of glucose, it rapidly malfunctions, causing interference with information processing and the development of cognitive dysfunction, which underlies the generation of neuroglycopenic symptoms such as difficulty concentrating, feelings of tiredness and drowsiness, faintness, dizziness, generalised weakness, confusion, difficulty speaking and blurring of vision.

Statistical techniques have also been used to classify the symptoms of hypoglycaemia. Applying methods such as Principal Components Analysis (PCA), the symptoms of hypoglycaemia segregate into three distinct factors or groups: *neuroglycopenic, autonomic* and *general malaise* [8]. This 'three-factor' validated model containing 11 common symptoms of hypoglycaemia (the 'Edinburgh Hypoglycaemia Scale'), has been used to classify symptoms objectively in various groups of subjects, and has shown age-specific differences in the nature of hypoglycaemic symptoms as classified by this statistical method (Table 21.1). Symptoms of hypoglycaemia are idiosyncratic and vary between individuals. They may also differ in intensity in different situations, and their perception can be influenced by distraction or other external influences. In perceiving the onset of hypoglycaemia (often described as subjective 'awareness'), the intensity of a few cardinal symptoms is of importance to the individual,

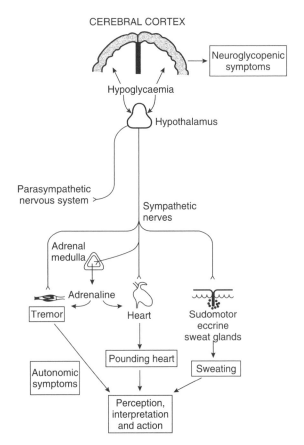

Figure 21.3 Activation of the autonomic nervous system and the sympathoadrenal system during hypoglycaemia. Reproduced with permission from Frier, B.M. and Fisher, B.M. (eds) (1993), *Hypoglycaemia and Diabetes*, Edward Arnold (Publisher) Ltd, London.

Table 21.1 Classification of symptoms of hypoglycaemia in patients with insulin-treated diabetes depending on age group.

Children (pre-pubertal)	Adults	Elderly
Autonomic/ Neuroglycopenic	Autonomic	Autonomic
	Neuroglycopenic	Neuroglycopenic
Behavioural	Non-specific malaise	Neurological

Reproduced with permission from Ref. [10].

rather than the number or nature of the symptoms generated. An assessment of the subjective reality of symptoms is therefore essential in attempting any form of measurement or devising a scoring system. Both autonomic and neuroglycopenic symptoms appear to be of equal value in warning people with type 1 diabetes of the onset of hypoglycaemia, provided that the symptoms peculiar to the individual are identified and interpreted correctly [11].

21.2.3 Glycaemic thresholds

Specific physiological responses occur when the declining blood glucose reaches different levels of hypoglycaemia. Although these glycaemic thresholds are readily reproducible in non-diabetic humans [12], they are plastic and dynamic and can be modified. In non-diabetic humans the glycaemic threshold at which the secretion of most counter-regulatory hormones is triggered is around 3.8 mmol l^{-1} (measured as arterialized blood glucose), so that counter-regulation is usually activated when blood glucose falls below the normal range. Counter-regulation therefore occurs at a blood glucose that is higher than that at which the symptomatic response to hypoglycaemia occurs (3.0 mmol l^{-1}) and before the onset of cognitive dysfunction (2.8 mmol l^{-1}) (Figure 21.1). The glycaemic threshold for autonomic symptoms coincides with the classical autonomic 'reaction' to hypoglycaemia, which can be identified by the sudden development of physiological changes [13].

In people with diabetes, glycaemic thresholds can be modified by the prevailing glycaemic state, and particularly by strict control (Figure 21.4), and can be influenced by metabolic perturbations such as preceding (antecedent) hypoglycaemia. Many studies in people with insulin-treated diabetes who have strict glycaemic control have demonstrated that the counter-regulatory

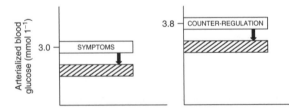

Figure 21.4 The glycaemic thresholds for counter-regulatory hormonal secretion and the onset of symptoms can vary depending on the prevailing level of glycaemic control in people with diabetes. Strict glycaemic control is associated with a higher glycaemic threshold (i.e. a lower blood glucose concentration is required), providing a more intense hypoglycaemic stimulus.

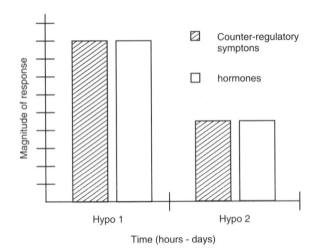

Figure 21.5 Schematic representation of the effect of antecedent hypoglycaemia on the neuroendocrine and symptomatic responses to subsequent hypoglycaemia. Reproduced with permission from BM Frier and M Fisher (eds) (2007), *Hypoglycaemia in Clinical Practice*, John Wiley & Sons Ltd, Chichester.

hormonal and symptomatic responses to hypoglycaemia do not occur until much lower blood glucose levels are reached, particularly when the glycated haemoglobin concentration is within the non-diabetic range [14]. Similarly, antecedent hypoglycaemia lasting for 1 h or more has been shown to diminish the magnitude of the symptomatic and neuroendocrine responses to any subsequent episode of hypoglycaemia occurring within the following 24–48 h [13] (Figure 21.5). This duration of untreated hypoglycaemia is not uncommon during sleep, and may be one of the mechanisms that induce impaired awareness of hypoglycaemia in people with type 1 diabetes.

21.3 Acquired hypoglycaemia syndromes in type 1 diabetes

21.3.1 Counter-regulatory deficiencies

In many people with type 1 diabetes, the glucagon secretory response to hypoglycaemia becomes diminished or absent within a few years of the onset of insulin-deficient diabetes. With glucagon deficiency alone, blood glucose recovery from hypoglycaemia is relatively unaffected because counter-regulation is maintained by the actions of epinephrine. However,

Table 21.2 Frequency of abnormal counter-regulatory responses to hypogly-caemia in patients with type 1 diabetes.

Duration of diabetes (years)	Glucagon (%)	Adrenaline (%)	Cortisol (%)	Growth hormone (%)
<1	27	9	0	0
1–5	75	25	0	0
5–10	100	44	11	11
>10	92	66	25	25

Reproduced with permission from Frier, B.M. and Fisher, B.M. (eds) (1999), *Hypoglycaemia and Diabetes*, Edward Arnold (Publisher) Ltd.

in up to 45% of people who have type 1 diabetes of long duration, a dual impairment of the secretion of glucagon and epinephrine is observed [15], predisposing them to serious deficiencies of glucose counter-regulation when exposed to hypoglycaemia, delaying the recovery of blood glucose, and allowing progression to more severe hypoglycaemia (Table 21.2). People with type 1 diabetes of long duration are therefore at increased risk of developing severe and prolonged hypoglycaemia, particularly when intensive insulin therapy is used [16]. Indeed, people with type 1 diabetes who have combined deficiencies of their glucagon and epinephrine responses to hypoglycaemia have been shown to be at 25-fold or even higher increased risk for severe iatrogenic hypoglycaemia if subjected to intensive insulin therapy compared to those whose glucagon response is absent but who retain their epinephrine response [16, 17]. These counter-regulatory deficiencies co-segregate with impaired awareness of hypoglycaemia in people with type 1 diabetes [18], suggesting that they share a common pathogenetic mechanism within the brain.

21.3.2 Impaired awareness of hypoglycaemia

This occurs when the symptomatic warning is diminished or inadequate in people with diabetes, and many factors can influence the awareness of hypoglycaemia (Table 21.3). Impaired awareness is not an 'all-or-none' phenomenon. Rather, a 'partial' impairment of awareness may develop, with the individual being aware of some episodes of hypoglycaemia, but not others. Alternatively, they may experience a reduction in the intensity or number of symptoms which varies between hypoglycaemic events, and progress to 'absent' awareness where the patient is no longer aware of the onset of hypoglycaemia. Several mechanisms underlying this problem have been proposed (Table 21.4).

Table 21.3 Factors influencing normal awareness of hypoglycaemia.

Internal	External
Physiological	*Drugs*
Recent glycaemic control	Beta-adrenoceptor blockers (non-selective)
Degree of neuroglycopenia	Hypnotics, tranquilizers
Symptom intensity/sensitivity	Alcohol
Psychological	*Environmental*
Arousal	Sleep
Focused attention	Posture
Congruence; denial	Distraction
Competing explanations	
Education	
Knowledge	
Symptom belief	

Reproduced with permission from Ref. [13].

Impaired awareness of hypoglycaemia is generally thought to result from diminished sympathoadrenal activation with a resultant reduction in the symptomatic response to a given level of hypoglycaemia [19]. This acquired syndrome of hypoglycaemia is common in type 1 diabetes, affecting around one-quarter of patients, becomes more prevalent with increasing duration of diabetes, and predisposes the patient to a much higher risk of severe hypoglycaemia than people who retain normal awareness [13]. It is much less common in insulin-treated patients with type 2 diabetes [20]. In some patients with type 1 diabetes, when impaired awareness of hypoglycaemia is associated with strict glycaemic control during intensive insulin therapy, or has followed episodes of recurrent severe hypoglycaemia [21], this syndrome may be reversible by relaxing glycaemic control or by avoiding further hypoglycaemia, but in many patients with type 1 diabetes of long duration, it appears to be a permanent defect [13].

Table 21.4 Possible mechanisms of impaired awareness of hypoglycaemia.

CNS adaptation

Chronic exposure to low blood glucose
Strict glycaemic control in diabetic patients
Insulinoma in non-diabetic patients

Recurrent transient exposure to low blood glucose
Antecedent hypoglycaemia

CNS glucoregulatory failure
Counter-regulatory deficiency (hypothalamic defect?)
Hypoglycaemia-associated central autonomic failure

Peripheral nervous system dysfunction
peripheral autonomic neuropathy
reduced peripheral adrenoceptor sensitivity

Reproduced with permission from Ref. [13].

21.3.3 Central autonomic failure

Because hormonal counter-regulatory deficiencies and impaired awareness of hypoglycaemia usually coexist, and are associated with an increased frequency of severe hypoglycaemia, the concept of a "Hypoglycaemia-Associated Autonomic Failure" (HAAF) was proposed [22], when it was argued that recurrent severe hypoglycaemia is the primary problem which provokes these acquired abnormal responses. The concept of HAAF deems that recent antecedent hypoglycaemia, in people with type 1 diabetes [22] and in patients with type 2 diabetes who have progressed to pancreatic beta-cell failure [23], causes defective glucose counter-regulation in the setting of an absent glucagon response. This occurs because the epinephrine response is then markedly attenuated during exposure to subsequent hypoglycaemia, while impaired awareness of hypoglycaemia develops through blunting of the sympathoadrenal response and reduced generation of autonomic symptoms [13, 24].

21.4 Effects of age on physiological responses to hypoglycaemia

21.4.1 Counter-regulatory mechanisms

Because, in humans, many physiological processes alter with advancing age, it is important to determine whether the ageing process *per se* may affect the nature and efficacy of the glucose counter-regulatory response to hypoglycaemia. In non-diabetic elderly subjects, a

study of the counter-regulatory hormonal responses to hypoglycaemia induced by an intravenous infusion of insulin suggested that diminished secretion of growth hormone and cortisol is a feature of advanced age, and a modest impairment of hormonal counter-regulatory secretion was associated with some attenuation of blood glucose recovery [25]. Insulin clearance was reduced, as was the secretion of glucagon, while the release of epinephrine was delayed; these abnormalities were unchanged following a period of physical training, suggesting that they were not secondary to a sedentary lifestyle [25]. However, a different study using the hyperinsulinaemic glucose-clamp technique has suggested that age *per se* has no effect [26]. Comparative analysis and interpretation of these studies are problematical because of differences between study groups with respect to the rate of onset and duration of hypoglycaemia and of the magnitude of the plasma insulin concentrations achieved – factors which can influence the nature of the counter-regulatory hormonal response.

A study in older non-diabetic subjects (mean age 76 years) [27], using a stepped glucose-clamp technique, demonstrated deficiencies in the secretion of glucagon and epinephrine. In another study [28], the counter-regulatory responses in 11 older, non-diabetic individuals (mean age 65 years) were compared to those of 13 young, healthy volunteers (mean age 24 years). Subtle differences were observed in the magnitude of the hormonal counter-regulatory responses in the older group (in whom the epinephrine, glucagon, pancreatic polypeptide and cortisol responses were lower) in response to modest hypoglycaemia (arterialized blood glucose 3.3 mmol l^{-1}). However, no such differences were demonstrated when the hypoglycaemic stimulus was more profound (arterialized blood glucose 2.8 mmol l^{-1}). Two further studies in non-diabetic elderly subjects, using similar designs and methodologies, failed to demonstrate any significant age-related impairment of the counter-regulatory hormonal responses to hypoglycaemia [29, 30].

21.4.2 Symptomatic response to hypoglycaemia

Differences between age groups in the symptom profiles in response to hypoglycaemia have been demonstrated in children and adults with type 1 diabetes [9], while older people with insulin-treated type 2 diabetes have been observed to experience a cluster of 'neurological' symptoms (unsteadiness, poor

Table 21.5 Symptoms of hypoglycaemia in the elderly [31].

Neuroglycopenic	Autonomic	Neurological
Weakness	Sweating	Unsteadiness
Drowsiness	Shaking	Poor coordination
Poor concentration	Pounding heart	Double vision
Dizziness	Anxiety	Blurred vision
Confusion		Slurred speech
Light-headedness		

Table 21.6 Hypoglycaemia in the elderly: effects of age.

1. Mild attenuation of blood glucose recovery may occur (hepatic glucose production is diminished)

2. Modest reductions demonstrable in counter-regulatory hormonal responses (but maximal response to more severe hypoglycaemia)

3. Symptom response is less intense with altered glycaemic threshold and reduced awareness of hypoglycaemia

Table 21.7 Hypoglycaemia in the elderly: symptoms.

1. Autonomic symptoms are not selectively diminished

2. Intensity of all symptoms (historical reports and experimental studies) is low

3. Glycaemic threshold for onset of symptoms is altered by age; lower blood glucose is required to initiate symptoms

4. Cognitive dysfunction induced simultaneously by hypoglycaemia may interfere with perception of symptoms

5. Awareness of hypoglycaemia may be reduced by ageing

coordination, slurring of speech and visual disturbances) [31], in addition to the classical autonomic and neuroglycopenic groups of symptoms recognized in young adults (Table 21.5). Age *per se* may therefore modify the nature and intensity of some symptoms of hypoglycaemia, possibly as a consequence of other age-related changes such as effects on cerebral circulation, and the presence of underlying cerebrovascular disease or degenerative abnormalities of the central nervous system (Table 21.6).

In a small group of non-diabetic subjects in whom hypoglycaemia was induced using a stepped glucose-clamp, lower symptom scores were recorded in the seven older subjects (mean age 72 years) than in the six younger subjects (mean age 30 years), and the usual haemodynamic responses to hypoglycaemia (particularly a rise in heart rate) were absent in the older group [29]. This suggests that the symptomatic awareness of hypoglycaemia may be reduced in the elderly, and is associated with an attenuated end-organ response to sympathoadrenal stimulation. As these responses generate many of the autonomic symptoms of hypoglycaemia, the perception of hypoglycaemia is affected.

In another study of older, non-diabetic subjects, the symptomatic response to hypoglycaemia commenced at a lower blood glucose (mean $\pm$ SD: 3.0 ± 0.2 mmol l^{-1}) compared to a younger group (3.6 ± 0.1 mmol l^{-1}), suggesting that the glycaemic threshold

for the generation of symptoms is modified by age, with a lower blood glucose being required to initiate a symptomatic response [30] (Table 21.7).

21.4.3 Cognitive function

The hierarchy of the cognitive changes in response to hypoglycaemia may change with age. In one study of non-diabetic subjects [30], the responses to moderate hypoglycaemia of seven elderly men were compared with those of seven young men. The four-choice reaction time, a measure of psychomotor coordination, deteriorated in the older men at a mean ($\pm$SD) plasma glucose of 3.0 ± 0.1 mmol l^{-1}, compared to 2.6 ± 0.1 mmol l^{-1} in the young group, and the abnormality was more profound (Figure 21.6). The symptomatic response to hypoglycaemia commenced at a lower blood glucose concentration in the older men than in the young adults (3.0 ± 0.2 versus 3.6 ± 0.1 mmol l^{-1}), while in the older subjects the glycaemic threshold for subjective symptomatic awareness of hypoglycaemia and that for the onset of cognitive dysfunction were

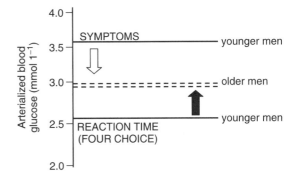

Figure 21.6 The difference between the glycaemic threshold for subjective awareness of hypoglycaemia and that for the onset of cognitive dysfunction may be absent in the elderly. Derived from data in Ref. [30].

coincidental. A similar difference has been observed in patients with type 1 diabetes who have an impaired awareness of hypoglycaemia, in whom the onset of the cognitive dysfunction induced by hypoglycaemia either preceded or was coincidental with the onset of a symptomatic response [13]. This observation suggests that elderly people may be at an intrinsically greater risk of developing neuroglycopenia because the onset of warning symptoms and cognitive impairment occur simultaneously, so interfering with their ability to recognize and take action to self-treat a fall in blood glucose.

21.5 Effects of type 2 diabetes on responses to hypoglycaemia

21.5.1 Counter-regulation

Good glycaemic control in type 2 diabetes limits the development and severity of vascular complications, but achieving this with insulin and many of the oral antidiabetic agents inevitably increases the risk of hypoglycaemia [1]. The counter-regulatory and symptomatic responses to hypoglycaemia have been studied in patients with type 2 diabetes, but earlier studies were performed using a variety of techniques and protocols which makes comparisons between studies either difficult or impossible. Problems included the study of heterogeneous groups of subjects with type 1 and type 2 diabetes [32], variations in the magnitude of the hypoglycaemic stimulus between subjects because the blood glucose differed at baseline [33, 34], and

disparate methods used to induce hypoglycaemia [17, 35–37]. In these early studies the counter-regulatory hormonal responses were either normal or only mildly impaired in people with type 2 diabetes. Epinephrine secretion was invariably preserved (Table 21.8).

More recent studies of counter-regulatory responses to hypoglycaemia in people with type 2 diabetes, treated either with diet or oral medication, have shown that counter-regulatory hormone release occurs at higher blood glucose levels than in non-diabetic control subjects. In one study [41], hypoglycaemia was induced using a stepped glucose-clamp in 11 subjects with type 2 diabetes (mean age 56 years) and in a group of eight age- and weight-matched, non-diabetic subjects. Other comparator groups comprised 10 subjects with type 1 diabetes and another non-diabetic control group. The secretion of counter-regulatory hormones occurred at a higher blood glucose level in the subjects with type 2 diabetes than in those with type 1 diabetes, irrespective of the quality of glycaemic control as measured by glycated haemoglobin (HbA$_1$). However, differences in the gender distribution and insulin infusion rates in some subjects may have introduced potential confounders that could have influenced the results [41]. Non-diabetic female subjects with type 1 diabetes have a lesser magnitude of counter-regulatory responses to hypoglycaemia than male subjects [42–44], so an over-representation of male subjects in the first study [41] might have influenced the results. Similarly, in non-diabetic and type 1 diabetic subjects, hyperinsulinaemia suppresses glucagon release and

Table 21.8 Studies of hormonal counter-regulation to hypoglycaemia in type 2 diabetes.

Study	No. of patients	Method of hypogly-caemia induction	Mean glucose nadir (mmol l^{-1})	Hormonal response
[33]	27	iv insulin bolus	2.0	Reduced glucagon
[35]	10	iv insulin bolus	1.8	No impairment
[36]	10	iv insulin infusion	1.7	No impairment
[34]	8	iv insulin infusion	1.9	No impairment
[17]	13	sc insulin bolus	3.4	Reduced glucagon, cortisol and growth hormone
[37]	10	iv insulin infusion	2.4	No impairment
[38]	10	iv insulin infusion	2.8	Reduced glucagon and growth hormone; increased adrenaline and cortisol
[39]	9	iv insulin infusion	3.4	Reduced glucagon and increased epinephrine (adrenaline)
[40]	7	iv insulin infusion	2.4	Glucagon response preserved in 5 patients; magnitude of adrenaline response increased if poor glycaemic control
[41]	11	iv insulin infusion	2.2	No impairment

increases the secretion of catecholamines and cortisol in response to hypoglycaemia [45–48], such that the higher rate of insulin infusion required in some of the subjects with type 2 diabetes might also have modified their results.

Although type 2 diabetes may confer some protection against hypoglycaemia, especially in those subjects with relatively poor glycaemic control, improving blood glucose control with insulin alters the threshold for the counter-regulatory response to hypoglycaemia [40, 41], in a manner similar to that observed in people with type 1 diabetes when their glycaemic control is improved [19].

As previously noted, counter-regulatory failure occurs with increasing duration of type 1 diabetes, despite an initial compensatory catecholamine response [15]. Does type 2 diabetes follow the same pattern? The glucagon response in type 2 diabetes was diminished in some studies [17, 38, 39] but preserved in others [36, 37, 40, 41], perhaps reflecting the heterogeneous nature of subjects with type 2 diabetes who would have exhibited varying levels of insulin resistance and deficiency depending on their body weight, duration of diabetes and the underlying genetic component of their condition. Most investigators have reported preservation of the glucagon response to hypoglycaemia in people with type 2 diabetes who were most unlikely to be insulin-deficient at the time of study [36, 37, 41, 49]. By contrast, those subjects with type 2 diabetes who were insulin-deficient were shown to have significant impairment of the glucagon response to hypoglycaemia (Figure 21.7) [23, 39]. Growth hormone secretion in response to hypoglycaemia was approximately 50% lower compared with non-diabetic subjects [50].

In conclusion, few counter-regulatory hormonal deficiencies of significance are present in people with type 2 diabetes who can be treated with diet or oral medication, in contrast to the pronounced counter-regulatory hormonal deficiencies that are exhibited by many individuals with type 1 diabetes (Table 21.9). However, this situation changes when patients with type 2 diabetes progress to a state of pancreatic beta-cell failure, when they then develop the counter-regulatory hormonal deficiencies characteristic of type 1 diabetes.

21.5.2 Symptoms of hypoglycaemia

Allowing for differences in age, the symptoms of hypoglycaemia do not appear to differ between people with type 1 and type 2 diabetes, nor does the agent inducing

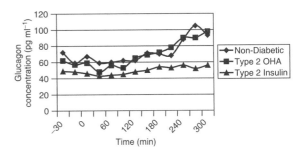

Figure 21.7 Mean plasma glucagon concentrations during hyperinsulinaemic stepped hypoglycaemic clamps in non-diabetic subjects (♦) and in patients with type 2 diabetes treated with OHA (■) or insulin (▲). P = 0.025 for non-diabetic versus type 2 diabetic insulin treatment contrast. Reproduced with permission from Ref. [23]; © 2002, American Diabetes Association.

Table 21.9 Combined effects of age and type 2 diabetes.

1. Modest attenuation of blood glucose recovery observed (no rise in hepatic glucose production and decline in peripheral utilization)

2. Some counter-regulatory hormonal responses are reduced, but not epinephrine (adrenaline)

3. Counter-regulatory hormonal response to profound hypoglycaemia is intact; subtle abnormalities are revealed by a slow decline in blood glucose

4. Some tests of cognitive function (psychomotor tests) are more abnormal than in controls

hypoglycaemia influence the nature of the symptoms. People with type 2 diabetes who were receiving treatment with insulin, reported a similar symptom profile associated with hypoglycaemia as a group with type 1 diabetes, who had been matched for duration of insulin therapy, but neither for age nor duration of diabetes [51]. By using the hyperinsulinaemic glucose-clamp technique [41], it could be shown that the hypoglycaemic symptoms experienced by subjects with type 2 and type 1 diabetes, who had a similar quality of glycaemic control, were identical. In a different study, the nature of the symptomatic response to a similar degree of hypoglycaemia, induced either by insulin or with tolbutamide, was compared in a group of non-diabetic subjects, and no differences were observed either in the nature or in the intensity of symptoms [52]. This would suggest that the agent inducing the hypoglycaemia is not important, as identical symptoms were produced when blood glucose was lowered by a similar amount. However, chronic treatment with a particular agent, such as a sulphonylurea, may influence symptomatic responses to hypoglycaemia, and this possibility remains to be elucidated.

21.5.3 Symptoms in elderly people with type 2 diabetes

Older people with type 2 diabetes have been shown to have a lower intensity, and more limited perception, of autonomic symptoms of hypoglycaemia than age-matched, non-diabetic elderly subjects [38]. In a descriptive study of 45 elderly patients with type 2 diabetes, who were receiving treatment either with insulin or a sulphonylurea, the symptoms of hypoglycaemia that were recognized most commonly were non-specific in nature and included weakness, unsteadiness, sleepiness and faintness [53]. In a retrospective study of people with type 2 diabetes treated with insulin [31], the hypoglycaemia symptoms that were reported with the greatest frequency and intensity were mainly 'neurological' in nature, and included unsteadiness, light-headedness and poor concentration (see Table 21.5). Trembling (71.2%) and sweating (75%) also featured prominently [31], contrasting with the results of a Canadian study in which it was claimed that the autonomic symptoms of hypoglycaemia in the elderly were attenuated [27]. However, the latter study did not use an age-specific symptom questionnaire, and differences in symptom questionnaires and in the scoring methods of inducing hypoglycaemia may account for the differences in symptom profiles that have been described.

Using the statistical technique of PCA, the hypoglycaemia symptoms of elderly people with type 2 diabetes could be separated into neuroglycopenic and autonomic groups, but the typical symptoms of a 'general malaise' group of symptoms, such as headache or nausea, were uncommon [31]. However, symptoms such as impaired motor coordination and slurring of speech were prominent. In elderly people, these symptoms may be misinterpreted as representing either cerebral ischaemia, intermittent haemodynamic changes associated with cardiac dysrhythmia, or as vasovagal and syncopal attacks. Health care professionals should be aware of the age-specific differences in hypoglycaemic symptoms (see Table 21.1), both from the need to identify and treat hypoglycaemia, and for educational purposes.

21.6 Epidemiology of hypoglycaemia in elderly people with diabetes

21.6.1 Determining the frequency of hypoglycaemia

The frequency of hypoglycaemia in people with diabetes is difficult to determine with accuracy, and many clinical studies have underestimated the total number of hypoglycaemic events. In subjects with type 1 diabetes, the retrospective recall of mild (self-treated) episodes of hypoglycaemia is inaccurate beyond a period of one week, and a prospective recording of hypoglycaemia is essential to obtain a precise measure [54]. The recall of severe hypoglycaemia may be affected by amnesia of the event, so that confirmation by observers and relatives is desirable to verify the accuracy of self-reporting. The frequency of hypoglycaemia among people with type 2 diabetes is even more difficult to ascertain and is prone to underestimation, partly because many are old with memory impairment and a limited knowledge of symptoms, and episodes may be attributed incorrectly to other conditions.

People with type 1 diabetes experience an average of two episodes of symptomatic hypoglycaemia per week, which amounts to thousands of such episodes over a lifetime of treatment with insulin [54]. However, many episodes of mild hypoglycaemia that occur in the community are either unrecognized, or are not documented, so that most assessments are likely to significantly underestimate the magnitude of this problem. By contrast, severe hypoglycaemia – defined as an event requiring external assistance to recover – occurs less frequently, with an estimated incidence that ranges from 1.0 to more than 3.0 episodes per patient per year, depending on the duration of the diabetes [55–58]. However, although some elderly patients will have an insulin-deficient type 1 diabetes, the majority will have type 2 diabetes so it is relevant to examine studies that have considered the latter.

21.6.2 Earlier studies of hypoglycaemia in type 2 diabetes

The earliest reports on subjects with type 2 diabetes who were treated with oral antidiabetic agents related mainly to sulphonylureas. One Swedish report of the annual incidence of sulphonylurea-induced hypoglycaemia of sufficient severity to require hospital treatment, recorded a rate of 4.2 per

1000 patients [59], but other European surveys have estimated this to be much lower, at 0.19 to 0.25 per 1000 patient-years (pt-yr) [60, 61]. This contrasts with the much higher incidence of *insulin-induced* hypoglycaemic coma, which has been estimated conservatively at 100 per 1000 pt-yr [62] and severe hypoglycaemia, defined as an episode requiring external assistance for recovery, is three times more frequent than coma. A two-year prospective trial that involved 321 subjects with type 2 diabetes receiving treatment with either chlorpropamide or glibenclamide, recorded an incidence of *symptomatic* hypoglycaemia of 19 per 1000 pt-yr [63]. Around one-fifth of a relatively young group of 203 patients with type 2 diabetes who were receiving treatment with oral sulphonylureas, had experienced symptoms suggestive of hypoglycaemia on at least one occasion during the previous 6 months [64]. Symptoms were reported most frequently with long-acting preparations such as glibenclamide, and in association with other medications recognized to potentiate their hypoglycaemic effect.

21.6.3 More recent studies of hypoglycaemia in type 2 diabetes

Interventional studies

With the increasing use of insulin to treat type 2 diabetes, the findings of a number of studies are now available to examine the effects of insulin-induced hypoglycaemia in type 2 diabetes. Many of these studies have also contributed more data on sulphonylurea-induced hypoglycaemia. As few large-scale studies have recorded the frequency of hypoglycaemic episodes in people with type 2 diabetes treated with insulin over a protracted period of treatment, the UK Prospective Diabetes Study (UKPDS) offered a valuable opportunity to contribute

to this area. Unfortunately, the UKPDS reported only the prevalence of hypoglycaemia, and missed the opportunity to provide more accurate information on this important complication of diabetes. The proportion of patients experiencing hypoglycaemia during the first 10 years of the UKPDS is shown in Table 21.10. Unsurprisingly, people in the intensively treated group of the UKPDS experienced significantly more episodes of hypoglycaemia than those in the conventionally treated group [1], but this was still much lower than estimated frequencies of severe hypoglycaemia, ranging from 1.1 to 1.7 episodes per patient per year in unselected cohorts of people with type 1 diabetes in whom strict glycaemic control was not an objective in specialist centres in Denmark [54] and in Scotland [55], while in a UK multicentre study, people with type 1 diabetes of more than 15 years' duration had an incidence in excess of 3.0 episodes per patient per year [58].

The Veterans Affairs Cooperative Study in the USA reported on the frequency of hypoglycaemia in insulin-treated type 2 diabetic patients. In this study, one group was treated with an intensive insulin regimen, while the other group was administered insulin once daily [65]. The results indicated a higher frequency of mild hypoglycaemia in the intensive group (intensive versus standard, 16.5 versus 1.5 episodes per patient per annum), but no difference was observed in the rate of severe hypoglycaemia between the groups (0.02 episodes per patient per annum). The standard treatment group were monitoring blood glucose less frequently, and the apparently large disparity between the groups may be an overestimate. Although these large interventional trials provide a wealth of information on diabetes and its treatments, they commenced more than a decade ago and do not represent the modern approach to diabetes care, with increasing

Table 21.10 Proportion of patients with type 2 diabetes experiencing hypoglycaemia per year in UK Prospective Diabetes Study over 10 years of the study by principal treatment regimen (mean figures are shown). Data derived from Ref. [1].

	One or more major[a] episodes of hypoglycaemia (%)	Any episode of hypoglycaemia (%)
Diet	0.1	1.2
Chlorpropamide	0.4	11.0
Glibenclamide	0.6	17.7
Insulin	2.3	36.5

[a]Major (severe) hypoglycaemia required third-party help or medical intervention.

use of insulin analogues and combination therapy to achieve glycaemic targets.

Observational studies

In the USA, a retrospective cohort study was undertaken of almost 20 000 elderly people with diabetes receiving treatment with either insulin or sulphonylureas, who were enrolling for health insurance [66]. The incidence of fatal hypoglycaemia and of 'serious hypoglycaemia' (defined as an emergency admission to hospital with a documented blood glucose concentration below 2.8 mmol l^{-1}) was approximately two per 100 pt-yr. People treated with insulin had a higher incidence of 'serious hypoglycaemia' than those treated with sulphonylureas (3 per 100 pt-yr versus 1 per 100 pt-yr). This restricted definition of serious hypoglycaemia differs considerably from the usual definition of severe hypoglycaemia, and so does not provide an accurate picture of the magnitude of the problem. The conclusion by the investigators of this study that sulphonylureas can be used safely in older people, without fear of inducing hypoglycaemia, is fallacious as it is not based on accurate measurement, and should be disregarded.

In a 6-month questionnaire study from Atlanta of African-American patients with type 2 diabetes treated with oral antidiabetic therapy or insulin, 25% had experienced one episode of hypoglycaemia during the study period [67]. Hypoglycaemia increased as treatment was escalated and severe hypoglycaemia occurred in 0.5% of patients, all of whom had been treated with insulin. In a study from Turkey, the frequency of severe hypoglycaemia in 165 patients treated with insulin, most of whom had type 2 diabetes, was reported to be very low at 0.15% episodes per patient per year [68], but this figure was derived solely by the retrospective examination of hospital case-notes; the significant underestimation of events associated with this approach makes this data highly dubious.

A number of studies from Scotland have reported on the frequency of hypoglycaemia in type 2 diabetes. In an early study, the prevalence of severe hypoglycaemia was estimated retrospectively in 104 people with type 2 diabetes of long duration who had progressed to pancreatic beta-cell failure and required insulin, and was not much lower than that of a group of patients with type 1 diabetes who were matched for duration of insulin therapy but not for age or duration of diabetes [51]. In another retrospective study from the same

centre, the incidence of severe hypoglycaemia was assessed in 600 insulin-treated patients. One in 10 of these patients had type 2 diabetes, and the reported incidences of severe hypoglycaemia were 0.73 episodes per patient per annum in type 2 diabetes compared to 1.7 episodes per patient per annum in type 1 diabetes [55]. In a study from Tayside, all episodes of severe hypoglycaemia that were attended by the emergency medical services were identified over 12 months [69]. During 244 episodes of severe hypoglycaemia, 7.1% had occurred in type 1 diabetes, 7.3% in insulin-treated type 2 diabetes, and 0.8% in patients taking oral medications. In a subsequent study, the same investigators undertook a short (1-month) prospective study of 267 patients with type 1 and insulin-treated type 2 diabetes to examine the frequency of hypoglycaemia [70]. The incidence of severe hypoglycaemia in insulin-treated type 2 diabetes was 0.35 episodes per patient per annum, which was one-third of the rate for patients with type 1 diabetes (1.15 episodes per patient per annum). Similarly, the incidence of all hypoglycaemia (mild and severe) in patients with insulin-treated type 2 diabetes was approximately one-third of that affecting those with type 1 diabetes (16.4 versus 42.9 episodes per patient per annum). Furthermore, the patients with type 2 diabetes were more likely to require treatment from the emergency services than their counterparts with type 1 diabetes.

The definitive study that is relevant to a Western European population with type 2 diabetes is an observational prospective multicentre study that was performed over one year in the UK. Here, the frequency of severe hypoglycaemia associated with treatment with sulphonylureas or with insulin alone (but not with combination regimens), was examined in groups of patients with type 2 diabetes, and compared to two groups of patients with type 1 diabetes of differing duration (<5 and >15 years) [58]. Patients with HbA_{1c} concentrations >9% were excluded, and the mean HbA_{1c} levels in the study groups ranged from 7.3 to 7.8%. This important study revealed that the annual prevalence of severe hypoglycaemia associated with sulphonylureas was 7% – a much higher than anticipated figure, and equivalent to the prevalence of severe hypoglycaemia recorded in people with type 2 diabetes who had been treated with insulin for up to two years. The prevalence of severe hypoglycaemia was always lower than that observed in type 1 diabetes of equivalent duration, but progressively increased with the *duration* of insulin therapy for type 2 diabetes (Figure 21.8).

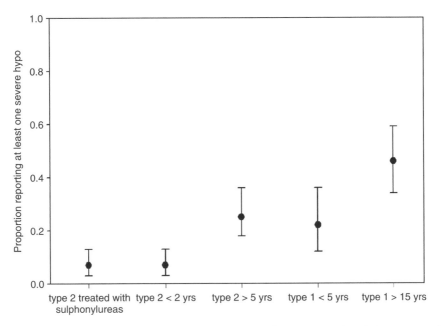

Figure 21.8 Prevalences of severe hypoglycaemia in patients with types 1 and 2 diabetes treated with different modalities. The proportion of each group experiencing at least one severe self-reported hypoglycaemic episode is shown during 9–12 months of follow-up. The vertical bars indicate 95% confidence intervals. Adapted from Ref. [58].

Because of its prospective design, this study has provided an accurate measure of the relative risk of developing severe hypoglycaemia with different treatment modalities and their duration. This has demonstrated that the prevalence of severe hypoglycaemia associated with sulphonylureas is higher than is generally appreciated, and that it is also a significant side effect of insulin treatment for type 2 diabetes that becomes greater the longer patients are treated with insulin.

21.7 Adverse effects of hypoglycaemia in the elderly

21.7.1 Mortality

Mortality associated with sulphonylurea-induced hypoglycaemia has been calculated as 0.014 to 0.033 per 1000 pt-yr [60, 61], contrasting with an estimated mortality from insulin-induced hypoglycaemia in the UK for diabetic patients aged <50 years of approximately 0.2 per 1000 pt-yr [71]. In one series, 10% of patients with severe sulphonylurea-induced hypoglycaemia who were admitted to hospital subsequently died [72]. Other reviews of the outcome of severe hypoglycaemia associated with sulphonylurea therapy have cited a mortality rate of approximately 10% [73],

although this high figure would appear to be an overestimation compared to the authors' recent clinical experience. In fact, the figure may have declined with the reduced use of long-acting sulphonylureas such as chlorpropamide and glibenclamide, that are most likely to induce severe hypoglycaemia.

21.7.2 Morbidity

The morbidity associated with hypoglycaemia in people with diabetes has been reviewed previously [74–76]. Because of increasing physical frailty and concomitant diseases such as osteoporosis, the elderly may be more susceptible to physical injury during hypoglycaemia, with fractures of the long bones, joint dislocations, soft tissue injuries, head injuries and occasionally burns being described as a direct consequence of accidents associated with hypoglycaemia. A trend towards an increase in fracture risk in people with diabetes who had a history of previous hypoglycaemia was observed in a large case-control study in Denmark; this was statistically significant for hip fractures, and is thought be the result of hypoglycaemia-induced falls [77]. Hypothermia may be a direct consequence of hypoglycaemic coma, and the fall in skin temperature during experimentally induced hypoglycaemia is significantly greater in the presence of the non-selective beta-blocker, propranolol [78], although this drug is now seldom used.

Acute hypoglycaemia provokes a profound haemodynamic response secondary to sympathoa-drenal activation and the secretion of epinephrine (adrenaline), causing an increase in cardiac output and the workload of the heart [75]. Although this degree of haemodynamic stress seldom causes any pathophysiological problem to the young person with normal cardiac function, in the older individual with diabetes – who may have underlying macrovascular disease – hypoglycaemia may have serious, or even fatal, consequences. Although the peripheral systolic blood pressure rises, the central pressure falls during hypoglycaemia, which may compromise coronary artery perfusion during diastole and promote my-ocardial ischaemia in people with diabetes of longer duration, in whom premature stiffening of arteries is common [79]. In diabetic patients who have coronary heart disease, cardiac arrhythmias may be induced. These have been described during experimentally induced hypoglycaemia and in anecdotal case reports, with atrial fibrillation, nodal rhythms and premature atrial and ventricular contractions all being observed during hypoglycaemia in diabetic patients who had no overt clinical evidence of heart disease [75, 80]. Sudden death during hypoglycaemia-induced cardiac arrhythmia has been described in individual case reports [81, 82]. Transient ventricular tachycardia has been observed during experimental hypoglycaemia in a non-diabetic subject with coronary heart disease, while acute myocardial infarction has also been reported in association with acute hypoglycaemia [75]. Acute hypoglycaemia can lengthen the QT interval on the electrocardiogram, both in non-diabetic and diabetic subjects [83]. QT dispersion is a marker of spatial difference in myocardial recovery time that, when increased, indicates a heightened risk of ventricular arrhythmias and sudden death. This was significantly higher during acute insulin-induced hypoglycaemia in 13 patients with type 2 diabetes aged 48–63 years [84]. When combined with the effects of catecholamine-mediated hypokalaemia and the profound haemodynamic changes associated with acute hypoglycaemia, the potential for inducing a serious cardiac arrhythmia is enhanced in elderly people, many of whom have coronary heart disease (Table 21.11).

Various psychological and neurological manifesta-tions of acute hypoglycaemia can cause variable loss

Table 21.11 Potential cardiac sequelae of acute hypo-glycaemia.

Prolongation of QT-interval
Cardiac arrhythmias
Silent myocardial ischaemia
Angina
Myocardial infarction
Cardiac failure

Table 21.12 Neuropsychological manifestations of severe hypoglycaemia.

Neurological
Focal or generalized convulsions
Coma
Hemiparesis; transient ischaemic attacks
Ataxia; choreoathetosis
Focal neurological deficits
Decortication

Psychological
Cognitive impairment
Behavioural/personal changes
Automatic or aggressive behaviour; psychosis

of sensory and motor functions (Table 21.12). Tran-sient ischaemic attacks and transient hemiplegia may be a feature of neuroglycopenia, and less commonly permanent neurological deficits have been described, especially in elderly patients. These are presumably caused by mechanisms such as direct focal cerebral damage from glucopenia, acute thrombotic occlusion secondary to the haemodynamic, haematological and haemorrheological effects of hypoglycaemia, or by cerebral ischaemia provoked by changes in regional blood flow in the brain [76]. Elderly people who ex-perience intermittent hypoglycaemia, particularly from the effect of long-acting oral antidiabetic agents, may be misdiagnosed as having transient ischaemic attacks. In a retrospective review of 778 cases of drug-induced hypoglycaemia, permanent neurological deficit was de-scribed in 5% of the survivors [85]. In a report of 102 cases of hypoglycaemic coma induced either by insulin or by glibenclamide, physical injury was re-ported in seven patients, myocardial ischaemia in two, and stroke in one patient [86].

21.8 Risk factors for hypoglycaemia in the elderly

Retrospective studies have identified advanced age and fasting as the two major risk factors associated with sulphonylurea-induced hypoglycaemia [66, 87–90]. However, the increasing number of elderly patients treated with insulin is exposing many to the traditional risk factors for hypoglycaemia. These include insulin administration errors, missed meals, increased insulin sensitivity through weight loss, and delayed insulin clearance, often from renal failure. A short prospective study demonstrated that treatment with insulin for longer than 10 years is an important predictor of severe hypoglycaemia in type 2 diabetes [70], while the progressive rise in frequency of severe hypoglycaemia with increasing duration of treatment with insulin was illustrated in a large multicentre study in the UK [58]. Although impaired awareness of hypoglycaemia appears to be uncommon in insulin-treated type 2 diabetes, it does increase the risk of severe hypoglycaemia ninefold [20]. The principal risk factors are listed in Table 21.13, and are most pertinent to the elderly.

Surveys conducted in Sweden [87, 88] of fatal and severe cases of sulphonylurea-induced hypoglycaemia revealed that severe hypoglycaemia was common during the first month of treatment, was not related to the dose of the drug used, and that coma and serious morbidity were common sequelae. A frequent problem in the elderly is intercurrent illness during which caloric intake is reduced substantially while the dose of sulphonylurea is maintained, so provoking severe hypoglycaemia. However, adherence to therapy is a common problem, particularly with increasing frequency of administration and numbers of drugs prescribed [91, 92]. Occasionally, hypoglycaemia is induced when older people with diabetes are admitted to hospital and their prescribed dose of oral hypoglycaemic medication is administered accurately, often in the setting of reduced carbohydrate intake. In a cohort of 20 000

Table 21.13 Risk factors for hypoglycaemia in elderly patients with type 2 diabetes mellitus.

Age (not dose of drug)
Impaired renal function
Poor nutrition or fasting
Intercurrent illness
Duration of diabetes >10 years
Alcohol ingestion
Polypharmacy
Use of long-acting sulphonylureas or insulin
Recent hospital admission
Endocrine deficiency (pituitary, thyroid, adrenal)
Deficient counter-regulatory hormonal responses
Impaired awareness of hypoglycaemia

elderly Americans, admission to hospital in the preceding 30 days was identified as the strongest predictor of severe hypoglycaemia [66]. In those persons aged ≥80 years, the risk of serious hypoglycaemia was increased further within 30 days of discharge from hospital.

21.8.1 Alcohol

Alcohol inhibits hepatic gluconeogenesis, even at blood alcohol concentrations that are not usually associated with intoxication, and in people with type 1 diabetes it also impairs the ability to perceive and interpret the symptoms of hypoglycaemia [93]. Small amounts of alcohol can increase the cognitive impairment caused by hypoglycaemia in people with type 1 diabetes [94], and will presumably have a similar effect in people with type 2 diabetes. In addition, hypoglycaemia may be mistaken as inebriation by observers, so delaying the initiation of appropriate treatment. Most research into the effects of alcohol has been carried out in people with type 1 diabetes. However, one group performed a prospective, double-blind, placebo-controlled trial in 10 older subjects with type 2 diabetes (mean age 68 years) to assess the effects of combining alcohol ingestion with fasting [95]. After a 14-h fast, the administration of glibenclamide and intravenous alcohol (equivalent to drinking one or two alcoholic beverages) resulted in a lower blood glucose nadir $(4.3 \pm 1.2$ mmol $1^{-1})$ compared to the group who did not receive alcohol $(5.0 \pm 1.4$ mmol $1^{-1})$. In one subject who developed hypoglycaemia (defined as blood glucose <2.8 mmol 1^{-1} with typical symptoms, or any blood glucose concentration <2.2 mmol $1^{-1})$ during both arms of the study, hypoglycaemia occurred earlier (at 5 h) in the ethanol study compared to the placebo arm (8.5 h). This observation is of practical importance, since the quantity of alcohol administered in the study was of a similar amount to that consumed on a regular basis by many people with type 2 diabetes.

21.8.2 Oral antidiabetic agents

Hypoglycaemia caused by oral antidiabetic agents occurs predominantly with insulin secretagogues. Although most sulphonylureas can cause fatal hypoglycaemia, this has been associated most frequently with chlorpropamide and glibenclamide [96].

Many studies have recorded higher rates of hypoglycaemia with long-acting sulphonylureas such as chlorpropamide and glibenclamide [90, 97, 98]. A community-based study conducted over a 12-year period in Basle, Switzerland, showed that the treatment of elderly subjects with type 2 diabetes with longer-acting sulphonylureas was threefold more likely to precipitate admission to hospital with severe hypoglycaemia than was the use of short-acting agents [90].

Almost all sulphonylurea drugs are metabolized in the liver to metabolites that are subsequently excreted in the urine. While most of these metabolites either have minimal or no metabolic activity, the two major hepatic metabolites of chlorpropamide do possess hypoglycaemic activity. In combination with its long half-life of approximately 36 h, chlorpropamide is more likely to induce prolonged hypoglycaemia in elderly people because of the normal age-related decline in the glomerular filtration rate (GFR).

Glibenclamide-induced hypoglycaemia may be more pronounced because the drug accumulates within pancreatic beta cells, and its metabolites retain some hypoglycaemic activity. Despite this, many elderly patients with type 2 diabetes who have accompanying risk factors for hypoglycaemia are still receiving these agents [86, 99]. In a review of 150 elderly people with type 2 diabetes, 40 of the 45 taking glibenclamide had one or more identifiable risk factors for hypoglycaemia [99]. In general, the use of long-acting sulphonylureas should be avoided in elderly patients with type 2 diabetes, and also in those with renal impairment.

However, not all long-acting sulphonylureas provoke hypoglycaemia. Glimepiride is administered once daily and stimulates insulin production primarily in response to meals, but the incidence of reported hypoglycaemia is low [100]. In randomized studies comparing glimepiride with glibenclamide and gliclazide, the incidence of symptomatic hypoglycaemia was lower in glimepiride-treated patients [101]. Furthermore, in a multi-centre, double-blind, controlled trial the modified release (MR) preparation of gliclazide was reported to cause less hypoglycaemia compared to glimepiride (3.7% and 8.9%, respectively). Importantly, in this latter study more than one-third of the subjects were aged >65 years [102].

21.8.3 Adverse drug interactions

Several adverse drug interactions between sulphonylureas and other commonly prescribed medications are recognized that increase the risk of sulphonylurea-induced hypoglycaemia. In a comprehensive review, 15% of patients with sulphonylurea-induced

Table 21.14 Drug interactions with sulphonylureas leading to hypoglycaemia.

Interaction	Drug
Displacement from albumin binding sites	Aspirin, fibrates, sulphonamides, warfarin, trimethoprim
Decreased renal excretion	Probenecid, aspirin, allopurinol
Decreased hepatic metabolism	Warfarin, monoamine oxidase inhibitors
Insulin secretagogues	Non-steroidal anti-inflammatory drugs; low-dose aspirin
Inhibition of gluconeogenesis	Alcohol
Increased peripheral glucose uptake	Aspirin

hypoglycaemia were simultaneously taking medications known to increase the risk of hypoglycaemia [89]. Many drugs can potentiate the effects of sulphonylurea agents via a variety of mechanisms; the important drug interactions promoting hypoglycaemia are summarized in Table 21.14.

21.9 Treatment

Hypoglycaemia is only one of a number of differential diagnoses in an elderly diabetic patient who presents in a comatose state. Although manifestations of cerebrovascular disease may be suspected, hypoglycaemia should be excluded by measuring blood glucose.

However, even when the blood glucose is low, other common causes such as stroke, intracerebral or subarachnoid haemorrhage, head injury and deliberate or accidental drug or alcohol overdose must not be overlooked. Failure to respond to treatment with parenteral glucose should immediately arouse suspicion that there might be another cause for the coma. Failure to recover consciousness following an episode of severe hypoglycaemia may be associated with cerebral oedema, which has a poor prognosis. Affected patients require management in hospital in an intensive care unit, with the use of agents such as mannitol, steroids and high-flow oxygen. This suspected presence of cerebral oedema must be confirmed, and other causes of coma excluded, by neuroimaging of the brain. Although most patients recover rapidly from an episode of hypoglycaemia, it can take up to an hour after blood glucose has been

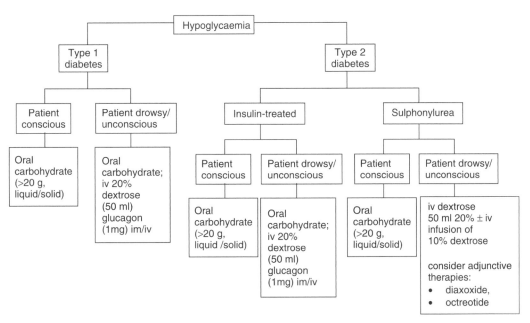

Figure 21.9 Treatment measures for acute hypoglycaemia.

restored to normal for all cognitive functions to be fully recovered [103–105]. Recovery may take longer in the elderly, although this point has not been studied in older people.

The treatment of hypoglycaemia in people with type 2 diabetes follows the same basic principles as for type 1 diabetes, but important differences are present between those treated with insulin and those treated with sulphonylureas (Figure 21.9). In the conscious individual, acute hypoglycaemia is treated with rapid-acting oral carbohydrate, usually in the form of glucose tablets or confectionery such as sweets or chocolate. Beverages with a high glucose content are also suitable, such as fresh orange juice. Following ingestion, some form of long-acting carbohydrate should be consumed to prevent recurrence of the hypoglycaemia. In the drowsy or unconscious patient who cannot swallow, an intravenous injection of dextrose (50 ml of a 20% solution) will cause a rapid reversal of neuroglycopenia. Glucagon is very effective if administered to people treated with insulin that are semi-conscious or in a hypoglycaemic coma. Glucagon (1 mg, intramuscular injection) can be administered either by a friend or relative who is familiar with the technique or by paramedical staff, but it may induce nausea and/or vomiting. It acts through promoting hepatic glycogenolysis to stimulate hepatic glucose output, so on occasion may

prove to be ineffective in patients with protracted hypoglycaemia whose stores of glycogen are exhausted, in people with advanced liver disease or alcohol abuse, and in those with malnutrition or inanition.

21.9.1 Sulphonylurea-induced hypoglycaemia

Mild sulphonylurea-induced hypoglycaemia is treated in a similar fashion to insulin-induced hypoglycaemia, by the ingestion of rapid-acting glucose followed by a longer-acting complex carbohydrate in the form of bread, biscuits, cereal or other alternatives. Sulphonylurea-induced hypoglycaemic coma requires inpatient management and, following the administration of intravenous dextrose, the patient should not be discharged immediately from hospital, despite apparent recovery, as hypoglycaemia from this cause is often associated with relapse and is therefore protracted [96, 106, 107]. Glucagon can stimulate insulin secretion in people with type 2 diabetes who have residual pancreatic beta-cell function [108], and is therefore said to be contraindicated in the treatment of sulphonylurea-induced hypoglycaemia, although the evidence for this supposition is very limited. Following a bolus intravenous injection of 50 ml of 20% dextrose, many patients require prolonged intravenous infusion of 10% (or even 20%) dextrose to maintain a blood glucose concentration above $5.0 \, \text{mmol} \, \text{l}^{-1}$.

The duration of the intravenous infusion will depend upon the half-life of the sulphonylurea ingested, and in cases of drug overdose it may be necessary to continue the dextrose infusion for several days.

21.9.2 Adjunctive therapies

Diazoxide has a direct inhibitory effect on insulin secretion, and has been used as an adjunct to dextrose infusion in the treatment of sulphonylurea-induced hypoglycaemia [109, 110]. In the unconscious patient, diazoxide can be infused intravenously (300 mg over 30 min, repeated 4-hourly if necessary), or in the conscious patient can be administered orally (300 mg every 4 h). Unfortunately, this is unlikely to be a practical option because this drug is no longer commercially available and is now very difficult to obtain. Octreotide, a long-acting synthetic analogue of somatostatin, was used to treat sulphonylurea-induced hypoglycaemia successfully in a non-diabetic patient who had taken an overdose of tolbutamide [111]. Octreotide reverses the hyperinsulinaemia induced by excessive administration of a sulphonylurea and, in contrast to diazoxide, reduces the amount of dextrose required to maintain euglycaemia [112].

21.10 Knowledge of symptoms

Many patients and their relatives are remarkably uninformed about the symptoms of hypoglycaemia [53, 113] and its emergency treatment. In one study, 9% of elderly people who were taking sulphonylureas or insulin were unable to state any of the symptoms associated with hypoglycaemia. Only 20% of the group said that they had been told about the symptoms of hypoglycaemia. Of particular concern, people who were living alone had no better knowledge of symptoms, despite being at greater risk from the consequences of hypoglycaemia [113]. Knowledge of the symptoms of hypoglycaemia was unrelated to the duration of diabetes and living alone, and did not differ between men and women. However, older people knew even less about hypoglycaemia than younger individuals with diabetes. Many people with diabetes taking sulphonylureas did not know about the potential risk of developing hypoglycaemia, whereas people treated with insulin were more knowledgeable on this subject. These findings were confirmed by a different study, in which 88% of elderly people taking sulphonylureas did not know the potential risk of hypoglycaemia, whereas

only 32% of those treated with insulin denied any knowledge of hypoglycaemia [53]. This lack of knowledge extends to the treatment of hypoglycaemia, with around 20% of elderly people with insulin-treated diabetes being unfamiliar with the appropriate measures required to treat symptomatic hypoglycaemia [114]. This reflects the problems of providing information about side effects of therapy and the putative deficiencies of the education for an elderly group with type 2 diabetes, some of whom have memory impairment and may have difficulty retaining information about the risk of drug-induced hypoglycaemia. Hence, regular reinforcement is required regarding potential symptoms and the treatment of hypoglycaemia [115]. Most elderly patients with type 2 diabetes are treated in primary care, and education about therapeutic side effects must not be overlooked, particularly on the mistaken assumption that hypoglycaemia is rarely a clinical problem.

21.11 Prevention of hypoglycaemia

All patients taking insulin or sulphonylureas should receive education about the symptoms of hypoglycaemia and the most appropriate form of self-treatment, and should be advised to eat regular meals so as to ensure an adequate intake of carbohydrate. All patients taking insulin should carry a card or other form of identification, stating that they have diabetes and what treatment they are taking. People who are self-administering insulin should carry a source of rapid-acting carbohydrate. Individuals at increased risk of hypoglycaemia should be identified, such as those aged >70 years and people with renal impairment. In the elderly type 2 diabetic, the longer-acting sulphonylurea agents such as chlorpropamide and glibenclamide should be avoided, and short-acting sulphonylureas such as glipizide and gliclazide used and commenced at the lowest dose, titrated against the patient's fasting or postprandial blood glucose level. Persistently low blood glucose values will require a reduction in dose.

Consideration should be given to the use of alternative oral antidiabetic agents that either do not cause or have a much lower risk of hypoglycaemia, such as metformin and the thiazolidinediones, and the newer incretin mimetics such as the gliptins, or the injectable GLP-1 agonist, exenatide. The utilization of fast-acting insulin analogues and fixed mixtures containing these insulin preparations may also be of value in elderly

Table 21.15 Prevention of hypoglycaemia.

1. Identify high-risk patients: advanced age, renal impairment
2. Avoid long-acting sulphonylurea preparations
3. Use short-acting sulphonylurea (e.g. gliclazide)
4. Be aware of drug interactions
5. Educate patients and relatives/carers about hypoglycaemia
6. Consider agents that do not cause hypoglycaemia

people treated with insulin, in particular to avoid nocturnal hypoglycaemia. Any oral agent may promote hypoglycaemia in situations where the patient is unable to eat normally, and the dose may have to be reduced, or the drug temporarily discontinued.

In order to improve adherence to a prescribed oral antidiabetic therapy, a dosette box is often used in elderly patients, although this might also reduce the risk of overdose due to forgetfulness and to the difficulties of coping with polypharmacy. Clinicians must be particularly aware of drug interactions with sulphonylureas, and anticipate and modify their prescribing patterns accordingly (see Table 21.14). It is important to provide adequate information to relatives and other carers who may be administering medications and monitoring blood glucose at home, because they may lack knowledge of the symptoms and consequences of hypoglycaemia (Table 21.15).

21.12 Summary and conclusions

To summarize:

- Hypoglycaemia in the elderly person with type 2 diabetes is a potentially serious and underestimated clinical problem that has a significant morbidity and mortality.

- Many symptoms of hypoglycaemia in the elderly are 'neurological' in type, the cause of which may be misinterpreted as representing a cerebrovascular event or cardiac arrhythmia.

- The effects of ageing and of type 2 diabetes on the hormonal counter-regulation, symptoms and awareness of hypoglycaemia should be considered when deciding upon targets for glycaemic control in elderly people with diabetes.

- Although most elderly people have type 2 diabetes, insulin therapy is increasingly being used. Although the counter-regulatory hormonal deficiencies and impaired awareness of hypoglycaemia that are common in people with type 1 diabetes are observed infrequently in elderly people with insulin-treated diabetes, these acquired hypoglycaemia syndromes may increase in prevalence.

- Although hypoglycaemia is a common side effect of insulin therapy, it occasionally may be a life-threatening problem in people taking long-acting sulphonylureas, especially those patients of advanced years who have concomitant renal impairment and/or inadequate caloric intake.

- Long-acting sulphonylureas, such as glibenclamide and chlorpropamide, should be avoided in the elderly. Adverse drug interactions with sulphonylurea agents can cause profound hypoglycaemia.

- If the treatment of hypoglycaemic coma with intravenous dextrose is unsuccessful, other causes of coma should be sought urgently, and the presence of cerebral oedema excluded by neuroimaging.

- People with diabetes who are treated with sulphonylureas or insulin, and their relatives or carers, must be fully informed of the symptoms and effects of hypoglycaemia and its emergency management. This should be reinforced with appropriate education at intervals.

References

1. UK Prospective Diabetes Study Group (1998) Intensive blood-glucose control with sulphonylureas or insulin compared with conventional treatment and risk of complications in patients with type 2 diabetes (UKPDS 33). *Lancet*, **352**, 837–53.
2. Cryer PE (1993) Glucose counterregulation: prevention and correction of hypoglycemia in humans. *Am J Physiol*, **264**, E149–55.
3. Gerich JE (1988) Glucose counterregulation and its impact on diabetes mellitus. *Diabetes*, **37**, 1608–17.
4. Cryer PE, Binder C, Bolli GB, Cherrington AD, Gale EAM, Gerich JE and Sherwin RS (1989) Hypoglycemia in IDDM. *Diabetes*, **38**, 1193–9.
5. Towler DA, Havlin CE, Craft S and Cryer P (1993) Mechanism of awareness of hypoglycemia. Perception of neurogenic (predominantly cholinergic) rather than neuroglycopenic symptoms. *Diabetes*, **42**, 1792–8.

6. Corrall RJM, Frier BM, Davidson NMcD, Hopkins WM and French EB (1983) Cholinergic manifestations of the acute autonomic reaction to hypoglycaemia in man *Clin Sci*, **64**, 49–53.

7. Macdonald IA and Maggs DA (1993) Cutaneous blood flow, sweating, tremor and temperature regulation in hypoglycaemia. In: *Hypoglycaemia and diabetes: Clinical and physiological aspects*, BM Frier and BM Fisher (eds), Edward Arnold, London, pp. 132–43.

8. Deary IJ, Hepburn DA, MacLeod KM and Frier BM (1993) Partitioning the symptoms of hypoglycaemia using multi-sample confirmatory factor analysis. *Diabetologia*, **36**, 771–7.

9. Frier BM and Fisher BM (eds) (1993) *Hypoglycaemia in Diabetes: Clinical and Physiological Aspects*, Edward Arnold (Publishers) Ltd, London.

10. Deary, I.J. (2007) Symptoms of hypoglycaemia and effects on mental performance and emotions. In: BM Frier and BM Fisher (eds) *Hypoglycaemia in Clinical Diabetes*, 2nd edition. John Wiley & Sons, Chichester, pp. 25–48.

11. McAulay V, Deary IJ, Frier BM (2001) Symptoms of hypoglycaemia in people with diabetes *Diabet Med*, **18**, 690–705.

12. Vea H, Jorde R, Sager G, Vaaler S and Sundsfjord J (1992) Reproducibility of glycaemic thresholds for activation of counterregulatory hormones and hypoglycaemic symptoms in healthy subjects. *Diabetologia*, **35**, 958–61.

13. Frier BM (2007) Impaired awareness of hypoglycaemia. In: *Hypoglycaemia in Clinical Diabetes*, 2nd edition. BM Frier and M Fisher (eds), John Wiley & Sons, Chichester, pp. 141–70.

14. Amiel SA (2007) Risks of strict glycaemic control. In: *Hypoglycaemia in Clinical Diabetes*, 2nd edition. BM Frier and M Fisher (eds), John Wiley & Sons, Chichester, pp. 171–89.

15. Gerich JE and Bolli GB (1993) Counterregulatory failure. In: *Hypoglycaemia and Diabetes: Clinical and Physiological Aspects*. BM Frier and BM Fisher (eds), Edward Arnold, London, pp. 253–67.

16. White NH, Skor DA, Cryer PE, Levandoski LA, Bier DM and Santiago JV (1983) Identification of type 1 diabetic patients at increased risk for hypoglycemia during intensive therapy. *New Engl J Med*, **308**, 485–91.

17. Bolli GB, Tsalikian E, Haymond MW, Cryer PE and Gerich JE (1984) Defective glucose counterregulation after subcutaneous insulin in non-insulin-dependent diabetes mellitus. *J Clin Invest*, **73**, 1532–41.

18. Ryder RE, Owens DR, Hayes TM, Ghatei MA and Bloom SR (1990) Unawareness of hypoglycaemia and inadequate hypoglycaemic counterregulation: no causal relation with diabetic autonomic neuropathy. *Br Med J*, **301**, 783–7.

19. Cryer PE (2002) Hypoglycaemia: the limiting factor in the management of type 1 and type 2 diabetes. *Diabetologia*, **45**, 937–48.

20. Henderson JN, Allen KV, Deary IJ and Frier BM (2003) Hypoglycaemia in insulin-treated type 2 diabetes: frequency, symptoms and impaired awareness. *Diabet Med*, **20**, 1016–21.

21. Cryer PE, Fisher JN and Shamoon H (1994) Hypoglycemia. *Diabetes Care*, **17**, 734–55.

22. Cryer PE (1992) Iatrogenic hypoglycemia as a cause of hypoglycemia-associated autonomic failure in IDDM. A vicious cycle. *Diabetes*, **41**, 255–60.

23. Segel SA, Paramore DA and Cryer PE (2002) Hypoglycemia-associated autonomic failure in advanced type 2 diabetes. *Diabetes*, **51**, 724–33.

24. Cryer PE (2004) Diverse causes of hypoglycemia-associated autonomic failure in diabetes. *N Engl*, **350**, 2272–9.

25. Marker JC, Cryer PE and Clutter WE (1992) Attenuated glucose recovery from hypoglycemia in the elderly. *Diabetes*, **41**, 671–8.

26. Meneilly GS, Minaker KL, Young JB, Landsberg L and Rowe JW (1985) Counterregulatory responses to insulin-induced glucose reduction in the elderly. *J Clin Endocrinol Metab*, **61**, 178–82.

27. Meneilly GS, Cheung E and Tuokko H (1994) Altered responses to hypoglycemia of healthy elderly people. *J Clin Endocrinol Metab*, **78**, 1341–8.

28. Ortiz-Alonso FJ, Galecki A, Herman WH, Smith MJ, Jacquez JA and Halter JB (1994) Hypoglycemia counterregulation in elderly humans: relationship to glucose levels. *Am J Physiol*, **267**, E497–506.

29. Brierley EJ, Broughton DL, James OWF and Alberti KGMM (1995) Reduced awareness of hypoglycaemia in the elderly despite an intact counterregulatory response. *Quart J Med* **88**, 439–45.

30. Matyka K, Evans M, Lomas J, Cranston I, Macdonald I and Amiel SA (1997) Altered hierarchy of protective responses against severe hypoglycemia in normal ageing in healthy men. *Diabetes Care*, **20**, 135–41.

31. Jaap AJ, Jones GC, McCrimmon RJ, Deary IJ and Frier BM (1998) Perceived symptoms of hypoglycaemia in elderly type 2 diabetic patients treated with insulin. *Diabet Med*, **15**, 398–401.

32. Reynolds C, Molnar GD, Horwitz DL, Rubenstein AH, Taylor WF and Jiang NS (1977) Abnormalities of endogenous glucagon and insulin in unstable diabetes. *Diabetes*, **26**, 36–45.

33. Nonaka K, Toyoshima T, Yoshida T, Matsuyama T, Trarni S and Nishikawa M (1977) The nature of hyperglucagonaemia in diabetes mellitus. In: *Glucagon: its Role in Physiology and Clinical Medicine*, TP Foa,

JS Jajos, NL Foa (eds), Springer-Verlag, New York, pp. 662–77.

34. Polonsky KS, Herold KC, Gilden JL, Bergenstal RM, Fang VS, Moossa AR and Jaspan JB (1984) Glucose counterregulation in patients after pancreatectomy. Comparison with other clinical forms of diabetes. *Diabetes*, **33**, 1112–19.

35. Levitt NS, Vinik AI, Sive AA, Child P and Jackson WPU (1979) Studies on plasma glucagon concentration in maturity-onset diabetics with autonomic neuropathy. *Diabetes*, **28**, 1015–21.

36. Boden G, Soriano M, Hoeldtke RD and Owen OE (1983) Counterregulatory hormone releases and glucose recovery after hypoglycemia in non-insulin-dependent diabetic patients. *Diabetes*, **32**, 1055–9.

37. Heller SR, Macdonald IA and Tattersall RB (1987) Counterregulation in type 2 (non-insulin-dependent) diabetes mellitus. Normal endocrine and glycaemic responses, up to ten years after diagnosis. *Diabetologia*, **30**, 924–9.

38. Meneilly GS, Cheung E and Tuokko H (1994) Counterregulatory hormone responses to hypoglycemia in the elderly patient with diabetes. *Diabetes*, **43**, 403–10.

39. Shamoon H, Friedman S, Canton C, Zacharowicz L, Hu M and Rossetti L (1994) Increased epinephrine and skeletal muscle responses to hypoglycemia in non-insulin-dependent diabetes mellitus. *J Clin Invest*, **93**, 2562–71.

40. Korzon-Burakowska A, Hopkins D, Matyka K, Lomas J, Pernet A, Macdonald I and Amiel S (1998) Effects of glycemic control on protective responses against hypoglycemia in type 2 diabetes. *Diabetes Care*, **21**, 283–90.

41. Levy CJ, Kinsley BT, Bajaj M and Simonson DC (1998) Effect of glycemic control on glucose counterregulation during hypoglycemia in NIDDM. *Diabetes Care*, **21**, 1330–8.

42. Amiel SA, Maran A, Powrie JK, Umpleby AM and Macdonald IA (1993) Gender differences in counterregulation to hypoglycaemia. *Diabetologia*, **36**, 460–4.

43. Davis SN, Fowler S and Costa F (2000) Hypoglycemic counterregulatory responses differ between men and women with type 1 diabetes. *Diabetes*, **49**, 56–72.

44. Sandoval DA, Ertl AC, Richardson MA, Tate DB and Davis SN (2003) Estrogen blunts neuroendocrine and metabolic responses to hypoglycemia. *Diabetes*, **52**, 1749–55.

45. Diamond MP, Hallerman L, Starick-Zych K, Jones TW, Connolly-Howard M, Tamborlane WV and Sherwin RS (1991) Suppression of counterregulatory hormone response to hypoglycemia in normal man. *J Clin Endocrinol Metab*, **73**, 1123–8.

46. Liu D, Moberg E, Kollind M, Lins PE and Adamson U (1991) A high concentration of circulating insulin suppresses the glucagon response to hypoglycemia in normal man. *J Clin Endocrinol Metab*, **73**, 1123–8.

47. Davis SN, Goldstein RE, Jacobs J, Price L, Wolfe R and Cherrington AD (1993) The effects of differing insulin levels on the hormonal and metabolic response to equivalent hypoglycemia in normal humans. *Diabetes*, **42**, 263–72.

48. Fanelli C, Pampanelli S, Epifano L, Rambotti AM, Ciofetta M, Modarelli F, et al. (1994) Relative roles of insulin and hypoglycaemia on induction of neuroendocrine responses to, symptoms of, and deterioration of cognitive function in hypoglycaemia in male and female humans. *Diabetologia*, **37**, 797–807.

49. Spyer G, Hattersley A, Macdonald IA, Amiel S and MacLeod KM (2000) Hypoglycaemic counterregulation at normal blood glucose concentrations in patients with well controlled type 2 diabetes. *Lancet*, **356**, 1970–4.

50. Israelian Z, Szoke E, Woerle J, Bokhari S, Schorr M, Schwenke DC, Cryer PE, Gerich JE and Meyer C (2006) Multiple defects in counterregulation of hypoglycemia in modestly advanced type 2 diabetes mellitus. *Metab Clin Exp*, **55**, 593–8.

51. Hepburn DA, MacLeod KM, Pell ACH, Scougal IJ and Frier BM (1993) Frequency and symptoms of hypoglycaemia experienced by patients with type 2 diabetes treated with insulin. *Diabet Med*, **10**, 231–7.

52. Peacey SR, George E, Rostami-Hodjegan A, Bedford C, Harris N, Hardisty CA, Tucker GT, Macdonald IA and Heller SR (1996) Similar physiological and symptomatic responses to sulphonylurea and insulin induced hypoglycaemia in normal subjects. *Diabet Med*, **13**, 634–41.

53. Thomson FJ, Masson EA, Leeming JT and Boulton AJM (1991) Lack of knowledge of symptoms of hypoglycaemia by elderly diabetic patients. *Age Ageing*, **20**, 404–6.

54. Pramming S, Thorsteinsson B, Bendtson I and Binder C (1991) Symptomatic hypoglycaemia in 411 type 1 diabetic patients. *Diabet Med*, **8**, 217–22.

55. MacLeod KM, Hepburn DA and Frier BM (1993) Frequency and morbidity of severe hypoglycaemia in insulin-treated diabetic patients. *Diabet Med*, **10**, 238–45.

56. ter Braak EWMT, Appleman AMMMF, van de Laak M, Stolk RP, van Haeften TW and Erkelens DW

(2000) Clinical characteristics of type 1 diabetic patients with and without severe hypoglycemia. *Diabetes Care*, **23**, 1467–71.

57. Pedersen-Bjergaard U, Pramming S, Heller SR, Wallace TM, Rasmussen AK, Jorgensen HV, Matthews DR, Hougaard P and Thornsteinsson B (2004) Severe hypoglycaemia in 1076 adult patients with type 1 diabetes: influence of risk markers and selection. *Diabetes Metab Res Rev*, **20**, 479–86.

58. UK Hypoglycaemia Study Group (2007) Risk of hypoglycaemia in types 1 and 2 diabetes: effects of treatment modalities and their duration. *Diabetologia*, **50**, 1140–7.

59. Dahlen M, Bergman U, Idman L, Martinsson L and Karlsson G (1984) Epidemiology of hypoglycaemia in patients on oral antidiabetic drugs in the island of Gotland, Sweden. *Acta Endocrinol*, **263** (Suppl. 21), Abstract.

60. Berger W (1985) Incidence of severe side-effects during therapy with sulfonylureas and biguanides. *Horm Metab Res*, **15** (Suppl.), 111–15.

61. Campbell IW (1985) Metformin and the sulphonylureas: the comparative risk. *Horm Metab Res* **15**, 105–11.

62. Gerich JE (1989) Oral hypoglycemic agents. *New Engl J Med*, **321**, 1231–45.

63. Clarke BF and Campbell IW (1975) Long-term comparative trial of glibenclamide and chlorpropamide in diet-failed, maturity onset diabetics. *Lancet*, **i**, 246–8.

64. Jennings AM, Wilson RM and Ward JD (1989) Symptomatic hypoglycemia in NIDDM patients treated with oral hypoglycemic agents. *Diabetes Care*, **12**, 203–8.

65. Abraira C, Colwell JA, Nuttall FQ, Sawin CT, Nagel NJ, Comstock JP, Emanuele NV, Levin SR, Henderson W and Lee HS (1995) Veterans Affairs Cooperative Study on glycemic control and complications in type II diabetes mellitus (VACSDM). Results of the feasibility trial. Veterans Affairs Cooperative Study in Type II Diabetes. *Diabetes Care*, **18**, 1113–23.

66. Shorr RI, Ray WA, Daugherty JR and Griffin MR (1997) Incidence and risk factors for serious hypoglycemia in older persons using insulin or sulfonylureas. *Arch Intern Med*, **157**, 1681–6.

67. Miller CD, Philips LS, Ziemer DC, Gallina DL, Cook CB and El-Kebbi IM (2001) Hypoglycemia in patients with type 2 diabetes mellitus. *Arch Intern Med*, **161**, 1653–59.

68. Gurlek A, Erbas T and Gedik O (1999) Frequency of severe hypoglycaemia in type 1 and type 2 diabetes during conventional insulin therapy. *Exp Clin Endocrinol Diabetes*, **107**, 220–4.

69. Leese GP, Wang J, Broomhall J, Kelly P, Marsden A, Morrison W, Frier BM, Morris AD, the

DARTS/MEMO Collaboration (2003) Frequency of severe hypoglycemia requiring emergency treatment in type 1 and type 2 diabetes: a population-based study of health service resource use. *Diabetes Care*, **26**, 1176–80.

70. Donnelly LA, Morris AD, Frier BM, Ellis JD, Donnan PT, Durrant R *et al.*, for the DARTS/MEMO Collaboration (2005) Frequency and predictors of hypoglycaemia in type 1 and insulin-treated type 2 diabetes: a population-based study. *Diabet Med* **22**, 749–55.

71. Tunbridge WMG (1981) Factors contributing to deaths of diabetics under fifty years of age. *Lancet*, **ii**, 569–72.

72. Seltzer HS (1972) Drug-induced hypoglycemia: a review based on 473 cases. *Diabetes*, **21**, 955–66.

73. Campbell IW (1993) Hypoglycaemia and Type II diabetes: sulphonylureas. In: *Hypoglycaemia and diabetes. Clinical and physiological aspects*, BM Frier and BM Fisher (eds), Edward Arnold, London, pp. 387–92.

74. Frier BM (1992) Hypoglycaemia - how much harm? *Hospital Update*, **18**, 876–84.

75. Fisher BM and Heller SR (2007) Mortality, cardiovascular morbidity and possible effects of hypoglycaemia on diabetic complications. In: *Hypoglycaemia in Clinical Diabetes*, 2nd edition, BM Frier and M Fisher (eds), John Wiley & Sons, Chichester, pp. 265–83.

76. Perros P and Deary IJ (2007) Long-term effects of hypoglycaemia on cognitive function and the brain in diabetes. In: *Hypoglycaemia in Clinical Diabetes*, 2nd edition, BM Frier and M Fisher (eds), John Wiley & Sons, Chichester, pp. 285–307.

77. Vestergaard P, Rejnmark L and Mosekilde L (2005) Relative fracture risk in patients with diabetes mellitus, and the impact of insulin and oral antidiabetic medication on relative fracture risk. *Diabetologia*, **48**, 1292–9.

78. Macdonald IA, Bennett T, Gale EAM, Green JH and Walford S (1982) The effect of propranolol or metoprolol on thermoregulation during insulin-induced hypoglycaemia in man. *Clin Sci*, **63**, 301–10.

79. Sommerfield AJ, Wilkinson IB, Webb DJ and Frier BM (2007) Vessel wall stiffness in type 1 diabetes and the central hemodynamic effects of acute hypoglycemia. *Am J Physiol Endocrinol Metab*, **293**, E1274–9.

80. Lindström T, Jorfeldt L, Tegler L and Arnqvist HJ (1992) Hypoglycaemia and cardiac arrhythmias in patients with type 2 diabetes mellitus. *Diabet Med*, **9**, 536–41.

81. Frier BM, Barr StCG and Walker JD (1995) Fatal cardiac arrest following acute hypoglycaemia in a diabetic patient. *Pract Diab Internat*, **12**, 284.

82. Burke BJ and Kearney TK (1999) Hypoglycaemia and cardiac arrest. *Pract Diab Internat*, **16**, 189–90.

83. Marques JLB, George E, Peacey SR, Harris ND, Macdonald IA, Cochrane T and Heller SR (1997) Altered ventricular repolarisation during hypoglycaemia in patients with diabetes. *Diabet Med*, **14**, 648–54.

84. Landstedt-Hallin L, Englund A, Adamson U and Lins PE (1999) Increased QT dispersion during hypoglycaemia in patients with type 2 diabetes. *J Intern Med*, **246**: 299–307.

85. Seltzer HS (1979) Severe drug-induced hypoglycaemia: a review. *Compr Ther*, **5**, 21–9.

86. Ben-Ami H, Nagachandran P, Mendelson A and Edoute Y (1999) Drug-induced hypoglycemic coma in 102 diabetic patients. *Arch Intern Med*, **159**, 281–4.

87. Asplund K, Wilholm BE and Lithner F (1983) Glibenclamide associated hypoglycaemia: a report on 57 cases. *Diabetologia*, **24**, 412–17.

88. Asplund K, Wilholm BE and Lundman B (1991) Severe hypoglycaemia during treatment with glipizide. *Diabet Med*, **8**, 726–31.

89. Seltzer HS (1989) Drug-induced hypoglycemia: a review of 1418 cases. *Endocrinol Metab Clin North Am*, **18**, 163–83.

90. Stahl M and Berger W (1999) Higher incidence of severe hypoglycaemia leading to hospital admission in type 2 diabetic patients treated with long-acting versus short-acting sulphonylureas. *Diabet Med*, **16**, 586–90.

91. Paes AHP, Bakker A and Soe-Agnie CJ (1997) Impact of dosage frequency on patient compliance. *Diabetes Care*, **20**, 1512–17.

92. Donnan PT, MacDonald TM and Morris AD (2002) Adherence to prescribed oral hypoglycaemic medication in a population of patients with type 2 diabetes: a retrospective cohort study. *Diabet Med*, **19**, 279–84.

93. Kerr D, Macdonald IA, Heller SR and Tattersall RB (1990) Alcohol causes hypoglycaemic unawareness in healthy volunteers and patients with type I (insulin-dependent) diabetes. *Diabetologia*, **33**, 216–21.

94. Cheyne EH, Sherwin RS, Lunt MJ, Cavan DA, Thomas PW and Kerr D (2004) Influence of alcohol on cognitive performance during mild hypoglycaemia: implications for type 1 diabetes. *Diabet Med*, **21**, 230–7.

95. Burge MR, Zeise TM, Sobhy TA, Rassam AG and Schade DS (1999) Low-dose ethanol predisposes elderly fasted patients with type 2 diabetes to sulfonylurea-induced low blood glucose. *Diabetes Care*, **22**, 2037–43.

96. Ferner RE and Neil HA (1988) Sulphonylureas and hypoglycaemia. *Br Med J*, **296**, 949–50.

97. Brodows RG (1992) Benefits and risks with glyburide and glipizide in elderly NIDDM patients. *Diabetes Care*, **15**, 75–80.

98. Tessier D, Dawson K, Tetrault JP, Bravo G and Meneilly GS (1994) Glibenclamide vs gliclazide in type 2 diabetes of the elderly. *Diabet Med*, **11**, 974–80.

99. Yap WS, Peterson GM, Vial JH, Randall CT and Greenaway TM (1998) Review of management of type 2 diabetes mellitus. *J Clin Pharm Ther*, **23**, 457–65.

100. Campbell RK (1998) Glimepiride: Role of a new sulfonylurea in the treatment of type 2 diabetes mellitus. *Ann Pharmacother*, **32**, 1044–52.

101. Schneider, J (1996) An overview of the safety and tolerance of glimepiride. *Horm Metab Res*, **28**: 413–18.

102. Schernthaner G, Grimaldi A, Di Mario U, Drzewoski J, Kempler P, Kvapil M, Shaw KM, the GUIDE Study (2004) Double blind comparison of once-daily gliclazide MR and glimepiride in type 2 diabetic patients. *Eur J Clin Invest*, **34**, 535–42.

103. Lindgren M, Eckert B, Stenberg G and Agardh CD (1996) Restitution of neurophysiological functions, performance, and subjective symptoms after moderate insulin-induced hypoglycaemia in non-diabetic men. *Diabet Med*, **13**, 218–25.

104. Evans ML, Pernet A, Lomas J, Jones J and Amiel SA (2000) Delay in onset of awareness of acute hypoglycemia and of restoration of cognitive performance during recovery. *Diabetes Care*, **23**, 893–7.

105. Fanelli CG, Pampanelli S, Porcellati F *et al.* (2003) Rate of fall of blood glucose and physiological responses of counterregulatory hormones, clinical symptoms and cognitive function to hypoglycaemia in type 1 diabetes mellitus in the postprandial state. *Diabetologia*, **46**, 53–64.

106. Gale EAM (1980) Hypoglycaemia. *Clin Endocrinol Metab*, **9**, 461–75.

107. Marks V (1981) Drug-induced hypoglycaemia. In: *Hypoglycaemia*, 2nd edition, V Marks and FC Rose (eds), Blackwell Scientific Publications, Oxford, pp. 357–86.

108. Marri G, Cozzolino G and Palumbo R (1968) Glucagon in sulphonylurea hypoglycaemia? *Lancet*, **i**, 303–4.

109. Johnson SF, Schade DS and Peake GT (1977) Chlorpropamide-induced hypoglycemia: successful treatment with diazoxide. *Am J Med*, **63**, 799–804.

110. Palatnick W, Meatherall RC and Tenenbein M (1991) Clinical spectrum of sulfonylurea overdose and experience with diazoxide therapy. *Arch Intern Med*, **151**, 1859–62.

111. Krentz AJ, Boyle PJ, Justice KM, Wright AD and Schade DS (1993) Successful treatment of severe

refractory sulfonylurea-induced hypoglycemia with octreotide. *Diabetes Care*, **16**, 184–6.

112. Boyle PJ, Justice K, Krentz AJ, Nagy RJ and Schade DS (1993) Octreotide reverses hyperinsulinemia and prevents hypoglycemia induced by sulfonylurea over-doses. *J Clin Endocrinol Metab*, **76**, 752–6.

113. Mutch WJ and Dingwall-Fordyce I (1985) Is it a hypo? Knowledge of symptoms of hypoglycaemia in elderly diabetic patients. *Diabet Med*, **2**, 54–6.

114. Pegg A, Fitzgerald F, Wise D, Singh BM and Wise PH (1991) A community-based study of diabetes-related skills and knowledge in elderly people with insulin-requiring diabetes. *Diabet Med*, **8**, 778–81.

115. Strachan MWJ, Deary IJ, Ewing FME and Frier BM (1997) Is type II diabetes associated with an increased risk of cognitive dysfunction? A critical review of published studies. *Diabetes Care*, **20**, 438–45.

22

Diabetes in Care Homes

Alan Sinclair[1] and Terry Aspray[2]

[1]*Bedfordshire and Hertfordshire Postgraduate Medical School, University of Bedfordshire, Putteridge Bury, Hitchin Road, Luton, UK*
[2]*Newcastle University, Campus for Ageing and Vitality, Newcastle upon Tyne, UK*

Key messages

- The quality of diabetes care within care homes and other assisted-living facilities needs to improve and this requires implementation of evidence-based guidelines and policy enforcement
- Screening for diabetes at the time of admission to a care home and regularly afterwards is an important measurable outcome
- Maintenance of health status and functional performance are key goals of care for all residents with diabetes

22.1 Introduction

For the United Kingdom, between the years 2000 and 2050, it is projected that the number of people aged over 65 years will continue to increase from 9.3 million to 17 million. In addition, a fourfold increase is anticipated in the number of over- 85-year-olds, from 1.1 million to 4.4 million! [1]. Independent living may be increasingly difficult for this older population as frailty and chronic ill-heath are accompanied by isolation. Diabetes is known to be an independent risk factor for admission to a care home [2] and is impicated in up to a quarter of admissions [3].

In the industrialized nations of the world, increasing numbers of older people continue to leave their own homes and move into institutions where their physical and social needs may be better met. In the United States, apart from chronic care settings such as nursing homes, there is a growing industry of assisted-living facilities where facilities such as the provision of a meal service, supervision, leisure and cleaning are provided. In other countries such as Australia, low-level hostels provide care services for many older patients. The organization and operation of such facilities affect the nature of the provision of health and social care to residents and as a consequence impact on the quality of care delivered, irrespective of the health condition.

22.2 The United Kingdom as a model of care home reform

In the United Kingdom, after World War II, the 1948 National Assistance Act established the local authority as the responsible body for overseeing the reform of public assistance institutions (the origins of which came from the Elizabethan Poor Law) and the creation of residential care homes for older people "...in need of care and attention".

Improvements to bed provision were slow and hampered by a lack of funds. Residents were more frail and increasingly dependent, but fewer hospital beds

Diabetes in Old Age. Third Edition. Edited by Alan J. Sinclair
© 2009 John Wiley & Sons, Ltd

for frail older people were being provided, putting continued pressure on local authority and social services to support the care of frail older people at home and in residential and nursing homes. During the 1980s, there was also an expansion of the independent sector to complement (or compete with) social services provision. Between 1982 and 1991, the number of beds in private care homes rose from 49 900 to 161 200 [4]. However, the free provision of care within these homes is dependent on residents having a low level of wealth. As increasing numbers of frail older people have moved into private care homes, National Health Service (NHS) long-stay hospital beds have also closed, so that more than 50% of all health care beds in the UK are now provided in nursing homes! [5].

As a result of these trends, more people are living in care homes and, indeed, UK estimates are that the current population of 450 000 will increase to 1 130 000 in the next 50 years. This will be associated with the social and health costs of providing care escalating from £13 billion to £55 billion by the year 2051 [6]. In the UK, Section 49 of the Health and Social Services Act, 2001, made care provided by registered nurses in care homes an NHS responsibility, and thus free of charge. Hence, the nomenclature is intimately linked with costs of care and eligibility for free care funded by the NHS.

Since 2004, the Commission for Social Care Inspection (CSCI) has incorporated the roles of the Social Services Inspectorate (SSI), the joint review team of the SSI, the National Care Standards Commission (NCSC) and the Audit Commission in the UK. Further reorganization of regulatory services is anticipated, incorporating the Healthcare Commission and the Mental Health act commission. However, the CSCI and its successor will have responsibility for the regulation, inspection and review of social care services. In particular, they inspect care homes and rate them, according to national standards, as well as reviewing local councils and their own provision of advice and purchase of services. According to the UK Commission for Social Care Inspection, the distinction between *Residential* and *Nursing* homes is that:

- *Residential care* (sometimes termed *personal care only*) is provided to people either short or long term, offering accommodation, meals and personal care (such as help with washing and eating).

- *Nursing care homes*, by comparison, offer the same as those without nursing care but they also have *registered nurses* who can provide care for more complex health needs.

This distinction between social and nursing care needs applies to individuals. Although residents may enter a home requiring only personal care assistance, they are likely to become increasingly frail, and health needs may increase requiring a *nursing* bed. While this may necessitate a move, many homes offer both residential and nursing care, allowing the resident to remain in the same home.

Other aspects of specialist care include the accommodation of residents with mental health disorder. The archaic term Elderly Mentally Infirm is abbreviated to EMI, which remains in common usage. For this group, both residential and nursing care is provided. Finally, there is an increasing population of older adults with learning disability, who have left their former long-term care in psychiatric hospitals to live in the community and present their own special challenges [7].

22.3 Epidemiology

A number of studies and surveys of diabetes prevalence have been performed, and the key references for this are presented in Table 22.1. In the US, the proportion of residents with diagnosed diabetes has increased from 14.5% to 24.6% between 1979 and 2004 [8]. This may represent an increase in prevalence of type 2 diabetes in the USA and possibly an increase in survival, but there has probably been an increase in screening and diagnosis of the condition to explain much of this trend. European estimates of self-reported diabetes are much lower; however, when studies have been augmented by the direct assessment of glucose tolerance, the estimated prevalence exceeds 20%. Such studies thus identify a large population who are unaware of their abnormal glucose tolerance.

There are important challenges highlighted by these data. If interested in diabetes prevalence, then we can be convinced that the condition is common and – at least in Europe – often undiagnosed. If we wish to identify cases for treatment, then widespread screening programmes for diabetes may not be practical, where such a large proportion are frail and unlikely to comply with a glucose tolerance test. The use of fasting glucose alone will miss cases, and a postprandial test may be helpful in increasing the numbers screened but will also miss cases.

Table 22.1 Estimates of diabetes prevalence among frail older care home residents.

Source	No. of patients	Criteria	Prevalence (%)	Comments
Wisconsin, USA, 1979 [9]	7850 (approx.)	Self reported	10	A community-based study: 0.9% of cases living in nursing homes. However, 17.5% of adults aged 80+ years were in nursing homes!
Toronto 1965–86 [10]	1177	Newly diagnosed	30–35	Longitudinal study of care home residents not diabetic at admission on oral glucose tolerance test.
US National Nursing Home survey, USA 1979		Self-report	14.5	Difficulty in collating data from this report.
Wales, 1997 ([11])	1514	Self-report	7.2	Study was not aimed at screening new cases but at looking at characteristics of known cases.
Liverpool, 1997 [12]	1611	Self-report	9.9	Primarily a description of the quality of care.
Germany, 2001 [13]	1936	Self-report	26.2	Study also examined the undiagnosed population, but used HbA_{1c} as diagnostic test. Data not considered here.
Birmingham UK [3]	636	Self-report Plus OGTT	12.0 26.7	The first study to use a screening test. WHO 1998 Criteria used. Details given of those unable to participate.
USA, 2004 [8]	549 125	Self-report	26.4	This review of all new admissions to care homes during 2002 suggests that diagnostic coverage has improved.
Newcastle, 2006 [14]	1461	Self-report Plus fasting/ postprandial glucose	11.4 19.9	Fasting and postprandial glucose used to increase coverage but may have resulted in underestimate of prevalence. Difference in prevalence between residential, nursing and EMI care homes found.
New Zealand, 2006 [15]	1567	Self-report	11.7	
Norway, 2006 [16]	788 186	Self-report HbA_{1c}/OGTT	20.2 0.5	Including frail older people in their own home BUT the majority (427) were unfit to participate. Patients had to have a raised HbA_{1c} in order to be eligible for OGTT screening.

OGTT = oral glucose tolerance test.

22.4 Complications and comorbidity

Chronic disease is common among care home residents, compared with older people living in the community. Despite this, the quality of care for older people living in nursing homes may be worse than for those living at home. For example, fewer residents have been found to receive vaccination or blood pressure monitoring [17]. In one large study of American nursing homes, diabetes, dementia, cancer, heart failure, renal failure, chronic pulmonary disease and anaemia were all associated with an increased risk of mortality at 12 months [18]. Susceptibility to infections, particularly pneumonia, has been highlighted in nursing homes [19–21] and, more recently, with concern about the risk of methicillin-resistant *Staphylococcus aureus* (MRSA) infection [22, 23].

Having diabetes is associated with a doubling of the risk of admission to nursing home from a subject's own home [2], and diabetes accounts for 12.3% of all admissions to nursing home care [24]. Disability associated with diabetes is characteristically progressive in those requiring long-term care [25]. Residents with diabetes are likely to be at greater risk from microvascular disease [26] and visual impairment, with cataract prevalent in 80% and diabetic retinopathy in 2.1% of all nursing home residents [27]. In the UK and the USA, diabetic residents are younger and at increased risk of hospital readmission, cognitive impairment, limb amputations and death, when compared to non-diabetic residents [12, 28]. Pressure sores are more common in diabetic residents: in one prospective study of 14 607 residents, the odds ratio for developing a pressure ulcer, adjusted for other comorbidities, was 1.4 (95% CI: 1.2–1.8) [29].

In addition, residents with diabetes have a range of other comorbidities. Although there are no studies of dementia specific to care homes, cognitive impairment is associated with diabetes in older age [30, 31]. One recent study of diabetes prevalence found the highest rates of undiagnosed diabetes in EMI residential care homes [14], and the diabetes care for these residents in particular failed to meet local and national standards. The impact of comorbidities on diabetes care warrants further study. For example, cognitive impairment may result in patients being less able to monitor their glucose levels or inject insulin; Parkinson's disease has been associated with an increase in cost of diabetes care by up to 300%! [32].

Obesity is a risk factor for diabetes and, in one US study, the proportion of obese residents newly admitted to nursing homes rose from 15% to 25% over a 10-year period [33]. Obesity in middle age is associated with a 30% increased risk of admission to nursing homes after 25 years [34]. The associated risks of diabetes may explain some of the secular trend in diabetes prevalence in US nursing homes, which have already been discussed [35]. However, for nursing home residents with diabetes, undernutrition is also commonly seen. Half of all subjects in one study received lower dietary energy intakes than recommended [36], while in a further study switching diabetic residents to the normal diet provided in the care home was not associated with any significant deterioration in glycaemic control [37].

22.5 Common management problems

Some common clinical management problems arise in the care of older adults, living in care homes (see Table 22.2):

- *Nutrition:* Weight loss and nutritional deficiency can occur through anorexic symptoms and reduced calorific intake. Other contributing factors include severe physical and cognitive impairment, as well as neurological and gastroenterological disorders associated with dysphagia, including stroke. In the future, increasing numbers of residents are also anticipated with obesity and associated problems, thus exacerbating function and mobility, as discussed above [34].

- *Increased risk of hypoglycaemia:* This condition may occur in residents receiving sulphonylureas or insulin, through several predisposing factors. These include: (i) nutritional deficiency and weight loss; (ii) cognitive impairment resulting in meals being missed through poor memory and orientation; (iii) anorexic conditions such as malignancy or infection; and (iv) a lack of awareness of the symptoms and signs of hypoglycaemia by residents themselves or by care staff. The latter may be compounded by a lack of monitoring of diabetes by residents and staff.

- *Infections:* Recurrent skin, chest and urinary infections may occur, especially if the control of blood glucose is not optimal. Infections themselves predispose the resident with diabetes to marked hyperglycaemia or metabolic decompensation, and even to hyperosmolar non-ketotic coma or ketosis.

Table 22.2 Management problems in care homes.

- Nutritional deficiency and weight loss
- Increased risk of hypoglycaemia
- Infections
- Urinary incontinence
- Pressure sores
- Leg and foot ulceration
- Communication difficulties
- Increased risk of adverse drug reactions

- *Urinary incontinence:* This may be secondary to hyperglycaemia, urinary infection, poor mobility or cognitive impairment.

- *Pressure sores and leg or foot ulceration:* These can lead to rapid deterioration and need for hospital admission.

- *Communication difficulties:* These can lead to un-recognized diabetes care needs. Predisposing factors include cognitive impairment, dysphasia and dysarthria from cerebrovascular or other neurological disease, and sensory impairments such as visual and hearing loss.

- *Increased risk of adverse drug reactions:* These can occur because residents are often taking multiple drugs for their diabetes and other coexisting diseases. Risks can be exacerbated by infrequent review of medication and lack of monitoring of renal and hepatic function.

22.6 Organization of diabetes care in residential settings

22.6.1 Setting standards for diabetes care

The American Diabetes Association (ADA) reviews its clinical practice recommendations, annually, and these are both comprehensive and up-to-date [38]. In Great Britain, the National Institute for Health and Clinical Excellence (NICE) and the National Service Framework (NSF) for diabetes identify the key components of diabetes care [39, 40], and similar guidelines are available from other organizations and countries. Overall, in the UK the introduction of standards has been credited with improvements in health care, especially when linked to payments to general practitioners through the Quality and Outcomes Framework (QOF) [41]. The Diabetes NSF identified a series of standards to be applied to the care of children and adults with diabetes, and their relevance (or lack of relevance) and/or implications for residents of care homes has been addressed in Table 22.3. These may be directly applicable to other health care organizations in different countries.

Appropriate standards of care should take into consideration, where feasible, with specific concerns for diabetes in frail, older care-home residents. The common clinical problems in this group, which may not be seen in younger adults with diabetes, are listed in Table 22.2. For example, there is an increased likelihood of undernutrition, risk of hypoglycaemia and recurrent urinary infection. With immobility comes the risk of ulceration of the lower limbs and perineum, the healing of which may be impaired by the presence of diabetes.

Although, both the ADA and the NSF include sections about adults living in institutions, these primarily relate to prisoners and not to care home residents. In response to such guidelines and standards, health services are bound to develop policies to implement change, and the danger of using such inappropriate standards has been highlighted as vulnerable older people may suffer in the absence of targets specific to their needs [42]. However, they can also act as important audit tools, allowing the priorities of older people to be highlighted. In one case study, a combination of national, local and care home-specific standards was used to develop an audit tool to evaluate services for older people [43].

22.6.2 Developing standards for care homes

There are two main barriers to optimizing diabetes care in care homes. First, there are some clinical issues (as already outlined above; see Table 22.2) which are specific to older people, and may not be included in local diabetes service design. Second, there are factors relating to the care home itself; for example, there is a well-recognized lack of sufficient staff training with few opportunities for continuing professional development in diabetes. There are high rates of staff turnover in many homes, compounded by a large proportion of unqualified staff with little experience or training to prepare them for looking after residents with diabetes. Finally, there is often a lack of available resources of staff time, catering services and equipment. In addition, there may be a lack of clear boundaries between medical and nursing responsibilities, which can be exacerbated by poor communication.

Staff preparing meals and supervising residents at meal time may lack a basic understanding of nutritional principles. Communication difficulties between staff and residents may exist, which prevent needs being met; these may be linguistic or cultural, or might reflect comorbidities, including neurological problems. Restrictive professional boundaries may prevent health care professionals from having specific inputs into care homes, especially within the independent sector. Quite clearly, the establishment of national standards

Table 22.3 UK National Service Framework Standards, 2001.

Standards	Summary	Comments with regard to implementation for Care Home Residents
Prevention of type 2 diabetes	• Reduce risk of developing type 2 diabetes • Population as a whole • Reduce inequalities	Focus on intervention has been on reducing prevalence of overweight and obesity in adults and children. Lifestyle interventions are often not appropriate to older subjects, especially those living in institutions.
Identification of people with diabetes	• Identify people who do not know they have diabetes	Strategy has been to increase awareness of symptoms, but these are less specific and relevant in frail older people. Follow-up, regular testing and opportunistic screening should be feasible. However, such services may not reach care home residents [17].
Empowering people with diabetes	• Encourage partnership in decision-making, self-management and maintain healthy lifestyle • Parents and carers should be fully engaged	Partnership may be difficult, where residents have lost autonomy and may be cognitively impaired. Structured education programmes (e.g. DESMOND XPERT) do not accommodate people living in institutions.
Clinical care of adults with diabetes	• High-quality care for patients throughout lifetime • Optimize control of blood glucose, blood pressure and other risk factors	There may be specific barriers to monitoring: residential homes without nursing staff may not monitor blood glucose, and there may be increasing dependence on district nurses. There may be difficulties in transporting frail residents to diabetes clinics in primary care and hospital settings.
Clinical care of children and young people with diabetes	• High-quality care and transition between paediatric and adult services	There is an analogy to be drawn here with transition between routine diabetes care and specialist care for older people living in institutions.
Management of diabetic emergencies	• Protocols for treatment of diabetic emergencies and acute complications • Minimize risk of recurrence	No specific mention is made of the management of hyperosmolar states, more common in older people and associated with adverse outcomes. Care-home staff will require specific training on the identification and treatment of hypoglycaemia.
Care of people with diabetes during admission to hospital	• Effective hospital care for diabetes • Continue to be involved in decisions	These apply equally to frail older people admitted to hospital.
Diabetes and pregnancy	• Optimize outcome of pregnancy for women	Hopefully, not applicable!
Detection and management of long-term complications	• Surveillance for long-term complications • Protocols to investigate and to treat reducing risk of disability and premature death	Retinopathy and podiatry surveillance may not reach care home residents. Less aggressive approaches to secondary prevention may be adopted, through inertia and/or lack of evidence. Long-term benefits may not be as relevant to frail older patients with a shorter life expectancy.

of diabetes care within care homes may be an important initiative to promote care within these settings.

There is a clear lack of diabetes-related experience and knowledge among care home staff, and appropriate education and training is needed to improve diabetes care. However, difficulties in providing education and training include a lack of staff training budget in many homes, resulting in a reliance on free advice and information. Many care staff are young and unskilled, with older members of staff often employed part time and unqualified. Many homes have a high staff turnover rate, with poor pay and conditions, which can lead to a low staff morale. Nursing staff work a rotating shift system which can lead to a poor continuity of care, and often precludes attendance at training events. In spite of these difficulties, diabetes training and education is provided to homes by many local diabetes care teams. These are usually welcomed by care home managers, and their success seems to relate to good local relationships being built up. It also requires the local diabetes team to feel a responsibility for these homes and to be allowed by their managers to go in and help.

In the United Kingdom, individual home proprietors and trade associations can assist in improving diabetes care. For example, the Independent Healthcare Association is the largest association in the independent sector, representing acute, psychiatric and long-term care providers across the UK. By facilitating the promotion and dissemination of best practice, research reports and quality control systems within care homes, they are well placed to liaise with care home owners, managers and staff to support education and training initiatives.

In response to such concerns, Diabetes UK has reviewed diabetes care in institutions and produced a guideline for care homes. The Diabetes UK guideline [44] synthesized available evidence to identify the clinical issues of particular relevance to this group:

- Lack of care plans and case management approaches for residents with diabetes.

- Inadequate nutritional guidance.

- Lack of specialist health professional input.

- Diabetes care not coordinated between primary and secondary care services.

- Inadequate review and poor metabolic control.

- Lack of knowledge relating to diabetes among staff working in care homes.

- Lack of structured education and training for staff.

Difficulties with diabetes care in institutional settings have been shown elsewhere. For example, in the United States Funnel and Herman examined the policies and practices in a group of 17 skilled nursing homes in Michigan [45]. Although, the ADA and the American Association for Diabetes Education first developed guidelines for diabetes care in skilled nursing homes in 1981 [46], the authors carried out their review using the 1995 version of less-specific criteria derived from the ADA [38]. The homes studied were generally large (mean number of beds 137) and the number of residents with diabetes per home ranged from 1 to 46 (mean 19). Almost all of the homes reviewed had some diabetes care protocols, plans or standing orders in place, although the standing orders usually consisted of guidelines relating to nutrition or some aspects of nursing care. Guidelines of care relating to parameters of metabolic control, when to call a physician, or the surveillance of complications, were least often present. In general, the care provided did not meet local or national standards of diabetes care, but care practices were better when registered dieticians were involved in meal planning and where written institutional policies were actually present.

More recently, a European Working Party devoted a section of its evidence-based diabetes guidelines specifically to care homes [47]. Such guidelines offer an important competing viewpoint to more generic guidelines such as the NSF, outlined in Table 22.3.

Examples of evidenced-based recommendations provided in the European Guidelines are as follows:

- At the time of admission to a care home, each resident requires to be screened for the presence of diabetes. Level of evidence 2++; Grade of recommendation B.

- Each resident should have an annual screen for diabetes. Level of evidence 2+; Grade of recommendation C.

- Each resident with diabetes should have an individualized diabetes care plan with the following minimum details: dietary plan, medication list, glycaemic targets, weight and nursing plan. Level of evidence 2+; Grade of recommendation C.

- Each care home with diabetes residents should have an agreed Diabetes Care Policy or Protocol which is regularly audited. Level of evidence 2++; Grade of recommendation B.

- Optimal blood pressure and blood glucose regulation may help to maintain cognitive and physical performance for each resident with diabetes. Level of evidence 2+; Grade of recommendation C (extrapolated data).

22.6.3 Improving care

If current guidelines and protocols fail to support appropriate diabetes care in institutional settings, then what should be the aims of optimal care? Residents with diabetes in care homes should receive a level of comprehensive diabetes care commensurate with their needs, and this should be on an equitable basis with those people with diabetes who do not live in an institutional setting. The two most important objectives are:

1. To maintain the highest degree of quality of life and well-being, without subjecting residents to unnecessary and inappropriate medical and therapeutic interventions.

2. To provide sufficient support and opportunity to enable residents to manage their own diabetes condition where this is a feasible and worthwhile option.

However, there are several additional processes of care which represent important goals to achieve for any resident with diabetes in a care home.

Metabolic Control

- Avoiding malaise and lethargy of hyperglycaemia

- Minimizing the risk of hypoglycaemia

- Promoting the greatest level of physical and cognitive function.

The European Guidelines [47] provide the following recommendation for glycaemic control:

"For frail (dependent; multisystem disease; care home residency including those with dementia) patients where the hypoglycaemia risk is high and symptom control and avoidance of metabolic decompensation is paramount, the target HbA1c range should be >7.5 to ≤.5%. Evidence level 3/4; Grade of recommendation D." (In the revision of Guidelines to be published in early 2009, a target range of <7.0% will be stated.)

Foot Care

- Preserving the integrity of the feet

- Promoting mobility where possible

- Preventing unnecessary hospital admissions for diabetic foot problems.

Eye Care

- Preserving vision, including screening for refractive error and cataract.

Screening for Neurovascular Complications

- Peripheral neuropathy and peripheral vascular disease which predispose to foot infection and ulceration.

Management of Coexisting Disease in a Structured Way

- Including the diagnosis and treatment of depressive illness, heart failure and hypertension.

Nutritional Assessment

- Provide a well-balanced individualized healthy eating

- Compatible with well-being

- Maintaining appropriate bodyweight.

22.6.4 Nutrition in diabetic residents

Residents are likely to have several reasons for being nutritionally at risk. These include a lack of nutritional knowledge and outdated ideas about diabetic diets that are held by some staff. It is vital that up-to-date information about diabetes and healthy eating be provided to care home staff, especially those who have responsibility for menu planning, food purchasing and cooking. Local dietetic services will usually be a good source of help and advice in implementing healthy-eating policies. They may often be able to help in staff training on the dietary aspects of diabetes care.

22.6.5 Responsibility of the physician

All residents of care homes in the UK are registered with a general practitioner (GP), and diabetes care is assumed to be delivered by GPs for the majority of patients. The increasing numbers of older people in care homes is having a significant impact on the workload of many GPs [48], and there is no recognition or encouragement for GPs to provide specialist diabetes care in residential settings. Many visits to care homes are 'reactive' in nature, taking place only when a problem has been identified by the home staff. Care home residents often have mobility problems, preventing them from visiting the GP's surgery for annual review, and few GPs provide a multidisciplinary annual review service in the care home. Diabetologists often have little experience of managing frail older people in the community, and geriatricians are doing less in continuing and community care. Meanwhile, commissioning priorities for older people focus on the management of long-term conditions by community matrons and other non-medical staff, concentrating on acute illness and the prevention of hospital admission. The transfer of long-term care from hospitals to care homes has not been accompanied by any significant transfer of medical resources to the community. In consequence, older people in care homes increasingly fall between primary, secondary and social care services, and all too often their needs are forgotten [49].

Since some concerns about care home medicine in the UK were highlighted over 10 years ago [50], there have been no significant national developments and no clear model has evolved. At the time, a number of options was envisaged: visiting medical officers; dedicated geriatric medical and psychiatric outreach services; integrated care by specialists, commissioned by primary care or a more formalized model of shared care between hospital and GP. Some studies have been conducted in the UK on chronic disease management using American-style Health Maintenance Organizations (HMOs), but they have not gone as far as employing their own medical staff. Rather perversely, the Evercare project used a model of care devised and implemented in the USA for the care of nursing home residents, but applied it to frail older people living in their own homes, with no evidence of beneficial effect [51].

Today, the GPs are still responsible for the medical care of individual residents registered with their practice. There remains no formal structure for the routine involvement of consultants in geriatric medicine or diabetes, nor other health care professionals to provide multidisciplinary diabetes care when required. In the absence of any formal national structure local, *ad hoc* arrangements are still being employed in an attempt to provide the best possible multidisciplinary care.

22.6.6 Multidisciplinary diabetes care

The elements of multidisciplinary diabetes care include the following:

- An individualized diabetes care plan, with each resident contributing to agreed objectives summarized in a care plan.

- The plan should include: (i) a series of metabolic targets; and (ii) an individualized dietary and nutritional plan.

- An annual review assessment should involve: (i) an eye check; and (ii) a foot check.

- Support and assistance in diabetes care from a named person who will be involved in metabolic monitoring with the resident.

- Inclusion of all residents with diabetes in the local diabetes registers at General Practice and/or district level, as appropriate

In the locally variable arrangements that exist in the UK, these elements may be provided by a number of health care professionals. The diabetes NSF covers all of these, but the targeting of this community is not well addressed, and there is the risk that QOF returns are not submitted for some of the more challenging tasks, resulting in older people being excluded from care.

22.6.7 Nursing care

Diabetes specialist nurses

These nurses, who have had special training and education in diabetes, are known to be an invaluable link between primary and secondary diabetes care for older people [52], and can provide a high-quality service to disadvantaged people with diabetes [53]. Increasingly, diabetes specialist nurses are employed to work in the community and, within the time constraints of their busy jobs, may become involved in diabetes education and support for home care staff, assisting in the development of the diabetes care policies for the home and individual care plans.

Primary care practice nurses

Increasingly, practice-based nurses who have had special training in diabetes are coordinating diabetes care in general practice. They may also be empowered to visit residents of the practice who are living in care homes, to assist in the delivery of the care objectives outlined above.

District (community) nurses

District nurses can play an immense supporting role in diabetes care in residential settings, despite many receiving little – if any – special training in this area. The major remit of the district nurse is in the provision of nursing support to residential homes, including advice to staff on diabetes care. They often administer insulin to residents unable to self-inject because of physical impairment, cognitive disability or behavioural disturbance. Specific arrangements can be made between care homes and District Nursing services with the delegation of specific diabetes care tasks to care home staff. However, care homes have been criticised over recent years for their medicines management policies, with insulin having attracted particularly heavy criticism [54]. There can also be tensions, where the residents' personal care needs alter to a point where they require *nursing* rather than personal care, with an expectation that the care home nursing staff will offer monitoring and insulin therapy.

22.6.8 Footcare

Published information from many countries worldwide testifies to the high prevalence of diabetic foot disease among the residents of care homes [26, 55–57]. The risk of *foot ulceration* is increased in those with advancing age, loss of protective pain sensation due to diabetic peripheral neuropathy, peripheral vascular disease, and bony foot abnormalities. Although residents should have access to free care from state-registered podiatrists, in some homes private podiatrists are employed to offer routine foot care, and residents maybe encouraged to pay fees for their footcare. Thus, a local state-registered podiatrist with an interest in diabetes is a very important member of a local multidisciplinary diabetes team, and his or her skills need to be utilized by care home staff in appropriate ways.

All people with diabetes should have an annual foot examination as part of the review process, and residents in care homes are not exempt from this recommendation [39]. This examination is to detect feet at risk of ulceration. At its simplest, this involves a brief history to discover any previous episodes of ulceration, an inspection of the feet to check for bony abnormalities, palpation of the dorsalis pedis and posterior tibial pulses to detect ischaemia, and the use of a 5.07 g nylon monofilament to detect the loss of protective pain sensation. This foot examination can be carried out by any member of the community diabetes team who has the relevant skills and experience and, if the foot is deemed to be at risk, it should be checked every 3 months by a podiatrist. It is also important to train care home staff to understand the importance of preventive footcare, and to alert them to the importance

of detecting early signs of foot ulceration and infection, so that urgent prompt referral and action can be taken. The local state-registered podiatrist with an interest in diabetes will usually be the best person to provide this help.

22.6.9 Provision of eye care

The lack of specialist eye care and regular ophthalmology review of residents with diabetes has been demonstrated in UK care homes [12, 56]. Many older people with diabetes have undetected refractive error, and screening of immobile residents in care homes is feasible, but costly [58].

The national standard for eye screening programmes in the UK are established, including exclusion criteria [59]. Where screening programmes are based on examinations carried out by experienced and specially trained optometrists, there may be a better service to older people, as refractive error, glaucoma and cataract can be checked at the same time as screening for diabetic retinopathy. The national standard is for diabetes eye screening using digital photography of the retina. However, immobile patients are excluded, which argues that they are unlikely to receive retinal surgery.

The barriers to optometrists working in care homes include:

- The funding of retinal screening at the exclusion of eye examinations in care homes.

- No financially viable option for the self-employed optometrists.

Thus, eye care for care home residents could be improved by an adequate funding of optometric assessment by contractual arrangements with the local commissioners resulting in:

- An improved and regular access of optometrists into care homes

- Visual screening of all new admissions who have diabetes.

This would require: (i) improved accommodation and facilities at each care home to allow full optometric assessment; (ii) the education of care staff about the visual health in residents; (iii) the identification of a member of care home staff responsible for organizing visits by the optometrist; and (iv) improved referral systems for residents with eye problems to specialist secondary care.

22.6.10 Assessing the efficacy and efficiency of diabetes care

Outcome measurements for diabetes in Primary Care have been incorporated into the audit tools supporting the NSF [39], and some of the gaps relating to the care of older people are outlined in Table 22.3. A uniform, comprehensive, standardized assessment for the routine long-term care of older people, the minimum dataset–resident assessment instrument (MDS-RAI), has been introduced into all nursing homes in the United States and Iceland, and also in three provinces in Canada. A US research group has combined data from the MDS-RAI instrument with other available data from Medicare and hospital discharge, to study treatment effects using valid measures of outcome in this frail population [60]. More recently, similar assessments have been carried out in the UK to assess nursing care needs [61].

Today, a number of national and international outcome measures are available for older adults with diabetes [47, 56], but these have not (yet) been adequately tested in care home settings. The purpose of outcome measures in care homes is to:

- Assess the quality of care delivered to each resident with diabetes.

- Assess the impact of diabetes on each resident in terms of personal well-being, functional disability, and rate of diabetes complications.

- Determine the impact of use of care home resources for residents with diabetes in terms of use of care staff time, dietary planning, monitoring equipment, and educational initiatives.

The potential outcome measures are summarized in Table 22.4. The data collection must be carried out by care staff and visiting health care professionals, and must represent the common objectives of diabetes care for all parties.

22.7 Sustaining effective diabetes care

Detailed recommendations for care are contained in both the BDA and the European Working Party reports [44, 47]. These are outlined below.

Table 22.4 Outcome measures for use in residential diabetes care.

1. The percentage of residents achieving agreed metabolic targets of HBA_{1c}, blood pressure, and weight during previous 12 months

2. Frequency and severity of hypoglycaemic episodes in previous 12 months

3. Frequency of hospital admissions for diabetes-related problems in previous 12 months

4. Complication rates of visual loss, foot ulceration, renal impairment, and angina

5. Changes in level of dependency and physical and mental function using the Barthel ADL (or extended ADL measures) and Mini-Mental State Examination Score (MMSE) during previous 12 months

6. Health-related quality of life and well-being of each resident with diabetes (e.g. using the SF 36 or sickness impact profile (SIP) measures); changes from admission to now, or changes within previous 12 months

7. The percentage of patients with completed diabetes care plans and annual reviews in the past 12 months

22.7.1 What the care home needs to provide

In order to sustain effective diabetes care, homes need to provide a suitable care environment in terms of staff, resources, equipment and facilities. These should include:

- Staff who have received appropriate training and education in the basic management diabetes in care home settings.

- Facilities to carry out blood glucose monitoring and staff trained in the use of the equipment.

- Accommodation for annual review examination of residents and foot care.

- A member of catering staff familiar with dietary planning for residents with diabetes.

- A protocol of diabetes care agreed by the staff of the home, visiting diabetes health care professionals and the GP.

- A method of collecting agreed diabetes outcome indicator data.

- Sufficient staff members trained to administer insulin.

- Educational resources on diabetes for residents and their families.

- Access to transport to enable residents to receive specialist treatment off site.

- An admission policy including a strategy for those with known diabetes and screening for diabetes.

Aspray and colleagues have shown that the use of a combination of such standards (generalized and age-environment-specific) can point to appropriate service changes [43].

22.7.2   What needs to be provided at the local level

Local diabetes services must encompass the special needs of care home residents with diabetes, including support and guidance for homes. In the UK, the general funding of care in residential and nursing homes will remain a subject of continued government debate for the foreseeable future. The joint commissioning of health and social services for older people would be a great step forward. Diabetes contracts within this context would support high-quality care for residents of care homes, and should include:

- Optometric services providing both on-site and clinic-based eye services.

- Podiatry services with time specifically dedicated to care home residents.

- Agreed criteria for referral to secondary and intermediate care specialist services.

- At least one diabetes specialist nurse specifically responsible for older people. He or she would play a prominent role in the effective organization and delivery of diabetes care to care homes in the area, including diabetes education.

- At least one community dietician in each locality, responsible for dietary and nutritional support of residents.

- The registration of all care home residents with diabetes on diabetes registers to ensure that they are involved in diabetes clinical audit projects.

- Diabetes educational and training programmes for care home staff at local, regional and national level to ensure that the staff are kept up to date.

22.8   Conclusions

Previously, diabetes care in residential settings has not attracted a great deal of scientific clinical enquiry, and consequently little has been known about the quality of diabetes care delivered; or the outcomes of care in residential settings. There are many important topics for future clinical research as the number of people with diabetes resident in care homes across the world continues to grow rapidly. The tremendous morbidity and disability of residents with diabetes within long-term care poses many complex and challenging problems for all health care professionals involved in delivering diabetes care. Some possible practical strategies to improve diabetes care have been proposed in this chapter.

References

1. Wittenberg, R., Comas-Herrera, A., Pickard, L. and Hancock, R. (2004) *Future demand for long-term care in the UK: A summary of projections of long-term care finance for older people to 2051.* The Joseph Rowntree Foundation, York.

2. Tsuji, I., Whalen, S. and Finucane, T. E. (1995). Predictors of nursing home placement in community-based long-term care. *J Am Geriatr Soc*, 43 (7), 761–6.

3. Sinclair, A.J., Gadsby, R., Penfold, S., Croxson, S.C. and Bayer, A.J. (2001) Prevalence of diabetes in care home residents. *Diabetes Care*, 24 (6), 1066–8.

4. Means, R., Morbey, H. and Smith, R. (2002) *From community care to market care?: the development of welfare services for older people.* Policy Press, Bristol.

5. Pollock, A.M., Player, S. and Godden, S. (2001) How private finance is moving primary care into corporate ownership. *Br Med J*, 322 (7292), 960–3.

6. *Paying for long-term care: Moving forward.* (2006) The Joseph Rowntree Foundation, York. Available at: www.jrf.org.uk.

7. Aspray, T.J., Francis, R.M., Tyrer, S.P. and Quilliam, S.J. (1999) Patients with learning disability in the community. *Be Med J*, 318 (7182), 476–7.

8. Travis, S.S., Buchanan, R.J., Wang, S. and Kim, M. (2004) Analyses of nursing home residents with diabetes at admission. *J Am Med Dir Assoc*, 5 (5), 320–7.

9. Klein, R., Klein, B.E., Moss, S.E., DeMets, D.L., Kaufman, I. and Voss, P.S. (1984) Prevalence of diabetes mellitus in southern Wisconsin. *Am J Epidemiol*, 119 (1), 54–61.

10. Grobin, W. (1989) A longitudinal study of impaired glucose tolerance and diabetes mellitus in the aged. *J Am Geriatr Soc*, 37 (12), 1127–34.

11. Sinclair, A.J., Allard, I. and Bayer, A. (1997) Observations of diabetes care in long-term institutional settings with measures of cognitive function and dependency. *Diabetes Care*, 20 (5), 778–84.

12. Benbow, S.J., Walsh, A. and Gill, G.V. (1997) Diabetes in institutionalised elderly people: a forgotten population? *Br Med J*, 314 (7098), 1868–9.

13. Hauner, H., Kurnaz, A.A., Haastert, B., Groschopp, C. and Feldhoff, K.H. (2001) Undiagnosed diabetes mellitus and metabolic control assessed by HbA(1c) among residents of nursing homes. *Exp Clin Endocrinol Diabetes*, 109 (6), 326–9.

14. Aspray, T.J., Nesbit, K., Cassidy, T.P., Farrow, E. and Hawthorne, G. (2006) Diabetes in British nursing and residential homes: a pragmatic screening study. *Diabetes Care*, 29 (3), 707–8.

15. Gill, E.A., Corwin, P.A., Mangin, D.A. and Sutherland, M.G. (2006) Diabetes care in rest homes in Christchurch, New Zealand. *Diabet Med*, 23 (11), 1252–6.

16. Jorde, R. and Hagen, T. (2006) Screening for diabetes using HbA1c in elderly subjects. *Acta Diabetol*, 43 (2), 52–6.

17. Fahey, T., Montgomery, A.A., Barnes, J. and Protheroe, J. (2003) Quality of care for elderly residents in nursing homes and elderly people living at home: controlled observational study. *Br Med J*, 326 (7389), 580.

18. van Dijk, P.T., Mehr, D.R., Ooms, M.E., Madsen, R., Petroski, G., Frijters, D.H., *et al.* (2005) Comorbidity and 1-year mortality risks in nursing home residents. *J Am Geriatr Soc*, 53 (4), 660–5.

19. Garibaldi, R.A. (1999). Residential care and the elderly: the burden of infection. *J Hosp Infect*, 43 (Suppl.), S9–18.

20. Loeb, M. (2005) Epidemiology of community- and nursing home-acquired pneumonia in older adults. *Expert Rev Anti Infect Ther*, 3 (2), 263–70.

21. Marrie, T.J., Durant, H. and Kwan, C. (1986) Nursing home-acquired pneumonia. A case-control study. *J Am Geriatr Soc*, 34 (10), 697–702.

22. Libert, M., Elkholti, M., Massaut, J., Karmali, R., Mascart, G. and Cherifi, S. (2008) Risk factors for meticillin resistance and outcome of *Staphylococcus aureus* bloodstream infection in a Belgian university hospital. *J Hosp Infect*, 68(1), 17–24.

23. Lucet, J.C., Grenet, K., Armand-Lefevre, L., Harnal, M., Bouvet, E., Regnier, B., *et al.* (2005) High prevalence of carriage of methicillin-resistant *Staphylococcus aureus* at hospital admission in elderly patients: implications for infection control strategies. *Infect Control Hosp Epidemiol*, 26 (2), 121–6.

24. Russell, L.B., Valiyeva, E., Roman, S.H., Pogach, L.M., Suh, D.C. and Safford, M.M. (2005) Hospitalizations, nursing home admissions, and deaths attributable to diabetes. *Diabetes Care*, 28 (7), 1611–17.

25. Ferrucci, L., Guralnik, J.M., Pahor, M., Corti, M.C. and Havlik, R.J. (1997) Hospital diagnoses, Medicare charges, and nursing home admissions in the year when older persons become severely disabled. *JAMA*, 277 (9), 728–34.

26. Mooradian, A.D., Osterweil, D., Petrasek, D. and Morley, J.E. (1988) Diabetes mellitus in elderly nursing home patients. A survey of clinical characteristics and management. *J Am Geriatr Soc*, 36 (5), 391–6.

27. Whitmore, W.G. (1989) Eye disease in a geriatric nursing home population. *Ophthalmology*, 96 (3), 393–8.

28. Duffy, R.E., Mattson, B.J. and Zack, M. (2005) Comorbidities among Ohio's nursing home residents with diabetes. *J Am Med Dir Assoc*, 6 (6), 383–9.

29. Berlowitz, D.R., Brandeis, G.H., Morris, J.N., Ash, A.S., Anderson, J.J., Kader, B., *et al.* (2001) Deriving a risk-adjustment model for pressure ulcer development using the Minimum Data Set. *J Am Geriatr Soc*, 49 (7), 866–71.

30. Korf, E.S., White, L.R., Scheltens, P. and Launer, L.J. (2006) Brain aging in very old men with type 2 diabetes: the Honolulu-Asia Aging Study. *Diabetes Care*, 29 (10), 2268–74.

31. Xu, W.L., Qiu, C.X., Wahlin, A., Winblad, B. and Fratiglioni, L. (2004) Diabetes mellitus and risk of dementia in the Kungsholmen project: a 6-year follow-up study. *Neurology*, 63 (7), 1181–6.

32. Pressley, J.C., Louis, E.D., Tang, M.X., Cote, L., Cohen, P.D., Glied, S., *et al.* (2003) The impact of comorbid disease and injuries on resource use and expenditures in parkinsonism. *Neurology*, 60 (1), 87–93.

33. Lapane, K. L. and Resnik, L. (2005) Obesity in nursing homes: an escalating problem. *J Am Geriatr Soc*, 53 (8), 1386–91.

34. Elkins, J.S., Whitmer, R.A., Sidney, S., Sorel, M., Yaffe, K. and Johnston, S.C. (2006) Midlife obesity and long-term risk of nursing home admission. *Obesity (Silver Spring)*, 14 (8), 1472–8.

35. Resnick, H.E., Heineman, J., Stone, R. and Shorr, R.I. (2008) Diabetes in U.S. nursing homes, 2004. *Diabetes Care*, 31 (2), 287–8.

36. Benbow, S.J., Hoyte, R. and Gill, G.V. (2001) Institutional dietary provision for diabetic patients. *Q J Med*, 94 (1), 27–30.

37. Coulston, A.M., Mandelbaum, D. and Reaven, G.M. (1990) Dietary management of nursing home residents with non-insulin-dependent diabetes mellitus. *Am J Clin Nutr*, 51 (1), 67–71.

38. American Diabetes Association. (2008) Clinical Practice Recommendations. *Diabetes Care*, 31(Suppl. 1), S1–108.

39. Great Britain. Department of Health. (2001) *National service framework for diabetes: standards*. Department of Health, London.

40. National Institute for Clinical Excellence. (2002) *Management of type 2 diabetes*. National Institute for Clinical Excellence, London.

41. Campbell, S., Reeves, D., Kontopantelis, E., Middleton, E., Sibbald, B. and Roland, M. (2007) Quality of primary care in England with the introduction of pay for performance. *N Engl J Med*, 357 (2), 181–90.

42. Holt, R.M., Schwartz, F.L. and Shubrook, J.H. (2007) Diabetes care in extended-care facilities: appropriate intensity of care? *Diabetes Care*, 30 (6), 1454–8.

43. Aspray, T.J., Nesbit, K., Cassidy, T.P. and Hawthorne, G. (2006) Rapid assessment methods used for health-equity audit: diabetes mellitus among frail British care-home residents. *Public Health*, 120 (11), 1042–51.

44. British Diabetes Association. (1999) *Guidelines of Practice for Residents with Diabetes in Care Homes*. British Diabetes Association, London.

45. Funnell, M.M. and Herman, W.H. (1995) Diabetes care policies and practices in Michigan nursing homes, 1991. *Diabetes Care*, 18 (6), 862–6.

46. Van Nostrand, J. (1985) Nursing home care for diabetes. In: *Diabetes in America: Diabetes data compiled by National Diabetes Data group*. US Government Printing Office, Washington, DC, NIH publication 85-1468.

47. Sinclair, A.J., Cromme, P.V.M., Rodriguez-Manas, L., Fasching, P., Muggeo, M. and Hader, C. (2004) *Clinical Guidelines for Type 2 Diabetes Mellitus in older people*. Retrieved 1st July, 2008, from http://www.eugms.org/index.php?pid=31.

48. Kavanagh, S. and Knapp, M. (1998) The impact on general practitioners of the changing balance of care for elderly people living in institutions. *Br Med J*, 317 (7154), 322–7.

49. Bowman, C., Johnson, M., Venables, D., Foote, C. and Kane, R.L. (1999) Geriatric care in the United Kingdom: aligning services to needs. *Br Med J*, 319 (7217), 1119–22.

50. Black, D. and Bowman, C. (1997) Community institutional care for frail elderly people. *Br Med J*, 315 (7106), 441–2.

51. Gravelle, H., Dusheiko, M., Sheaff, R., Sargent, P., Boaden, R., Pickard, S., *et al.* (2007) Impact of case management (Evercare) on frail elderly patients: controlled before and after analysis of quantitative outcome data. *Br Med J*, 334 (7583), 31.

52. Sinclair, A.J., Turnbull, C.J. and Croxson, S.C. (1996) Document of care for older people with diabetes. Special Interest Group in Diabetes, British Geriatrics Society. *Postgrad Med J*, 72 (848), 334–8.

53. Norman, A., French, M., Hyam, V. and Hicks, D. (1998) Development and audit of a home clinic service. *Journal of Diabetic Nursing*, 2 (2), 51–4.

54. Great Britain. Commission for Social Care Inspection. (2006) *Handled with care? Managing medicines for residents of care homes and children's homes – a follow up study*. CSCI, London.

55. Cantelon, J.F. (1972) Diabetic residents of homes for the aged: observations for an eleven-year period. *J Am Geriatr Soc*, 20 (1), 17–21.

56. Sinclair, A.J., Turnbull, C.J. and Croxson, S.C. (1997) Document of diabetes care for residential and nursing homes. *Postgrad Med J*, 73 (864), 611–12.

57. Wolffenbuttel, B.H., van Vliet, S., Knols, A.J., Slits, W.L., Sels, J.P. and Nieuwenhuijzen Kruseman, A.C. (1991) Clinical characteristics and management of diabetic patients residing in a nursing home. *Diabetes Res Clin Pract*, 13 (3), 199–206.

58. Anderson, S., Broadbent, D.M., Swain, J.Y., Vora, J.P. and Harding, S.P. (2003) Ambulatory photographic screening for diabetic retinopathy in nursing homes. *Eye*, 17 (6), 711–16.

59. UK National Screening Committee. (2006) *Excluding patients from the NHS Diabetic Retinopathy Screening Programme temporarily or permanently: Good practice guide version 2.0*, from http://www.nscretinopathy.org.uk/exclusions.html

60. Carpenter, G.I., Bernabei, R., Hirdes, J.P., Mor, V. and Steel, K. (2000) Building evidence on chronic disease in old age. Standardised assessments and databases offer one way of building the evidence. *Br Med J*, 320 (7234), 528–9.

61. Carpenter, I., Perry, M., Challis, D. and Hope, K. (2003) Identification of registered nursing care of residents in English nursing homes using the Minimum Data Set Resident Assessment Instrument (MDS/RAI) and Resource Utilisation Groups version III (RUG-III). *Age Ageing*, 32 (3), 279–85.

23

Primary and Community Care of Diabetes in Older People

Roger Gadsby

Warwick Medical School, University of Warwick, Coventry, UK

Key messages

- Today, with rising numbers of older people living with diabetes, there is a shift from secondary to primary care delivery in many countries.
- Multidisciplinary teamwork and pay-for-performance schemes have been developed to provide incentives for better care.
- Care must be individualized, and issues of polypharmacy and medication adherence addressed.

23.1   Introduction

The number of people worldwide who are living with diabetes is rapidly increasing, with numbers expected to rise from today's figure of 194 million – equal to 5.1% of the adult population – to a total of 333 million in 2025, or 6.3% of the adult population [1]. Since people in general are living longer, the number of older people living with diabetes is likely to increase significantly in most countries of the world. Inevitably, this will place a severe strain on healthcare resources and healthcare provision. Consequently, systems of care will need to evolve in order to cope with this increasing diabetes population, and in many countries this has resulted in a shift in care status, from secondary to primary.

23.1.1   Definitions of primary, secondary and tertiary care

- *Primary care* is defined as the first-contact, continuous, comprehensive, coordinated care provided to people undifferentiated by age, gender, disease or organ system [2] In most countries it is provided by primary care physicians – often termed general practitioners (GPs) – and their associated teams.

- *Secondary care* is hospital care, either as an inpatient or as an outpatient. Such care is often consultative, short-term in nature, and provides assistance in the diagnosis and management for primary care physicians. Secondary care is provided by specialist doctors (often termed consultants) and their specialist teams.

- *Tertiary care* is very specialized care for those people with specific conditions that are often complex and rare, and require specific expertise. Tertiary care is usually based at regional or subregional hospitals, and provided by specialist doctors and their teams.

23.1.2   The funding and organization of healthcare

Different countries have different models by which health care is funded and organized. In the United Kingdom, care is free at the point of delivery and paid

Diabetes in Old Age. Third Edition. Edited by Alan J. Sinclair
© 2009 John Wiley & Sons, Ltd

for by the government out of taxation. Primary care is delivered by GPs, usually working in partnership with one another in small groups called 'practices'. The GPs employ their own staff and practice nurses. In other countries, however, funding is provided by health insurance companies, and patients may pay via a fee for service payment which is reimbursed by the insurance company.

Funding issues may influence the mode of provision of healthcare, the two central features of many primary care-driven healthcare systems being the concepts of:

- All people being registered with an individual primary care physician or practice which provides the first-contact care for all conditions.

- A 'gatekeeper function' which restricts access to more expensive and invasive secondary care services for those people referred from primary care [3].

23.2 The shift of diabetes care from the hospital to the community

During the 1950s and 1960s, diabetes was seen in many countries to be a condition that was dealt with by secondary care. Consequently, many hospitals had large diabetes outpatient clinics which people with diabetes attended, often on an annual basis.

During the 1970s, some family doctors in the UK and in some other countries began to assume responsibility for the routine review of their patients with diabetes. This came about when the hospital doctors developed a policy of trying to discharge patients to general practice in order to reduce the size of their clinics. Occasionally this occurred by agreement and planning, but in other situations it just 'happened'.

Over the past 20–30 years, increasing numbers of people have been diagnosed with diabetes, and this led to the hospital specialist model coming under considerable strain. In the UK, this was highlighted in a report from the audit commission entitled 'Testing Times', which reviewed secondary care diabetes services and concluded that many services were under considerable strain. One way forward proposed in the report was for primary care to provide more of the routine care, so that hospitals could concentrate on specialist care and professional support and training, while allowing patients to receive continuity of care closer to home [4].

Continuity of care with the same doctor and nurse team is especially important for elderly people with diabetes, and this may be more easily provided in primary care (Figure 23.1).

There is an evidence base to support this secondary to primary care shift. In 1998, a study was conducted which aimed to identify and evaluate all published randomized trials of hospital versus general practice care

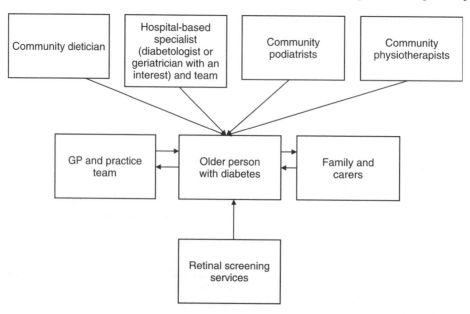

Figure 23.1 Healthcare professionals involved in the care of older people with diabetes in the community.

for people with diabetes, so as to compare the effectiveness of general practice and hospital care through the use of meta-analysis of the identified trials [5]. Five trials that included a total of 1058 patients were identified that fulfilled the inclusion criteria; three of these were from the UK, and two from Australia. The overall mean age of the patients was 58.4 years, and the results were found to be heterogeneous between the trials. In shared care schemes featuring more intensive support through a computerized prompting system for GPs and patients, there was no difference in mortality between care in hospital and care in general practice. The glycated haemoglobin (HbA$_{1c}$) level tended to be lower in primary care, and losses to follow up were significantly lower in primary care. Schemes with less well-developed support for family doctors were associated with adverse outcomes for patients.

The review concluded that unstructured care in the community was associated with a poorer follow up, worse glycaemic control and a greater mortality than hospital care. Computerized central recall, with prompting for patients and their family doctors, can achieve standards of care as good as – or even better than – hospital outpatient care, at least in the short term. The evidence supported the provision of a regular, prompted recall and the review of selected people with diabetes by willing GPs. Moreover, this goal could be achieved if a suitable organization were in place.

23.3 The primary care diabetes team

This should consist of a motivated GP (primary care physician) with access to a team of health care professionals including a practice nurse, dietician, podiatrist and a diabetes nurse or district (community) nurse with well-defined responsibilities for each team member [6].

The practice should operate a dedicated record-keeping system, with quality assessment and a recall system to enhance clinic attendance.

There should also be a structured protocol to include criteria for referral to a hospital specialist. This should include [6]:

- Patients with severe vascular complications.

- Patients who require treatment for diabetes eye disease, foot ulceration or nephropathy.

- Patients with increasing dependency and immobility.

- Patients with unstable cardiovascular disease (CVD).

- Patients with poor metabolic control where it is proving very difficult to control HBA$_{1c}$, lipids or blood pressure to agreed targets.

23.4 Routine care of people with diabetes by the primary care diabetes team

In a number of countries, the health economies have introduced – or are considering the introduction of – financial incentives for providing good quality care for people with chronic diseases. Payments are often made when processes of care are shown to reach a pre-specified standard. Some systems also reward the achievement of good quality care in specific areas. In diabetes, 'pay for performance' systems can reward the achievement of pre-specified target levels of blood pressure, HBA$_{1c}$ levels and lipids in a pre-specified percentage of patients. Although a number of pay for performance incentive schemes have been launched in the USA, the best-developed is in the UK, where it is referred to as a 'Quality and Outcomes framework'. In this system, points are achieved for both process and outcome achievement; the points then attract a payment figure which depends on the number of patients in the practice and the square root of the disease prevalence.

When it was launched as part of the new GP contract in the UK, the Department of Health stated that the Quality and Outcomes Framework (QOF) represented – for the first time in any large health system in any country – that GP practices would be rewarded systematically on the basis of the quality of care delivered to patients [7]. The basis for the Quality and Outcomes framework is a series of clinical domains which contain 10 disease areas, for which there are a maximum of 550 points.

For the first two years of the new GP contract in 2004/5 and 2005/6, the diabetes area had a maximum of 99 points (approximately 10% of the total available), spread across 18 clinical indicators.

23.4.1 Quality diabetes clinical indicators relevant to older people

These indicators insist that:

- a comprehensive diabetes review, including vision and footcare is undertaken annually;

- metabolic targets for blood pressure, HBA1c, and cholesterol are individualized and agreed with the older person, their families and carers; and

- issues of polypharmacy and concordance with medications are discussed, and agreed.

There has been an increase in the average number of points scored in 2005/6 as compared to the previous year (2004/5), and also an increase in the register prevalence of diabetes, from 3.4% to 3.6%. There is evidence therefore that health care professionals – when provided with an incentive – will strive to achieve that incentive as they will achieve more income. A recently published study described changes in performance of a random sample of 42 UK general practices in 1998, 2003 and 2005 [8]. This reported that, although the quality of care of people with diabetes was improving before the introduction of the 'pay for performance' scheme in 2004, there was an acceleration in improvement after its introduction.

In a review of six reports on the quality of diabetes care in the UK conducted since 1999, there was a trend towards improvement in both process and outcome of care relating to the period 1999–2004 [9]. The quality of both process and outcomes of care in the Quality and Outcomes framework results for 2004/5 and 2005/6 was significantly greater than that found in the published studies from previous years, and there was improvement in the scores for all clinical indicators for diabetes from 2004/5 to 2005/6 (see Table 23.1). The report authors concluded that modest financial incentives paid to primary care physicians might represent a successful strategy for improving the care of people with diabetes.

23.5 Which strategies to prevent CVD are appropriate for older people with diabetes?

One of the main questions in such incentive schemes is how hard should health care professionals strive so that old and very old people achieve the quality targets for glycaemic control, blood pressure and cholesterol. The concern is that, by zealous striving after blood pressure, cholesterol and HBA$_{1c}$ targets, there will be an impairment of the quality of life of older people with diabetes by increasing the risks of hypotension, the adverse side effects of medication and hypoglycaemia

that would 'outweigh' any benefits gained in increasing the quantity of life.

This balance between striving for targets and providing the best care for an individual older person with diabetes can be one of the most difficult judgements to make in the primary and community care of older people with diabetes.

The quality and outcomes targets in the UK system are based on evidence from randomized controlled trials and guidelines; there is, however, a judgement to be made as to whether this evidence applies to older people.

23.5.1 Primary prevention of adverse events: The evidence base

Glycaemic control

In the United Kingdom Prospective Diabetes Study of glycaemic control [10], newly diagnosed patients with type 2 diabetes were enrolled up to the age of 65 years and followed for mean of 10 years. The intensively treated group attained a mean HBA$_{1c}$ of 7% compared to the standard control group (mean 7.9%). This 0.9% reduction resulted in a 12% reduction for any diabetes-related endpoint, and 25% reduction for microvascular endpoints. There was also a 16% reduction in macrovascular events, which just failed to reach the level of statistical significance. Thus, it might be suggested that there is an evidence base for tight glycaemic control up to the age of 75 years. Studies conducted specifically in older people tend to be descriptive rather than true randomized controlled trials, and have shown an association between poor glycaemic control and mortality [11], cardiovascular events [12] and retinopathy [13].

Cholesterol control

In the Heart Protection Study (HPS) [14], patients aged up to 80 years were recruited and followed for a mean of 4 years. Hence, it could be suggested that there is an evidence base for cholesterol lowering with a statin up to 84 years. In the HPS, treatment with simvastatin (40 mg per day) resulted in a 27% reduction in the incidence of first non-fatal myocardial infarction, and a 25% reduction in first incidence of fatal or non-fatal stroke as compared to placebo.

In the CARDS study [15], a total of 2838 people aged 40–75 years with type 2 diabetes and no coronary heart disease (CHD) but who had one other risk

Table 23.1 Quality and outcomes framework (QOF) scores for diabetes; clinical indicators for 2004/5 and 2005/6.

Diabetes Mellitus (Diabetes)

Quality indicator	2005/06 Denominator	2005/06 Numerator	2005/06 %	2004/05 %	Difference
DM2 The percentage of patients with diabetes whose notes record BMI in the previous 15 months	1,835,480	1,726,599	94.1	90.6	3.5
DM3 The percentage of patients with diabetes in whom there is a record of smoking status in the previous 15 months except those who have never smoked where smoking status should be recorded once	1,870,940	1,821,376	97.4	95.9	1.5
DM4 The percentage of patients with diabetes who smoke and whose notes contain a record that smoking cessation advice has been offered in the last 15 months	277,317	265,623	95.8	93.2	2.6
DM5 The percentage of diabetic patients who have a record of HbA1c or equivalent in the previous 15 months	1,841,571	1,776,415	96.5	94.4	2.1
DM6 The percentage of patients with diabetes in whom the last HbA1C is 7.4 or less (or equivalent test/reference range depending on local laboratory) in last 15 months	1,674,231	1,034,293	61.8	58.8	3.0
DM7 The percentage of patients with diabetes in whom the last HbA1C is 10 or less (or equivalent test/reference range depending on local laboratory) in last 15 months	1,786,114	1,633,981	91.5	89.4	2.1
DM8 The percentage of patients with diabetes who have a record of retinal screening in the previous 15 months	1,781,716	1,580,830	88.7	83.4	5.3
DM9 The percentage of patients with diabetes with a record of presence or absence of peripheral pulses in the previous 15 months	1,785,322	1,574,374	88.2	78.9	9.3
DM10 The percentage of patients with diabetes with a record of neuropathy testing in the previous 15 months	1,782,667	1,558,411	87.4	77.6	9.8
DM11 The percentage of patients with diabetes who have a record of the blood pressure in the past 15 months	1,874,539	1,840,954	98.2	97.0	1.2
DM12 The percentage of patients with diabetes in whom the last blood pressure is 145/85 or less 17 55%	1,753,856	1,313,740	74.9	70.3	4.6
DM13 The percentage of patients with diabetes who have a record of micro-albuminuria testing in the previous 15 months (exception reporting for patients with proteinuria)	1,684,327	1,396,760	82.9	70.9	12.0
DM14 The percentage of patients with diabetes who have a record of serum creatinine testing in the previous 15 months	1,857,309	1,777,422	95.7	93.0	2.7
DM15 The percentage of patients with diabetes with proteinuria or micro-albuminuria who are treated with ACE inhibitors (or A2 antagonists)	161,211	138,292	85.8	82.1	3.7
DM16 The percentage of patients with diabetes who have a record of total cholesterol in the previous 15 months	1,849,405	1,764,280	95.4	92.7	2.7
DM17 The percentage of patients with diabetes whose last measured total cholesterol within previous 15 months	1,703,389	1,345,409	79.0	71.8	7.2
DM18 The percentage of patients with diabetes who have had influenza immunisation in the preceding 1 September to 31 March	1,651,515	1,477,561	89.5	85.2	4.3
Diabetes Prevalence (registered)	53,211,253	1,890,663	3.6	3.4	0.2

factor for CHD (e.g. hypertension or smoker) were randomized to atorvastatin (10 mg per day) or placebo. The trial was stopped earlier than expected because the pre-specified early stopping rule for efficacy had been met; hence, the median duration of follow-up was 3.9 years. Compared with placebo, the risk reduction in the atorvastatin group for a CHD event was 37%, and for death was 27%.

Blood pressure-lowering

The United Kingdom Prospective Diabetes Study (UKPDS) [16] began as a study of glycaemic control in people newly diagnosed with type 2 diabetes, but subsequently had a blood pressure control study embedded into it. People were recruited up to the age of 75 years and followed for a mean of 10 years.

In the blood pressure study, 1148 people with hypertension and type 2 diabetes were randomized to a tight control arm or a less-tight control arm. The final mean difference between the two groups was 10/5 mmHg (144/82 mmHg with tight control, 154/87 mmHg with less-tight). Over nine years, patients in the tight control group showed significant reductions in morbidity and mortality, with: (i) a 32% reduction in diabetes-related death; (ii) a 44% reduction in fatal and non-fatal stroke; (iii) a 56% reduction in congestive cardiac failure; and (iv) a 37% reduction in developing microvascular complications. The tightly controlled patients were treated with the beta-blocker atenolol or the ACE-inhibitor captopril, but the study was not sufficiently powered to determine which agent was superior [1].

In the Hypertension Optimal Treatment Trial [17], a total of 18 790 patients with hypertension were randomized into three groups, the aim being to achieve diastolic pressures less than 90 mmHg, 85 mmHg and 80 mmHg in each group. The trial included about 1500 people with type 2 diabetes, who were aged up to 80 years. There were significant reductions in cardiovascular morbidity and mortality in the tightest controlled group, with a relative risk reduction of 50% [2].

Based on the results of these studies, it can be suggested that there is an evidence base for blood pressure lowering up to the age of about 80 years in people with type 2 diabetes.

Unfortunately, the people enrolled into clinical trials tend to be relatively fit and healthy, with a single specific disease that is the 'target' of the trial. But this does not correlate with many of the old and very old people with type 2 diabetes seen in primary care.

There is, therefore, a significant question as to the applicability of these trials to older people with type 2 diabetes who consult in primary care.

23.5.2 Applying the evidence to independent and frail older people

It is possible to divide old and very old people into two broad categories:

- Those who have type 2 diabetes as their only significant disease and are otherwise fit, healthy and living independently. Approximately one-third of individuals fall into this group, based on data obtained from a large community study in Wales conducted during the 1990s, where the objective measures of dependency were based on Barthel Activities of Daily Living (ADL) score, Extended ADL score and Mini-Mental State Examination score [18]. The recommendation for primary prevention in these subjects, where the precise evidence is lacking, would be to treat to targets set for younger people, in consultation with the individual. Thus there would be striving to obtain all the QOF targets for that individual.

- Those who are frail and elderly and have significant comorbidities, such as arthritis, high dependency levels or significant dementia. Approximately two thirds of individuals fall into this group. The practical care for people in this group would be to ensure symptomatic control, avoid hypoglycaemia and intensive monitoring, in consultation with the individual and their carers.

The GP contract QOF allows individuals to be excluded for varying reasons, and exception reporting can therefore be used for older people if the clinician feels that achieving targets is not in the individual patient's best interests.

23.5.3 Exception reporting

Exception reporting allows the practice to exclude individual patients from the disease indicators in particular circumstances. These are:

- Patients excepted from the whole clinical area:
  ○ Those who have been recorded as refusing to attend a review, having been invited on at least three occasions during the preceding 12 months.
  ○ Those for whom it is not appropriate to review the chronic disease parameters due to specific circumstances, such as extreme frailty or terminal illness or severe dementia.

- Where a patient does not agree to investigation and treatment and, after a reasonable discussion or written advice, has given their informed dissent; it is essential that such dissent has been recorded in the medical notes.

- Patients exempted from one clinical indicator only (if a valid Read code is used):
  - Patients on maximum tolerated doses of medication whose level of outcome remains suboptimal.
  - Patients for whom prescribing a medication is not clinically appropriate; for example, those who have an allergy, another contraindication, or who have experienced an adverse reaction.
  - Where a patient has not tolerated a medication.
  - Where a patient does not agree to investigation and treatment and, after a reasonable discussion or written advice, they have given their informed dissent; this dissent must be recorded in the medical notes.
  - Where the patient has a supervening condition which makes treatment of their condition inappropriate, for example cholesterol reduction where the patient has liver disease.
  - Where an investigative service or secondary care service is unavailable.

- Patients exempted automatically from any of the indicators by reporting software:
  - Patients newly diagnosed within the practice with diabetes or who have recently registered with the practice, who should have measurements made within 3 months and delivery of clinical standards within 9 months; for example, blood pressure or cholesterol measurements within target level.

23.6 Preventive health care in older people: Further debate

The whole problem of preventive health care in older people has been recently highlighted in a report in the *British Medical Journal* [19]. In an analysis of the PROSPER trial, in which older people aged 70–82 years were randomized to pravastatin or placebo, there was a clear but small benefit on mortality and morbidity from CVD in the group given pravastatin. However, all-cause mortality was not altered. The reduction in cardiovascular-related deaths was countered by an increase in deaths from cancer. A meta-analysis of all statin trials has failed to show any increase in cancer deaths in people treated with statins [20].

As none of the studies (apart from PROSPER) included elderly people, Mangin *et al.* concluded that the more likely reason for the results seen in elderly people was a substitution of the cause of death. These authors argued that the best interests of elderly people might lie in investing money in health care to relieve suffering, such as cataract operations, dementia care and joint replacements, rather than the primary prevention of CVD. Mangin *et al.* considered this the reason why GPs in the UK during the first year of the Quality and Outcomes framework were reluctant to follow the guidelines for cholesterol measurement and lipid lowering in people aged >75 years [21].

In a large cohort study in Canada of people aged ≥66 years with newly diagnosed type 2 diabetes, 21.8% received an antiplatelet drug, 39.6% an antihypertensive drug, and 21% a lipid-lowering drug within one year of initiation on antidiabetic oral therapy [22]. Only 7.6% received all three agents. Whether this was a suboptimal use of cardioprotective drugs, or whether it was appropriate prescribing clearly depended on the perceived risk:benefit ratio of these interventions in this population.

Mangin *et al.* argued that many patients fear the manner of their dying rather than death itself, and despite the distressing nature of some cardiac deaths many people regard death from a heart attack as a "good way to go". By using treatments for primary prevention, it is suggested that the GP is selecting for another cause of death unknowingly, and doing this without the patient's informed consent.

The argument continues that a way is needed to assess prevention and treatment of risk factors in the elderly that takes a wider perspective when balancing benefits and harms. Rather than consider absolute risk and death prevention, consideration should be given to an overall life extension and a reduction in overall morbidity, taking the duration of treatment into account.

23.7 Delivering appropriate diabetes care

Today, primary care organizations in most developed countries play a significant part in the chronic disease management of people with diabetes. Pay for performance schemes provide an added incentive to deliver high-quality care. However, care delivery is usually structured around the patient with diabetes attending the practice premises. For those people who are house-bound, or who live in care homes, the unstructured, largely reactive care received results in poor levels of the collection and processing of data, and reduced lev-els of diabetes care. In the author's practice, a review of non-attenders at the practice diabetes clinic showed that a significant number were housebound or living in institutional settings [23].

In a recent re-audit of the 452 people on the practice diabetes register, a 'housebound' person was defined as somebody for whom the last three GP contacts were home visits, and who the practice would expect to visit at home if such a request were made. The subgroup totalled 38 people, representing 8.2% of the practice diabetes register. Of these patients, six lived in resi-dential or nursing homes (1.3% of the practice diabetes register), three lived in sheltered housing complexes and 29 lived in private housing.

Among the 38 housebound patients, two had ter-minal illness and four had severe dementia (and were living in care homes), four were younger people with chronic psychiatric illness and 26 were frail elderly in the age range 78–90 plus years.

In order for those people who are housebound to receive optimal diabetes care, they either need special-ized support and transport to allow them to be taken from their homes to the site of care delivery, or they need to receive diabetes care in their homes.

There is a trend towards a reduction in home visiting among primary care teams in the UK (www.statistics 2002/3) which is being replicated in other developed countries. Most home visits now take place because a request is made by the patient, their family or carer because a health problem has developed.

When such visits take place they often concentrate on the presenting problem, and a review of any chronic conditions such as diabetes may be overlooked. Visits to patients in care homes are usually made in a similar way, in response to an acute problem.

One solution proposed in the UK in a review of care home diabetes [24] was for the appointment of a Diabetes Specialist Nurse, who would have respon-sibility for older people with diabetes and who were housebound or in a care home. The nurse would proac-tively visit these people to provide diabetes care and review their diabetes management. The nurse would then be in a position to suggest appropriate changes in diabetes management to the GP. However, this idea has not been taken up by health communities in the UK.

23.7.1 Optimizing care and reducing hospital admissions in the frail elderly

Many health economies in the developed world have realized that reducing the number of admissions to hospital of frail elderly patients with multiple chronic conditions (which includes diabetes) is a vital step in trying to stem the rapid escalation in health care costs. One model is based on a system from the USA, which uses nurses in a managed-care programme called 'Ev-ercare'. In one evaluation study directed specifically at long-stay nursing home residents [25], the provi-sion of a case manager reduced hospital admissions by 50% over a 15-month period compared to controls. The Evercare programme is currently being trialled in the UK, with a plan to recruit 3000 case managers, called 'community matrons'. The system combines elements of proactive nurse-led assessment and intensive case management, but located in the community rather than in a nursing home setting.

A recent study examined the rates of emergency ad-mission, emergency bed days and mortality between 2001 and 2005 in nine Primary Care Trusts in the UK, who piloted the intervention [26]. A total of 62 Ever-care practices was compared with between 6960 and 7695 control practices in England (depending on the analysis being carried out). The intervention showed no significant effect on rates of emergency admission, emergency bed days and mortality for a high-risk pop-ulation aged over 65 years with a history of two or more emergency medical admissions in the preceding 13-month period. The authors concluded that the case management of frail elderly people introduced an addi-tional range of services into primary care, without any associated reduction in hospital admissions.

23.7.2 Integration of diabetes care into the community

In many health care systems the GP who has re-sponsibility for a defined number of patients is cen-tral to the delivery of health care in the community (see Figure 23.1). In many health economies, GPs now work alongside practice nurses, district nurses and case managers for frail elderly patients. In car-ing for older people with diabetes, community dieti-cians, community diabetes specialist nurses, commu-nity physiotherapists, community podiatrists and those working in retinal screening programmes are also vi-tal members of the care team. They also need to work alongside hospital-based specialists in geriatric medicine, and their teams. Sharing information and working together is vital if such a large, diverse group of health care professionals is to function effectively so as to provide optimal care and reduce hospital admissions. In many health economies it is the GP and their primary health care team that provide the focus for this integration, with the other associated health care professionals feeding in their expertise. Good-quality computer-based records that can be read by, and receive input from, all health care professionals providing support for older people with diabetes are important to facilitate the integration.

23.8 Problems of polypharmacy and medication concordance in older people with diabetes

The importance of polypharmacy in older people has been recognized in the UK by the Royal College of Physicians (RCP) [27], which confirmed that polypharmacy affects 16–17% of such patients. Many older people with diabetes will be receiving a number of different medications for the control of blood glucose, blood pressure and lipids. But they may also have other comorbidities such as osteoarthritis, constipation and respiratory problems, all of which may require drug therapy. Hence, the older diabetic patient may well be receiving six or more medications simultaneously.

Older patients are more prone to problems related to their medicines because of the higher number they use, and because of a decline in cognitive and physical functioning [28]. A study of these problems found that two-thirds of all older people had problems using their medicines correctly, and that these problems could lead to a deterioration in a clinical condition for one in four older people [29]. Community pharmacists in a number of countries are being trained and equipped to perform treatment reviews on patients taking multiple therapeutic agents. In some countries, such as the UK, community pharmacists may receive a financial incentive for doing this work [30]. Published studies from the USA [31] and UK [32] have shown that such treatment reviews can be helpful. The components of a treatment review would include:

- A review of the patient's dug history.

- A review of all currently administered medications both prescribed and any bought 'over-the-counter'.

- A drug 'education' – the reasons for taking each therapy, the frequency of administration and a review of any side effects.

- Appropriate monitoring, for example renal function when prescribed ACE inhibitors.

In a recent study [28] conducted in the Netherlands, two procedures for treatment were reviewed by a team consisting of a community pharmacist and a GP. In one group (the 'case conference' group), the pharmacist and GP personally discussed problems as identified in the pharmacotherapy of the patient, and together drew up a care plan. In the other group (the 'written feedback' group), the pharmacist passed the results of their treatment review back to the GP as written feedback. The effects and cost differences were determined at 6 and 9 months, and the yearly savings in medicine costs for each year that the medication change persisted were determined.

In the case conference group, significantly more medication changes were initiated than in the written feedback group; this difference was present at 6 months after treatment reviews, but was no longer significant after 9 months. The authors concluded that performing treatment reviews with case conferences between the community pharmacist and GP would lead to a greater uptake of clinically relevant recommendations than would a written feedback, while the extra costs incurred seemed to be covered by the related savings. However, as the effect of the intervention declined over time, the performance of treatment reviews for older people should be integrated into the routine collaboration between GPs and community pharmacists, and should occur at 6-month intervals.

23.8.1 Improving medication concordance in primary care

The problem of patients not complying with treatment was first recorded over 2000 years ago, when Hippocrates advised the physician "... to be alert to the faults of the patients which make them lie about their taking of the medicines prescribed and when things go wrong, refuse to confess that they have not been taking their medicine" [33]. In a retrospective cohort study from Scotland [34], a total of 2920 subjects with at least 12 months' prescriptions for oral hypoglycaemic agents was identified, and their adherence to treatment estimated using data gathered from dispensed prescriptions.

An adequate adherence to treatment – defined as dispensed doses of at least 90% of doses prescribed – was identified in only 31% of patients receiving sulphonylurea monotherapy, and 34% with metformin monotherapy. There were significant linear trends of poorer adherence with each increase in daily number of tablets taken, and increase in co-medication

Several reasons have been proposed why elderly people may not take their tablets as prescribed, including:

- A lack of education or understanding regarding appropriate self-administration and the importance of daily treatment.

- Confusion over which tablets to take, and when; this may occur especially in older people with developing memory loss.

- Any changes in the drug or dose regimen.

- Unpleasant side effects.

- Physical problems opening the packaging, or problems reading the label.

- The demands of a busy lifestyle.

A systematic review of interventions to enhance medication adherence in chronic medical conditions, conducted in 2007 [35], identified 37 eligible trials, in 12 of which the intervention was informational, in 10 behavioural, and in 15 combined informational, behavioural and/or social investigations.

Twenty of these studies reported a significant improvement in at least one adherence measure. Adherence was increased most consistently with behavioural interventions that reduced dosing demands, and those involving monitoring and feedback. Adherence was also improved in six multi-sessional information trials and eight combined interventions. The authors concluded that several types of intervention may be effective in improving medication adherence in chronic medical conditions, but few had any significant effect on the clinical outcome.

A simple strategy can be developed to try to improve medication concordance in older people with diabetes:

- Carefully explaining to people what each tablet is for, when it should be taken, and the importance of remembering to take each treatment as prescribed.

- Trying to minimize the number of tablets to be taken, and the frequency with which they need to be taken. Once-daily tablet treatments are ideal from the adherence perspective, and combination preparations should also be considered to reduce the tablet load.

- Using treatments that have few, if any, side effects wherever possible.

- Ensuring that treatments are appropriately packaged and the labelling is clear.

- Considering the use of a pre-filled tablet dispensing system if forgetting whether tablets have been taken, or not, is becoming an issue.

23.9   Conclusions

As the numbers of older people in society with diabetes continues to increase, there will be a shift in care from the hospital to the community, and improved systems of primary care will be required to provide optimal care. Today, there is evidence that multidisciplinary team working, pay-for-performance incentives, the individualization of care and dealing with issues of polypharmacy and medication concordance, may all play their part in helping to deliver optimal to the person with diabetes in the community.

References

1. Diabetes Atlas (2003), 2nd edition. IDF, Belgium.
2. Starfield B 1992 Primary Care. Oxford University Press, New York, USA.
3. Forrest CB. Primary care gatekeeping and referrals: effective filter or failed experiment. *Br Med J* 2003, 326: 692–5.
4. Testing Times: A review of diabetes services in England and Wales. The Audit Commission, London, 2000.
5. Griffin S. Diabetes care in general practice: a meta-analysis of randomised controlled trials. *Br Med J* 1998, 317: 390–6.
6. Clinical Guidelines for Type 2 Diabetes: European Diabetes Working Party for Older People 2001-2004 (www.eugms.org) (last accessed 20 October 2007.)
7. British Medical Association (2003) Investing in General Practice: The New General Medical Services Contract. British Medical Association, London, UK. Available at: www.bma.org.
8. Campbell S, Reeves D, Kontopantelis E *et al.* Quality of primary care in England with the introduction of pay for performance. *N Engl J Med* 2007, 357: 181–90.
9. Khunti K, Gadsby R, Millett C *et al.* (2007) Quality of diabetes care in the UK: comparison of published

quality of care reports with results from the Quality and Outcomes Framework for Diabetes. *Diabetic Medicine* 24, 1436–41.

10. United Kingdom Prospective Diabetes Study (UKPDS 33). (1998) Intensive blood glucose control with sulphonylureas or insulin compared with conventional treatment and risk of complications in patients with type 2 diabetes. *Lancet*, 352; 837–53.

11. Muggeo M, Verlato G, Bonara E, *et al*. Long-term instability of fasting plasma glucose predicts mortality in elderly NIDDM patients: the Verona Diabetes Study. *Diabetologia* 1995, 38, 672–8.

12. Kuusisto J, Mykkanen L, Pyorla K and Laakso M. NIDDM and its metabolic control predict coronary heart disease in elderly subjects. *Diabetes* 1994, 43, 960–7.

13. Nathan DM, Singer DE, Godine JE *et al*. Retinopathy in older type 2 diabetics: association with poor control. *Diabetes* 1986, 35, 797–801.

14. Heart Protection Study Group. (2002) MRC/BHF Heart Protection Study of cholesterol lowering with simvastatin in 20,536 high-risk individuals: a randomised placebo-controlled trial. *Lancet*, 360, 7–22.

15. Colhoun HM, Betteridge DJ, Durrington PN *et al*. (2004) Prevention of cardiovascular disease with Atorvastatin in type 2 diabetes The CARDS multicentre randomized, placebo controlled trial. *Lancet* 2004, 4: 685–96.

16. United Kingdom Prospective Diabetes Study (UKPDS 38). (1998) Tight blood pressure control and risk of macrovascular and microvascular complications in type 2 diabetes (UKPDS 38). *Br Med J*, 317; 703–13.

17. Hansson L, Zanchetti A, Carruthers SG *et al*. (1998) Effects of intensive blood pressure lowering and low dose aspirin therapy in patients with hypertension. Principal results of the Hypertension Optimal Treatment (HOT) randomised trial. *Lancet*, 351; 1755–62.

18. Sinclair AJ, Bayer AJ and the All Wales Research in Elderly (AWARE) Diabetes Study (1998) UK Government Report 121/3040, Department of Health, London.

19. Mangin D, Sweeney K and Heath I. Preventive health care in elderly people needs rethinking. *Br Med J* 2007, 335: 285–7.

20. Bjerre LM and LeLorier J. Do statins cause cancer? A meta-analysis of large randomised controlled clinical trials. *Am J Med*, 2001, 110: 716–23.

21. Hippisley-Cox J, Pringle M and Carter R. Coronary heart disease prevention and age inequalities: the first year of the national service framework for CHD. *Br J Group Pract*, 2006, 11, 27–31.

22. Sirois C, Moisan J, Poirer P and Gregoire J-P. Sub-optimal use of cardioprotective drugs in newly treated elderly individuals with type 2 diabetes. *Diabetes Care* 2007, 30, 1880–2.

23. Gadsby R. Care of people with diabetes who are housebound or in nursing and residential homes. *Diabetes in General Practice* 1994, 4, 30–1.

24. British Diabetic Association, (1999) Guidelines of Practice for Residents with Diabetes in Care Homes. British Diabetic Association, London.

25. Kane RL, Keckhafer G, Flood S *et al*. The effect of Evercare on hospital use. *J Am Geriatr Soc* 2003, 51, 1427–34.

26. Gravelle H, Dusheiko M, Sheaff R *et al*. Impact of case management (Evercare) on frail elderly patients: controlled before and after analysis of quantitative outcome data. *Br Med J* 2007, 334: 31–4.

27. Royal College of Physicians (RCP) (1997) Medications for Older people. Royal College of Physicians, London.

28. Denneboom W, Dautzenberg MG, Grol R and Smet PA. Treatment reviews of older people on polypharmacy in primary care. *Br J Gen Pract*, 2007, 57, 723–31.

29. Denneboom W, Dautzenberg MG, Grol R and Smet PA. User-related pharmaceutical care problems and factors affecting them: the importance of clinical relevance. *J Clin Pharm Ther*, 2005, 30, 215–23.

30. Pharmaceutical Services Committee 2007 (www.psnc. org.uk; last accessed 28 November 2007).

31. Hanlon IT, Weinberger M, Samsa GP *et al*. A randomised controlled trial of a clinical pharmacist intervention to improve inappropriate prescribing in elderly outpatients with polypharmacy. *Am J Med*, 1996, 100, 428–37.

32. Zermansky AG, Petty DR Raynor DK *et al*. Randomised controlled trial of clinical medication review by a pharmacist of elderly patients receiving repeat prescriptions in general practice. *Br Med J*, 2001, 323, 1340–3.

33. Sawyer S. Adherence: Whose Responsibility? http:// www.nationalasthma.org.au/html//management/ adherence/adh009 (accessed 14 December 2008).

34. Donnan PT, MacDonald TM, Morris AD for the DARTS/MEMO Collaboration. Adherence to oral hypoglycaemic agents prior to insulin therapy in Type 2 diabetes. *Diabetic Medicine*, 2002, 19, 279–84.

35. Kripalani S, Yao X and Haynes B. Interventions to enhance medication adherence in chronic medical conditions. *Arch Int Med*, 2007, 167, 540–50.

24

Diabetes Care in Special Circumstances

I Acute Hospital Admission
II Serious Infections
Jay Chillala
Trafford General Hospital, Manchester, UK
III Minor Ethnic Populations
Gurch Randhawa
University of Bedfordshire, Putteridge Bury, Luton, UK

I Acute Hospital Admissions

Key messages
- Hospital admissions are higher in elderly patients with diabetes.
- Comorbidities increase the length of stay.
- Discharge planning can be complex and should start early.

24.1 Introduction

Patients with diabetes have an increased frequency of hospitalization compared to patients without diabetes. Over 50% of patients with diabetes are admitted at least once for any cause. Compared to patients without diabetes, there is an excess risk of 30% [1]. The rates are higher in patients with comorbid conditions such as congestive cardiac failure, cardiomyopathy, coronary atherosclerosis and hypertension (see Table 24.1).

Non-cardiovascular comorbidities in elderly patients with diabetes, such as chronic obstructive pulmonary disease (COPD), asthma and lower respiratory disorders, Alzheimer's disease/dementia, personality disorders, depression and osteoporosis, also increase the likelihood of a hospital admission (see Table 24.1) [2]. Comorbidities increase the length of stay in hospital, with the stay doubling if five are present. The presence of nephropathy, coronary/peripheral artery disease, higher glycated haemoglobin (HbA$_{1c}$) level, insulin treatment and older age all predict a higher rate of hospitalization [3].

24.2 Hyperosmolar hyperglycaemic state and diabetic ketoacidosis insulin regimes

The following three conditions are described in greater detail elsewhere in this book, and so will be dealt with only briefly at this point. Treatment consists of insulin, fluids and potassium. The regimes suggest the use of a syringe pump with 50 units soluble insulin and 50 ml saline, starting at 0.1 U/kg/h [4]. A sliding scale is subsequently followed, which should be modified according to response, and 5% dextrose started when the glucose level is <12 mmol/l. When the patient

Diabetes in Old Age. Third Edition. Edited by Alan J. Sinclair
© 2009 John Wiley & Sons, Ltd

Table 24.1 Reasons for acute hospital admissions in patients with diabetes.

Acute metabolic complications	• Hyperosmolar hyperglycaemic state • Diabetic ketoacidosis • Hypoglycaemia
Poor diabetes control	• For monitoring and correction of cause and modification of therapy
Infections	• Chest, cystitis, pyelonephritis, septicaemia, cellulitis
Cardiac causes	• Chronic heart failure, arrhythmias, ischaemic heart disease, hypertension
Ophthalmic complications	• Cataract, glaucoma, blindness leading to complications (e.g. falls)
Renal complications	• End-stage renal failure
Neurological	• Cerebrovascular disease
Tissue diseases	• Amputation, foot and lower limb ulcers, pressure sores

is eating and the ketone level is $\leq 1+$ (as per the dipstick scale), then subcutaneous insulin treatment can be started.

In diabetic ketoacidosis (DKA), fluid depletion is 3–6 litres, and the aim should be replacement over a 24-h period. Care is needed when replacing fluids in patients with heart failure so as not to fluid overload. The rapid replacement of fluids may also lead to cerebral oedema; consequently, it is also important to monitor levels of consciousness.

24.2.1 Hyperosmolar hyperglycaemic state (HHS)

In HHS, the fluid loss is 8–10 l, and normal saline should be administered until the patient is rehydrated. When the blood glucose level is <12 mmol/l, dextrose may be administered instead of saline. If the plasma sodium level is >160 mmol l^{-1}, 0.45% (w/v) saline can be used for the first 3 litres of replacement fluid.

24.2.2 Hypoglycaemia

Autonomic symptoms start at glucose levels of 3.3–3.6 mmol l^{-1}, and neuroglycopenia at <2.6 mmol/l [5]. Autonomic symptoms include sweating, tremor and palpitations, with neuroglycopenia presenting as confusion and drowsiness leading on to seizures and coma if not treated. Treatment is with 50 ml of 50% dextrose or intramuscular/intravenous glucagon (1 mg).

24.3 Factors which affect management

Older patients may be admitted with conditions that occur secondary to their diabetes, such as falls or leg ulcers occurring as a consequence of their neuropathy or retinopathy. Their functional status may then be affected by this, leading to higher care requirements and possibly a care home on discharge.

Elderly diabetic patients in care homes have a higher level of cognitive impairment and an already existing high level of dependency [6]. These factors would delay the time for recovery.

Other factors affecting management include depression, social problems, poor vision and difficulties with activities of daily living (see Table 24.2).

24.4 Discharge planning

Discharge planning should begin at an early stage, preferably on admission, with information being collected about care packages and other help received by patients. Both, relatives and patients should be encouraged to highlight areas where additional input may be required.

Multi-disciplinary input on a regular basis is very important, with involvement of the doctor, physiotherapist, occupational therapist and social worker. In view

Table 24.2 Summary of key in-patient criteria for managing older people with diabetes.

Management	Reason for consideration
Assessment of preadmission status	Aim to achieve preadmission status at time of discharge
Early use of antibiotics	Infections can escalate rapidly and be severe. Signs may be subtle
Early use of insulin	Infections can be severe, blood sugars very variable, good control needed rapidly. Patients may be admitted with HHS.
Check renal function regularly	Rapid deterioration can occur with some antibiotics. Monitor to check for correction of dehydration.
Daily review of fluids and antibiotics	Fluid overload/dehydration can occur rapidly. Complications related to antibiotics can occur
Review of diabetes control and other modifiable risk factors	Patients may not have attended their annual review
Review of current medication	Check for drug interactions, ability to take medications
Early multidisciplinary assessment	Important to maintain physical abilities and cognitive function as soon as possible
Weekly goal setting	Patient condition may improve or decline. Realistic goals need to be set.
Early discharge planning	Discharge may be complex. Consider timescale and people involved e.g. social services, family
Post-discharge review	Follow-up of elderly patients with complex problems important. Establish where review will be done and by whom. Possibly outpatients/own home/day hospital. Review can be by doctor/diabetes nurse/community nurse

of the comorbidities and general frailty, elderly patients may require a period of rehabilitation, and so the timing of discharge becomes very important. The aim should be to achieve the predischarge status.

Communication with relatives needs to be effective, with discussion about the patient's needs and the care packages that social services can provide. Patients may require modifications to their home prior to discharge, or step up to residential/nursing care. These discussions must be started as early as possible.

Discharge planning can be very complicated and time-consuming, but with the appropriate specialist input it can be successful, allowing patients to remain at home and reduce the risk of readmission.

Follow-up and the continuation of care is extremely important, and continues with the GP and consultant, with additional input from district nurses and health visitors. Some areas will have a specialist input from a diabetes nurse specially trained in treatment of the elderly, who will monitor blood sugars and visit those patients in care homes.

II Serious Infections

Key messages

- Serious infections in the elderly may present atypically.
- Consequences of infections may be serious due to comorbidities.
- Care is required for the dosing and the route used when administering antibiotics.

24.5 Introduction

Serious infections in the elderly frequently present in an atypical manner (e.g. falls, incontinence), and with very few clinical signs. It is therefore crucial that investigations are conducted promptly and appropriate treatment instituted at an early stage.

The consequences of infections may be serious due to the patient's comorbidities, although the organisms may be the same as those encountered in the younger population. This, combined with immune system deficits, may lead to patients being susceptible to life-threatening complications (Table 24.3).

24.6 How is the treatment of elderly patients different?

Clinical signs may be subtle or atypical, with patients presenting with symptoms such as poor mobility, confusion or lethargy. This may occur on a background of cognitive impairment, making the diagnosis very challenging. The usual signs of infection such as fever may not occur, and in fact in severe infections temperatures may drop below baseline.

Changes in the immune system make elderly patients more susceptible to bacterial and viral infections. The immune system undergoes changes with age [8]. Due to thymic involution, the T cells that respond to new antigens decrease in number (naive T cells), such that most of the T cells are memory T cells that respond to the exposure of previous antigens; however, the response to new antigens is poor. Humoral immunity is also mildly affected, but only where the T helper cells mediate B-cell functions. Immunoglobulin levels are constant, although the levels of IgG, IgM and/or IgA may change.

Table 24.3 Common and more serious infections in patients with diabetes [7].

Site of infection	Infection
Head and neck	• Rhinocerebral mucormycosis • 'Malignant otitis externa' • Ophthalmic infections
Mouth and oesophagus	• Oral candidiasis, • Oesophageal candidiasis
Chest	• Community-acquired infections • Pneumococcal and influenza infections • Tuberculosis, *Staphylococcus aureus, Klebsiella pneumoniae* and other Gram-negative organisms
Abdomen	• Emphysematous cholecystitis, retroperitoneal abscess, hepatic abscess and pelvic abscess
Renal	• Bacteriuria, cystitis, pyelonephritis, renal/perinephric abscess, emphysematous cystitis/pyelonephritis
Skin, soft tissue and bone	• Cellulitis, wound infections, foot ulcers, osteomyelitis, Fournier's gangrene, necrotising fasciitis/cellulitis

Elderly patients may already have symptoms of illnesses, which makes the diagnosis very difficult. Many patients have incontinence or an indwelling catheter that may mask the signs of infection. Although asymptomatic bacteriuria is very common, it should not be treated unless the symptoms of a urinary tract infection develop.

Elderly patients with diabetes are more prone to certain infections, especially skin infections. They are also likely to have peripheral vascular disease and neuropathies, which makes ulcers and skin lesions more likely.

Patients may already be taking several medications, and care is needed to ensure that any antibiotic treatment does not interact with existing tablet regimes. It is also important to ensure that drug levels are kept within limits, especially when renal impairment exists.

24.7 Management

Treatment is along standard lines, although classical signs are often not seen and antibiotics are used at an early stage with therapy often given empirically. Details of the suggested management are as follows:

- Oropharyngeal infections
  - Oral candidiasis: nystatin or oral fluconazole
  - Oesophageal candidiasis: oral fluconazole

- Chest infections
  - *Streptococcus pneumoniae*: penicillin or a macrolide if penicillin-allergic
  - Gram-negative bacilli: *Klebsiella/Pseudomonas aeruginosa*: third-generation cephalosporin plus macrolide
  - *Legionella pneumophilia*: macrolide ± rifampicin
  - *Chlamydia* and *Mycoplasma*: macrolide
  - Influenza/parainfluenza/RSV: oseltamivir and zanamivir can be given within 48 h of onset of symptoms

The following infections are more common in patients with diabetes:

- Tuberculosis

- *Klebsiella*

- *Staphylococcus aureus*

24.7.1 Rare infections (see Table 24.4)

- *Rhinocerebral mucormycosis [10]:* This infection occurs due to inhalation of the fungus (several different fungi can be involved, including *Rhizopus, Absidia* and *Mucor*) into the paranasal sinuses. From there it may spread to the palate, sphenoid sinus, cavernous sinus, orbits and the brain. Presentation can be by fever, confusion, a visible black eschar or cranial nerve palsies. Treatment is with amphotericin B and debridement.

- *Malignant otitis externa:* This is an invasive infection of the external auditory canal and skull base. Treatment is with a quinolone.

- *Emphysematous cystitis/pyelonephritis:* Patients present with symptoms of a urinary tract infection with X-rays showing the presence of air in the bladder lumen, bladder wall, the renal parenchyma or perinephric space. Treatment for the former is with antibiotics, and the latter with antibiotics and relief of the obstruction. In some cases nephrectomy is necessary. The antibiotics of choice would be cephalosporin or quinolone.

- *Fournier gangrene:* the male genitalia are affected by necrotizing fasciitis. Treatment is debridement, combined with antibiotics active against *Streptococcus* sp., *Clostridium* sp. and Gram-negative organisms.

- *Necrotizing cellulitis/fasciitis:* treat with debridement and antibiotics.

24.8 Precautions for the medical management of infections in the elderly

Elderly patients with an infection can deteriorate rapidly, and attempts should be made to identify the source of sepsis with blood, urine cultures or wound swabs. Broad-spectrum antibiotics should be started at an early stage, with the appropriate changes when organism sensitivities are available.

The renal function and glomerular filtration rate decreases with age; consequently, the dose levels of drugs that are normally excreted via the renal route will need to be adjusted.

For example, the aminoglycosides are adjusted according to the patient's renal function and their body weight. In patients with a normal renal function, the dose levels should be monitored after three to four doses and adjustments made accordingly to the

Table 24.4 Summary of treatment of infections in elderly diabetes patients. (Adapted in part from Ref. [9]).

Head and neck	
• Rhinocerebral mucormycosis	• Surgical debridement and amphotericin B
• Malignant otitis externa	• Quinolone
Mouth and oesophagus	
• Oral candidiasis	• Nystatin or fluconazole
• Oesophageal candidiasis	• Fluconazole
Chest	
• Community-acquired infections	• Amoxicillin or a macrolide if penicillin allergic
• Atypical pathogen	• Erythromycin or clarithromycin
• Severe *Legionella*	• Add rifampicin
• Staphylococcal e.g. in influenza	• Add flucloxacillin
• Staphylococcal, if MRSA suspected	• Add vancomycin
• Gram-negative bacilli	• Cefuroxime (or cefotaxime) plus macrolide
Abdomen	
• Emphysematous cholecystitis,	• Tazocin, or aminoglycoside/quinolone with clindamycin or metronidazole
• Hepatic abscess and pelvic abscess	• Tazocin or third-generation cephalosporin, or fluroquinolone plus metronidazole. Antibiotics given whilst awaiting results of Gram stain and culture
Renal	
• Bacteruria, cystitis, pyelonephritis, renal/perinephric abscess, emphysematous cystitis/pyelonephritis	• Cephalosporin or quinolone
Skin, soft tissue, bone	
• Necrotizing cellulitis/fasciitis	• Surgical debridement and broad spectrum antibiotics (e.g. penicillin, clindamycin)
• Fournier's gangrene	• Treatment similar to above, addition of quinolone or aminoglycoside plus surgical debridement

dosage. In those patients with a once-daily regime, local guidelines on monitoring drug serum levels should be followed. Aminoglycosides should also (preferably) not be co-administered with ototoxic diuretics (e.g. furosemide), although if this is unavoidable then the dose interval been the two drugs must be as long as possible.

The route of drug administration must also be considered, with the oral route being ideal (if possible). If a patient is confused, or compliance at home is likely to be poor, they may require to be admitted to hospital for intravenous treatment.

If tablets are large and difficult to swallow, liquid preparations may provide an alternative, although the doses may be less accurate. All tablet bottles must be accessible and easily opened; if necessary dosette boxes may need to be issued.

24.9 When should the microbiologist be called?

Microbiologists should be contacted at an early stage when diabetic patients have complicated or rare infections. If a patient's condition is deteriorating despite appropriate antibiotics, it is useful to discuss changes in antibiotics. There may also be uncertainty regarding the source of infection, and the microbiologist can suggest the best broad-spectrum regime.

The serum levels of antibiotics such as the aminoglycosides have a narrow therapeutic margin, and the microbiologist may well wish to be involved closely in the dosing and monitoring of these patients.

Serious infections represent a major challenge, and especially so in the elderly diabetic patient. Hence, it is important to be aware of their atypical presentations, and take rapid actions.

III Minority Ethnic Populations

Key messages

- The increased rate of type 2 diabetes among minority ethnic groups compared to Caucasians in the UK is well documented.
- Diabetes complications, such as end-stage renal failure, are much more prevalent among the UK's South Asian and African-Caribbean population.
- Inequalities currently exist in diabetes and renal services; the solutions to rectifying this situation are complex, and involve focusing both upon disease prevention and disease management.
- The financial and human burden of not addressing these inequalities should encourage some immediate action.

24.10   Introduction

The UK Government's Cross Cutting Review of Health Inequalities published earlier this decade reminded us not only that health gaps still exist in the UK but also, in some cases, they are growing ever wider:

"There are wide geographical variations in health status, reflecting the multiple problems of material disadvantage facing some communities. These differences begin at conception and continue throughout life. Babies born to poorer families are more likely to be born prematurely, are at greater risk of infant mortality and have a greater likelihood of poverty, impaired development and chronic disease in later life. This sets up an inter-generational cycle of health inequalities." [11].

This statement reflects the shift in the focus of policy during the past 20 years, in which there has been a growing interest in the health of minority ethnic populations in the UK. (For the purposes of this chapter and availability of data, the term 'minority ethnic groups' is used to refer to South Asian and African-Caribbean populations in the UK.)

Throughout this period, the provision of diabetes services for minority ethnic groups has become a particularly important area of debate. This is in part due to the observation of high rates of type 2 diabetes among South Asian (those originating from the Indian subcontinent, India, Sri Lanka, Pakistan and Bangladesh) and African-Caribbean populations in the UK, and the disproportionately higher numbers of South Asians and African-Caribbeans progressing towards diabetic nephropathy.

According to the Census, 4.6 million people are from minority ethnic groups. This represents a total of 7.9% of the total population of the UK. Some 75% of the minority ethnic populace are classified as either Black/Black British (24.8%) or Asian or Asian British (50.2%) [12].

Diabetes is becoming one of the greatest health problems facing the UK today. The recent 'All Parliamentary Group' for Diabetes and Diabetes UK reported that over three million people are expected to be diagnosed with diabetes by the year 2010, and that half of these cases will be people from disadvantaged communities. According to the Diabetes National Service Framework, people of South Asian, African and African-Caribbean descent have a higher than average risk of developing type 2 diabetes, as compared with the white population [13]. Type 2 diabetes is up to sixfold more common in people of South Asian descent, and up to threefold more common in those of African-Caribbean descent. It has been estimated [14] that 15.2% of the South Asian population had diabetes, as compared to 3.8% of the white population. The risk of death resulting from the complications of diabetes is between three- and sixfold higher within minority ethnic groups [14].

24.11   Epidemiology of diabetes among minority ethnic groups in the UK

Both, South Asian and African-Caribbean communities have a high prevalence of type 2 diabetes, with recent studies having indicated a prevalence rate fourfold greater than that in Whites (Table 24.5). It has been reported that 20% of South Asians aged 40–49 years have type 2 diabetes, and that by the age of 65 years that proportion will have risen to one-third [15]. Clearly, this has significant consequences for planning diabetes services for the elderly in areas of the UK where there are higher proportions of minority ethnic groups.

Table 24.5 Relative risk of diabetes and diabetic nephropathy among South Asians and African-Caribbeans in the UK population.

Condition	Relative risk
Diabetes	>4
Diabetic nephropathy	>6

A further complication is that diabetic nephropathy is the major cause of end-stage renal failure (ESRF) in South Asian and African-Caribbean patients receiving renal replacement therapy (RRT), either by dialysis or transplantation. Nationally, this higher relative risk, when corrected for age and gender, has been calculated in England as 4.2 for the South Asian community and 3.7 for those with an African-Caribbean background [16]. Data acquired from Leicester show that South Asians with diabetes have a 13-fold higher risk of developing ESRF than do 'White' Caucasians [17]. Thus, not only are South Asians and African-Caribbeans more prone to diabetes than Whites, they are more likely to develop ESRF as a consequence.

Importantly, the South Asian and African-Caribbean populations in the UK are relatively young compared to the White population. Since the prevalence of ESRF increases with age, this has major implications for the future need for RRT, and highlights the urgent need for preventive measures [18]. The incidence of ESRF has significant consequences for both local and national NHS resources. The National Renal Review has estimated an increase over the next decade of 80% in the 20 000 or so patients receiving RRT, and a doubling of the current cost – to about £600 million per year – of providing renal services [15].

Consequently, there is an urgent need to invest in renal services as well as diabetes services, given the greater propensity of diabetes complications among diabetics from minority ethnic groups.

24.12 Improving access to services

The Diabetes National Service Framework highlights the importance of access to services, in particular to meet the needs of minority ethnic groups [13]. The Renal Services NSF also focuses on 'renal disease complicating diabetes', and emphasizes inequalities experienced by minority ethnic groups [19]. However, there is evidence that knowledge of diabetes and its complications is poor among South Asians and African-Caribbeans [20, 21]. Preliminary evidence also suggests that the quality of health care for South Asians and African-Caribbeans is inadequate and the compliance poor [15, 21]. There is also a low-uptake of hospital-based diabetes services, with growing evidence that South Asians are subsequently referred later for renal care, and are more likely to be lost to follow-up [22]. Late referral may reduce opportunities to implement measures to slow the progression of renal failure, or to prepare adequately for RRT, thus adding to both morbidity and mortality.

The World Health Organization (WHO) study group on diabetes has noted that resources should be directed towards improving the quality of preventive care in primary care settings and to public health interventions for controlling diabetes. Education, early diagnosis and effective management of diabetes is important for safeguarding the health of susceptible populations and for long-term savings for the NHS [15]. Most encouragingly, recent studies from the United States and Finland have demonstrated that modest lifestyle changes can reduce the risk, by more than 58%, of developing overt type 2 diabetes in susceptible groups [23, 24]. Furthermore, various interventions, such as tight blood pressure control, and the effective use of angiotensin-converting enzyme (ACE) inhibitors or angiotensin receptor (ATR) blockers and tight blood sugar control can significantly delay the progression of diabetic nephropathy [25–30].

24.13 Looking to the future

It is clear that minority ethnic groups are disproportionately affected by diabetes and consequent renal health problems, both in terms of access to appropriate services and the higher prevalence of diabetes and renal complications.

A major undertaking for researchers and clinicians in the UK will be to explore *access to* and the *progression through* the diabetes and 'renal disease complicating diabetes' care pathways, and to identify health beliefs and experiences associated with diabetes and diabetic renal complications among African-Caribbean and South Asian groups. A systematic exploration of these would provide a valuable resource for health professionals working with these groups, and allow for the development of a culturally competent diabetic and renal service, which is sensitive to the needs of minority ethnic groups [31].

Specifically, these gaps are:

- The identification of cultural beliefs and practices relevant to diabetes and diabetic renal disease self-management, including attitudes to medication and attendance to GPs, diabetic services and nephrology services for routine monitoring.

- The examination of referral patterns to hospital-based diabetic services, and subsequent attendance.

- The exploration of referral patterns to nephrology services.

- The exploration of the relevance of current renal complications education programmes for minority ethnic groups [32].

Kidney Research UK have recently launched the ABLE – "A better life through education and empowerment" – campaign, which aims to redress some of the above issues by education and raising personal awareness of kidney health issues among minority ethnic groups. Professor Randhawa is leading a national pilot study (with colleagues from Imperial College and the University of Leicester) to explore the above issues, and the study is to due to be completed in 2009.

Concomitantly, there needs to be a reduction in the incidence of diabetes among the African-Caribbean and South Asian population in order to alleviate the human and economic costs of this condition. This process can only begin if the public are in an informed position to consider and debates the issues of disease prevention, healthy living and self-management. Central to attaining this goal are increased levels of health education and awareness of the specific problems within the African-Caribbean and South Asian population. This is a difficult challenge as many of these communities live within the most deprived (and difficult-to-reach) communities in the UK [12].

24.14 Conclusions

Inequalities do currently exist in diabetes services in the UK, and the solutions to rectifying this situation are complex. They also require an holistic approach that considers both the short-term requirement to manage diabetes and its complications among minority ethnic groups, and the longer-term focus to decrease the incidence of diabetes among minority ethnic groups via preventive strategies.

There has been substantial recognition of the need to improve diabetes care among minority ethnic groups, as evidenced by a number of new initiatives launched by the NHS National Diabetes Support Team and Diabetes UK. Many of these initiatives are recognized to be at the forefront worldwide in the development of culturally competent diabetes education materials. However, the success of these initiatives has been limited by the lack of a focused strategy that brings together the various strands of a multi-faceted problem that would lead to a coherent implementation plan. It is hoped that this chapter will contribute to beginning and shaping this process, not only in the UK but also for many other countries who have a multi-ethnic and multi-faith society.

On a final note, it is worth remembering that the relatively young minority ethnic population ages, the burden of diabetes and its complications will become unsustainable in many parts of the UK, given the disproportionate incidence of diabetes among these communities. It is also worth noting that detailed debates concerning diabetes and ethnicity are relatively new, and are limited by the quality of data available not only in the UK but also worldwide. In future, it is imperative that data are collected on a wide range of variables including age, ethnicity, social class, gender and religion. The potential interaction of these variables will be an important area of research in future to identify more effective methods in targeting resources to those populations most in need [33].

It is only when these issues are addressed adequately that a diabetes service might emerge that can truly meet the needs of a multi-ethnic and multi-faith population within the UK.

References

1. Bo S, Ciccone G, Grassi G, Gancia R and Rosato R. Patients with type 2 diabetes had higher rates of hospitalization than the general population. *J Clin Epidemiology* 2004, 57 (11), 1196–201.

2. Aro S, Kangas T, Reunanen A, Salinto M and Kovisto V. Hospital use among diabetic patients and the general population. *Diabetes Care* 1994, 17 (11), 1320–9.

3. Rosenthal MJ, Fajardo M, Gilmore S, Morley JE and Nailboff BD. Hospitalization and mortality of diabetes in older adults. A 3 year prospective study. *Diabetes Care* 1998, 21 (2), 231–5.

4. Lebovitz HE. Diabetic ketoacidosis. *Lancet* 1995, 345, 767–72.

5. Kearney T and Dang C. Diabetic and endocrine emergencies. *Postgrad Med J* 2007, 83, 79–86.

6. Sinclair AJ, Allard I and Bayer A. Observations of diabetes care in long-term institutional settings with measures of cognitive function and dependency. *Diabetes Care* 1997, 20 (5), 778–84.

7. Calvet CM and Yoshikawa TT. Infections in diabetics. *Infect Dis Clin North Am* 2001; 15: 407–21.

8. Weksler ME. Senescence of the immune system. *Med Clin North Am* 1983; 67: 263–72.

9. Rajagopalan S. Serious infections in elderly patients with diabetes mellitus. *Clinical Infectious Diseases* 2005; 40: 990–6.

10. Tierney MR and Baker AS. Infections of the head and neck in diabetes mellitus. *Infect Dis Clin North Am* 1995; 9: 195–216.

11. Department of Health (2002) *Tackling health inequalities: Cross Cutting Review*. Department of Health, London.

12. Randhawa G (2008) Organ donation and transplantation – The realities for minority ethnic groups in the UK. In: W. Weimar, M.A. Bos, J.J. van Busschbach (eds). *Organ Transplantation: Ethical, Legal and Psychosocial Aspects. Towards a Common European Policy*. Pabst Publishers, Lengerich, Germany.

13. Department of Health. (2002) *National Service Framework for Diabetes: Standards*. Department of Health, London.

14. Burden, A.C. (2001) Diabetes in Indo-Asian people. *The Practitioner*: 245 (1622): 445–51.

15. Raleigh VS. (1997) Diabetes and hypertension in Britain's ethnic minorities: implications for the future of renal services. *Br Med J*; 314: 209–12.

16. Roderick PJ, Raleigh VS, Hallam L and Mallick NP. (1996) The need and demand for renal replacement therapy amongst ethnic minorities in England. *J Epidemiol Community Health*; 50: 334–9.

17. Burden AC, McNally PG, Feehally J and Walls J. (1992) Increased incidence of end-stage renal failure secondary to diabetes mellitus in Asian ethnic groups in the United Kingdom. *Diabetic Medicine*; 9: 641–5.

18. Randhawa G. (1998) The impending kidney transplant crisis for the Asian population in the UK. *Public Health*, 112: 265–8.

19. Department of Health. (2004) *National Service Framework for Renal Services*. Department of Health, London.

20. Nazroo, J.Y. (1997) *The Health of Britain's Ethnic Minorities*. Policy Studies Institute, London.

21. Johnson M., Owen D. and Blackburn, C. (2000) *Black and minority ethnic groups in England: The second health and lifestyles survey*. Health Education Authority, London.

22. Jeffrey RF, Woodrow G, Mahler J, Johnson R and Newstead CG. (2002) Indo-Asian experience of renal transplantation in Yorkshire: results of a 10year survey. *Transplantation*; 73: 1652–7.

23. Diabetes Prevention Program Research Group (DPPRG). (2002) Reduction in the incidence of Type 2 diabetes with lifestyle intervention or metformin. *N Engl J Med*, 346: 393–403.

24. Tuomilehto J, Lindström J, Eriksson JG, Valle TT, Hämäläinen H, Ilanne-Parikka P, Keinänen- Kiukaanniemi S, Laakso M, Louheranta A, Rastas M, Salminen V and Uusitupa M; Finnish Diabetes Prevention Study Group. (2001) Prevention of type 2 diabetes mellitus by changes in lifestyle among subjects with impaired glucose tolerance. *N Engl J Med*, 344: 1343–50.

25. UK Prospective Diabetes Study (UKPDS) Group. (1998) Intensive blood-glucose control with sulphonylureas or insulin compared with conventional treatment and risk of complications in patients with type 2 diabetes (UKPDS 33). *Lancet*, 352: 837–53.

26. Feest, T.G., Dunn, E.J. and Burton, C.J. (1999) Can intensive treatment alter the progress of established diabetic nephropathy to end-stage renal failure? *Q J Med*, 92: 275–82.

27. Brenner BM, Cooper ME, de Zeeuw D, Keane WF, Mitch WE, Parving HH, Remuzzi G, Snapinn SM, Zhang Z and Shahinfar S; RENAAL Study Investigators. (2001) Effects of losartan on renal and cardiovascular outcomes in patients with type 2 diabetes and nephropathy. *N Engl J Med*, 345: 861–9.

28. Cinotti, G.A. and Zucchelli, P.C. (2001) Effect of lisinopril on the progression of renal insufficiency in mild proteinuric non-diabetic nephropathies. *Nephrol Dial Transplant*, 16: 961–6.

29. Lewis EJ, Hunsicker LG, Clarke WR, Berl T, Pohl MA, Lewis JB, Ritz E, Atkins RC, Rohde R and Raz I; Collaborative Study Group (2001) Renoprotective effect of the angiotensin-receptor antagonist irbesartan in patients with nephropathy due to type 2 diabetes. *N Engl J Med*, 345: 851–60.

30. Lightstone, L. (2001) *Preventing kidney disease: The ethnic challenge*. National Kidney Research Fund, Peterborough, UK.

31. Randhawa, G. (2000) Increasing the donor supply from the UK's Asian Population: the need for further research. *Transplantation Proceedings*, 32: 1561–62.

32. Randhawa, G. (2003) Developing culturally competent renal services in the United Kingdom: Tackling inequalities in health. *Transplantation Proceedings*, 35: 21–3.

33. Randhawa, G. (2007) Tackling health inequalities for minority ethnic groups: Challenges and Opportunities. Better Health Briefing Paper 6. Race Equality Foundation, London.

Managing Surgery in the Elderly Diabetic Patient

Geoffrey Gill and Susan Benbow

Department of Diabetes and Endocrinology, Aintree University Hospitals, Liverpool, UK

Key messages

- Diabetes *per se* is in general not a barrier to surgery in the elderly person.
- A thorough preoperative assessment is an essential prerequisite in the management of older people about to undergo surgery.
- Excessively high blood glucose levels should be avoided during surgery; hypoglycaemia must be avoided at ALL costs.
- Locally agreed protocols for the treatment of diabetes during surgery should be available in every hospital.

25.1   Introduction

During their lifetime, most patients with diabetes will require some form of surgery, and the likelihood increases as age advances. Nowadays, a considerable amount of major surgery is undertaken in the elderly (e.g. coronary artery bypass grafts, peripheral vascular and aneurysm surgery, removal of malignancies), of whom more are proportionally likely to have diabetes than at the earlier stages of their lives. Even during the past few years in England, there has been a 16% increase in coronary artery bypass grafts and a similar increase in hip replacements in the elderly. Surgical practice is also changing in many countries, with an increasing number of day-case procedures and shorter postoperative hospital stays. Diabetes management in the elderly is also changing with the increasing use of insulin, and sometimes with more complicated multiple injection regimens and even occasionally the use of insulin pumps [1].

Although carefully planned and executed surgery is highly successful in the elderly, such patients with diabetes may tolerate metabolic and infective complications less well than younger subjects. Diabetes *per se* should never be a reason to decide *not* to operate on an elderly patient, but it *is* a reason for careful planning and management – whether preoperatively, perioperatively or postoperatively. In this chapter the potential problems, the basis of current management systems, and the practical methods of treatment will be examined.

25.2   Metabolic and other problems induced by surgery

Anxiety, anaesthetic drugs and possibly also the underlying condition requiring surgery, may all contribute to metabolic destabilization in the diabetic surgical patient. The most important factors, however, are starvation and the pathophysiological metabolic and humoral

Diabetes in Old Age. Third Edition. Edited by Alan J. Sinclair
© 2009 John Wiley & Sons, Ltd

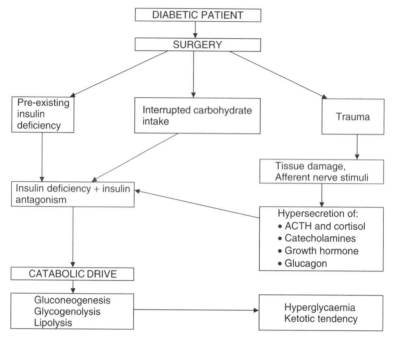

Figure 25.1   Diagram outlining the hormonal and metabolic effects of surgery in the diabetic patient.

response to trauma. All but the most minor of operations involve some interruption of normal food intake, and this may not infrequently last for several days. This poses obvious practical difficulties for diabetic patients whose tablets or insulin injections must be accompanied by the intake of food. Of a more sinister note, however, is that starvation leads to catabolism and, in the presence of insulin deficiency – that is, the diabetic state – ketosis becomes likely and eventually inevitable [2, 3].

Such problems are greatly enhanced by the well-known humoral and metabolic changes associated with trauma, which also greatly enhance catabolism. Surgical trauma disturbs the usual fine balance between anabolism (which effectively is controlled only by insulin) and catabolism (which is driven by a variety of hormones, notably cortisol, catecholamines, growth hormone and glucagon). These latter hormones are often collectively known as the 'stress' or 'counter-regulatory' hormones, and they are hypersecreted in traumatic states. Cortisol and adrenaline levels in particular rise promptly (within minutes or hours after the initiation of trauma), and often massively (to some extent in proportion to the degree of trauma). In addition, insulin secretion is relatively reduced, and a state of insulin resistance ensues [2–4]. Many of these changes are neurally mediated via

afferent nerves from the injured tissue; cortisol, for example, is secreted secondarily to the release of adrenocorticoptrophic hormone (ACTH) [5]. The result of these changes is a massive catabolic drive (see Figure 25.1), with increased gluconeogenesis and glycogenolysis leading to glucose release into the circulation. Lipolysis and protein breakdown also occur, although in the non-diabetic even small amounts of insulin ('basal') secretion are sufficient to contain dangerous hyperglycaemia and lipolysis. This of course is not true in the insulin-deficient or diabetic state. The danger of this metabolic scenario to the diabetic depends on its degree (as mentioned above, this is roughly proportional to the severity of the trauma), and to the level of insulin reserves available.

25.3   Implications for management of surgery in diabetic patients

These basic principles can be translated logically into principles of management for diabetic patients undergoing surgery [6]. The major requirement is to ensure adequate insulinization, with the important variables being the degree of surgical trauma and the individual level of endogenous insulin reserves. In practical terms, patients can be grouped into those receiving insulin

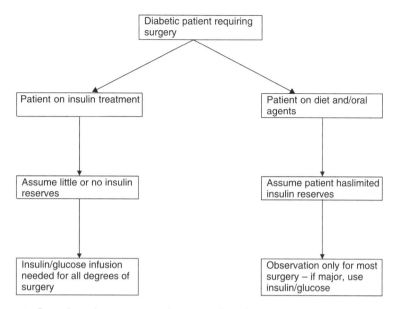

Figure 25.2 Schematic flow chart demonstrating the principles of managing diabetes during surgery.

treatment, and those treated with dietary control and/or oral hypoglycaemic agents (OHAs). The insulin-treated group may or may not be truly insulin-dependent (type 1 diabetes), but even if they are insulin-treated type 2 patients they can be assumed to have little or no insulin reserves, and deemed to require such treatment. In fact, these patients require continuous exogenous insulin treatment for all types of surgery.

Those not receiving insulin must have at least limited insulin reserves, and for minor to moderate degrees of surgical trauma can usually be monitored simply by close observation. Major surgery, however, will require continuous insulin (as for the first group above). These principles are summarized in Figure 25.2.

25.4 Potential risks of surgery in diabetic patients

Surprisingly few studies have been conducted to investigate postoperative mortality and morbidity, comparing diabetic with non-diabetic subjects. Diabetes has certainly been considered a major risk factor for surgery during past decades. An American study conducted in 1963 reported a 5% postoperative mortality in a large (n = 487) group of surgical diabetic patients, the major causes of death being ketoacidosis, infection and myocardial infarction [7]. It is likely, however, that the methods of management were highly suboptimal compared to modern management principles. In a more

recent study, Hjortrup *et al.* [8] used modern treatment methods but failed to show any difference in mortality between diabetic and non-diabetic subjects (2.2% versus 2.7%). Some specific surgical procedures – notably vascular – may have an increased risk in diabetic patients. Thus, aortic and lower-limb revascularization procedures carry an increased mortality risk in diabetic compared to non-diabetic patients [9]. However, this was clearly a selected diabetic group with established advanced large-vessel disease, and such an outcome difference may therefore not be surprising. Nevertheless, such results are of relevance to surgery in the elderly, as in this study the mean age of the diabetic group was 68 years. More recently, no increased cardiac morbidity or overall mortality was reported in a similarly aged group of patients with diabetes undergoing major vascular surgery when compared to a non-diabetic group [10].

On the subject of morbidity, there is little conclusive evidence available that diabetes *per se* causes any increased risk. Diabetic patients with pre-existing cardiac or renal problems may have increased morbidity, but not if relatively uncomplicated and properly managed [11, 12]. The results of a recent study showed a worse outcome for patients with diabetes following hip fracture [13], though this was not due to the diabetes itself but rather to a reduced functional status prior to the fracture, such as stroke. This is an important point, as there appears to be an increased risk of hip fracture in the older person with diabetes [14]. Neither did the risk of postoperative infection appear definitely increased, in contrast to normally accepted clinical dogma [8, 12]. In the Danish study conducted by Hjortrup *et al.* [8], the wound infection rate was identical among both diabetic (13/224; 5.8%) and non-diabetic (12/224; 5.4%) patients. A recent study of diabetic patients undergoing coronary artery surgery showed an increased risk of post-surgical infections, but that was accounted for by excessive postoperative hyperglycaemia [15].

Overall, a critical assessment of the available literature does not support a generally increased risk for diabetic patients undergoing surgery, in terms of both mortality and postoperative complications.

25.5   Special problems in the elderly

Increased age is known to increase postoperative morbidity, and possibility also mortality, in general. Whilst this includes diabetics, again there is no convincing evidence that the effect is significantly greater among such patients. In general, however, diabetic surgical patients are frequently older and 'sicker' than their non-diabetic counterparts [12] (typically amputees, coronary bypass surgery, etc.), but when these factors are taken into account any increased morbidity amongst diabetics becomes insignificant, or at least much less significant.

When preparing the elderly for surgery, any preoperative assessment should be particularly thorough because of comorbidity and polypharmacy. The patient may not be able to provide an accurate history because of memory problems or communication difficulties. Likewise, ischaemic heart disease may be underestimated as the patient may not provide a typical history of chest pain on exertion if their level of exercise is limited by another pathology such as osteoarthritis. Pressure area management is important in the elderly throughout the period of immobility, and particularly so if the individual has diabetes, where peripheral vascular disease and peripheral neuropathy both increase the risks. The nutritional status can already be compromised in the elderly hospitalized patient, and further exacerbated by surgery. Prophylaxis against venous thromboembolic disease must also be considered. An assessment of pain during the postoperative period can again be difficult in the elderly, due to communication problems or secondary to dementia. Postoperative confusion thus requires a thorough assessment of the whole patient, their drugs and fluid

balance, remembering that they may well present differently from a younger patient; for example, in the elderly patient constipation or even a simple urinary tract infection may cause confusion.

The potential iatrogenic complications of diabetes management during surgery will be discussed at a later point. Elderly diabetic patients tolerate hypoglycaemia poorly [16], and are less efficient at maintaining water homeostasis than their younger counterparts [17]; consequently the risk of fluid and electrolyte imbalance is increased during the postoperative period. Renal impairment can be precipitated or exacerbated by these changes, while hydration may already be compromised by drugs, vomiting, preparation for the operation (e.g. bowel clearance), preoperative starvation, or simply by an inability to obtain or reach fluids.

25.6   New diabetes therapies and surgical management

The past 5–10 years has witnessed a rapid and extensive increase in therapies for both type 1 and type 2 diabetes. Some discussion of these treatments are necessary at this point, as they may lead to concerns regarding both preoperative and perioperative management of the diabetic patient.

25.6.1   Insulins

Analogue insulins are non-human synthetic insulins which have more favourable absorption characteristics than the traditional insulins. They are currently in widespread use, and include short-acting (e.g. Lispro, Aspart), long-acting (Glargine and Detemir) and premixed formulations (e.g. Humalog 25, Novomix 30). Those patients receiving the short-acting or premixed analogues pose no problem for surgical management, as the short-acting component does not have a greatly altered time course of action. However, the long-acting analogues are often administered during in the evening, and their theoretical 24-h action could mean that, when given the night before surgery their absorption may continue into the next day, and potentially affect the patient's perioperative insulin requirements. One option would be to move the Glargine or Detemir injection to earlier in the day prior to surgery, or alternatively simply to be aware of the problem and (depending on the dose level) possibly reduce the operative insulin delivery. In fact, a prolonged absorption of these insulins is not always the case and there is evidence that, for both Glargine [18] and Detemir [19], twice-daily administration provides smoother absorption profiles than once-daily. So, the next day 'hangover' effect may be an exaggerated problem.

Although *inhaled insulin* was introduced in 2006, its use has been limited and the manufacturers recently withdrew this formulation for commercial reasons [20]. Other companies, however, are planning its reintroduction, and the preparation may in time return to use. Inhaled insulin has absorption characteristics similar to those of subcutaneous short-acting insulin, and does not therefore have implications for surgical management.

25.6.2 Type 2 diabetes preparations

The glitazones – rosiglitazone and pioglitazone – are insulin receptor sensitizers were introduced during the recent past and are now widely used, most commonly in combination with either sulphonylureas or metformin, but increasingly as 'triple therapy' with both drugs [21]. For patients established on these drugs, there are no implications for surgery other than those which apply to other oral agents. That is, unless glucose/insulin infusions are required the drugs should be stopped on the day of surgery and restarted when food intake is resumed.

Two novel agents for type 2 diabetes treatment have been recently introduced. *Exanetide* is an incretin mimetic, or a GLP-1 (glucagon-like peptide 1) agonist. It is administered twice-daily, subcutaneously, and lowers the blood glucose level without causing weight gain. The mode of action of exanetide is to slow gastric emptying, enhance glucose-dependent insulin secretion, and suppress glucagon secretion [22].

Sitagliptin inhibits DDP-4, the enzyme involved in the metabolism of incretin hormones such as GLP-1. Consequently, sitagliptin has similar effects to exanetide, but it is given orally rather than subcutaneously [23]. Although current experience with both of these drugs is limited, neither has a prolonged action and so should not have any significant implications for surgery.

25.7 The practical management of surgery in diabetic patients

25.7.1 The aims of treatment

The obvious aims of treatment are avoidance of excess mortality and morbidity. As discussed above, with

modern management there should nowadays be little or no excess mortality or postsurgical infection risk. Ideally, the period of hospitalization should not be unduly prolonged, although admission a day or two earlier than usual is often required (see later). Postoperative ketoacidosis should no longer occur, but hypoglycaemia is always a risk with intravenous insulin delivery. The avoidance of hypoglycaemia is very important – the surgical patient may be unable to perceive or report hypoglycaemia, and low blood glucose levels may therefore be allowed to become profound and serious before detection and treatment. Elderly diabetic patients in general may present atypically with hypoglycaemia and, for instance, appear to be confused. Additionally, there is no evidence that over-zealous attempts at achieving normoglycaemia are of benefit in the surgical situation. Indeed, it was found, paradoxically [8], that patients with particularly 'good' control appeared to be at greater risk of postoperative complications, although this has not been confirmed by others [15].

Over recent years, there has been a concerted move to tightly control hyperglycaemia in critically ill diabetic and non-diabetic surgical patients [24]. However, this is not without some controversy [25, 26], and has been associated with troublesome hypoglycaemia.

Glycaemic aims during surgery should, therefore, be to avoid hypoglycaemia at all costs, but in addition to not allow excessive hyperglycaemia, nor to risk ketoacidosis. In numerical terms, plasma glucose levels in the region of 6.0–12.0 mmol l^{-1} would be a reasonable compromise target, although below 10 mmol l^{-1} is preferable.

25.7.2 Preoperative assessment

The preoperative assessment of elderly diabetic patients is aimed at checking general fitness for surgery, ensuring that the diabetic management is appropriate, and that glycaemic control is reasonable. By 'inappropriate' management is meant potentially hazardous drugs such as the potent and/or long-acting sulphonylureas glibenclamide and chlorpropamide. Regrettably, a number of older diabetic persons may still be receiving such preparations, and their treatment may need to be updated prior to surgery. There are theoretical reasons for avoiding metformin also, if possible (because of lactic acidosis risk), although this is not strictly evidence-based [27]. Increasingly, metformin is being used in combination with insulin both in type 1 and 2 diabetes, and patients should be advised accordingly on which of their drugs to avoid preoperatively. This is also important with the new long-acting metformin preparations.

Any assessment of glycaemic control should be made using 'bedside' blood glucose monitoring with reagent strips, although the potential inaccuracies of such measurement must be borne in mind [28]; the occasional laboratory plasma glucose level should also be checked and, if possible, the preoperative glycosylated haemoglobin (HbA$_{1c}$) level. As mentioned previously, 'excellent control' is not necessary, but significant hyperglycaemia (e.g. consistently $>10.0\,\mathrm{mmol\,l^{-1}}$) will require action to be taken. This may involve moving patients from diet to sulphonylureas, increasing tablet doses if already receiving oral agents, or perhaps introducing insulin on a temporary basis. If the latter step is required, thrice-daily short-acting insulin (e.g. Actrapid, Humulin S) or short-acting analogues, insulin lispro (Humalog) or insulin aspart (Novorapid), with or without evening isophane insulin, or twice-daily 30/70 premixes (e.g. Humulin M3, Human Mixtard 30, Novomix 30, Humalog Mix 25) are usually suitable. Such patients will of course require preoperative treatment as for 'insulin -requiring' diabetic patients.

Other preoperative assessments in the elderly should include checking for autonomic neuropathy. This can be achieved with simple electrocardiography testing (e.g. R-R ratio standing and lying – the '30:15 ratio'; or during deep breathing) [29]. However, postural hypotension in the elderly diabetic patient does not always indicate autonomic neuropathy, as it can be secondary to a wide variety of precipitants, especially drugs. This is important because autonomic neuropathy (which is more common in the elderly) may occasionally be associated with sudden perioperative death [30], as well as increased intraoperative morbidity [31]. The anaesthetist must be aware of such information, so that patients can receive close cardiac monitoring.

It can be appreciated that much of the standard preoperative assessment can be carried out prior to admission, either by liaison with the patient's physician or at a pre-admission anaesthetic clinic. Although this has been advocated for many years [6], regrettably it rarely occurs, and patients continue to need admission at least a day or two earlier than usual. Moreover, surgery may need to be further delayed if unforeseen problems are discovered following admission.

A summary checklist of the preoperative diabetic assessment is provided in Table 25.1 (note the important final step of liaising with the anaesthetist).

Table 25.1 Checklist for preoperative diabetic assessment

1. Assess as outpatient and/or admit 2–3 days earlier than usual.

2. Full medical assessment. Chest X-ray and ECG, electrolytes, serum creatinine.

3. Full diabetic assessment. Four times daily bedside blood glucose levels, HbA$_{1c}$, autonomic function, etc.

4. Optimize diabetic management; avoid excessively long-acting hypoglycaemic agents.

5. Ensure reasonable glycaemic control.*

6. Liaise closely with the anaesthetist.

*See Section 25.7.2 for suggested target blood glucose levels

25.7.3 Management in non-insulin-requiring diabetes

There is general agreement that diabetic patients *not* receiving insulin treatment, undergoing surgery of less than major severity, can be managed conservatively by observation only [2, 32–35]. Surprisingly, there has been very little critical evaluation of this presumed optimal therapy, although the information that is available does support a conservative approach. Thus, Thompson and colleagues [36] measured plasma glucose and metabolite responses in three groups of male patients undergoing transurethral surgery to the bladder or prostate gland. The groups were non-diabetic, type 2 diabetic patients treated with intravenous glucose and insulin ('GKI infusion') [37], and type 2 patients treated conservatively. There was no significant difference between the two diabetic groups in terms of perioperative and postoperative blood glucose levels. The plasma insulin and metabolite levels were actually closer to the non-diabetic group in the diabetic patients *not* treated with insulin. The authors concluded that 'GKI' in this situation induced an abnormal metabolic state, with no overall glycaemic benefit. The results of this study were of general importance, but especially so for those caring for elderly diabetic patients requiring surgery. The patients studied had a mean age of about 65 years, and type 2 disease – by far the most common type of diabetes among the elderly.

Guidelines for the conservative management of diabetes in surgery for type 2 patients are listed in Table 25.2. It must again be emphasized that *major* surgery in such patients (e.g. opening the abdominal or thoracic cavity) should be managed as

Table 25.2 Guidelines for surgical care in diabetics *not* receiving insulin treatment.*

1. Operate in the morning if possible.

2. Frequently monitor bedside blood glucose levels (e.g. 2-hourly).

3. If receiving oral agents, omit on morning of surgery, and restart with first postoperative meal.

4. Avoid glucose and lactate-containing fluids intravenously.

5. Liaise with the anaesthetist.

*Unless surgery is of major severity, or preoperative control poor – in which case GKI infusion is advisable.

for insulin-treated patients. Also of note is the importance of avoiding glucose-containing intravenous solutions, which can greatly destabilize glycaemic control. Lactate-containing fluids (e.g. Ringer's lactate and Hartmann's fluid) should also not be used as they can have hyperglycaemic effects [38]. Close plasma glucose monitoring is of course essential, and again liaison with the anaesthetist important – it is often in operating theatre that the dextrose or Ringer's drip is erected! Surgery in the morning is advisable for all types of diabetes; there are no special metabolic reasons for this but, from a practical point of view, it is much easier (and safer) to manage postoperative control problems in the afternoon rather than the middle of the night!

These simple management principles are successful in almost all type 2 patients. Very rarely, excessive postoperative hyperglycaemia may occur, and this should be managed with subcutaneous, short-acting insulin with meals. Alternatively, if the patient cannot tolerate food, a GKI infusion (if the blood glucose is very high, an insulin infusion may initially be required to bring the glucose levels down to about $10–12 \, \text{mmol} \, l^{-1}$), following which a GKI infusion can be used.

25.7.4 Management in insulin-requiring diabetes

This group includes true type 1 diabetes patients, type 2 patients on insulin treatment (including those on a combination of oral hypoglycaemics and insulin), and patients with type 2 diabetes requiring temporary peroperative insulin because of poor glycaemic control or planned major surgery. Historically, a confusing number of systems have been advocated at various times; these include early bizarre systems such as the complete omission of insulin, or insulin with no subsequent

glucose [27, 39]. Not surprisingly, these systems did not work well! Later systems involved subcutaneous insulin with subsequent intravenous glucose infusions. Many such systems were complex, with widely varying types, amounts and proportions of insulin, and equally varied concentrations and rates of glucose infusion. The results with such methods were variable, although in good hands they were comparable with more modern methods [40, 41].

Subcutaneous methods of insulin delivery have, however, now been generally abandoned because they are awkward and inflexible. Continuous intravenous insulin and glucose delivery was introduced during the late 1970s [42], and became rapidly popular because of its flexibility and simplicity. There are two major methods of use:

- The 'separate-line' system (see Figure 25.3). Here, insulin is infused continuously via a syringe pump, with glucose infused separately. The glucose infusion is usually 10% dextrose, delivered at a rate of $100 \, \text{ml} \, h^{-1}$ ($10 \, \text{g} \, h^{-1}$) via an electric drip counter. Insulin is usually delivered via a 50 ml syringe driver – 50 units of soluble insulin (e.g. Acrapid, Humulin S) in 50 ml of 0.9% saline. Thus, $1 \, \text{ml} \, h^{-1}$ is equivalent to 1 unit h^{-1}, and an average starting infusion rate is 3 units h^{-1}. The glucose infusion rate is kept constant throughout, and the insulin rate varied according to frequent (e.g. 1–2-hourly) bedside blood glucose measurements, aiming to maintain levels in the range of $6–12 \, \text{mmol} \, l^{-1}$. Whilst it can be appreciated that this system is highly flexible and simple, it is very 'high-tech', and requires expensive equipment which may not always be available. There is also a potential for 'metabolic disaster' if one of the lines comes adrift. The interruption of glucose will lead to dangerous hypoglycaemia, while the cessation of insulin will conversely lead to hyperglycaemia and possibly ketosis.

- The GKI infusion (see Figure 25.3). A simpler and more 'user-friendly' version of the above method is to combine glucose and insulin in the same infusion bag, and give them together. A small amount of potassium is added to avoid hypokalaemia – hence the term 'GKI' (glucose–KCl–insulin). Interestingly, this method was first advocated in 1963 by Galloway and Shuman [7], but did not become popular until re-described by Alberti and Thomas in 1979 [39], and modified by the same group in 1982 [37]. The present most widely used 'mix' is 500 ml of 10% dextrose with 15 units of soluble insulin and

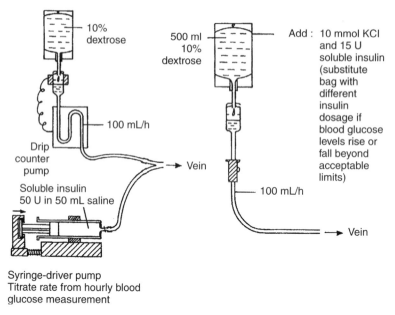

Figure 25.3　The 'separate line' (left) and 'GKI infusion' (right) systems of delivering intravenous insulin and glucose to diabetic patients undergoing surgery. (Reproduced by kind permission of Blackwell Scientific Publications Ltd.) [to be reproduced from 2nd edition].

10 mmol KCl, delivered at $100\,\mathrm{ml\,h^{-1}}$. This will provide 3 units of insulin and 10 g glucose per hour, as does the 'separate-line' technique described above, but without the need for pumps and drip counters. The current (1999) report of the European Diabetes Policy Group [43] suggests that 16 units of soluble insulin be used in the 10% dextrose bag, and that the infusion is run at $80\,\mathrm{ml\,h^{-1}}$. No reason is given for the variation but either system will work, as the differences are inconsequential. Of course if the patient has a tendency to hyperkalaemia (e.g. with renal impairment), then the potassium content of the bags must be adjusted, or potassium avoided altogether.

Because the insulin and glucose in GKI infusions are delivered together, the potential metabolic problems of rate alterations, line blockages, and so on, do not exist. The main disadvantage of GKI is that if dose changes are needed, the whole bag must be discarded and a fresh one prepared and erected. In practice, however, this occurs in only 10–20% of cases [37].

As well as being practically effective, glucose–insulin infusion systems have advantageous metabolic effects, reducing the counter-regulatory hormone stress response, and improving insulin sensitivity [44]. The actual method of delivering insulin and glucose

(whether GKI or 'separate line'; see Figure 25.3), is of no metabolic consequence, and it is a matter of practicalities as to which is chosen. Many hospitals use GKI in the general ward situation, and 'separate lines' in high-dependency or intensive care situations. The GKI system certainly works well in practice and is supported by a study of 85 episodes of surgery using GKI, in which mean plasma glucose levels ranged from 8.3 to $10.2\,\mathrm{mmol\,l^{-1}}$ during the operative day and first two postoperative days [45]. A summary algorithm for management of the surgical diabetic patient is shown in Figure 25.4. This includes a suggested scheme for altering GKI infusions if necessary according to bedside blood glucose monitoring. When the GKI and 'separate line' systems were compared in a random fashion [46], the separate lines were generally preferred by nursing staff, and resulted in more blood glucose levels within the target range. The length of hospital stay, duration of insulin infusion and numbers of untoward incidents were similar with both systems. Importantly, the study report did not provide details of the level of nursing care available – a major advantage of GKI is that it is relatively safe on busy, low-dependency wards.

Electrolytes should be measured daily in patients on GKI infusion, in case hyponatraemia develops. Finally,

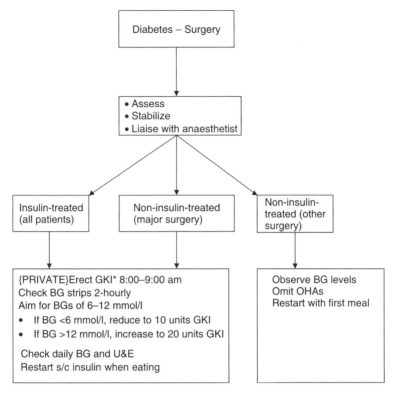

*Standard GKI: 500 ml 10% dextrose + 15 units soluble + 10 mmol KCl. The solution is infused at 100 mlh⁻¹.

Abbreviations: BG = blood glucose; OHA = oral hypoglycaemic agents; U&E = urea and electrolytes; GKI = glucose–potassium–insulin infusion; s/c = subcutaneous.

Figure 25.4 Summary chart for managing diabetes during surgery.

it should be noted that both systems described here can be used with 5% dextrose if desired, halving the insulin dose delivered as appropriate. Similarly, if the infused volume needs to be reduced – as may be the case in elderly patients with cardiac problems, or patients with other causes of fluid overload such as renal failure – then 20% dextrose at half the volume can be used, or a standard 10% GKI system used at $50 \, \text{ml h}^{-1}$ rather than $100 \, \text{ml h}^{-1}$ (this would be equivalent to a 5% dextrose system).

The management of insulin-requiring diabetic patients being fed preoperatively or postoperatively via a nasogastric tube, or with parenteral nutrition, may cause some management difficulties. Insulin infusions are safe if the patient is in a high-dependency or intensive care area, but in general wards subcutaneous insulin can be used. There is little trial evidence available examining the various insulin regimens under these circumstances [47]. Provided that the feed has

a continuous carbohydrate provision, 12-hourly subcutaneous isophane insulin, or possibly long-acting analogues once or twice daily [48], may be satisfactory. Potential problems exist with both of these regimens, however [47]. With intermittent feeds, once-daily subcutaneous insulin may be initially introduced, although again twice-daily insulin may be necessary [49].

25.7.5 Special surgical situations

Emergency surgery

Truly urgent surgery is, fortunately, relatively rare in diabetic patients. However, it does occur and is perhaps more common in the elderly; examples include peripheral and mesenteric embolization, ruptured aneurysms and trauma. Urgent plasma glucose, urea and electrolyte estimates are of course mandatory, and if the glycaemic and metabolic status is adverse it is best to correct this as far as possible prior to surgery. The urgency of the surgical situation will, of course, need to be assessed carefully in each case, and no 'blanket' rules can be made. Similarly, as regards the method of peroperative glycaemic control, this too must be decided on an individual basis. Generally, a GKI system will be advisable in these unplanned situations, but the amounts of insulin needed cannot always be predicted. For example, if the patient requiring urgent surgery has received a sulphonylurea drug or insulin injection with the past 12 hours, the amount of insulin in the GKI infusion may need to be reduced. Each situation must be judged individually, and very frequent bedside blood glucose monitoring is necessary. In many cases, it may be judged that a 'separate line' system of delivery may be indicated to provide extra flexibility.

Open-heart surgery

Cardiac surgery is today very common, and coronary artery bypass grafting (CABG) in particular is well established as a symptom-relieving and sometimes life-prolonging operation of low mortality. As such, it is now being offered to many relatively elderly patients. Compared with other forms of surgery, CABG is unusual in that it is a long and unusually traumatic operation. Moreover, the patients are also rendered hypothermic and later given large doses of inotropic agents after the restoration of cardiac activity. All of these factors will promote increased insulin demands. Additionally, however, it has been traditional to use a dextrose 'priming solution' to fill the cardiopulmonary pump, often amounting to a glucose load of about 75 g at the start of surgery [50]. Not surprisingly, the initial results using standard GKI systems in this situation were poor [50, 51], but changing to a non-glucose priming solution greatly improved the peroperative glycaemic control [51, 52]. A 'separate line' system for glucose and insulin provision is essential, with frequent blood glucose monitoring. Relatively large insulin doses are needed [53], but the results are good and algorithms have been produced to aid insulin delivery decisions [54]. When using modern systems such as these, the results of open-heart surgery in diabetic patients have been comparable with those in non-diabetic counterparts [55, 56]. Hence, the most important aims of diabetes management during surgery have been fulfilled – acceptable glycaemic control by a simple and logical system, without excess mortality or morbidity.

During recent years, the use of GKI in diabetic patients undergoing CABG has resulted in an improvement in outcome measures such as length of hospital stay, risk of arrhythmias and ventilation duration, when compared to those managed without GKI [57]. Recently, a combination of intravenous and then subcutaneous insulin was shown to result in similar levels of morbidity and mortality in diabetic and non-diabetic patients following CABG [58].

25.8   Conclusions

Although few centres are currently investigating the practical and theoretical aspects of the operative care of the diabetic patient, the subject remains a popular topic for review articles [33, 59]. Perhaps this is not surprising. As a clinical problem it is very common, and although current management procedures are well accepted, their detailed application continues to cause confusion.

Safe and effective perioperative diabetic care requires the acceptance of hospital-based agreed protocols of care which must be widely distributed. Transferring these protocols to safe and effective patient treatment, depends on a team approach by physician, surgeon and anaesthetist.

The importance of an appropriate management of inpatients with diabetes has been recognized nationally in England by the diabetes National Service Framework (NSF). The NSFs are long-term government strategies for improving specific areas of care, and the diabetes NSF was launched in 2001. The equally important NSF for older people (published in the same year as the diabetes NSF) includes standard 4 which covers 16 core topics in areas such as nutrition, fluid balance and pressure area care. Despite these two strategies, much remains to be done to optimise the perioperative care of elderly people with diabetes, in England and elsewhere.

References

1. Kamoi K. Good long-term quality of life without diabetic complications with 20 years of continuous subcutaneous insulin infusion therapy in a brittle diabetic elderly patient. *Diabetes Care* 2002; 25: 402–3.
2. Allison SP, Tomlin PJ and Chamberlain MJ. Some effects of anaesthesia and surgery on carbohydrate and fat metabolism. *Brit J Anaesth* 1979; 41: 588–93.

3. Elliott MJ and Alberti KGMM. Carbohydrate metabolism – effects of preoperative starvation and trauma. *Clin Anaesthesiol* 1983; 1: 527–50.

4. Nordenstrom J, Sannenfield J and Arner P. Characterisation of insulin resistance after surgery. *Surgery* 1989; 105: 28–35.

5. Hume DM and Egdahl RH. The importance of the brain in the endocrine response to injury *Ann Surg* 1959; 150: 697–712.

6. Gill GV and Alberti KGMM. Surgery and diabetes. *Hospital Update* 1989; 15: 327–36.

7. Galloway JA and Shuman CR. Diabetes and surgery. *Am J Med* 1963; 34: 177–91.

8. Hjortrup A, Sorenson C, Dynemose E, Hjortso NC and Kehlet H. Influence of diabetes mellitus an operative risk. *Brit J Surg* 1985; 72: 783–5.

9. Melliere D, Berrahal D, Desgranges P *et al.* Influence of diabetes on revascularisation procedures of the aorta and lower limb arteries: early results. *Eur J Vasc Endovasc Surg* 1999; 17: 438–41.

10. Hamdan AD, Saltzberg SS, Sheahan M *et al.* Lack of association of diabetes with increased postoperative mortality and cardiac morbidity. *Arch Surg* 2002; 137: 417–21.

11. MacKenzie CR and Charlson ME. Assessment of perioperative risk in the patient with diabetes mellitus. *Surg Gynaecol Obstet* 1988; 167: 293–9.

12. Sandler RS, Maule WF and Baltus ME. Factors associated with post-operative complications in diabetics after biliary tract surgery. *Gastroenterology*, 1986; 91: 157–62.

13. Lieberman D, Friger M and Lieberman D. Rehabilitation outcome following hip fracture surgery in elderly diabetics: A prospective cohort study of 224 patients. *Disability and Rehabilitation* 2007; 29: 339–45.

14. Lipscombe LL, Jamal SA, Booth GL and Hawker GA. The risk of hip fractures in older individuals with diabetes. *Diabetes Care* 2007; 30: 835–41.

15. Golden SH, Kao WHL, Peart-Vigilance C and Broncati FL. Perioperative glycemic control and the risk of infectious complications in a cohort of adults with diabetes. *Diabetes Care* 1999; 22: 1408–14.

16. Jennings AM, Wilson RM and Ward JD. Symptomatic hypoglycaemia in NIDDM patients treated with oral hypoglycaemic agents. *Diabetes Care* 1989; 12: 203–8.

17. Faull CM, Holmes V and Baylis PH. Water balance in elderly people: is there a deficiency of vasopression? *Age and Ageing* 1993; 22: 114–20.

18. Ashwell SG, Gebbie J and Home PD. Twice-daily compared with once-daily insulin glargine in people with type 1 diabetes using meal-time insulin aspart. *Diabetic Medicine* 2006; 23: 879–86.

19. Bott S, Tusek C, Jacobsen LV *et al.* Insulin detemir under steady-state conditions: no accumulation and constant metabolic effect over time with twice daily administration in subjects with type 1 diabetes. *Diabetic Medicine* 2006; 23: 522–8.

20. Mathieu C and Gale EAM. Inhaled insulin: gone with the wind? *Diabetologia* 2008; 51: 1–5.

21. Rosenstock J, Saltes-Rak E, Sugimoto D *et al.* Triple therapy in type 2 diabetes. *Diabetes Care* 2006; 29: 554–9.

22. DeFronzo RA, Kim DD, Ratner RE, Fineman MS, Han J and Baron AD. Effects of exanetide (Exendin-4) on glycaemic control and weight over 30 weeks in metformin-treated patients with type 2 diabetes. *Diabetes Care* 2005; 28: 1092–100.

23. Goldstein BJ, Johnson J, Feinglos MN, Williams-Herman DE and Lunceford JK. Effect of initial combination therapy with sitagliptin, a dipeptidyl peptidase-4 inhibitor, and metformin on glycemic control patients with type 2 diabetes. *Diabetes Care* 2007; 30: 1979–87.

24. Van den Berghe G, Wouters P, Weekers F *et al.* (2001) Intensive insulin therapy in critically ill patients. *New Engl J Med*, 345, 1359–67.

25. Coursin DB and Murray MJ. How sweet is euglycaemia in critically ill patients? *Mayo Clin Proc* 2003; 78: 1460–2.

26. Watkinson P, Barber VS and Young JD. Strict glucose control in the critically ill. *Br Med J* 2006; 332: 865–6.

27. Gill GV and Alberti KGMM. (1992) The care of the diabetic patient during surgery. In: *International Textbook of Diabetes Mellitus.* KGMM Alberti, RA deFronzo, H Keen and P Zimmet (eds). John Wiley & Sons, Chichester, pp. 1173–83.

28. Hutchison ASA and Shenkin A. BM strips: how accurate are they in general wards? *Diabetic Medicine* 1984; 1: 225–6.

29. Ewing DJ, Martyn CN, Young RJ and Clarke BF. The value of cardiovascular autonomic function: 10 years' experience in diabetes. *Diabetes Care* 1985; 8: 491–8.

30. Page MM and Watkins PJ. Cardiorespiratory arrest with diabetic autonomic neuropathy. *Lancet* 1978; i: 14–16.

31. Burgos LG, Ebert TJ, Asiddao C, Turner LA, Pattison CZ, Wang-Cheng R and Kampine JP. Increased intra-operative cardiovascular morbidity in diabetics with autonomic neuropathy. *Anaesthesiology* 1989; 70: 591–7.

32. Podolsky S. Management of diabetes in the surgical patient. *Med Clin North America* 1982; 66: 1361–72.

33. Hirsch IB, McGill JB, Cryer PE and White PF. Perioperative management of surgical patients with diabetes mellitus. *Anaesthesiology* 1991; 74: 346–59.

34. Alberti KGMM and Marshall SM. (1988) Diabetes and surgery. In: *The Diabetes Annual* Ed KGMM Alberti

and LP Krall (eds). Elsevier Publishers, Amsterdam, pp. 248–71.

35. Schade DS. Surgery and diabetes. *Med Clin of North America* 1988; 72: 1531–43.

36. Thompson J, Husband DJ, Thai AC and Alberti KGMM. Metabolic changes in the non-insulin dependent diabetic undergoing minor surgery: effect of glucose-insulin-potassium infusion. *Brit J Surg* 1986; 73: 301–4.

37. Alberti KGMM, Gill GV and Elliott MJ. Insulin delivery during surgery in the diabetic patient. *Diabetes Care* 1982; 5: 65–77.

38. Thomas DJB and Alberti KGMM. The hyperglycaemic effects of Hartmann's solution in maturity-onset diabetics during surgery. *Brit J Anaesth* 1978; 50: 185–8.

39. Alberti KGMM and Thomas DJB. The management of diabetes during surgery. *Brit J Anaesth* 1979; 51: 693–710.

40. Thomas DJB, Platt HS and Alberti KGMM. Insulin-dependent diabetes during the peri-operative period. *Anaesthesia* 1984; 39: 629–37.

41. Gill GV. Surgery and diabetes mellitus. In *Textbook of Diabetes* J. Pickup and G. Williams (eds). Blackwell Publishers, London, 1991, pp. 820–6.

42. Taitelman U, Reece EA and Bessman AN. Insulin in the management of the diabetic surgical patient. Continuous intravenous administration versus subcutaneous administration. *JAMA* 1977; 237: 658–60.

43. European Diabetes Policy Group 1998. A desktop guide to Type 1 (insulin-dependent) diabetes mellitus. *Diabetic Medicine* 1999; 16: 253–66.

44. Nygren JO, Thorell A, Soop M *et al.* Perioperative insulin and glucose infusion maintains normal insulin sensitivity after surgery. *Amer J Physiol* 1998; 275: E140–8.

45. Husband DJ, Thai AC and Alberti KGMM. Management of diabetes during surgery with glucose-insulin-potassium infusion. *Diabetic Medicine* 1986; 3: 69–74.

46. Simmons D, Morton K, Laughton S and Scott DJ. A comparison of two intravenous insulin regimens among surgical patients with insulin-dependent diabetes mellitus. *Diabetes Educator* 1994; 20: 422–7.

47. Clement S, Braithwaite SS, Magee MF *et al.* Management of diabetes and hyperglycaemia in hospitals. *Diabetes Care* 2004; 27: 553–91.

48. Putz D and Karabadi UM. Insulin glargine in continuous enteric tube feeding. *Diabetes Care* 2002; 25: 1889–90.

49. Jain N, John LJ, McGlinchey L *et al.* Audit of the management of glycaemia in hospitalised enterally fed patients with diabetes. *Diabetic Med* 2008; 25 (Suppl. 1): 101.

50. Gill GV, Sherif IH and Alberti KGMM. Management of diabetes during open heart surgery. *Brit J Surg* 1981; 68: 171–2.

51. Stephens JW, Krause AH, Petersen CA *et al.* The effect of glucose priming solutions in patients undergoing coronary artery bypass grafting. *Ann Thorac Surg* 1988; 45: 544–7.

52. Crock PA, Ley CJ, Martin IK *et al.* Humoral and metabolic changes during hypothermic coronary artery bypass surgery in diabetic and non-diabetic subjects. *Diabetic Medicine* 1988; 5: 47–52.

53. Elliott MJ, Gill GV, Home PD *et al.* A comparison of two regimens for the management of diabetes during open-heart surgery. *Anaesthesiology* 1984; 60: 364–8.

54. Watson BG, Elliott MJ, Pay DA *et al.* Diabetes mellitus and open heart surgery. A simple practical closed loop insulin infusion system for blood glucose control. *Anaesthesia* 1986; 41: 250–7.

55. Lawrie GM, Morris GC and Glaeser DH. Influence of diabetes mellitus on the results of coronary bypass surgery. Follow-up of 212 diabetic patients 10 to 15 years after surgery. *JAMA* 1986; 256: 2967–71.

56. Devinen R and McKenzie FN. Surgery for coronary artery disease in patients with diabetes mellitus. *Can J Surg* 1985; 28: 367–70.

57. Lazar HL, Chipkin S, Philippides G *et al.* Glucose-insulin-potassium solutions improve outcomes in diabetics who have coronary artery operations. *Ann Thorac Surg* 2000; 70: 145–50.

58. Schmeltz LR, DeSantis AJ, Thiyagarajan V *et al.* Reduction of surgical mortality and morbidity in diabetic patients undergoing cardiac surgery with a combined intravenous and subcutaneous insulin glucose management strategy. *Diabetes Care* 2007; 30: 823–8.

59. Anonymous. Drugs in the peri-operative period: corticosteroids and therapy for diabetes mellitus. *Drug and Therapeutics Bulletin* 1999; 37: 68–70.

SECTION V

Management of Associated Complications

26

The Implications of the Evolving Diabetes Epidemic for Disability in Older Adults

Edward W. Gregg and Linda Geiss

Division of Diabetes Translation, Centers for Disease Control and Prevention, Atlanta, GA, USA

Key messages

- Diabetes leads to a variety of vascular and neuropathic complications which increase the likelihood of disability.
- In older people, because of the increased risk of other geriatric syndromes, diabetes may be associated with further disability.
- The excess disability risk associated with diabetes may lead to a higher prevalence of falls and fractures and may underpin the development of frailty.

26.1 Diabetes and older adults: The magnitude and character of the problem

The increase in diabetes prevalence in the United States, western Europe and many areas of the developing world in recent decades is an ominous threat to public health [1–3]. While the threat of increased diabetes incidence in young adults and adolescents associated with obesity has garnered much attention [4–6], these observations may have overshadowed some of the realities of the diabetes epidemic. Namely, diabetes remains largely a disease of ageing, and this is likely to be even more the case in the future [7–9]. Both, the incidence and prevalence of diabetes have increased substantially in relative terms among the young and middle-aged adults. Age is one of most important risk factors for diabetes, roughly equivalent to the body mass index (BMI) as a continuous, graded risk factor. The prevalence of total diabetes (diagnosed and undiagnosed diabetes combined) among persons aged >65 years in the US was 31% in 2005–2006 [9]. However, these estimates hide considerable variation across ethnic groups, as more than one-third of older Mexican-Americans and African-Americans have diabetes. Furthermore, prevalence has been estimated at 25% in studies of nursing homes in both the US and United Kingdom [10, 11].

The results of multi-national studies conducted during the mid- to late 1990s in Europe suggested that the prevalence of diabetes among Northern European populations (e.g. UK, Netherlands, Poland, Sweden) was only slightly lower than the American estimates, whereas estimates from Southern European populations (e.g. Italy, Spain, Malta) were even higher [12]. In a multi-national study of Asian cohorts, older adults in China and Japan had a total diabetes prevalence

Diabetes in Old Age. Third Edition. Edited by Alan J. Sinclair
© 2009 John Wiley & Sons, Ltd

similar to that of the US (i.e. approximately one in five), whereas prevalence exceeded one in three in many areas of India [13].

The steep association between age and type 2 diabetes has practical implications for future projections of diabetes burden in older adults. Because the absolute prevalence is so high among older adults, the gradual increases in prevalence of diabetes observed across the entire age range has a much more substantial absolute impact among the prevalence of the old than the young. For example, among adults age 65–74 years, the prevalence of diagnosed diabetes has doubled during the past 25 years, adding nine prevalent cases per 100 to the population (i.e. from 9.1 to 18.5%) (Figure 26.1). Prevalence also increased by 125% among persons aged 0–44 years, but this increase added less than one case per 100 to the population (i.e. from 0.6 to 1.4%) (8). As a result, within 25 years, most cases of diagnosed diabetes will be among the population age ≥65 years, and the total number of cases is expected to triple [7]. Accordingly, many of the developed countries of the world will see the most substantial increases in total numbers of diabetes cases among older adults [14].

Diabetes presents a unique problem for older adults, because it leads to a variety of vascular and neuropathic complications that are likely to be further compounded by age. Diabetes is the leading cause of blindness, non-traumatic amputation and end-stage renal disease, and more than doubles the risk of coronary heart disease (CHD), stroke and peripheral arterial disease

[3]. Because these complications are a function of diabetes duration and are also influenced by age, older adults with diabetes are likely to have several of these conditions simultaneously.

In addition to the traditional diabetic complications, diabetes increases the risk for several components of the geriatric syndrome, including cognitive decline and Alzheimer's disease, sarcopenia, depression, osteoporotic fractures and incontinence [15, 16]. The end result of this convergence of vascular, neuropathy and geriatric conditions is a complex of functional disabilities that are of *higher* prevalence in people with diabetes (Figure 26.2). These functional disabilities emanate from impairments in mobility, cognitive decline, depression and other emotional or affective disorders, and social isolation. For the older adult with diabetes, the implications of these impairments for early loss of independence and quality of life are as concerning as the more traditionally recognized clinical implications of diabetes [17]. Diabetes may contribute to functional disabilities through the multiple complications of diabetes or, alternatively, it may influence functional disability through the more direct effects on glycaemic lability, such as through symptom distress associated with hyperglycaemia or hypoglycaemia.

In addition to the obvious implications for the individual, disability prevalence associated with diabetes is important from the perspective of understanding the trends of health status of the population, as well as the

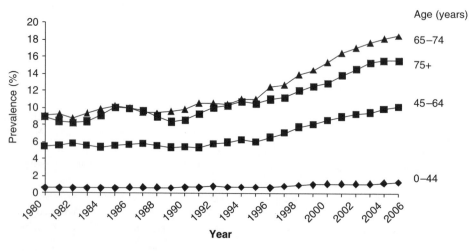

National Diabetes Surveillance System, 2008;

Figure 26.1　Prevalence of diagnosed diabetes in the United States, by age, between 1980 and 2006.

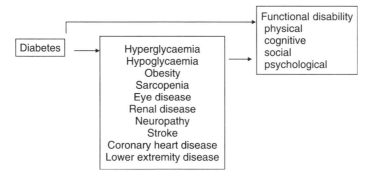

Figure 26.2 Model of potential long-term impact of diabetes on aging-related morbidity.

effectiveness of public health interventions in the diabetic population [18, 19]. Fries et al. have described the compression of morbidity as the ultimate objective of public health efforts for the adult population [19]. For population morbidity to be compressed, medical and public health efforts will have to lead to reductions in disability incidence that are even more rapid than mortality reductions. The end result would be a reduced average number of years that the average person spends in a disabled state.

In this chapter, the relationship between diabetes and functional disability is described, and the prominent explanatory factors and modifiable risk factors for functional decline summarized and prioritized. In addition, the most promising modifiable risk factors and interventions are outlined.

26.2 Diabetes and functional disability

Several epidemiological studies have examined the association of diabetes with functional disabilities, with most focusing on physical impairments. During the 1990s, diabetes was shown to be an important predictor of maintenance of independence and successful aging in diverse cohorts, including adults up to the age of 75 years in the Alameda County Study, the Framingham Study, and the US Longitudinal Study of Aging and the Established Population for the Epidemiologic Study of the Elderly Survey [20–24]. The steep rise in diabetes prevalence during the 1990s in turn led to more detailed and comprehensive examinations of the particular role of diabetes on physical disability. In an examination of the US non-institutionalized population, women and men with diabetes consistently had twice

the prevalence of inability to perform key tasks of mobility, including walking 0.4 km (quarter-mile), doing housework and walking up stairs [25]. For example, 32% of women with diabetes reported being unable to walk 0.4 km, compared to about 14% of non-diabetic women. A similar excess disability existed for climbing steps and doing housework. The excess prevalence of mobility problems extended to objective measures of physical functioning, including tests of balance, gait speed and lower-extremity function, as reflected in chair stands. Diabetes was associated with a similar risk for mobility impairments in men, although the absolute prevalence of impairments tended to be lower. These findings were corroborated by another nationally representative survey, the National Health Interview Survey, which showed that diabetes was associated with about twice the prevalence of inability to perform diverse mobility tasks, with the greatest excess risk observed for lower-extremity tasks [26]. These cross-sectional studies have the important caveat of not being able to determine whether diabetes preceded disability, or *vice versa*. Nevertheless, they played an important role in defining the extent of morbidity in the population with diagnosed diabetes.

Prospective studies further support the association between diabetes and the development of disability, demonstrating a 100–150% increased incidence of disability among older women with diabetes relative to their non-diabetic peers [27]. In the Study of Osteoporotic Fractures (SOF), highly functioning community dwelling women with diabetes developed an inability to walk 0.4 km mile at the rate of 4% per year, an inability to do housework at a rate of 8% per year, and 10% per year developed an inability to do at least one task (Figure 26.3) [27]. For example, the 5-year cumulative incidence of disability – defined by onset of inability to perform major physical tasks – was about

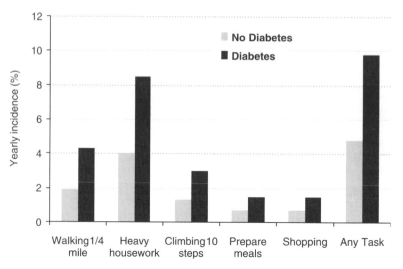

Figure 26.3 Yearly incidence of inability to do physical and household tasks among women aged ≥65 years, with and without diabetes. Data taken from the Study of Osteoporotic Fractures [28].

40% for 65–80-year old women with diabetes, compared to about 20% in their same age non-diabetic counterparts. In the SOF, having diabetes was equivalent to about 7 years of aging in terms of functional status. The Women's Health and Aging Study (WHAS) found similar findings in a cohort of older women with mild to moderate impairments. Women with diabetes had a 78% increased risk of mobility-related disability and a 65% increased risk of ADL disability [37].

The results of several studies have suggested that the excess disability risk associated with diabetes extends to an increased risk of falls and osteoporotic fractures. In NHANES III, diabetic women had a 45% higher prevalence of falls (35% in the past year) compared to non-diabetic women (25%), and a 69% increased risk of an injurious fall in the previous year. In the WHAS, women with diabetes had a 50% increased risk of falls. The increased frailty and risk of falls is sufficient to increase hip fracture risk even though people with type 2 diabetes tend to have a higher bone mineral density (BMD) than their non-diabetic peers [28–30]. People with type 1 diabetes, on the other hand, have both a decreased BMD and an increased risk of falls, creating a double jeopardy in terms of fracture risk [31, 32].

26.3   Modifiable factors explaining diabetes and disability

Diabetes could lead to physical disability through a variety of pathophysiological pathways, including some that occur before the onset of diabetes, such as obesity, insulin resistance, inflammation, CHD and peripheral arterial disease. Other disabilities that follow may result from diabetes, such as peripheral neuropathy, diabetic nephropathy, vision loss, cardiovascular disease and stroke, while other factors are directly associated with glycaemic status (e.g. hyperglycaemia symptoms, hypoglycaemia). Among the US population, CHD was a dominant factor, explaining about one-third of the excess disability in diabetic women and about one-quarter in diabetic men. The BMI also explained a large portion of disability, but only in women (24%), as the BMI and CHD combined explained 52% of the excess disability [25]. In men, the BMI was relatively unimportant but was offset somewhat by stroke, which explained about one-fifth of the excess disability. About one-third of the excess disability risk remained unexplained by all complications included in the statistical analyses. The observation that BMI was a more important intervening factor in women than in men was also consistent with a study of national sample of older community-dwelling adults (diabetic and non-diabetic combined) [33]. Men with class III obesity (BMI >40) had an 83% increased disability risk, but there was no excess disability risk associated with overweight or moderate obesity (i.e. BMI 30–35). In women, there were 15%, 54% and 83% increases in the risk of disability associated with class I, II and III obesity, respectively.

Subsequent studies with a better assessment of lower-extremity conditions showed that the ankle:brachial index and sensory and motor nerve function each had strong correlations with objective measures of mobility and balance, and were potent predictors of incident disability [34–36]. Analyses of the Womens Health and Aging Study (a cohort with moderate physical impairment at baseline) found that peripheral arterial disease, peripheral neuropathy and depression were all important predictors, each accounting for up to one-fifth of the excess disability in older diabetic women [37]. Again, a large proportion of excess mobility and activities of daily living (ADL) disability, and about 40% of excess walking limitations and performance measures, remained unexplained by all factors combined. These findings were further supported by subclinical assessments of functioning, defined by objective physical performance tests such as walking speed, balance and chair stands [38]. A follow-up of the Health ABC Study showed that older adults with type 2 diabetes have a greater decline in leg muscle mass, strength and muscle quality (strength per unit of mass) than those without diabetes. Of note, this difference in the rate of decline was limited to lower-extremity strength, which the authors speculated may be due to neuropathy, which affects the lower extremities more dramatically than upper extremities [39].

Whereas, the studies described above examined factors explaining the difference in disability risk between diabetic and non-diabetic population, other studies have examined the predictors of poor physical function and disability specifically within the diabetic population. In a sample of over 1000 managed-care patients with diabetes, obesity, lack of exercise, depression symptoms and lower formal education were each associated with disability [40]. In the SOF, physical activity and obesity were each prominent modifiable risk factors for incident disability [27]. Obese women developed an inability to perform physical tasks at twice the rate of lean women, while women in the highest quintile of physical activity had a 39% lower disability risk compared to sedentary women. In a detailed examination of the association of diabetes with risk of falls among diabetic older women, those who used insulin and had a glycated haemoglobin (HbA_{1c}) level of <6% had a fourfold higher risk of falls than women with higher HbA_{1c} levels [40]. Peripheral nerve dysfunction, poor vision, poor renal function and weight loss were each associated with a 40–60% increased risk of falls.

In summary, the route between diabetes and physical disability is multifactorial. Lower-extremity diseases,

of both atherosclerotic and neuropathic origin, appear to be among the most dominant factors because they exact a large magnitude of increased disability risk. Yet, at the same time they are fairly common among the population with diabetes, with lower-extremity disease (either peripheral arterial disease or peripheral neuropathy) being present in 38% of adults aged 70–80 years, in 45% of those aged >80 years, and likely in an even higher proportion of the subset with diabetes [41]. Here, CHD plays a similar role, at least doubling the incidence of disability and affecting perhaps one-quarter of the older diabetic population. Other factors such as stroke and hip fracture have profound effects on disability when they occur, but fortunately are less common than lower-extremity conditions on the whole and thus may act as secondary factors. Further research is required into the intervening factors in disability, and how interventions can be developed to exploit them.

26.4 Interventions to reduce disability risk

Observational studies have pointed to a wide range of potentially effective interventions to reduce the risk of disability in diabetic populations, but have rarely been tested using randomized clinical trials. The strongest evidence exists for exercise, strength and balance training among persons with moderate impairments. Studies conducted during the 1990s showed that older adults at a high risk of falls can improve their physical performance and reduce their risk of falling when randomized to structured programmes of lower-extremity strength, balance training, walking and tai chi [42–44]. These programmes have typically been aimed at people who already have an established functional impairment. More recent studies of overweight and obese adults with arthritis symptoms have shown that structured exercise programmes also reduce symptoms, improve mobility and maintain independence [45]. The fact that exercise also improves functional capacity in persons with lower-extremity arterial disease, and is also an aide to weight maintenance, are further justification to recommend structured, moderate exercise programmes. While such studies have not been conducted specifically among adults with diabetes, suitable evidence for collateral benefits on glycaemic control without adverse events exists to justify the generalization of exercise programmes to older adults with diabetes [46]. Accordingly, the American College of

Sports Medicine and the American Heart Association have revised their recommendations for physical activity, suggesting that older adults should have an activity plan that includes appropriate levels of regular aerobic, muscle-strengthening, flexibility and balance exercise, and also integrates preventive and therapeutic recommendations specific to individual chronic conditions present with the individual patient [47].

Depression is common, underdiagnosed and undertreated in adults with diabetes [48, 49]. The fact that depression was a factor explaining excess disability in diabetic patients suggests that better identification and treatment could also reduce disability [27, 37]. Improved glycaemic control has been shown to reduce symptom distress and improve physical functioning over the short term. However, despite the clear benefits of glycaemic control in terms of reduced microvascular complications, the impact on long-term disability remains unclear. In addition, the recent controversial findings of the ACCORD study, in which intensively managed older adults had a higher risk of death than those under simply good control, will likely lead to a further review of the optimal levels of glycaemic control among men [58]. Structured weight-loss programmes have been suggested as a means of reducing disability in high-risk populations, based on observations of the impact of obesity on disability risk combined with the collateral benefits of weight loss in terms of exercise capacity and reduced cardiovascular risk. On the other hand, the potential for loss of lean mass associated with weight loss could conceivably negate the advantages of fat loss. Observational studies have associated weight loss with either no benefit or increased disability and mortality, pointing to the need for randomized controlled trials [50–52]. The ongoing Look AHEAD study, which ostensibly was designed to examine the impact of intensive long-term weight loss in obese diabetic adults, should also provide important information on the impact of weight loss on disability [53, 54].

Given the role of CHD, stroke and lower-extremity disease on the development of disability over the long term, cardiovascular risk factor management including smoking cessation, lipid and lipid and blood pressure control, aspirin use and early screening for diabetic complications, may have long-term effects on disability. However, such interventions may be far upstream from effects on disability, and both clinical trial and observational studies have not (yet) demonstrated any effects on disability. Nevertheless, recent attempts to tailor guidelines and implications to the needs of older adults are a positive step in the reduction of disability [15].

26.5   Trends in disability among the diabetic population

Population trends in the prevalence and incidence of disability over time will help to evaluate the cumulative effects of public health efforts to reduce morbidity among the diabetic population. Meta-analyses of US national surveys have suggested that the prevalence of disability has declined consistently among adults aged >65 years during the past 20 years [55]. Such decline in disability prevalence has been attributed to a combination of wide-scale improvements in medical care, key health behaviours such as smoking, the availability of assistive devices and general improvements in the socioeconomic status of the population [56]. However, whether these improvements have also occurred among the US population with diabetes remains unclear.

Data from the US National Diabetes Surveillance System suggest that there have been modest reductions in disability prevalence over the past decade. Declines in the prevalence of mobility limitation among the diabetes population have been greatest among black men (i.e. a decline from 60% to 38%) and Hispanic men (52% to 36%) [57] (Figure 26.4). These findings are consistent with reduced rates of hospitalization associated with complications among the diabetic population [57]. However, part of the decline in disability prevalence may have been driven by an increased incidence of diabetes diagnosis and an accompanying lower average duration of diabetes in the overall diabetic population. Disability prevalence has also declined in black and Hispanic women by 7 percentage points, but has been flat in white women [57].

26.6   Summary

Disability is a central complication of diabetes in older adults, and represents the cumulative impact of the numerous chronic, acute and transient complications of diabetes. Since the prevalence of diabetes is also heavily influenced by demographic and mortality trends in the population, an understanding of the trends in morbidity and disability will require novel and more sensitive approaches to measuring disability among the population. The reduction in disability among people

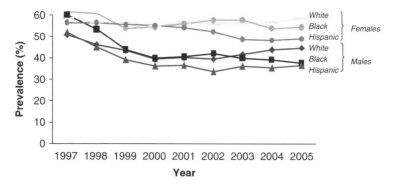

Figure 26.4 Trends in age-adjusted prevalence of any mobility limitation per 100 adults with diabetes, by race/ethnicity and gender in the United States, 1997–2005. Data available from the US national diabetes surveillance system.

with diabetes will continue to depend on the development and implementation of new interventions at individual, health system and health policy levels.

References

1. Wild S, Roglic G, Green A, Sicree R and King H. Global prevalence of diabetes: estimates for the year 2000 and projections for 2030. Diabetes Care 2004; 27 (5): 1047–53.

2. Zimmet P, Alberti KG and Shaw J. Global and societal implications of the diabetes epidemic. Nature 2001; 414 (6865): 782–7.

3. Engelgau MM, Geiss LS, Saaddine JB, Boyle JP, Benjamin SM, Gregg EW et al. The evolving diabetes burden in the United States. Ann Intern Med 2004; 140 (11): 945–50.

4. Dabelea D, Pettitt DJ, Jones KL and Arslanian SA. Type 2 diabetes mellitus in minority children and adolescents. An emerging problem. Endocrinol Metab Clin North Am 1999; 28 (4): 709–29, viii.

5. Olshansky SJ, Passaro DJ, Hershow RC, Layden J, Carnes BA, Brody J et al. A potential decline in life expectancy in the United States in the 21st century. N Engl J Med 2005; 352 (11): 1138–45.

6. Williams DE, Cadwell BL, Cheng YJ, Cowie CC, Gregg EW, Geiss LS et al. Prevalence of impaired fasting glucose and its relationship with cardiovascular disease risk factors in US adolescents, 1999-2000. Pediatrics 2005; 116 (5): 1122–6.

7. Boyle JP, Honeycutt AA, Narayan KM, Hoerger TJ, Geiss LS, Chen H et al. Projection of diabetes burden through 2050: impact of changing demography and disease prevalence in the US. Diabetes Care 2001; 24 (11): 1936–40.

8. Centers for Disease Control and Prevention. Prevalence of Diagnosed Diabetes by Age, United States, 1980–2000. http://www.cdc.gov/diabetes/statistics/prev/national/fig2 2003. Available from: URL: www.cdc.gov/diabetes/statistics/prev/national/fig2

9. Cowie CC, Rust KF, Ford ES, Eberhardt MS, Byrd-Holt DD et al. Full accounting of diabetes and pre-diabetes in the U.S. population in 1988–1994 and 2005–2006. Diabetes Care 2009; 32: 287–294.

10. Resnick HE, Heineman J, Stone R and Shorr RI. Diabetes in U.S. nursing homes, 2004. Diabetes Care 2008; 31 (2): 287–8.

11. Sinclair AJ, Gadsby R, Penfold S, Croxson SC and Bayer AJ. Prevalence of diabetes in care home residents. Diabetes Care 2001; 24 (6): 1066–8.

12. Age- and sex-specific prevalences of diabetes and impaired glucose regulation in 13 European cohorts. Diabetes Care 2003; 26 (1): 61–9.

13. Qiao Q, Hu G, Tuomilehto J, Nakagami T, Balkau B, Borch-Johnsen K et al. Age- and sex-specific prevalence of diabetes and impaired glucose regulation in 11 Asian cohorts. Diabetes Care 2003; 26 (6): 1770–80.

14. King H, Aubert RE and Herman WH. Global burden of diabetes, 1995–2025: prevalence, numerical estimates, and projections. Diabetes Care 1998; 21 (9): 1414–31.

15. Brown AF, Mangione CM, Saliba D and Sarkisian CA. Guidelines for improving the care of the older person with diabetes mellitus. J Am Geriatr Soc 2003; 51 (5 Suppl. Guidelines): S265–80.

16. Gregg EW and Brown A. Cognitive and physical disabilities and aging-related complications of diabetes. Clinical Diabetes 2003; 21: 113–18.

17. Phelan EA, Anderson LA, La Croix AZ and Larson EB. Older adults' views of 'successful aging' – how do they compare with researchers' definitions? J Am Geriatr Soc 2004; 52 (2): 211–16.

18. Fried LP, Tangen CM, Walston J, Newman AB, Hirsch C, Gottdiener J et al. Frailty in older adults: evidence for a phenotype. J Gerontol A Biol Sci Med Sci 2001; 56 (3): M146–56.

19. Fries JF. Measuring and monitoring success in compressing morbidity. Ann Intern Med 2003; 139(5Pt 2): 455–9.

20. Black SA, Ray LA and Markides KS. The prevalence and health burden of self-reported diabetes in older Mexican Americans: findings from the Hispanic established populations for epidemiologic studies of the elderly. Am J Public Health 1999; 89 (4): 546–52.

21. Boult C, Kane RL, Louis TA, Boult L and McCaffrey D. Chronic conditions that lead to functional limitation in the elderly. J Gerontol 1994; 49 (1): M28–36.

22. Guccione AA, Felson DT, Anderson JJ, Anthony JM, Zhang Y, Wilson PW et al. The effects of specific medical conditions on the functional limitations of elders in the Framingham Study. Am J Public Health 1994; 84 (3): 351–8.

23. Moritz DJ, Ostfeld AM, Blazer D, Curb D, Taylor JO and Wallace RB. The health burden of diabetes for the elderly in four communities. Public Health Rep 1994; 109 (6): 782–90.

24. Strawbridge WJ, Cohen RD, Shema SJ and Kaplan GA. Successful aging: predictors and associated activities. Am J Epidemiol 1996; 144 (2): 135–41.

25. Gregg EW, Beckles GL, Williamson DF, Leveille SG, Langlois JA, Engelgau MM et al. Diabetes and physical disability among older U.S. adults. Diabetes Care 2000; 23 (9): 1272–7.

26. Ryerson B, Tierney EF, Thompson TJ, Engelgau MM, Wang J, Gregg EW et al. Excess physical limitations among adults with diabetes in the U.S. population, 1997–1999. Diabetes Care 2003; 26 (1): 206–10.

27. Gregg EW, Mangione CM, Cauley JA, Thompson TJ, Schwartz AV, Ensrud KE et al. Diabetes and incidence of functional disability in older women. Diabetes Care 2002; 25 (1): 61–7.

28. Lipscombe LL, Jamal SA, Booth GL and Hawker GA. The risk of hip fractures in older individuals with diabetes: a population-based study. Diabetes Care 2007; 30 (4): 835–41.

29. Robbins J, Aragaki AK, Kooperberg C, Watts N, Wactawski-Wende J, Jackson RD et al. Factors associated with 5-year risk of hip fracture in postmenopausal women. JAMA 2007; 298 (20): 2389–98.

30. Schwartz AV, Nevitt MC, Brown BW, Jr and Kelsey JL. Increased falling as a risk factor for fracture among older women: the study of osteoporotic fractures. Am J Epidemiol 2005; 161 (2): 180–5.

31. Ivers RQ, Cumming RG, Mitchell P and Peduto AJ. Diabetes and risk of fracture: The Blue Mountains Eye Study. Diabetes Care 2001; 24 (7): 1198–203.

32. Strotmeyer ES and Cauley JA. Diabetes mellitus, bone mineral density, and fracture risk. Curr Opin Endocrinol Diabetes Obes 2007; 14 (6): 429–35.

33. Imai K, Gregg EW, Chen YJ, Zhang P, de RN and Williamson DF. The association of BMI with functional status and self-rated health in US adults. Obesity (Silver Spring) 2008; 16 (2): 402–8.

34. Dolan NC, Liu K, Criqui MH, Greenland P, Guralnik JM, Chan C et al. Peripheral artery disease, diabetes, and reduced lower extremity functioning. Diabetes Care 2002; 25 (1): 113–20.

35. Resnick HE, Stansberry KB, Harris TB, Tirivedi M, Smith K, Morgan P et al. Diabetes, peripheral neuropathy, and old age disability. Muscle Nerve 2002; 25 (1): 43–50.

36. Brach JS, Solomon C, Naydeck BL, Sutton-Tyrrell K, Enright PL, Jenny NS et al. (2008) Incident physical disability in people with lower extremity peripheral arterial disease: the role of cardiovascular disease. J Am Geriatr Soc, 56 (6), 1037–44.

37. Volpato S, Blaum C, Resnick H, Ferrucci L, Fried LP and Guralnik JM. Comorbidities and impairments explaining the association between diabetes and lower extremity disability: The Women's Health and Aging Study. Diabetes Care 2002; 25 (4): 678–83.

38. de Rekeneire N, Resnick HE, Schwartz AV, Shorr RI, Kuller LH, Simonsick EM et al. Diabetes is associated with subclinical functional limitation in nondisabled older individuals: the Health, Aging, and Body Composition study. Diabetes Care 2003; 26 (12): 3257–63.

39. Park SW, Goodpaster BH, Strotmeyer ES, Kuller LH, Broudeau R, Kammerer C et al. Accelerated loss of skeletal muscle strength in older adults with Type 2 diabetes: the health, aging, and body composition study. Diabetes Care 2007; 30 (6): 1507–12.

40. Schwartz AV, Vittinghoff E, Sellmeyer DE, Feingold KR, de RN, Strotmeyer ES et al. Diabetes-related complications, glycemic control, and falls in older adults. Diabetes Care 2008; 31 (3): 391–6.

41. Gregg EW, Sorlie P, Paulose-Ram R, Gu Q, Eberhardt MS, Wolz M et al. Prevalence of lower-extremity disease in the US adult population>=40 years of age with and without diabetes: 1999-2000 national health and nutrition examination survey. Diabetes Care 2004; 27 (7): 1591–7.

42. Campbell AJ, Robertson MC, Gardner MM, Norton RN, Tilyard MW and Buchner DM. Randomised controlled trial of a general practice programme of home based exercise to prevent falls in elderly women. Br Med J 1997; 315 (7115): 1065–9.

43. Gregg EW, Pereira MA and Caspersen CJ. Physical activity, falls, and fractures among older adults: a review of the epidemiologic evidence. J Am Geriatr Soc 2000; 48 (8): 883–93.

44. Province MA, Hadley EC, Hornbrook MC, Lipsitz LA, Miller JP, Mulrow CD *et al*. The effects of exercise on falls in elderly patients. A preplanned meta-analysis of the FICSIT Trials. Frailty and Injuries: Cooperative Studies of Intervention Techniques. JAMA 1995; 273 (17): 1341–7.

45. Messier SP, Loeser RF, Miller GD, Morgan TM, Rejeski WJ, Sevick MA *et al*. Exercise and dietary weight loss in overweight and obese older adults with knee osteoarthritis: the Arthritis, Diet, and Activity Promotion Trial. Arthritis Rheum 2004; 50 (5): 1501–10.

46. Boule NG, Haddad E, Kenny GP, Wells GA and Sigal RJ. Effects of exercise on glycemic control and body mass in Type 2 diabetes mellitus: a meta-analysis of controlled clinical trials. JAMA 2001; 286 (10): 1218–27.

47. Nelson ME, Rejeski WJ, Blair SN, Duncan PW, Judge JO, King AC *et al*. Physical activity and public health in older adults: recommendation from the American College of Sports Medicine and the American Heart Association. Circulation 2007; 116 (9): 1094–105.

48. Anderson RJ, Freedland KE, Clouse RE and Lustman PJ. The prevalence of comorbid depression in adults with diabetes: a meta-analysis. Diabetes Care 2001; 24 (6): 1069–78.

49. Dealberto MJ, Seeman T, Mcavay GJ and Berkman L. Factors related to current and subsequent psychotropic drug use in an elderly cohort. J Clin Epidemiol 1997; 50 (3): 357–64.

50. Launer LJ, Harris T, Rumpel C and Madans J. Body mass index, weight change, and risk of mobility disability in middle-aged and older women. The epidemiologic follow-up study of NHANES I. JAMA 1994; 271 (14): 1093–8.

51. Lee JS, Kritchevsky SB, Tylavsky FA, Harris T, Everhart J, Simonsick EM *et al*. Weight-loss intention in the well-functioning, community-dwelling elderly: associations with diet quality, physical activity, and weight change. Am J Clin Nutr 2004; 80 (2): 466–74.

52. Lee JS, Kritchevsky SB, Tylavsky F, Harris T, Simonsick EM, Rubin SM *et al*. Weight change, weight change intention, and the incidence of mobility limitation in well-functioning community-dwelling older adults. J Gerontol A Biol Sci Med Sci 2005; 60 (8): 1007–12.

53. Rejeski WJ, Lang W, Neiberg RH, Van DB, Foster GD, Maciejewski ML *et al*. Correlates of health-related quality of life in overweight and obese adults with Type 2 diabetes. Obesity (Silver Spring) 2006; 14 (5): 870–83.

54. Wadden TA, West DS, Delahanty L, Jakicic J, Rejeski J, Williamson D *et al*. The Look AHEAD study: a description of the lifestyle intervention and the evidence supporting it. Obesity (Silver Spring) 2006; 14 (5): 737–52.

55. Manton KG, Corder L and Stallard E. Chronic disability trends in elderly United States populations: 1982–1994. Proc Natl Acad Sci USA 1997; 94 (6): 2593–8.

56. Cutler DM. The reduction in disability among the elderly. Proc Natl Acad Sci USA 2001; 98 (12): 6546–7.

57. Centers for Disease Control and Prevention. Diabetes Surveillance System: Health Status and Disability. Diabetes Surveillance System 2004. Available from: URL: http://www.cdc.gov/diabetes/statistics/health_status_national.htm.

58. Gerstein HC, Miller ME, Byington RP *et al*. Action to Control Cardiovascular Risk in Diabetes Study Group. The Effects of Intensive Glucose Lowering in Type 2 Diabetes. N Engl J Med 2008; 358: 2545–59.

Diabetes and Cognitive Dysfunction

Alan J. Sinclair[1] and Koula G. Asimakopoulou[2]

[1]*Bedfordshire and Hertfordshire Postgraduate Medical School, University of Bedfordshire, Luton, UK*
[2]*King's College London Dental Institute, Oral Health Services Research and Dental Public Health, London, UK*

Key messages

- Diabetes mellitus and cognitive dysfunction are likely to be interrelated, and often coexist in the same individual.
- There is an increasing evidence base linking a greater likelihood of cognitive dysfunction in subjects with diabetes, especially of long duration.
- The assessment of cognitive function using standard cognitive screening tests is recommended in the routine assessment of all older people with diabetes.
- The detection of cognitive dysfunction may provide an early opportunity to consider drug-based intervention strategies and care packages that provide more effective management, and may delay the need for early dependency.

27.1 Introduction

Since the early 1920s, when Miles and Root [1] first proposed a link between diabetes and cognitive dysfunction, knowledge concerning the relationship between these two states – as well as the methods of investigation of such a relationship – have progressed enormously.

The idea that diabetes may be related to cognitive dysfunction makes intuitive sense. The brain relies on a steady supply of glucose in order to function optimally, but at the same time is unable to store glucose in situations of over-supply (e.g. hyperglycaemia). Equally, it cannot rely on stored facilities in situations of under-supply (hypoglycaemia). It follows that a condition associated with abnormalities in glucose availability to the brain, such as diabetes, might lead to brain processes becoming compromised.

Cognitive function is a short descriptive term for the multitude of mental processes that people engage in in everyday life, from paying attention to and perceiving information, to remembering it, organizing it into meaningful chunks, retrieving it and using it to solve abstract or practical problems. Cognitive psychologists refer to such processes as 'cognitive domains', and classify them – among others – in terms of attention, speed and amount of information processing (mental flexibility), and memory. A trauma or insult to the brain such as that posed by hyper- or hypoglycaemia, can affect any or all of these processes selectively. Older patients with diabetes (either type 1 or 2) have an increased risk of developing cognitive dysfunction by virtue of their increasing age, irrespective of other factors such as diabetes itself. Practising clinicians must expect to see patients with both diabetes and cognitive dysfunction, as both conditions are highly prevalent

Diabetes in Old Age. Third Edition. Edited by Alan J. Sinclair

Table 27.1 Background to the relationship between diabetes and cognitive disorders [2].

- Professional and public concern about the impact of diabetes on cognition
- Long-term influence of hyperglycaemia and hypoglycaemia on cerebral function unknown
- Pathophysiological mechanisms involved uncertain, but may involve both vascular, inflammatory and neuronal mechanisms
- No current agreement on the most optimum method to detect/assess cognitive deficits in diabetes
- Clinical relevance of the changes observed uncertain.

chronic disease states in today's' communities. The development of dysfunction may have several important consequences for the patient and his/her family and carers in terms of the complexity of care, adherence to therapy, ability to self-manage, and the need for assisted care. Many of the important elements which have provided a background to this area are listed in Table 27.1.

27.2 Evidence of association between diabetes and cognitive dysfunction

In a recent editorial published in the *British Medical Journal* [3], it was argued that

"...diabetes, cognitive impairment and dementia are strongly linked, but the precise mechanisms are unclear."

This apt conclusion describes the findings of a, now substantial, body of literature on the subject spanning 15 years or so, and which has attempted to identify, what (if any) cognitive processes are mostly affected by diabetes, in what ways, and the factors that seem to be moderating the diabetes–cognitive dysfunction relationship. It is likely that further research will demonstrate that both vascular dementia (VaD) and Alzheimer's disease (AD) are possible outcomes of long-duration diabetes in a vulnerable individual [4].

The vast majority of studies in this field have been cross-sectional, often comparing a small sample of diabetes patients with diabetes-free individuals, on a battery of various cognitive tests, and reporting moderate differences in some – but usually not all – cognitive

measures used [5]. Such studies have varied not only in the sensitivity, specificity, reliability and validity of the tests they have employed, but also in the degree of methodological vigour they have adopted, with the tendency of studies revealing more diabetes-related cognitive deficits the less well-controlled they have been [6]. Nevertheless, the overall consensus based on a review of the vast majority of such studies seems to be that:

"...patients with type 2 diabetes have moderate impairments across all cognitive domains...a diminished ability to efficiently process unstructured information, particularly when the cognitive task at hand requires speed of response." [7]

Given the shortcoming of cross-sectional investigations, however, and the reported consensus that such studies are probably ill-equipped [3, 7, 8] to answer the question as to whether diabetes patients are cognitively impaired, the remainder of this section relies on the findings of reviews (e.g. [9]) and systematic reviews (e.g. [10]) of longitudinal studies in demystifying the relationship between diabetes and cognition.

In one of the first prospective studies of cognitive decline in diabetes [11], the investigators examined an all-female North American sample of women as part of a wider study on osteoporotic fractures. Using a modified Mini-Mental State Examination (MMSE; [12], measuring dementia), Digit Symbol Substitution (DSS; [13] a measure of psychomotor speed) and Trail Making B (TMB; [14]) measuring sustained visual attention and mental shift, it was reported that women with diabetes were twice more likely than their diabetes-free counterparts to show major cognitive decline.

A year later, Fontbonne *et al.* [15] reported from a French sample as part of the Epidemiology of Vascular Aging Study. Having classified the study participants in terms of glycaemic profile at baseline [normal fasting blood glucose, impaired (6.1–6.9 mmol l^{-1}) fasting glucose and diabetes], they were followed up for 4 years and then assessed for a sizeable battery of cognitive tests. These tests included the TMB and DSS, as well as measures of mental flexibility and auditory attention (Paced Auditory Serial Addition Test, PASAT; [16]), psychomotor speed (Finger Tapping Test; [17]), verbal memory (Auditory Verbal Learning Test, AVLT; [18]), visual memory (Benton Visual Retention Test, BVRT; [19]) and facial recognition (Facial Recognition Test, FRT; [20]). The authors reported a greater than twofold rate of cognitive impairment in people with diabetes, having controlled for confounding factors such as age, education and gender.

In a similar set-up, Kanaya *et al.* [21] reported 4-year follow-up data from a subset of participants in the Rancho Bernardo Study, a prospective trial which had been running in California since 1972. Both men and women (n = 999) were classified in terms of glycaemic status (normal, impaired glucose tolerance and diabetes) and assessed on three cognitive tests, namely the MMSE, TMB and a verbal fluency test assessing semantic memory (VF). The authors reported no age-adjusted differences in baseline cognitive function scores as a function of glycaemic group. Four years later, however, the women with diabetes had a fourfold increased risk of major cognitive decline, as evidenced in impaired verbal fluency test scores.

At about the same time, a study was conducted to assess the risk of cognitive dysfunction and development of AD in a prospective study of aging and AD in 824 older (age >55 years) Catholic nuns, priests and brothers (this was a subsample of the Religious Orders Prospective Study) [22]. The participants were followed-up for approximately 5.5 years, and had their cognitive performance assessed by a robust collection of global and specific tests. These included the MMSE, DSS, Logical Memory A (assessing ability to remember logical sequences [13]), items from the National Adult Reading Test (NART; a measure of pre-morbid intelligence and verbal fluency [23]), Digits Forward and Backward (assessing working memory and mental control [13]), items from the Standard Progressive Matrices (assessing visuospatial ability [24]), and many others. In appropriately adjusted analyses, the authors reported that, not only did the diabetes group have lower cognitive function scores at baseline in most of the cognitive domains assessed, but that diabetes was also associated with a more rapid (by ca. 44%) rate of cognitive decline in perceptual speed and a 65% increase in the risk of developing AD.

The trials reviewed above represent a small subset of several studies evaluating the link between diabetes and cognitive dysfunction, and are indicative of the overall pattern of results reported in the majority of published studies in the field. The same results have been echoed in a systematic review of prospective studies aiming to evaluate the extent to which diabetes is associated with cognitive decline and dementia [10]. This systematic review concluded that, compared to diabetes-free individuals, people with diabetes have:

- a 1.5-fold greater risk of cognitive decline;

- a 1.6-fold greater risk of developing dementia; and

- a greater rate of decline in cognitive function.

Interestingly, the authors noted that their results had probably underestimated the deleterious effects of diabetes on cognitive function, and cited two reasons. First, the reviewed studies tended to exclude people who already had some form of cognitive impairment at baseline, and as such, selectively sampled 'healthier' individuals with a lower subsequent risk of cognitive decline. Second, most of the data that they reviewed failed to include information on people who died or were lost at follow-up; it is argued that success in being followed-up may in itself be a result of better cognitive function and, as such, discounting people who could not be followed-up may have simply masked the true rate of cognitive decline in people with diabetes.

So, how might diabetes be related to cognitive decline? In type 1 diabetes, the amount and extent of exposure to hypoglycaemia have been argued to be predictive of cognitive decline [25], although a meta-analysis examining the effects of type 1 diabetes on cognition failed to find evidence for this association [26].

In type 2 diabetes the picture is much more complicated; patients with the illness tend to be older and present with other comorbidities such as hypertension, atherosclerotic vascular disease, obesity and depression – which in themselves are independent risk factors for cognitive dysfunction. In addition, disease duration, glycaemic control, socioeconomic status, age, gender, microvascular complications, insulin resistance and the presence of ApoE $\varepsilon4$ allele, may all moderate the relationship between diabetes and cognitive dysfunction (for helpful and detailed reviews on these, the reader is referred to Refs [7, 27, 28]). It is likely that the aetiology is multifactorial in origin, with varying contributions from repeated hypoglycaemia, long-duration hyperglycaemia, amyloid deposition, insulin resistance, cerebrovascular disease, changes in the hypothalamo-pituitary axis and inflammatory disease.

Another important factor which may exacerbate the influence of diabetes on cognitive performance is blood pressure control. Data from both the Framingham study [29] and the OCTO-Twin Study from Sweden [30] have demonstrated that, in patients with type 2 diabetes, cognitive performance is worse in the presence of hypertension or an increase in blood pressure. The Framingham cohort included patients aged 55–89 years who, over a long duration, demonstrated poorer results in logical memory scores and word fluency after an

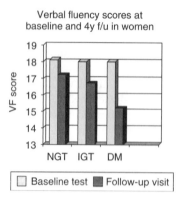

Verbal fluency scores at baseline and 4y f/u in women

- VF Scores adjusted for age, education, depression, lipids, blood pressure, HbA1c, and vascular disease

- Significant correlation with HbA1c and baseline (r= −0.08; p= 0.08) and follow-up (r = −0.10; p = 0.04) VF tests in women only

- NGT, normal glucose tolerance; IGT, impaired glucose tolerance; DM, diabetes mellitus

□ Baseline test ■ Follow-up visit

Figure 27.1 Association of verbal memory with glucose status: the rancho bernardo study. DM = diabetes mellitus; IGT = impaired glucose tolerance; NGT = normal glucose tolerance; VF = verbal fluency. Reproduced with permission from Ref. [21].

independent increase in blood pressure of 10 mmHg. In the OCTO-Twin Swedish population-based study, sequential MMSE scores over 8 years were significantly lower in the cohort of patients with both diabetes and hypertension than in the cohorts of either condition alone, or in those without either condition. This relationship between cognitive decline and with the presence of either diabetes and hypertension was also observed in the Atherosclerosis Risk in Communities (ARIC) study [31] in a 6-year follow-up of almost 11 000 individuals aged 47–70 years at the initial assessment.

The fact that people with diabetes are at an increased risk of cognitive dysfunction is now accepted unequivocally. However, the precise direction of this relationship – as well as its major constituent parts – remains unexplored and hence undetermined. Is it the case that diabetes causes cognitive decline independently of the moderating factors noted above? Could cognitive decline predispose to developing diabetes? Could it be that a combination of some (or all) of the comorbidities noted above may cause diabetes *per se*, cognitive decline *per se*, or perhaps both? Or, finally, is the presence of other comorbidities a moderator/mediator of a diabetes–cognitive dysfunction relationship? The jury is still out.

27.3 Cognitive dysfunction and glycaemic control

There is evidence that impaired glucose tolerance (IGT) is associated with poorer performance in certain cognitive function scores (lower Mini-Mental State examination, reduced verbal fluency) and in an increased risk of developing a dementing syndrome [32], although this has not been a consistent finding [33, 34]. In the Rancho Bernardo study, which included 999 Caucasian subjects aged 42–89 years with varying degrees of glucose tolerance who were followed over 4 years (see Figure 27.1), a significant correlation with HbA$_{1c}$ level and baseline and follow-up verbal fluency scores were observed, but in women only [21].

Various studies have demonstrated a relationship between measures of glycaemia and performance in cognitive assessment. The Stanford (USA) Studies in patients with type 2 diabetes showed that cognitive deficits involving verbal learning and complex perceptual-motor domains were worse in those with poorer glycaemic control, and that treatment with a sulphonylurea for 7 months led to significant improvements in metabolic control and tests of learning and memory [35, 36]. In another study, diabetic patients aged ≥70 years presenting to a geriatric diabetes clinic were screened for cognitive dysfunction with the MMSE and a clock-drawing test (CDT) [37]. The CDT scores were inversely correlated with HbA$_{1c}$ levels, which suggested that cognitive dysfunction was associated with poor glycaemic control (r = −0.38, p < 0.004).

The relationship between postprandial hyperglycaemia (PPG) and cognitive performance was recently studied in two groups of older patients with diabetes who were treated with either rapaglinide or glibenclamide [38]. The coefficient of variation of PPG was found to be associated with MMSE scores (r = −0.3410; p < 0.001) and a composite score of executive and attention functioning (r = −0.3744; p <

0.001) after adjusting for multiple confounders. The results suggested that a tighter control of PPG might influence the degree of cognitive decline in older patients with diabetes.

In a study of 1983 postmenopausal women (mean age 67 years) the association between HbA_{1C} level and risk of developing cognitive impairment was determined [39]. Mild cognitive impairment (MCI) or dementia was seen subsequently to develop over a 4-year period. For each 1% increase in HbA_{1C} level the women showed a greater age-adjusted likelihood of developing MCI (OR = 1.50; 95% CI: 1.14–1.97) and of developing dementia (OR = 1.40; 95% CI: 1.08–1.83). For those in whom the HbA_{1C} level was $\geq 7\%$, the age-adjusted risk for developing MCI was increased almost fourfold (OR = 3.70; 95% CI: 1.51–9.09) and for developing dementia was increased almost threefold (OR = 2.86; 95% CI: 1.17–6.98). These results clearly suggest that, in older patients with IGT or diabetes, the levels of glycaemia and cognitive status are linked.

27.4 The importance of detecting cognitive dysfunction

Several benefits may be acquired from the early recognition of cognitive impairment in older people with diabetes (see Table 27.2), and this places emphasis on the importance of tests of cognition as part of the functional assessment of older patients. Depending on its severity, cognitive dysfunction in older diabetic subjects may have considerable implications which include increased hospitalization, less ability for self-care, less likelihood of specialist follow-up, and an increased risk of institutionalization [40].

Table 27.2 Benefits of early recognition of cognitive dysfunction in diabetes.

- Prompts the clinician to consider the presence of cerebrovascular disease and to review other vascular risk factors.

- May be an early indicator of Alzheimer's disease and provides early access to medication.

- Allows patients and families to benefit early with social and financial planning and access to information about support groups and counselling.

- Creates opportunities to consider interventions for diabetes-related cognitive impairment: optimizing glucose control; controlling blood pressure and lipids.

Impaired cognitive function may result in poorer adherence to treatment, worsen glycaemic control due to erratic taking of diet and medication, and increase the risk of hypoglycaemia if the patient forgets that he or she has taken the hypoglycaemic medication and repeats the dose.

27.4.1 Methods of detection

Cognitive dysfunction has been traditionally assessed through cognitive tests, using many different procedures ranging from single global estimates of cognitive functioning (e.g. the MMSE) to substantial batteries of neuropsychological assessments spanning the major cognitive domains of language, perception, attention, memory, visuoconstruction ability, speed of information processing and executive (complex) functioning [20]. Some of these domains have been less well examined than others, and some tests – such as the MMSE and DSS – appear to have been used extensively when comparing people with diabetes with healthy controls. Whilst it is beyond the purpose of this chapter to describe the myriad of tests currently available to assess cognitive performance in older adults, the reader is referred to Lezak's [20] Neuropsychological Assessment for a compendium of hundreds of such tests.

What is of interest here is a distinction that needs to be drawn in terms of 'why' health care professionals might wish to cognitively assess people with diabetes. Until now, only those studies which assess cognitive function by comparing the performance of people *with* diabetes to that of diabetes-free controls have been considered. However, by adopting a case-control method of assessment, conclusions can be drawn regarding the extent to which diabetes patients are in some way impaired in the respective test domain, by comparing mean numerical scores in the diabetes sample with those in controls. In the absence of any established test 'norms', such a process allows the assessment of cognitive performance in order to compare functioning *between* a diabetes group and an appropriately matched control sample. So the answer to 'why assess' here is to establish cross-group differences.

Informative though such comparisons may be, they are not particularly useful in a clinical setting, where it is impractical to obtain appropriate control groups or indeed standardized norms for batteries of cognitive tests. Here, clinicians might be assessing cognition to determine whether their patient is currently cognitively compromised but, given the test setting, will not have access to a control group. In such cases, the 'why' behind the cognitive assessment is to establish whether further testing, referral or increased future cognitive monitoring might be necessary. In these cases, it can be argued that a significant proportion of cognitive tests which discuss the literature on diabetes and cognitive functioning renders itself beyond use, as such tests rely on comparing the patient's performance with that of others.

There are two notable exceptions to this general observation – the MMSE and the CDT. The MMSE, as the most widely used dementia screening, takes only 5–10 min to administer, and consists of questions relating to attention, orientation, memory, calculation and language. It has been criticised as being heavily reliant on language (and as such may not be suitable for non-English speakers), but it is available in different languages. Typical tasks on the MMSE involve patients being asked to recall the year, month, date, day and time, and to spell the word 'world' backwards. They are also asked to name three objects that are in the examination room and, a few minutes later, unexpectedly to recall them. Although the MMSE is a reliable indicator of moderate to severe cognitive impairment, it is not sensitive enough to detect MCI. This may not necessarily be an issue, however, as MCI is not thought to be related to diabetes self-care activities in any significant way [41]. The MMSE is scored out of 30, with higher scores being indicative of better cognitive performance. Specifically, scores of 27–30 are regarded normal, whiles scores <26 indicate various degrees of cognitive impairment.

The CDT is another popular measure that is quick and easy to administer. Participants are given a circle (no bigger than 4–10 cm in diameter) and are told that it represents a clock face. They are then instructed to put in the numbers so that the circle now looks like a clock and, when they have done so, to 'set the time' to 10 minutes past 11. The test assesses executive function and, in particular, the patient's ability to plan ahead, their visuospatial ability, ability to engage in abstract reasoning and, of course, their concentration. The CDT can be scored in several ways ranging in amount of detail and precision. An extensive discussion on CDT administration and scoring is provided by Shulman *et al.* [42]. Of the several scoring methods proposed, four-point [43] or five-point [44] systems are probably the quickest and easiest. For example, when using a five-point scoring system, the patient's drawing is assessed from being perfect (score 5), to showing inaccurate representation of 10 past 11 when the overall visuospatial organisation is good (score 3),

down to 0 for an inability to make any reasonable representation of a clock (for details, see Ref. [44]).

Nishiwaki *et al.* [45] have shown that, in isolation, the MMSE might not detect MCI, whilst the CDT might produce a large number of false positives. When used together, however, these tests can be reliable predictors of moderate to severe cognitive decline. Given that their administration and scoring make minimal demands in terms of time and resources, it has been argued [46] that, from a clinical point of view, they are ideal cognitive functioning screening tests for older people with diabetes.

27.4.2 Influence on diabetes self-care

Although many investigations have been conducted on ways to improve the patient's diabetes self-care and on their cognitive function, the relationship between the two states remains under-researched. The question here is whether cognitive functioning in diabetes patients predicts their efforts to self-manage the illness, with the implication that perhaps a poorer cognitive performance may be related to poorer self-management skills.

In one of the few studies in this area, [40] an investigation was conducted as to whether cognitive impairment was associated with changes in self-care behaviour and the use of health and social services in a community-based case control study of older patients with diabetes. Cognitive function was assessed using the MMSE and CDT, while self-care was assessed in two ways: (i) by counting the number of patients that were solely responsible for self-medication and blood glucose (BG) monitoring; and (ii) by monitoring their attendance at a specialist diabetes clinic. Performance on the CDT showed that respectively, 65% and 72% of diabetes patients placed the numbers and hands correctly, compared to 76% and 84% of controls. Age was found to interact with cognitive dysfunction and self-management, in that older diabetes patients were found to have worse cognitive test performance, a higher dependency and poorer diabetes self-management.

In another study [41], 51 people with type 2 diabetes completed a battery of cognitive tests and the Summary of Diabetes Self-Care Activities questionnaire [47]; however, only a few associations between cognitive functioning and self-management were observed. This lack of association might have been due to the limited statistical power of the study for detecting relationships, or to the absence of any significant practical association between self-reported self-care and specific cognitive skills. One of the few significant associations that were found was the inverse relationship between self-reported memory problems (as assessed by the Subjective Memory Questionnaire [48]) and the number of diabetes problem-solving strategies (as assessed by Toobert and Glasgow's Diabetes Problem-Solving Interview), although self-reported memory complaints were not a reliable indicator of objective cognitive function. A better dietary self-management was predicted by a better general (Modified Wisconsin Card Sorting Test [49]) and diabetes-specific abstract reasoning. Better exercise self-management was predicted by better scores on a test of mental flexibility, the Serial Subtractions of 7s [20], and generating more diabetes-specific problem-solving strategies was predicted by fewer subjective memory problems. The researchers assessed self-reported self-care through the Summary of Diabetes Self Care Activities (SDSCA [47]). In a later study, however, Asimakopoulou and Hampson [50] showed that the SDSCA may be prone to recall biases in people with diabetes and, as such, it is suggested that self-reported self-care as assessed by instruments such as the SDSCA should be confirmed by clinical interview and opinion.

Other groups have examined self-care on the basis of medication adherence and glycaemic control. For example, Rosen et al. [51] assessed the association between cognitive performance and adherence to oral hypoglycaemic medication, HbA$_{1c}$ level and missed appointments. Cognitive function was assessed among other measures with the MMSE, TMB and the Stroop test (this provides a measure of attention and mental flexibility, with patients being asked to read out the ink colour of words spelling out incongruent colour words [20]). Adherence to metformin was measured using pill bottle caps which contained a microprocessor that recorded the date and times of bottle openings; the caps were placed on the patients' prescribed antihyperglycaemic medication. Age was the best predictor of medication adherence, and accounted for just under 10% of the variance in this behaviour. Medication adherence was also predicted by performance on the Stroop word test and with TMB completion time, where a worse cognitive performance predicted poorer medication taking, although the amount of variance explained was only small (<10%). Interestingly, neuropsychological performance was not associated with HbA$_{1c}$ levels, but a poor MMSE score predicted missed appointments. These results suggested that, although

cognitive performance may play a role in medication taking, it fails to explain a substantial amount of patients' variability in this behaviour.

More recently, Trimble et al. [52] assessed the ability of the CDT to predict problematic insulin administration skills in older adults with diabetes. A group of 30 patients who had not used insulin before were taught to self-administer a sham insulin injection with an insulin pen, using a standardized protocol. The injections were continued for 7 days, after which self-administration was re-tested. An abnormal CDT was significantly associated with more problems in learning to perform the sham injections (measured as those who were unable to correctly complete all steps of the protocol, or those who omitted all or part of a step), although a small number of patients with a normal CDT also demonstrated major problems. The results were in line with those of other studies, which noted the frequency of abnormal CDTs in older patients [40], and the frequency of errors in older people self-administering insulin [53]; the suggested was made that "... the CDT is a valuable predictor of potential problems with insulin administration skills in elderly patients".

Finally, Munshi et al. [54] assessed the relationship between global cognitive function as measured by the MMSE, CDT and Clock in Box (CIB [55]) tests, as well as glycaemic control (measured by HbA$_{1C}$) in older adults with diabetes. Some 34% of patients had low scores on the CIB, and 38% had low scores on the CDT. Both, the CIB and CDT were superior at identifying patients with cognitive dysfunction, compared to the MMSE. The CIB test was more sensitive in predicting poor glycaemic control than the CDT; however, both clock tests were inversely correlated with HbA$_{1C}$ levels, which suggested that cognitive function might play a role in the control of diabetes.

It appears that the few studies which have assessed the relationship between diabetes self-management and cognition have argued for a relationship between cognitive dysfunction and impaired self-care, in patients with diabetes. The amount of variance in self-care behaviours that cognitive tests seem to predict seems rather low, however, and additional patient-centred research is required in order to elucidate the relationship between cognitive dysfunction and diabetes self-management behaviours. This is particular true with regards to the extent to which modest differences in cognitive testing might predict practical diabetes self-care skills.

27.5   The importance of excluding depression

The presence of a depressive illness may influence the outcome of any cognitive assessment in older patients with diabetes. Cognitive performance scores are likely to be diminished and create difficulties of interpretation for the clinician. Since it can be a chronic disorder with frequent relapse, patients often have difficulty in maintaining a stable level of glycaemia, and the consequent burden on caregivers can be increased substantially.

Diabetes appears to be significantly associated with depression, independent of age, gender or the presence of chronic disease [56], while the presence of diabetes appears to double the odds of developing depression [57]. In one study, the finding of depression had important implications for a group of in-patients as it was the single most important indicator of subsequent death [58]. Failure to recognize depression can be serious, since it is a long-term, life-threatening, disabling illness and can have a significant impact on the patient's quality of life [59]. Depression may be associated with worsening diabetic control and decreased treatment compliance [60].

It is important that, at the initial assessment, patients undergo a thorough history and examination and in particular are asked about any symptoms of depression. They should then undergo a mood screening test such as the four-item Geriatric Depression Score [61] or even shorter instruments. If a significant mood disorder is detected, the opportunity presents itself to offer appropriate treatment, or a referral to other specialist services.

27.6   Further investigations

The decision to investigate patients with diabetes who have observed deficits in cognition needs to be taken on the basis of history, examination, impact (if any) of deficits or behaviour, personality, normal social and professional functioning, and ability for diabetes self-care management.

Whilst a full neuropsychological battery of tests will prove helpful, it is not essential in everyday clinical practice. Special techniques such as visual and somatosensory evoked potentials are too sophisticated in routine care, as is electroencephalography. Techniques such as magnetic resonance imaging (MRI), functional MRI, single photon emission computed tomography and offer exciting opportunities to equate cognitive performance with definitive evidence of structural and physiological functioning [28, 32].

A scheme for the routine screening and detection of cognitive dysfunction is shown in Figure 27.2, and this should serve as a basis for other centres to develop this approach.

27.7   Conclusions

In view of the high prevalence of both diabetes and dementing syndromes in aged subjects, every physician/clinician involved in providing diabetes care to

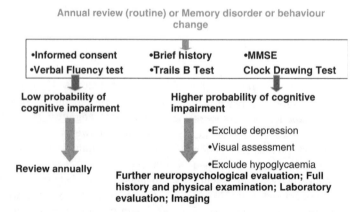

Figure 27.2   Scheme for the detection of cognitive dysfunction in type 2 diabetes mellitus.

this group should be familiar with this association and be skilled in the initial assessment of cognitive performance. Although the pathogenesis of cognitive dysfunction remains unclear, it can be regarded as a complication of long-duration diabetes and is likely to have an important vascular basis.

Older subjects may be particularly prone in view of other comorbidities, which makes it essential that a cognitive assessment should form part of an initial assessment of a newly diagnosed patient with diabetes, and also part of any routine, annual review.

In this respect, a familiarity with common screening methods of cognitive function would be of great help – as would the recognition that these individuals require greater specialist care, not less! [62].

References

1. Miles, W.R. and Root, H.F. 1922. Psychologic tests applied to diabetic patients. *Archives of Internal Medicine*, 30, 767–77.

2. Sinclair AJ 2004. European Diabetes Working Party for Older People 2001–2004. Clinical Guidelines for Type 2 Diabetes Mellitus. Available on: www.eugms.org.

3. Strachan, M.W., Price, J.F. and Frier, B.M. (2008) Diabetes, cognitive impairment, and dementia. *Br Med J* 336 (7634), 6.

4. Biessels GJ, Staekenborg S, Brunner E, Brayne C and Scheltens P. (2006) Risk of dementia in diabetes – a systematic review. *Lancet Neurology*, 5: 64–74.

5. Cosway, R., Strachan, M.W. *et al.* (2001) Cognitive function and information processing in type 2 diabetes. *Diabet Med* 18 (10): 803–10.

6. Asimakopoulou, K.G., S.E. Hampson, *et al.* (2002) Neuropsychological functioning in older people with type 2 diabetes: the effect of controlling for confounding factors. *Diabet Med* 19 (4): 311–16.

7. van den Berg, E., R.P. Kessels, *et al.* (2007) Type 2 diabetes, cognitive function and dementia: vascular and metabolic determinants. *Timely Top Med Cardiovasc Dis* 11: E7.

8. Strachan, M.W., I.J. Deary, *et al.* (1997) Is type II diabetes associated with an increased risk of cognitive dysfunction? A critical review of published studies. *Diabetes Care* 20 (3): 438–45.

9. Allen, K.V., B.M. Frier, *et al.* (2004) The relationship between type 2 diabetes and cognitive dysfunction: longitudinal studies and their methodological limitations. *European Journal of Pharmacology* 490 (1-3): 169–75.

10. Cukierman, T., H.C. Gerstein, *et al.* (2005) Cognitive decline and dementia in diabetes–systematic overview of prospective observational studies. *Diabetologia* 48 (12): 2460–9.

11. Gregg, E.W., Langlois, J.A., Beckels, G.L.A., Engelgau, M.M., Williamson, D.F., Narayan, K.M.V. and Leveille, S.G. (2000) Is diabetes associated with cognitive impairment and cognitive decline among older women? Study of Osteoporotic Fractures Research Group. *Archives of Internal Medicine* 160 (2): 174.

12. Folstein MF, Folstein, SE and McHugh PR (1975) Mini-Mental State: A practical method for grading the state of patients for the clinician. *Journal of Psychiatric Research*, 12: 189–98.

13. Weschler, D. (1997) *Weschler Adult Intelligence Scale - III.* The Psychological Corporation, San Antonio, Texas.

14. Reitan, R.M. and Wolfson, D. (1993) *The Halstead-Reitan neuropsychological test battery: Theory and clinical interpretation.* 2nd edition. Neuropsychology Press, South Tucson, AZ.

15. Fontbonne, A., Ducimetière, P., Berr, C. and Alperovitch, A. (2001) Changes in cognitive abilities over a 4-year period are unfavorably affected in elderly diabetic subjects: results of the Epidemiology of Vascular Aging Study. *Diabetes Care* 24 (2): 366.

16. Gronwall, D.M.A. (1977) Paced auditory serial-addition task: A measure of recovery from concussion. *Perceptual and Motor Skills* 44, 367–73.

17. Mitrushina, M.N., Boone, K.B. and D'Elia, L.F. (1999) *Handbook of Normative Data for Neuropsychological Assessment.* Oxford University Press, New York.

18. Spreen, O. and Strauss, E. (1991) *A compendium of neuropsychological tests: Administration, norms and commentary.* Oxford University Press, New York.

19. Benton AL. (1963) *The Revised Visual Retention Test*, 3rd edition. The Psychological Corporation, New York, pp. 1–74.

20. Lezak, M.D. (1995) *Neuropsychological Assessment.* Oxford University Press, New York.

21. Kanaya AM, Barrett-Connor E, Gildengorin G and Yaffe K (2004) Change in cognitive function by glucose tolerance status in older adults: a 4-year prospective study of the Rancho Bernardo study cohort. *Arch Intern Med* 164, 1060–5.

22. Arvanitakis, Z., R.S. Wilson, *et al.* (2004) Diabetes mellitus and risk of Alzheimer disease and decline in cognitive function. *Arch Neurol* 61 (5): 661–6.

23. Nelson, H.E. and Willison, J. (1991) *National Adult Reading Test Manual.* 2nd edition. NFER-Nelson, Windsor.

24. J. Raven, J.C. Raven and J.H. Court (1998) *Manual for Raven's progressive matrices and vocabulary scales. Section 1: General overview.* Oxford Psychologists Press, Oxford.

25. Deary, I.J. and Frier, B.M. (1996) Severe hypoglycaemia and cognitive impairment in diabetes. *Br Med J*, 313 (7060): 767–8.

26. Brands, A.M., G.J. Biessels, *et al.* (2005) The effects of type 1 diabetes on cognitive performance: a meta-analysis. *Diabetes Care* 28(3): 726–35.

27. Ryan, C.M. (2006) Diabetes and brain damage: more (or less) than meets the eye? *Diabetologia* 49 (10): 2229–33.

28. Kodl CT and Seaquist ER. (2008) Cognitive dysfunction and diabetes mellitus. *Endocrine Reviews* 29 (4): 494–511.

29. Elias PK, Elias MF, D'Agostino RB, Cupples LA, Wilson PW, Silbershatz H and Wolf PA. (1997) NIDDM and blood pressure as risk factors for poor cognitive performance: The Framingham Study. *Diabetes Care* 20: 1388–95.

30. Hassing LB, Hofer SM, Nilsson SE, Berg S, Pedersen NL, McClearn G and Johansson B. (2004) Comorbid type 2 diabetes mellitus and hypertension exacerbates cognitive decline: evidence from a longitudinal study. *Age Ageing*, 33 (4), 355–61.

31. Knopman D, Boland LL, Mosley T, Howard G, Liao D, Szklo M, McGovern P, Folsom AR for the Atherosclerosis Risk in Communities (ARIC) Study Investigators. (2001) Cardiovascular risk factors and cognitive decline in middle-aged adults. *Neurology*, 56 (1), 42–8.

32. Kodl, C.T. and E.R. Seaquist (2008) Cognitive dysfunction and diabetes mellitus. *Endocrine Reviews* 29 (4), 494–511.

33. Scott RD, Kritz-Silverstein D, Barrett-Commor E and Wiederholt WC (1998) The association of non-insulin-dependent diabetes mellitus and cognitive function in an older cohort. *J Am Geriatr Soc* 46, 1217–22.

34. Lindeman RD, Romero LJ, LaRue A, Yau CL, Schade DS, Koehler KM, Baumgartner RN and Garry PJ. (2001) A biethnic community survey of cognition in participants with type 2 diabetes, impaired glucose tolerance, and normal glucose tolerance: the New Mexico Elder Health Survey. *Diabetes Care* 24, 1567–72.

35. Reaven GM, Thompson LW, Nahum D and Haskins E. (1990) Relationship between hyperglycaemia and cognitive function in older NIDDM patients. *Diabetes Care* 13, 16–21.

36. Gradman TJ, Laws A, Thompson LW and Reaven GM. (1993) Verbal learning and/or memory improves with glycemic control in older subjects with non-insulin-dependent diabetes mellitus. *J Am Geriatr Soc*, 41 (12): 1305–12.

37. Munshi M, Grande L, Hayes M, Ayres D, Suhl E, Capelson R, Lins S, Milberg W and Weinger K. (2006) Cognitive dysfunction is associated with poor diabetes control in older adults. *Diabetes Care* 29, 1794–9.

38. Abbatecola AM, Rizzo MR, Barbieri M, Grella R, Arciello A, Laieta MT, Acampora R, Passariello N, Cacciapuoti F and Paolisso G. (2006) Postprandial plasma glucose excursion s and cognitive functioning in aged type 2 diabetics. *Neurology* 67: 235–40.

39. Yaffe K, Blackwell T, Whitmer RA, Krueger K and Barrett-Connor E. (2006) Glycosylated haemoglobin level and development of mild cognitive impairment or dementia in older women. *J Nutr Health Aging* 10, 293–5.

40. Sinclair AJ, Girling AJ and Bayer AJ. (2000) Cognitive dysfunction in older subjects with diabetes mellitus: impact on diabetes self-management and use of care services. All Wales Research into Elderly (AWARE) Study. *Diabetes Res Clin Pract* 50 (3): 203–12.

41. Asimakopoulou, K. and Hampson, S.E. (2002) Cognitive functioning and self-management in older people with diabetes. *Diabetes Spectrum* 15(2): 116.

42. Shulman, K.I. (2000). Clock drawing: Is it the ideal cognitive screening test?, *International Journal of Geriatric Psychiatry* 15: 548–61.

43. Death, J., Douglas, A. and Kenny, R.A. (1993) Comparison of clock drawing with Mini Mental State Examination as a screening test in elderly acute hospital admissions. *Postgraduate Medical Journal* 69: 696–700.

44. Shulman K.I., Gold, D.P., Cohen, C.A. and Zucchero, C.A. (1993) Clock drawing and dementia in the community: A longitudinal study. *International Journal of Geriatric Psychiatry* 8: 487–96.

45. Nishiwaki, Y., Breeze, E., Smeeth, L., Bulpitt, C.J., Peters, R. and Fletcher, AE. (2004) Validity of the Clock-Drawing test as a screening tool for cognitive impairment in the elderly. *American Journal of Epidemiology* 160 (8): 797–807.

46. Asimakopoulou K, Tomlin A and Sinclair A (2008) Cognitive function and self-care in type 2 diabetes. *Diabetes and Primary Care* 10 (2): 70–82.

47. Toobert, D.J. and Glasgow, R.E. (1994) Assessing diabetes self-management: the Summary of Diabetes Self-Care Activities questionnaire. In: C. Bradley (ed.), *Handbook of Psychology and Diabetes*. Harwood Academic, Chur, Switzerland.

48. Bennett-Levy J and Powell GE (1980) The subjective memory questionnaire (SMQ). An investigation into the self-reporting of 'real-life' memory skills. *Br J Social and Clinical Psychology*, 19, 177–88.

49. Hart RP, Kwentus JA, Wade JB and Taylor JR. (1988) Modified Wisconsin Sorting Test in elderly normal, depressed and demented patients. *Clin Neuropsychologist* 2: 49–56.

50. Asimakopoulou, K. and Hampson, S.E. (2005) Biases in self reports of self care in type 2 diabetes. *Psychology Health and Medicine* 11, 305–15.

51. Rosen, M.I., Beavais, J.E., Rigsby, M.O., *et al.* (2003) Neuropsychological correlates of suboptimal adherence to metformin. *Journal of Behavioral Medicine* 26 (4): 349–60.

52. Trimble, L.A., Sundberg, S., Markham, L., Janicijevic, S., Beattie, B.L. and Meneilly, G.S. (2005) Value of the Clock Drawing Test to predict problems with insulin skills in older adults. *Canadian Journal of Diabetes* 29 (2): 102–4.

53. Coscelli, C., Calabrese, G., Fedele, D., Pisu, E., Calderini, C., Bistoni, S., Lapolla, A., Mauri, M.G., Rossi, A. and Zappella, A. (1992) Use of premixed insulin among the elderly. Reduction of errors in patient preparation of mixtures. *Diabetes Care* 15 (11): 1628–30.

54. Munshi, M., Capelson, R., Grande, L., *et al.* (2006) Cognitive dysfunction is associated with poor diabetes control in older adults. *Diabetes Care* 29 (8): 1794–9.

55. Grande, L., Milberg, W., Rodolph, J., Gaziano, M. and McGlinchey, R. (2005) A timely screening for executive functions and memory. *J Int Neuropsychol Soc*, 11 (Suppl. 1), 9–10.

56. Amato L, Paolisso G, Cacciatore F, Ferrara N, Canonico S, Rengo F and Varricchio M. (1996) Non-insulin-dependent diabetes mellitus is associated with a greater prevalence of depression in the elderly. The Osservatorio Geriatrico of Campania Region Group. *Diabetes Metab* 22 (5): 314–18.

57. Anderson RJ, Freedland KE, Clouse RE and Lustman PJ. (2001) The prevalence of comorbid depression in adults with diabetes: a meta-analysis. *Diabetes Care* 24 (6): 1069–78.

58. Rosenthal MJ, Fajardo M, Gilmore S, Morley JE and Naliboff BD. (1998) Hospitalization and mortality of diabetes in older adults. A 3-year prospective study. *Diabetes Care* 21 (2): 231–5.

59. Egede LE, Zheng D and Simpson K. (2002) Comorbid depression is associated with increased health care use and expenditures in individuals with diabetes. *Diabetes Care* 25 (3): 464–70.

60. Lustman PJ, Anderson RJ, Freedland KE, de Groot M, Carney RM and Clouse RE. (2000) Depression and poor glycemic control: a meta-analytic review of the literature. *Diabetes Care* 23 (7): 934–42.

61. Burke WJ, Roccaforte WH and Wengel SP. (1991) The short form of the Geriatric Depression Scale: a comparison with the 30-item form. *J Geriatr Psychiatry Neurol* 4 (3): 173–8.

62. Sinclair AJ and Woodhouse K (1994) Meeting the challenge of diabetes in the aged. *J Roy Soc Med* 87 (10): 607.

Depression and Diabetes in Older Adults

Arie Nouwen and Jan R. Oyebode

School of Psychology, University of Birmingham, Birmingham, UK

Key Messages

- Depression in diabetes is a serious comorbidity associated with poor outcome and high health care expenditure.
- Clinicians should be alert to signs of depression in all older people with diabetes, but especially those with known risk factors.
- Depression in diabetes can be treated successfully with pharmacotherapy, and/or psychological therapy, but blood glucose levels should be monitored closely, especially with pharmacotherapy.

28.1 Defining depression

Feeling 'depressed' or 'low' does not necessarily indicate the existence of a depressive disorder. Depressive symptoms and feelings of unhappiness often occur as a transient mood state experienced by almost all individuals at some time in their life. These symptoms and feelings may be due to disappointments, or to difficulty in adapting to life events such as bereavement or disability. However, when depressive symptoms extend across affect, cognition, psychomotor activity and neurovegetative domains (i.e. appetite, ability to sleep and sex drive), and interfere with normal functioning, they are considered pathological and an individual with such a presentation may receive a diagnosis of depression.

There is currently no objective test to confirm the existence of a depressive disorder, and any diagnosis is based on clusters of signs and symptoms. The International Classification of Diseases (ICD-10) [1] and the Diagnostic and Statistical Manual of Mental Disorders-IV (DSM-IV) [2] detail several types of depression based on symptom duration, the number of symptoms and the degree of interference with normal activities. The essential features of (uni-polar) depression are a persistent lowering of mood, a loss of ability to enjoy usual activities and reduced energy levels (see Table 28.1).

While to some degree arbitrary, distinctions are made between *Depressive Episodes/Major Depressive Disorder* and *Persistent Affective Disorders/Dysthymia*. The former is characterized by a loss of pleasure in almost any activity for at least a 2-week period, while dysthymia is a milder but more chronic form of depression, with a depressed mood occurring for most of the day on more days than not, for at least two years. Two other diagnostic categories included in ICD-10 that may have relevance for people with diabetes are *Mild* or *Moderate Depressive Episodes* (with mild being equivalent to *Minor Depressive Disorder* in DSM-IV), which involve symptoms identical to severe depressive episodes but with fewer symptoms and less impairment, and *Adjustment*

Diabetes in Old Age. Third Edition. Edited by Alan J. Sinclair
© 2009 John Wiley & Sons, Ltd

Table 28.1   Criteria for a Major Depressive Episode* according to the DSM-IV-R and ICD-10.

DSM-IV-R	ICD-10
Clinical significance Symptoms represent a change from previous functioning and cause clinically significant distress or impairment in social, occupational, or other important areas of functioning	Symptoms cause distress or impairment of functioning
Duration of symptoms Most of the day, nearly every day for at least 2 weeks	Most of the day, almost every day, for at least 2 weeks, largely unaffected by circumstances
Severity Five or more symptoms of which at least one a 'key' symptom Mild: five or six symptoms with mild disability or capacity to function normally albeit with substantial effort Severe: presence of most symptoms and clear-cut and observable disability Moderate: in between mild and severe	Mild: Four symptoms of which at least two are key symptoms; probably able to continue most activities with increased effort Moderate: Six symptoms of which at least two are key symptoms; great difficulty in continuing with ordinary activities Severe: eight symptoms including all three key symptoms; marked distress and impairment
Key symptoms (a) Depressed mood most of the day (b) Diminished interest or pleasure in all or almost all activities	(a) Depressed mood most of the day (b) Loss of interest or pleasure in activities that are normally pleasurable (c) Decreased energy or increased fatiguability
Associated symptoms 1. Significant weight loss or gain or decrease or increase in appetite unrelated to dieting 2. Insomnia or hypersomnia 3. Psychomotor agitation or retardation nearly every day (observable by others) 4. Fatigue or loss of energy 5. Feelings of worthlessness or excessive or inappropriate guilt 6. Diminished ability to think or concentrate, or indecisiveness 7. Recurrent thoughts of death, recurrent suicidal ideation without a specific plan, or a suicide attempt or a specific plan for committing suicide	 1. Change in appetite (decrease or increase) with corresponding weight change 2. Sleep disturbance 3. Change in psychomotor activity, with agitation or retardation 4. Unreasonable feelings of self-reproach and inappropriate guilt 5. Diminished ability to think or concentrate, such as indecisiveness or vacillation 6. Recurrent thoughts of death or suicide, or any suicidal behaviour 7. Loss of confidence or self-esteem

*Note: For a DSM-IV-R diagnosis of Minor Depressive Disorder, a total of at least two but less than five symptoms is required.

Disorders (ICD-10), which consist of states of subjective distress and emotional upset, which interfere with social functioning, and arise in the period of adaptation to a significant life change or as a consequence of a stressful life event (including the presence or possibility of serious physical illness).

Adjustment Disorders in the WHO framework are similar to the DSM-IV diagnosis of *Mood Disorder Due to a General Medical Condition*, which consists of a prominent and persistent mood disturbance that is judged to be a direct effect of a general medical condition through a physiological mechanism. A key feature of the latter is the presence of a temporal relationship between the onset, exacerbation, or remission of the medical condition and the mood disturbance.

One condition that may cause mood symptoms is cerebrovascular disease (e.g. stroke), and this may have particular relevance for older adults with diabetes as they are susceptible to cerebrovascular disease [3–6].

28.2   Depression in older people

Although growing old is often accompanied by many new and often difficult challenges, depression is not a part of normal ageing [7, 8]. It is estimated that 1–3% of people aged >65 years suffer from major depression [9, 10]. These rates are relatively low compared with younger age groups [11], where approximately 15% of the general population is at risk of experiencing a (major) depressive episode [1, 2].

However, prevalence rates of severe depressive episodes/major depressive disorder (MDD) are higher amongst certain groups of older people, in particular, individuals with a comorbid medical illness, and those in residential [12] or nursing homes [13] and in people with a history of psychiatric illness [14] or previous depression [15].

Of relevance to working with diabetes, increased depression has also been found in older people with visual loss (36%) [16] and with cerebrovascular accident (CVA) or stroke [17]. Although these numbers concern individuals with a diagnosis of major depression, much larger numbers report experiencing clinically significant depressive symptoms that do not reach the threshold for a clinical diagnosis of severe depressive episode or MDD; typically reported patient proportions are 8–16% [10, 18], 16% [19] and 27% [20].

28.3   Epidemiology of depression in diabetes

28.3.1   General population

It is now commonly accepted that the prevalence of depression – that is, the total number of cases in a population at a given time – is increased in individuals with diabetes. In a systematic review/meta-analysis of 42 eligible studies [21], it was found that overall the odds of depression in patients with diabetes were double those of non-diabetic controls (OR = 2.0, 95% CI:

1.8–2.2). When diagnostic criteria are used (DSM-IV, ICD-10), the pooled point prevalence of depressive disorders has been estimated at about 10%. The pooled prevalence of depressive symptoms when self-report questionnaires are used is higher at 26%, which suggests that there are high levels of subthreshold, clinically significant psychological distress in diabetes populations. In a more recent systematic review and meta-analysis [22], a slightly lower odds ratio was found (OR = 1.59, 95% CI: 1.5–1.7). However, the studies included in these meta-analyses were based on cross-sectional data that precluded conclusions about cause and effect. The finding of an increase in the point prevalence of depression in diabetes has been reported not only from Western countries but also from various non-Western regions such as Pakistan [23], Iran [24] and Hong-Kong [25]. Although, the level of depression may vary from country to country, people with diabetes consistently have higher levels than the general population. However, the prevalence of depression in diabetes does not appear to be increased in comparison with other medical conditions such as heart disease and chronic obstructive pulmonary disease (COPD) [26, 27].

In addition to an increased prevalence, persistent or recurrent clinical and subclinical depression is present in a substantial number of adults with diabetes. In a sample of 245 patients with diabetes [28], depressive symptoms were assessed at the beginning and end of a comprehensive outpatient diabetes education programme, and at a 6-month follow-up. The rate of depression at follow-up was 10% for those without depressive symptoms at either of the earlier time points. However, 36% of the people who were depressed at one earlier time point, and 73% of those depressed at both earlier time points, reported depressive symptoms at follow-up. Likewise, Lustman *et al.* [29] found that the likelihood of symptomatic affective disorder was only 10% over a 5-year time period in a group of people with diabetes but without depression at time 1, whereas a recurrence or persistence of clinical depression occurred in 92% of cases with an average of 4.8 depressive episodes over a 5-year period.

28.3.2   Older population

A number of studies have specifically examined depression in elderly people with diabetes. For example, in one study [30] it was found that while depressive symptoms were not more prevalent in an elderly diabetic population, those who had diabetes-related complications were more depressed. Similar results were found in a study conducted in Hong-Kong [25]. This seems to suggest that, when the burden of living with diabetes is increased, so too is the level of depression. However, as these studies were cross-sectional in design it is impossible to determine whether depression increases the chance of developing diabetes-related complications, or whether diabetes-related complications lead to an increase in depression.

More recently, a number of longitudinal studies have examined the incidence (i.e. number of new cases in a population) of depression in type 2 diabetes, but the findings have been equivocal. Some studies identified an increased incidence of depression in older people with type 2 diabetes. For example, in a prospective longitudinal study in a well-functioning cohort of 70–79-year-old persons in the US [31], diabetes was found to be associated with a 30% increased risk of incident depressed mood (OR = 1.31; 95% CI: 1.07–1.61). An adjustment for diabetes-related comorbidities reduced this relationship (OR = 1.20, 95% CI: 0.97–1.48). The increased risk for developing depressive symptoms was mainly found in those with uncontrolled diabetes. Participants with a serum HbA_{1c} level >8.1% had the highest risk of developing recurrent depressive symptoms. Using a diagnosis of depression rather than self-reported depressive symptoms [32], a large community-based study in Spain found that elderly people with diabetes (age >55 years) had both a higher prevalence (OR = 1.47; 95% CI: 1.16–1.83) and incidence (OR = 1.40; 95% CI: 1.03–1.90) of depressive disorder than a non-diabetic control group. Controlling for potential confounders (demographics, cardiovascular risk factors, comorbid medical illness, cognitive functioning and disability) somewhat attenuated these results (prevalent depression: OR = 1.41, 95% CI: 1.08–1.83; incident depression: OR = 1.26, 95% CI: 0.90–1.77).

In contrast, no increase was found in the incidence of depressive symptoms in a Dutch cohort of people aged 55–85 years [33]. Although studying a slightly younger cohort (age range 50–89 years) in California, Palinkas et al. [34] also reported that diabetes did not result in a higher incidence of depressive symptoms.

None of the above studies excluded people with a history of depressive disorder. However, as people with a previous depressive episode are more likely to experience further episodes independently of diabetes [29], the results may have been different had the studies controlled for previous episodes.

One possible explanation for these divergent results is that, in the above-mentioned studies, no differentiation was made between early-onset (first episode <60 years) or late-onset (first episode >60 years) depression. A large body of research suggests that, while the phenomenology of early-onset and late-onset depression may be indistinguishable [35], late-onset depression is more likely to be associated with structural brain abnormalities [36] and psychosis [37], and less likely to be associated with a family history of depression [38]. This suggests different underlying aetiological processes in depression.

28.4 Depression in diabetes: Associated problems

28.4.1 Self-management

Clinical depression has been associated with poor diabetes self-care. Both clinical and subclinical depression were found to be associated with impaired adherence to diabetes medication [39, 40] and to anti-depressant medication [41]. This negative association was found even at mild levels of depression [42]. Adjustment for alcohol use, cognitive impairment, age and other medication use did not significantly alter this negative association. Others have shown that, in elderly samples, depression is associated with less-frequent self-monitoring of blood glucose [42] and dietary self-care activities [40, 42]. Interestingly, in the latter study it was found that while the consumption of fruit and vegetables and spacing of carbohydrates were affected, the consumption of high-fat foods was not increased. The results of a recent study conducted in Korea showed that depressed people with diabetes are also less likely to participate in diabetes education programmes [43].

28.4.2 Metabolic control

Both clinical and subclinical depression in diabetes have been associated with increased symptom reporting [44] and poorer metabolic control. In a meta-analytic review of 24 studies [45], it was found that depression was significantly associated with hyperglycaemia in both type 1 and type 2 diabetes. Larger effect sizes were found when diagnostic criteria rather than self-report questionnaires were used, suggesting that the relationship between depression and hyperglycaemia is stronger in patients with clinical rather than subclinical depression. However, the direction of this association remained unclear as the studies included were cross-sectional in nature and precluded the drawing of any cause-and-effect conclusions.

28.4.3 Diabetes complications

Depression has also been associated with increased risk of developing diabetes-related complications, especially cardiovascular complications [46, 47]. A significant association between depression and complication of diabetes, including diabetic retinopathy, nephropathy, neuropathy, macrovascular complications and sexual dysfunction, was reported in a meta-analysis of 27 studies [48]. Effect sizes ranged from small ($r = 0.17$ for retinopathy) to moderate ($r = 0.32$ for sexual dysfunction). More recently, in a population-based study of older people in Amsterdam [30], the rate of depressive disorder was found to be higher in diabetes patients with related complications than in those without complications.

28.4.4 Health care expenditure

It is not surprising that depression in people with diabetes increases health care expenditure. For example, in a US study it was found that among individuals with diabetes, the total health care expenditure for individuals diagnosed with depression was 4.5-fold higher than that for individuals without depression [49].

28.4.5 Mortality

A number of cohort studies have reported increased mortality in people with diabetes [50, 51], including in older adults [52]. It is not surprising that the mortality rates are also increased in depressed people. For example, in a longitudinal cohort study [53] it was found that, over a 2-year period, depression contributed as much to mortality as did myocardial infarction (MI) or diabetes in older primary care patients. The treatment of depression reduces such risk [54]. By following a large group of people ($n = 4154$) with diabetes for a period of up to 3 years [55], it was found that both minor and major depression were strongly associated with increased mortality, even when controlling for significant predictors of mortality.

Although many of the studies cited above were cross-sectional in nature, thus precluding conclusions about cause and effect, it would seem plausible that the control of depressive symptoms might help to improve diabetes self-management, diabetes control and also to reduce complications and health care costs, and even mortality rates.

28.5 Possible mechanisms for the aetiology of depression

28.5.1 Multiple pathways

To date, the aetiology of clinical depression remains poorly understood. However, several models have been proposed, including genetic, biochemical, psychological and social processes and environmental stressors [56]. There is consensus that there is no single explanation for the pathogenesis of depressive disorder. Rather, it is believed that the biochemical and psychosocial changes associated with type 2 diabetes interact with those of clinical depression [57], resulting in more severe depression with more frequent and longer-lasting episodes [29, 58]. Yet, the results from two large population-based studies – one in the US [59] and one in the Netherlands [60] – have suggested that disturbed glucose homeostasis is not associated with depressive symptoms. In fact, in both studies it was found that people with diabetes, but who were unaware of having the condition, did not have an increased risk of depressive symptoms. Those people diagnosed with type 2 diabetes (and who therefore were aware of having the condition) had an increased risk of developing depressive symptoms compared to subjects with normal glucose concentrations. Also, as the adjustment for the number of chronic diseases attenuated the risk of depressive symptoms in patients with diagnosed diabetes, these results may indicate that depressive symptoms in diabetes might be a consequence of its burden rather than a consequence of high glucose levels.

28.5.2 Stress-vulnerability model

One aetiological model of depression that may account for the epidemiological findings described above is a stress-vulnerability model. This model posits that individuals having specific depressogenic vulnerabilities or defects may suffer depression when these vulnerabilities or defects become activated, usually during stressful situations [61]. When applied to a diabetes population, this model predicts that the stresses associated with living with diabetes and its ramifications would increase the chances of developing depressive episodes in people with specific vulnerabilities.

28.5.3 Stresses associated with diabetes

Stresses associated with diabetes may vary from significant losses (e.g. bodily functions, amputations, loss of vision) to minor hassles (e.g. having to inject insulin in social gatherings). At the same time, many older adults are likely to experience a range of other stresses associated with ageing, including other physical illnesses, loss of roles (e.g. through retirement), bereavements and social difficulties (e.g. housing or financial problems). All of these have been found to be associated with greater levels of depression [62]. In one study [30] it was found that the rate of depressive disorder was higher in patients with diabetes complications than in those without complications; this may suggest that a higher burden of diabetes-related conditions is associated with more depression. It is also possible that enduring the negative sequelae of stresses related to diabetes accounts for the effects of life events on depression [63]. For example, 25% of patients with diabetes forego social activities because of social embarrassment related to insulin injections [64]. It is important to note that major life events occur quite infrequently, while relatively minor hassles of diabetes are probably daily events. Yet daily hassles, though small in themselves, may lead to a cumulative impact of stress over time.

28.6 The assessment of depression in older adults with diabetes

28.6.1 The aim of assessment

Based on the assumption that diabetes will lead to an increase in depressed mood, either as a result of the biochemical changes directly due to type 2 diabetes, or resulting from the burden of living with diabetes [57], it is not surprising that clinical guidelines (e.g. [65–67]) now recommend that all patients with diabetes undergo regular screening for depression. In particular, attention must be paid to the routine screening of those with known vulnerability factors, such as a previous history of depression, diabetes-related complications, poorly controlled diabetes, diagnosis of dementia and psychological stress.

There is evidence that depression among older people attending primary care health services goes undetected [68], perhaps because it is assumed that it is natural for an older person who has chronic health problems to feel somewhat depressed; consequently, the condition is not fully assessed, labelled and treated. The overlap of symptoms of depression with age-related changes (e.g. feeling slowed down; interrupted sleep), diabetes-related symptoms (e.g. tiredness, loss of libido) and the side effects of medication makes the assessment of depression in older people very complex.

The aim of an assessment, therefore, is to clearly establish whether an older person with diabetes is also experiencing depressive symptoms, thoughts or feelings. If so, it becomes important to further assess its extent, severity and impact, so that an appropriate level of intervention can be provided.

28.6.2 The process of assessment

A stepped approach is likely to be the most efficient and effective approach to the identification of depression in diabetes. The steps included comprise a brief screening during routine appointments, a full assessment in primary care, and a specialist assessment by mental health professionals.

Brief screening

Of three possible screening instruments used to identify depression, Henkel et al. [69] found that the WHO-5 Well-Being Index had the best sensitivity and specificity among 431 adults aged 18–88 years attending Primary Care Services in Germany. Various four-item versions of the Geriatric Depression Scale (GDS) [70, 71] have also been found to be reasonably accurate in the detection of depression specifically among older people with acute physical illness [72, 73] and those in primary care [74] (see Table 28.2 for details of these instruments). One of these short scales can easily be built into the conduct of routine appointments with primary care staff or specialist diabetes nurses.

Assessment of depression in primary care

Where a simple brief screen indicates possible depression, then a fuller assessment should be carried out which may lead to either intervention within primary care or referral on to mental health services for specialist assessment and treatment.

The assessment should preferably combine clinical observation, information about the patient's history, current functioning, thoughts and feelings and a standardized questionnaire. High levels of successful suicide among older people with multiple physical

Table 28.2   Screening Tools for Depression.

The WHO-5 Well-Being Index
Respondents are asked to indicate the frequency of their experience in relation to each of five questions over the past 2
   weeks on a six-point Likert scale which ranges from 'All of the time' to 'At no time'.

1. I have felt cheerful and in good spirits

2. I have felt calm and relaxed

3. I have felt active and vigorous

4. I woke up feeling fresh and rested

5. My daily life has been filled with things that interest me

4-item versions of the Geriatric Depression Scale
Respondents are asked to answer 'yes' or 'no' to whether they have felt like this over the past week.

1. Are you basically satisfied with your life?

2. Do you feel that your life is empty?

3. Are you afraid that something bad is going to happen to you?

4. Do you feel happy most of the time?

   [72, 131, 132]

Or

1. Are you basically satisfied with your life?

2. Have you dropped many of your activities and interests?

3. Do you feel happy most of the time?

4. Do you prefer to stay at home, rather than going out and doing new things?

   [74]

illnesses [75] mean that questions about the presence of suicidal ideas should always be asked if moderate to severe depression is present.

28.6.3   Measures specific to older people: The geriatric depression scale

One of the most widely used measures for depression in older people is the Geriatric Depression Scale (GDS) [70, 71]. The original version has 30 items concerning thoughts and feelings typical of depression in older people, and the respondent is asked to answer *yes* or *no* to whether they have experienced these during the past week. The questions do not include the somatic and physical symptoms that may fail to discriminate depression from other conditions in older people. The yes/no scale is easier for many older people to answer than the four- or five-point Likert scales that are used in general adult questionnaires, and there is also an informant version. The scheme is not subject to copyright, and is readily available from the Internet.

Shorter versions have also been developed with 15 items [76, 77], ten items, four items and one item [73]. The 15-item version has been found to be highly correlated with the total score from the longer version, and to have high internal consistency, good sensitivity and specificity among 198 older people attending primary care services [73]. Both sensitivity and specificity fall when even shorter versions are used [72, 73] although, as noted above, briefer versions may still be helpful in initial screening.

Scores on the GDS correlate highly with clinical diagnoses of depression [78]. Various research studies have indicated that the GDS is applicable across a wide variety of clinical populations, including primary care settings [74], medical outpatients and inpatients, nursing home residents and older people in mental health services [79]. A recent review of assessment for depression in older people identified nine studies evaluating use of the 15- and 30-item GDS systems in primary care settings [80]. These reported that sensitivity and specificity ranged from 79–100% and 67–80%, respectively. The GDS has also been specifically evaluated and found to be valid in a British African-Caribbean patient sample [81, 82].

28.6.4   Measures for people with dementia

Whilst the GDS-15 may be the scale of choice for older people without cognitive impairment, it does not perform as well in those with dementia. A direct comparison of the GDS with the Cornell Scale for Depression in Dementia (CSDD) [83] in a sample of patients aged >65 years, which included people with depression alone, dementia alone, depression and dementia and neither, found the CSDD to retain its specificity and sensitivity among people with depression and dementia better than the GDS [84].

The CSDD involves collecting information from both the older person with dementia and an informant. It includes 19 items on mood, physical and behavioural indicators, ideological symptoms and changes in diurnal patterns, with a three-point response scale. It has been used in samples of older people in both nursing homes [85] and community settings [84], and should be used in place of the GDS when it is thought that the subject might have cognitive impairment (e.g. a Mini Mental State Examination score <27).

28.6.5   General population measures

The most common general population measures of depression in diabetes research and practice include the Centre for Epidemiological Studies Depression scale (CES-D) [86] and the Beck Depression Inventory (BDI) [87].

The BDI is a very widely used and readily available scale, and the indications are that it is probably valid with older populations. However, it is a little longer (21 items) and is more complex (4-point Likert scale) to complete than the GDS. Research with the BDI has shown that items concerned with physiological signs of depression are minimally confounded with symptoms of diabetes [88], and it was found that eliminating the somatic symptoms did not improve the accuracy of this measure [89]. Nonetheless, the BDI was found to have satisfactory sensitivity and specificity to detect clinical depression in a mixed sample of type 1 and type 2 diabetes patients [90].

The CES-D has been used in a wide range of people in different situations and settings, and is now the most commonly used self-report measure of depressive symptoms in diabetes research [52]. The CES-D is often used in older populations [91–93], and has been shown to have wide cross-cultural use in the USA with Black and White older adults [91].

The CES-D consists of 20 items answered on a 4-point Likert scale, and enquires about symptoms experienced over the past week. A review of its properties in use with older populations found it to have sensitivity and specificity ranging from 75–93% and 73–87%, respectively, for the detection of severe depressive episodes/major depression. However, it may be less effective for identifying minor, subclinical levels of depression [94]. These authors noted that the CES-D was reported as being difficult to administer to those in nursing homes, where the respondents found it difficult to remember and answer the questions. Although the sensitivity of the CES-D to detect clinical depression was lower than that of the BDI, its specificity was higher [90].

28.6.6   Summary

Clinicians should be alert to the signs of depression in all older people with diabetes, but especially those with known risk factors. For these people, brief screening questions – as listed in Table 28.2 – should be routinely included in primary care appointments. Where these indicate possible depression, or where this is otherwise suspected, a fuller assessment should be carried out in primary care or, where there are complicating factors, in specialist mental health services. For those patients without significant cognitive impairment, the 15-item version of the GDS seems to be the instrument of choice to assess depression in primary care, hospital or residential settings. The CSDD should be used in preference where the diabetic patient has significant cognitive deficits. However, where data are being collected, or need to be compared across the adult age range, then the BDI or CES-D may be preferable. Where scores indicate possible depression, and this is supported by clinical information and observation, treatment can be undertaken in primary care, or the patient may be referred to a specialist mental health service. The guidelines issued by organizations such as the UK National Institute for Health and Clinical Excellence [95] suggest that mild depression be treated in primary care, whilst moderate to severe depression may be treated in either primary or secondary care, depending on the patient's particular circumstances and history.

28.7 The treatment of clinical depression

The goals for treating depressed diabetes patients are two-fold: (i) remission or improvement of depressive symptoms; and (ii) improvement of the often poor glycaemic control, which is generally considered as fundamental to the management of diabetes, in order to prevent or delay long-term complications.

The treatment of depression may have a positive effect on levels of motivation to manage activities of daily living, to take physical exercise, and to adhere to dietary management and medication regimes. However, only a handful of randomized control trials have been conducted examining the treatment of depression in people with diabetes, and these have been small-scale in design. Even fewer studies have specifically targeted an older population. However, the results to date appear to suggest that cognitive behaviour therapy and antidepressant medication are as effective in people with major depressive disorder (MDD) and diabetes as in those with MDD without diabetes with, in some instances, additional beneficial effects on glycaemic control [96]. Older depressed primary care patients with diabetes in practices that implement depression care management [monitoring, antidepressants such as serotonin reuptake inhibitors (SSRIs) or inter-personal therapy and follow-up sessions] have been found to have lower mortality levels over the course of a 5-year interval than depressed patients with diabetes in usual-care practices (adjusted hazard ratio 0.49, 95% CI: 0.24–0.98) [54].

28.7.1 Pharmacotherapy

According to the expert consensus guideline on the treatment of depressive disorders in older people [97], it is important to identify coexisting medical conditions, such as diabetes mellitus, which may contribute to depression itself or complicate its treatment. The preferred first-line treatment is a SSRI or a serotonin norepinephrine reuptake inhibitor (SNRI), and psychotherapy [97]. A Cochrane Database systematic review on the use of antidepressant versus placebo treatment in depressed elderly people [98] found that SSRIs, tricyclic antidepressants (TCAs) and monoamine reuptake inhibitors (MAOIs) were all effective for the treatment of depression in older people, and emphasized the need to wait for at least 6 weeks to ensure

optimal therapeutic effect. A more recent Cochrane review confirmed that SSRIs and TCAs were of similar efficacy, but that TCAs had a higher withdrawal rate due to their side effects [99].

In all age groups there is evidence that patients with depression and comorbid medical illness are significantly more likely to improve if treated with antidepressants compared to placebo or no treatment [100, 101]. Specifically, however, although the TCA nortriptyline was shown to improve depression, it was more likely to worsen the control of diabetes [100, 101] and to have an adverse effect on glucose control [102]. In fact, TCAs have been shown to increase serum glucose levels by up to 150%, causing hyperglycaemia as well as increasing appetite and reducing metabolic rate, resulting in weight gain [102–105]. In view of the above, TCAs such as nortriptyline would not be the first-line treatment for depression in diabetes.

Consistent with the guidance for treatment of older adults cited above, in those with diabetes SSRIs have been shown to be effective, with most data supporting the use of *fluoxetine*, as this improves both mood and glycaemic control [106, 107]. There is also promising evidence of the efficacy of *sertraline* [108, 109]. Fluoxetine improves HbA$_{1c}$ levels, reduces insulin requirements, and is associated with weight loss and enhanced insulin sensitivity [110]. Moreover, its effects on insulin sensitivity are independent of its effect on weight loss [111]. Despite these advantages, it has been reported that patients with diabetes may become hypoglycaemic during treatment with fluoxetine [112]. Furthermore, the side effects of fluoxetine include tremor, nausea, sweating and anxiety, and these may be mistaken by patients for an episode of hypoglycaemia. It has therefore been advised that patients are informed of these possible effects [113].

SNRIs such as *venlafaxine* do not appear to disrupt glycaemic control, although only limited data are available on the efficacy of this drug [103]. *Duloxetine* has been shown to be effective in the treatment of diabetic peripheral neuropathic pain and, given that it is also an antidepressant, it would be a suitable treatment for depression in diabetes. It has little influence on glycaemic control, but has been shown to be both safe and well-tolerated, with few adverse side effects [114].

Other available antidepressants include MAOIs and newer agents (mirtazapine, reboxetine and trazadone). Unfortunately, the MAOIs have been found to cause not only weight gain [108, 115] but also hypoglycaemic episodes [108], and there is little evidence as yet of the effectiveness of these newer agents [116, 117]. Were either to be used, they would probably best be administered under specialist psychiatric care.

In all patients with diabetes being treated with antidepressants, it is important to monitor blood sugar levels closely at the start of treatment, when the dose in changed, or after discontinuation [104].

28.7.2 Maintenance therapy

Current clinical guidelines [118] recommend that, following a first episode of depression, treatment should continue for 4–6 months. Maintenance treatment beyond 6 months is recommended for individuals who have had two or more episodes, have a comorbid physical illness, or have failed to make a complete recovery from their depressive episode. Other risk factors to take into consideration include age and ongoing psychosocial difficulties.

A number of studies have focused specifically on those with diabetes. In patients with diabetes, maintenance therapy with sertraline has been found to prolong the depression-free interval following recovery from major depression [109]. Depression recovery with sertraline, as well as sustained remission with or without treatment, is associated with improvements in HbA$_{1c}$ levels for at least 1 year [109].

A recent trial of maintenance pharmacotherapy for the prevention of depression recurrence showed a benefit of sertraline in younger patients with diabetes (aged <55 years) compared to placebo in patients who initially responded to sertraline, but not in the older population (>55 years). However, this was mainly due to a higher response to non-specific treatment factors in this group [119].

Although pharmacotherapy is the most likely prescribed treatment for MDD in primary care [120], it should be noted that in 50% of depressed diabetes patients pharmacotherapy does not lead to a full remission of depression [58, 121, 122]. Therefore, new approaches to the treatment of depression in diabetes seem warranted.

28.7.3 Psychological interventions

Psychological interventions may be provided within a stepped care model in which self-help or low-intensity work is provided in primary care. Where further intervention is indicated, higher intensity psychological therapy is then recommended either in primary or secondary care [123]. There is some evidence for the effectiveness of both these levels of psychological intervention for depression in diabetes.

In primary care, interventions such as 'depression care management' (which consists of patient education, support with adherence to medication, and assistance with coordination of primary and secondary care) [124] and 'depression case management' (education, medication support or problem-solving therapy) [125] have been found to reduce depression and increase exercise [124], or to reduce depression and increase satisfaction with care [125], with effects continuing at the 12-month follow-up.

Higher intensity psychological interventions such as counselling [126] and cognitive behavioural therapy (CBT) [121] have provided positive results regarding the improvement of depression, and have shown moderate to good positive effects with regards to glycaemic control.

A recent systematic review and meta-analysis of the effectiveness of psychological interventions (including counselling, CBT and psychodynamic psychotherapy) to improve glycaemic control in those with type 2 diabetes [127], concluded that these therapies led to long-term improvements in psychological distress and in glycaemic control. However, it should be noted that the studies included were not aimed primarily at the treatment of depression.

28.7.4 Treatment for mild to moderate depression

Studies exploring the effects of treatment of mild to moderate depression in diabetic patients are rare, although this subthreshold form of depression is highly prevalent in the diabetic population [21] and increases the risk of subsequent major depression [128]. To date, only a small randomized, placebo-controlled trial of *paroxetine* in mildly depressed postmenopausal women with type 2 diabetes (age >50 years) [129] has been carried out, and has shown beneficial treatment effects on insulin sensitivity and glycaemic control.

Self-help strategies for early intervention against subclinical depression, though proven to be beneficial in the general population [130], remain to be examined in persons with diabetes.

28.8 Case studies

28.8.1 Case study 1

Presentation

EH, a woman in her mid-70s who lives alone, is well known to the Practice having a history of both physical and mental health problems. Her postnatal depression many years ago was treated by her GP and a later episode of depression, after her husband died 20 years ago, was treated through inpatient psychiatric care. She has had no problems with depression since that time. However, she has some chronic health problems including heart failure treated with diuretics, COPD and type 2 diabetes treated through medication. Her diabetes is poorly controlled. She attends the surgery looking thin, frail and unkempt.

Commentary The indicators of possible depression on this occasion are EH's lack of self care and loss of weight, although her poorly controlled diabetes may also contribute to the weight loss. Taking these in conjunction with vulnerability factors (her known history of depression and her physical health problems) an assessment for possible depression is warranted.

Assessment

Her GP sees EH at the surgery and asks how she is. She says that over the past 2–3 weeks, she has been sleeping badly and is too breathless to go out, so is confined to the house. She cannot bring herself to put effort into cooking and cleaning as it seems pointless when she cannot do it to her usual high standard. She complains that the days seem very long being at home on her own. She no longer finds any pleasure in watching TV or reading. She does not ring friends as she feels she is not good company and her diet will be a trouble to them. She cannot see things getting better and expresses the view that her current state is a punishment for an extra-marital affair she had much earlier in life. She is convinced that no-one can do anything to improve her health and sometimes wonders if life is worth living.

Commentary EH gives evidence of having seven of the symptoms of depression that are outlined in ICD-10, including the three that are viewed as core

(depressed mood, loss of interest and enjoyment and reduced energy) as well as a number of others (reduced self-esteem and self-confidence, ideas of guilt, a bleak and pessimistic view of the future and disturbed sleep). This fulfils the criteria for a diagnosis of severe depressive episode.

Treatment

In view of her score on the GDS-15, her clinical picture and her history, the GP offers EH antidepressants and also refers her to the specialist Mental Health Service for further assessment and treatment. That Service supports the introduction of the antidepressants and is able to arrange for her to have a series of appointments for cognitive-behavioural therapy (CBT). The CBT therapist focuses with her on: (i) combating learned helplessness through re-introducing pleasant activities; (ii) helping her to learn to challenge negative thinking about her lack of control over her health and her life; (iii) helping her to build self-esteem by contacting friends; and (iv) helping her to consider alternative ways that her friends might see her dietary needs. The GP also refers her to a local programme of Physical Rehabilitation for COPD as exercising reduces depressive symptoms as well as improving diabetes control and COPD. As a result of these interventions, EH's depression improves, her sense of guilt reduces and her optimism returns, along with better self-care and dietary management.

Commentary In line with clinical guidelines, EH's treatment involves both medication and psychological therapy. Typical of work with older people, a multi-pronged approach is used to address a range of physical health (lack of exercise), mental health (negative thinking) and social (lack of social contact) issues. Following her initial improvement, consideration will now need to be given to its maintenance.

28.8.2 Case study 2

Presentation

BC is a 65-year-old recently retired plumber who was diagnosed with type 2 diabetes at the age of 52. He manages his diabetes through insulin (two injections per day), but is considerably overweight. He has hypertension, which is currently being controlled with medication, and has sustained diabetes-related damage to his vision. On a recent visit to the surgery he complains of lack of energy, a pervasive sense of tiredness and a loss of interest in his usual past-times.

Commentary BC's fatigue and withdrawal may be linked directly to physical health, but could equally be manifestations of depression.

Assessment

The Practice Nurse becomes aware of BC's situation and state of mind when she sees him for routine monitoring of blood pressure. She books a double appointment time with him for the following week when she establishes more about his current thoughts and feelings and completes the GDR-15.

Commentary BC's score on the GDS-15 is 7, which is at the lower end of the range and suggestive of mild depression. He is complaining of the three core symptoms of depression (reduced energy, loss of interest and enjoyment and depressed mood) as well as disturbed sleep and reduced self-esteem and self-confidence. This is sufficient for him to receive a formal diagnosis of a mild depressive episode.

Treatment

The Practice Nurse and GP in consultation decide to ask the Primary Care Mental Health Worker (PCMHW) who is based in the Practice to see BC. She sees him for six appointments over the following 10 weeks. She and he agree that his current feelings of uselessness may be exacerbated by his recent retirement and his deteriorating vision. They use a problem-solving approach and elements of CBT to consider ways of finding purpose and structure in life following retirement. As a result, BC turns the manual dexterity he formerly used in plumbing to use in a new hobby of model building. The PCMHW also directs him to a local charity that offers expert assessment and loans of aids to those with low vision. He visits the charity, and as a result joins a walking group designed to build confidence in those with acquired visual impairment. This gives him exercise, enables him to lose weight and introduces him to new acquaintances, one of whom becomes a good friend. Following the intervention, BC reports feeling more energetic and more satisfied with his life. His score on the GDS-15 has reduced to 2, which is a level typical of those who are not depressed.

Commentary In line with best practice, BC's mild depression is dealt with in Primary Care, through brief therapy focused on helping him to help himself through establishing satisfying activities and finding solutions to current problems. His loss of weight subsequent to joining the walking group may help in the longer term control of his diabetes as well as in keeping depression away.

28.8.3 Case study 3

Presentation

DW is a woman in her mid-80s who has mild vascular dementia and diabetes, managed through dietary control. She has recently moved into a Residential Home as she was unable to look after herself at home, but staff are finding her difficult to manage. She is not mixing with others and her personal hygiene is poor. She shouts aggressively at staff when they try to encourage her to wash.

Commentary Withdrawal, lack of self-care and irritability may all be signs of depression or of dementia. In addition, Miss W has a number of vulnerability factors for depression (diabetes, dementia and in Residential Care).

Assessment

The Diabetes Specialist Nurse, who has known DW for some time, visits the Home to find out more from the staff and to ascertain how Miss W feels she is settling in and managing. She fills out the CSDD and discovers a total score of 21.

Commentary The score of 21 in the CSDD is within the range typical of the presence of definite 'major depression'.

Treatment

The Specialist Nurse refers Miss W to the Community Mental Health team for Older People. The Associate Specialist in the team prescribes appropriate anti-depressants for DW. The CPN provides the staff of the Home with information about depression in dementia and helps them to work with DW to draw up a person-centred care plan that involves reconnecting her with some of her friends in the community. These measures lead to a relief of her depression and DW becomes less irritable.

Commentary As with EH, treatment involves more than one approach, in this case medication and psychosocial intervention. The backdrop of cognitive impairment means that the intervention is carried out with the collaboration of those staff who are in day-to-day contact with the patient.

28.9 Summary

In summary, there have been encouraging findings that depression can be treated successfully in diabetes patients, with at least good short-term results. As in the general population, there is no evidence that either pharmacotherapy or psychological therapy is superior to the other, and the choice of treatment may ultimately depend on patient preference.

References

1. World Health Organisation. *ICD-10 Classification of Mental and Behavioural Disorders*. World Health Organisation, Geneva; 1992.

2. American Psychiatric Association. *Diagnostic and Statistical Manual of Mental Disorders*, Fourth Edition. Washington, DC: American Psychiatric Association; 1994.

3. Alexopoulos GS, Meyers BS, Young RC, Campbell S, Silbersweig D, Charlson M. 'Vascular depression' hypothesis. Arch Gen Psychiatry 1997; 54 (10): 915–22.

4. Bruce DG, Casey G, Davis WA, Starkstein SE, Clarnette RC, Foster JK, *et al*. Vascular depression in older people with diabetes. Diabetologia 2006; 49 (12): 2828–36.

5. Krishnan KR, Hays JC, Blazer DG. MRI-defined vascular depression. Am J Psychiatry 1997; 154 (4): 497–501.

6. Robinson RG. Poststroke depression: prevalence, diagnosis, treatment, and disease progression. Biol Psychiatry 2003; 54 (3): 376–87.

7. Lewinsohn PM, Rohde P, Seeley JR, Fischer SA. Age and depression: unique and shared effects. Psychol Aging 1991; 6(2): 247–60.

8. Roberts RE, Kaplan GA, Shema SJ, Strawbridge WJ. Does growing old increase the risk for depression? Am J Psychiatry 1997; 154 (10): 1384–90.

9. Chapman DP, Perry GS. Depression as a major component of public health for older adults. Prev Chronic Dis. 2008; 5(1): http://www.cdc.gov/pcd/issues/2008/jan/07_0150.htm (accessed December 2007).

10. Blazer D. The epidemiology of depression in late life. J Geriatr Psychiatry 1989; 22: 35–52.

11. Weissman MM, Leaf PJ, Tischler GL, Blazer DG, Karno M, Bruce ML, *et al*. Affective disorders in five United States communities. Psychol Med. 1988; 18 (1): 141–53.

12. Ames D. Epidemiological studies of depression among the elderly in residential and nursing homes. Int J Geriatr Psychiatry 1991; 6, 347–54.

13. Parmalee P, Katz I, Lawton M. The design of special environments for the aged. In: J. Birren and K. Schaie (eds), *Handbook of the Psychology of Aging*, 3rd edition. Academic Press, San Diego; 1992, pp. 464–88.

14. Van Ojen R, Hooijer C, Jonker C, Lindeboom J, van Tilburg W. Late-life depressive disorder in the community, early onset and the decrease of vulnerability with increasing age. J Affect Disord. 1995; 33 (3), 159–66.

15. Cole MG, Dendukuri N. Risk factors for depression among elderly community subjects: a systematic review and meta-analysis. Am J Psychiatry 2003; 160: 1147–56.

16. Zarit S, Zarit J. *Mental Disorders in Older Adults: Fundamental of Assessment and Treatment*. Guilford, New York; 1998.

17. Sharpe M, Hawton K, Seagroatt V, Bamford J, House A, Molyneux A, *et al*. Depressive disorders in long term survivors of stroke: associations with demographic and social factors, functional status and brain lesion volume. Br J Psychiatry 1994; 164 (3), 380–6.

18. National Institute of Health Consensus Development conference. Diagnosis and treatment of depression in late life. JAMA 1992; 268 (8): 1018–24.

19. Livingstone G, Hawkins A, Blizard B, Mann A. The Gospel Oak study: prevalence rates of dementia, depression and activity limitation among elderly residents in inner London. Psychol Med. 1990; 20 (1): 137–46.

20. Blazer D, Hughes D, George L. The epidemiology of depression in an elderly community population. Gerontologist 1987; 27: 281–7.

21. Anderson RJ, Freedland KE, Clouse RE, Lustman PJ. The prevalence of comorbid depression in adults with diabetes: a meta-analysis. Diabetes Care 2001; 24 (6), 1069–78.

22. Ali S, Stone MA, Peters JL, Davies MJ, Kunti K. The prevalence of co-morbid depression in adults with type 2 diabetes: a systematic review and meta-analysis. Diabet Med. 2006; 23 (11): 1165–73.

23. Zahid N, Asghar S, Claussen B, Hussain A. Depression and diabetes in a rural community in Pakistan. Diabet Res Clin Prac. 2008; 79 (1): 124–7.

24. Khamseh ME, Baradaran HR, Rajabali H. Depression and diabetes in Iranian patients: a comparative study. Int J Psychiatry Med. 2007; 37 (1): 81–6.

25. Chou KL, Chi I. Functional disability related to diabetes mellitus in older Hong Kong Chinese adults. Gerontologist 2005; 51: 334–9.

26. Egede LE. Major depression in individuals with chronic medical disorders: prevalence, correlates and association with health resource utilization, lost productivity and functional disability. Gen Hosp Psychiatry 2007; 29 (5): 409–16.

27. Patten SB, Beck CA, Kassam A, Williams JV, Barbui C, Metz LM. Long-term medical conditions and major depression: strength of association for specific conditions in the general population. Can J Psychiatry 2005; 50 (4): 195–202.

28. Peyrot M, Rubin RR. Persistence of depressive symptoms in diabetic adults. Diabetes Care 1999; 22 (3): 448–52.

29. Lustman PJ, Griffith LS, Clouse RE. Depression in adults with diabetes. Results of 5-yr follow-up study. Diabetes Care 1988; 11 (8): 605–12.

30. Pouwer F, Beekman AT, Nijpels G, Dekker JM, Snoek FJ, Kostense PJ, et al. Rates and risks for co-morbid depression in patients with Type 2 diabetes mellitus: results from a community-based study. Diabetologia 2003; 46 (7): 892–8.

31. Maraldi C, Volpato S, Penninx BW, Yaffe K, Simonsick EM, Strotmeyer ES, et al. Diabetes mellitus, glycemic control, and incident depressive symptoms among 70- to 79-year-old persons: the health, aging, and body composition study. Arch Intern Med. 2007; 167 (11): 1137–44.

32. De Jonghe P, Roy J, Saz P, Marcos G, Lobo A, ZARADEMP investigators. Prevalent and incident depression in community dwelling elderly persons with diabetes mellitus: results from the ZARADEMP project. Diabetologia 2006; 49 (11): 2627–33.

33. Bisschop MI, Kriegsman DM, Deeg DJ, Beekman AT, van Tilburg W. The longitudinal relation between chronic diseases and depression in older persons in the community: the Longitudinal Aging Study Amsterdam. J Clin Epidemiol. 2004; 57: 187–94.

34. Palinkas LA, Lee PP, Barrett-Connor E. A prospective study of Type 2 diabetes and depressive symptoms in the elderly: the Rancho Bernardo Study. Diabet Med. 2004; 21 (11): 1185–91.

35. Janssen J, Beekman AT, Comijs HC, Deeg DJ, Heeren TJ. Late-life depression: the differences between early- and late-onset illness in a community-based sample. Int J Geriatr Psychiatry 2006; 21 (1): 86–93.

36. Simpson S, Baldwin R, Jackson A, Burns A, Thomas P. Is the clinical expression of late-life depression influenced by brain changes? MRI subcortical neuroanatomical correlates of depressive symptoms. Int Psychogeriatr. 2000; 12 (4): 425–34.

37. Kessing LV. Differences in diagnostic subtypes among patients with late and early onset of a single depressive episode. Int J Geriatr Psychiatry. 2006; 21 (12): 1127–31.

38. Mendlewicz J. The age factor in depressive illness: some genetic considerations. J Gerontol. 1976; 31 (3): 300–3.

39. Kalsekar ID, Madhaven SS, Amonkar MM, Makela EH, Scott VG, Douglas SM, et al. Depression in patients with type 2 diabetes: impact on adherence to oral hypoglycemic agents. Ann Pharmacother. 2006; 40 (4): 605–11.

40. Ciechanowski PS, Katon WJ, Russo JE. Impact of depressive symptoms on adherence, function, and costs. Arch Intern Med. 2000; 160: 3278–85.

41. Kilbourne AM, Reynolds CF, Good CB, Sereika SM, Justice AC, Fine MJ. How does depression influence diabetes medication adherence in older patients? Am J Geriatr Psychiatry. 2005; 13 (3): 202–10.

42. Gonzalez J, Safren S, Cagliero E, Wexler D, Delahanty L, Wittenberg E, et al. Depression, self-care, and medication adherence in type 2 diabetes: relationships across the full range of symptom severity. Diabetes Care 2007; 30 (9): 2222–7.

43. Park H, Hong Y, Lee H, Ha E, Sung Y. Individuals with type 2 diabetes and depressive symptoms exhibited lower adherence with self-care. J Clin Epidemiol. 2004; 57 (9): 978–84.

44. Ciechanowski PS, Katon WJ, Russo JE, Hirsch IB. The relationship of depressive symptoms to symptom reporting, self-care and glucose control in diabetes. Gen Hosp Psychiatry 2003; 25: 246–52.

45. Lustman PJ, Anderson RJ, Freedland KE, de Groot M, Carney RM, Clouse RE. Depression and poor glycemic control: a meta-analytic review of the literature. Diabetes Care 2000; 23 (7): 934–42.

46. Carney R, Freedland K, Lustman P, Griffith L. Depression and coronary disease in diabetic patients: a 10-year follow-up (Abstract). Psychosom Med. 1994; 56: 149.

47. Lloyd CE, Kuller LH, Ellis D, Becker DJ, Wing RR, Orchard TJ. Coronary artery disease in IDDM. Gender differences in risk factors but not risk. Arterioscler, Thromb Vasc Biol. 1996; 16 (6): 720–6.

48. de Groot M, Anderson R, Freedland KE, Clouse RE, Lustman PJ. Association of depression and diabetes complications: a meta-analysis. Psychosom Med. 2001; 63 (4): 619–30.

49. Egede LE, Zheng D, Simpson K. 2002 Comorbid depression is associated with increased health care use and expenditures in individuals with diabetes. Diabetes Care 2002; 25 (3): 464–70.

50. Zhang X, Norris SL, Gregg EW, Cheng YJ, Beckles G, Kahn HS. Depressive symptoms and mortality

among persons with and without diabetes. Am J Epidemiol. 2005; 161 (7): 652–60.

51. Egede LE, Nietert PJ, Zheng D. Depression and all-cause and coronary heart disease mortality among adults with and without diabetes. Diabetes Care 2005; 28 (6): 1339–45.

52. Black SA, Markides KS, Ray LA. Depression predicts increased incidence of adverse health outcomes in older Mexican Americans with type 2 diabetes. Diabetes Care 2003; 26: 2822–8.

53. Gallo JJ, Bogner HR, Morales KH, Post EP, Ten Have T, Bruce ML. Depression, cardiovascular disease, diabetes, and two-year mortality among older, primary-care patients. Am J Geriatr Psychiatry. 2005; 13 (9): 748–55.

54. Bogner HR, Morales KH, Post EP, Bruce ML. Diabetes, depression, and death: a randomized controlled trial of a depression treatment program for older adults based in primary care (PROSPECT). Diabetes Care 2007; 30: 3005–10.

55. Katon WJ, Rutter C, Simon G, Lin EH, Ludman E, Ciechanowski P, Kinder L, et al. The association of comorbid depression with mortality in patients with type 2 diabetes. Diabetes Care 2005; 28 (11), 2668–72.

56. Southwick SM, Vythilingam M, Charney DS. The psychobiology of depression and resilience to stress: implications for prevention and treatment. Annu Rev Clin Psychol. 2005; 1: 255–91.

57. Talbot F, Nouwen A. A review of the relationship between depression and diabetes in adults: is there a link? Diabetes Care 2000; 23 (10): 1556–62.

58. Lustman PJ, Griffith LS, Freedland KE, Clouse RE. The course of major depression in diabetes. Gen Hosp Psychiatry 1997; 19 (2): 138–43.

59. Palinkas LA, Barrett-Connor E, Wingard DL. Type 2 diabetes and depressive symptoms in older adults: a population-based study. Diabet Med. 1991; 8 (6): 532–9.

60. Knol MJ, Heerdink ER, Egberts AC, Geerlings MI, Gorter KJ, Numans ME, et al. Depressive symptoms in subjects with diagnosed and undiagnosed type 2 diabetes. Psychosom Med. 2007; 69 (4): 300–5.

61. Banks SM, Kerns RD. Explaining high rates of depression in chronic pain: A Diathesis-stress framework. Psychological Bulletin 1996; 119, 95–110.

62. Murphy E. Social origins of depression in old age. Br J Psychiatry 1982; 141, 135–42.

63. Kessler RC. The effects of stressful life events on depression. Annu Rev Psychol. 1997; 48: 191–214.

64. Wikblad KF, Wibell LB, Montin KR. Health and unhealth in chronic disease. Scand J Caring Sci. 1991; 5 (2): 71–7.

65. National Institute of Clinical Excellence. Depression. Management of depression in Primary and Secondary Care. Clinical Guideline 23. NICE, London, 2004.

66. American Diabetes Association. Standards of Medical Care in Diabetes. Diabetes Care 2005; 28 (Suppl. 1): S4–36.

67. International Diabetes Federation. Global Guideline for type 2 diabetes. International Diabetes Federation, Brussels, Belgium; 2005, pp. 19–21.

68. Iliffe S, Haines A, Gallivan S, Booroff A, Goldenberg E, Morgan P. Assessment of elderly people in general practice. 1. Social circumstances and mental state. Br J Gen Pract. 1991; 41 (342), 9–12.

69. Henkel V, Mergl R, Kohnen R, Maier W, Möller HJ, Hegerl U. Identifying depression in primary care: a comparison of different methods in a prospective cohort study. Br Med J. 2003; 326 (7382): 200–1.

70. Brink T, Yesavage J, Lum O, Heersuma P, Adey M, Rose T. Screening tests for geriatric depression. Clinical Gerontologist 1982; 1: 37–43.

71. Yesavage J, Brink T, Rose T, Lum O, Huang V, Adey M, et al. Development and validation of a geriatric depression screening scale: a preliminary report. J Psychiatric Res. 1983; 17 (1): 37–49.

72. Shah A, Herbert R, Lewis S, Mehendran R, Platt J, Bhattacharyya B. Screening for depression among acutely ill geriatric inpatients with a short Geriatric Depression Scale. Age Ageing 1997; 26 (3): 217–21.

73. D'Ath P, Katona P, Mullan E, Evans S, Katona C. Screening, detection and management of depression in elderly primary care attenders. I: The acceptability and performance of the 15 item Geriatric Depression Scale (GDS15) and the development of short versions. Fam Pract. 1994; 11 (3): 260–6.

74. van Marwijk H, Wallace P, de Bock G, Hermans J, Kaptein A, Mulder JD. Evaluation of the feasibility, reliability and diagnostic value of shortened versions of the geriatric depression scale. Br J Gen Pract. 1995; 45 (393): 195–9.

75. Juurlink D, Herrmann N, Szalai J, Kopp A, Redelmeier D. Medical illness and the risk of suicide in the elderly. Arch Intern Med. 2004; 164 (11), 1179–84.

76. Sheikh J, Yesavage J. Geriatric Depression Scale: recent findings and development of a short version. In: T. Brink (ed.). Clinical Gerontology: A guide to assessment and intervention. Howarth Press, New York; 1986, pp. 165–73.

77. Yesavage J. Geriatric Depression Scale. Psychopharmacol Bull. 1988; 24 (4): 709–10.

78. Wall J, Lichtenberg P, MacNeill S, Deshpande S, Walsh P. Depression detection in geriatric rehabilitation: Geriatric Depression Scale Short Form vs. Long Form. Clin Gerontol. 1999; 20 (1): 13–21.

79. Stiles P, McGarrahan J. The Geriatric Depression Scale: a comprehensive review. J Clin Geropsychol. 1998; 4 (1), 89.

80. Watson L, Pignone M. Screening accuracy for late-life depression in primary care: A systematic review. J Fam Pract 2003; 52 (12), 956–64.

81. Abas M, Phillip C, Carter J, Walter S, Banerjee S, Levy R. Culturally sensitive validation of screening questionnaires for depression in older African-Caribbean people living in South London. Br J Psychiatry. 1998; 173; 249–54.

82. Rait G, Burns A, Baldwin R, Morley M, Chew-Graham C, St Leger AS, et al. Screening for depression in African Caribbean elders. Fam Pract. 1999; 16 (6): 591–5.

83. Alexopoulos G, Abrams R, Young R, Shamoian C. Cornell Scale for depression in dementia. Biol Psychiatry. 1988; 23 (3): 271–84.

84. Kørner A, Lauritzen L, Abelskov K, Gulmann N, Brodersen AM, Wedervang-Jensen T, et al. The Geriatric Depression Scale and the Cornell Scale for Depression in Dementia. A validity study. Nord J Psychiatry 2006; 60 (5): 360–4.

85. Kurlowicz L, Evans L, Strumpf N, Maislin G. A Psychometric Evaluation of the Cornell Scale for Depression in dementia in a frail, nursing home population. Am J Geriatr Psychiatry 2002; 10 (5): 600–8.

86. Radloff LS. The CES-D scale: A self-report depression scale for research in the general population. Appl Psychol Measurement. 1977; 1: 385–401.

87. Beck AT, Ward, CH, Mendelsohn M, Mock J, Erbaugh J. An inventory for measuring depression, Arch Gen Psychiatry 1961; 4: 561–71.

88. Lustman PJ, Clouse RE, Griffith LS, Carney RM and Freedland KE. Screening for depression in diabetes using the Beck Depression Inventory. Psychosom Med. 1997; 59 (1), 24–31.

89. Lustman PJ, Clouse RE, Griffith LS, Carney RM, Freedland KE. Screening for depression in diabetes using the Beck Depression Inventory. Psychosom Med. 1997; 59 (1): 24–31.

90. Hermanns N, Kulzer B, Krichbaum M, Kubiak T, Haak T. How to screen for depression and emotional problems in patients with diabetes: comparison of screening characteristics of depression questionnaires, measurement of diabetes-specific emotional problems and standard clinical assessment. Diabetologia 2006; 49 (3): 469–77.

91. de Rekeneire N, Rooks RN, Simonsick EM, Shorr RI, Kuller LH, Schwartz AV, et al. Health, Aging and Body Composition Study. Diabetes is associated with subclinical functional limitation in nondisabled older individuals: the Health, Aging, and Body Composition study. Diabetes Care 2003; 26 (7): 3257–63.

92. Wu JH, Haan MN, Liang J, Ghosh G, Gonzalez HM, Herman WH. Diabetes as a predictor of change in functional status among older Mexican Americans: A population-based cohort study. Diabetes Care 2003; 26 (2): 314–19.

93. Black SA, Goodwin JS, Markides KS. The association between chronic diseases and depressive symptomatology in older Mexican Americans. J Gerontol. 1998; 53A: M188–94.

94. Papassotiropoulos A, Heun R, Maier W. The impact of dementia on the detection of depression in elderly subjects from the general population. Psychol Med. 1999; 29 (1), 113–20.

95. UK National Institute for Health and Clinical Excellence (NICE) Depression. Management of depression in Primary and Secondary Care. Clinical Guideline 23 (amended). NICE, London; 2007.

96. Jacobson AM, Weinger K. Treating depression in diabetic patients: is there an alternative to medications? Ann Intern Med. 1998; 129 (8): 656–7.

97. Alexopoulos G, Katz I, Reynolds C, Carpenter D, Docherty JP. Expert consensus panel for pharmacotherapy of depressive disorders in older patients. The expert consensus guideline series. Pharmacotherapy of depressive disorders in older patients. Postgrad Med. 2001; Special No. Pharmacotherapy: 1–86.

98. Wilson K, Mottram P, Sivanranthan A, Nightingale A. Antidepressant versus placebo for depressed elderly. Cochrane Database of Systematic Reviews 2001; (2): CD000561.

99. Mottram P, Wilson K, Strobl J. Antidepressants for depressed elderly. Cochrane Database of Systematic Reviews 2006; (1): CD003491.

100. Gill D, Hatcher S. Antidepressants for depression in medical illness. Cochrane Database of Systematic Reviews 2000; (4): CD001312.

101. Gill, D. Hatcher, S. Antidepressants for depression in medical illness: Update. Cochrane Database of Systematic Reviews 2007; (4): CD001312.

102. Lustman PJ, Griffith LS, Clouse RE, Freedland KA, Eisen SA, Rubin EH, et al. Effects of nortriptyline on depression and glycemic control in diabetes: results of a double-blind, placebo controlled trial. Psychosom Med. 1997; 59 (3): 241–50.

103. McIntyre R, Soczynska J, Konarski J, Kennedy S. The effect of antidepressants on glucose homeostasis and insulin sensitivity: synthesis and mechanisms. Expert Opin Drug Saf. 2006; 5 (4): 157–68.

104. Taylor D, Paton C, Kerwin R. *The South London and Maudsley & Oxleas Foundation Trust Prescribing Guidelines*, 9th edition. Informa Healthcare, London; 2007.

105. Bazire S. *Psychotropic Drug Directory*. Fivepin Publishing, Wiltshire; 2003.

106. Lustman PJ, Freedland KE, Griffith LS, Clouse RE. Fluoxetine for depression in diabetes: a randomized double-blind placebo-controlled trial. Diabetes Care 2000; 23 (5): 618–23.

107. Gulseren L, Gülseren S, Hekimsoy Z, Mete L. Comparison of fluoxetine and paroxetine in type II diabetes mellitus patients. Arch Med Res. 2005; 36 (2): 159–65.

108. Goodnick P. Use of antidepressants in treatment of comorbid diabetes mellitus and depression as well as in diabetic neuropathy. Ann Clin Psychiatry 2001; 13 (1): 31–41.

109. Lustman PJ, Clouse RE, Nix BD, Freedland KE, Rubin EH, McGill JB, *et al.* Sertraline for prevention of depression recurrence in diabetes mellitus: a randomized, double-blind, placebo-controlled trial. Arch Gen Psychiatry 2006; 63 (5): 521–9.

110. Gray D, Fujioka K, Devine W, Bray G. A randomized double-blind clinical trial of fluoxetine in obese diabetics. Int J Obes Relat Metab Dis. 1992; 16 (Suppl. 4): S67–72.

111. Maheux P, Ducros F, Bourque J, Garon J, Chiasson J-L. Fluoxetine improves insulin sensitivity in obese patients with non-insulin-dependent diabetes mellitus independently of weight loss. Int J Obes Relat Metab Disord. 1997; 21 (2): 97–102.

112. Andrew, J.E., Prescott, P., Smith, T.M.F., Inman, W.H.W. and Kubota, K. Fluoxetine: another new antidepressive. Drug and Therapeutics Bulletin 1990; 28, 33.

113. Bazire S. *Psychotropic Drug Directory*. 7th edition. Fivepin Publishing, Wiltshire; 2007.

114. Raskin J, Smith T, Wong K, Pritchett Y, D'Souza D, Iyengar S, *et al.* Duloxetine versus routine care in the long-term management of diabetic peripheral neuropathic pain. J Palliat Med. 2006; 9 (1): 29–40.

115. McIntyre R, Mancini D, Pearce M, Silverstone P, Chue P, Misener VL *et al.* Mood and psychotic disorders and Type 2 diabetes: a metabolic triad. Can J Diabet. 2005; 29, 122–32.

116. Himmerich H, Fulda S, Schaaf L, Beitinger P, Schuld A, Pollmächer T. Changes in weight and glucose tolerance during treatment with mirtazapine. Diabetes Care 2006; 29 (1): 170.

117. Musselman D, Betan E, Larsen H, Phillips L. Relationship of depression to diabetes types 1 and 2: epidemiology, biology, and treatment. Biol Psychiatry 2003; 54 (3): 317–29.

118. UK National Institute for Health and Clinical Excellence (NICE) *Depression. Management of depression in Primary and Secondary Care*. Clinical Guideline 23 (amended). NICE, London; 2007.

119. Williams MM, Clouse RE, Nix BD, Rubin EH, Sayuk GS, McGill JB, *et al.* Efficacy of sertraline in prevention of depression recurrence in older versus younger adults with diabetes. Diabetes Care 2007; 30 (4): 801–6.

120. Valenstein M, Vijan S, Zeber JE, Boehm K, Buttar A. The cost-utility of screening for depression in primary care. Ann Intern Med. 2001; 134 (5): 345–60.

121. Lustman PJ, Griffith LS, Freedland KE, Kissel SS, Clouse RE. Cognitive behavior therapy for depression in type 2 diabetes. A randomized controlled trial. Ann Intern Med. 1998; 129 (8): 613–21.

122. Lustman PJ, Clouse RE, Freedland KE. Management of major depression in adults with diabetes: implications of recent clinical trials. Sem Clin Neuropsychiatry 1998; 3 (2): 102–14.

123. UK National Institute for Health and Clinical Excellence (NICE) *Depression. Management of depression in Primary and Secondary Care*. Clinical Guideline 23 (amended). NICE, London; 2007.

124. Williams JW Jr, Katon W, Lin EH, Nöel PH, Worchel J, Cornell J, *et al.* The effectiveness of depression care management on diabetes-related outcomes in older patients. Ann Intern Med. 2004; 140 (12): 1015–24.

125. Katon W, Von Korff M, Lin E, Simon G, Ludman E, Russo J, *et al.* The Pathways Study: a randomized trial of collaborative care in patients with diabetes and depression. Arch Gen Psychiatry 2004; 61 (10): 1042–9.

126. Huang X, Song L, Li T. The effect of social support on type II diabetes with depression. Chin J Clin Psychol. 2001; 9, 187–9.

127. Ismail K, Winkley S, Rabe-Hesketh. Systematic review and meta-analysis of randomised controlled trials of psychological interventions to improve glycaemic control in patients with type 2 diabetes. Lancet 2004; 363 (9421): 1589–97.

128. Cuijpers P, Smit F. Subthreshold depression as a risk indicator for major depressive disorder: a systematic review of prospective studies. Acta Psychiatr Scand. 2004; 109 (5): 325–31.

129. Paile-Hyvarinen M, Wahlbeck K, Eriksson JG. Quality of life and metabolic status in mildly depressed women with type 2 diabetes treated with paroxetine: A single-blind randomised placebo controlled trial. BMC Fam Pract. 2003; 4, 7.

130. Christensen H, Griffiths KM, Jorm AF. Delivering intervention for depression by using the internet: randomised controlled trial. Br Med J. 2004; 328: 625.

29

Diabetes and Falls

Christine T. Cigolle [1] and Caroline S. Blaum [2]

[1]*Department of Family Medicine, University of Michigan, Ann Arbor and the Ann Arbor VA Healthcare System Geriatric Research, Education and Clinical Center, Ann Arbor, MI, USA*
[2]*Department of Internal Medicine, University of Michigan, Ann Arbor and the Ann Arbor VA Healthcare System Geriatric Research, Education and Clinical Center, Ann Arbor, MI, USA*

Key messages

- Falling may be the presenting sign of diabetes and other serious medical problems, and may result in considerable morbidity, disability and mortality.
- Diabetes, via a number of different mechanisms including hyperglycaemia, hypoglycaemia, sensory impairment, medication use, as well as balance, mobility and gait disorders, may cause a substantial increase in the risk of falls.
- All older adults with diabetes should be screened annually for falls.

Diabetes has its greatest incidence and prevalence in the older adult population, and diabetes and its treatments, complications and comorbid conditions affect the functioning of nearly all organ systems in the body. Falling, likewise, has its greatest incidence and prevalence among older adults, and nearly all organ systems can be implicated in the pathophysiology underlying falls. Thus, it is not surprising that the relationship between diabetes and falling is interconnected and complex. Compared to those without the disease, older adults with diabetes are at increased risk for falling, with diabetes contributing multiple causal factors for falls.

29.1 Introduction

Falling has been long recognized as a geriatric condition (or geriatric syndrome). It is common in the older adult population and is generally multifactorial in aetiology. Falling may be the presenting sign of serious medical problems, and falls themselves result in considerable morbidity, disability and mortality. They are also responsible for substantial economic costs. For example, health care expenditures for fall-related injuries in adults aged ≥ 65 years totalled more than $US 19 billion in the United States in 2000 [1, 2].

29.2 Definition

The definition of a fall includes several criteria. First, there is a change in body position, such that the individual comes to rest at a lower level, not necessarily on the floor or ground. Next, the change in body position is unintentional or inadvertent. Last, most authorities agree that a fall occurs without loss of consciousness (in contrast to syncope and seizures) or trauma (such as a motor vehicle-pedestrian accident). Physically, a fall results when the individual's centre of gravity moves beyond his or her base of support, and there is inadequate effort to maintain or restore balance [3].

Diabetes in Old Age. Third Edition. Edited by Alan J. Sinclair

Falls are frequently described with reference to their frequency, their outcome, and their association with balance or movement disorders. Falls in older adults are most concerning when the individual has multiple falls, has falls resulting in injury, or has an associated balance or gait disorder. Falling is often accompanied by an associated condition, a fear of falling. Here, an individual self-limits his activity due to a fear of and a desire to avoid falling and fall-related injury.

29.3   Epidemiology

29.3.1   Falls

The prevalence of falling in the older adult population is approximately 30% for adults aged ≥65 years [4]. Falling may be more prevalent among older adults having diabetes compared to those without the disease. Data from the Health and Retirement Study, a nationally representative, longitudinal health interview survey, have revealed falls to be more common across the age spectrum for older adults with diabetes, as compared to those without diabetes (Figure 29.1) [5]. Falling has similarly been shown to be more prevalent in older women with diabetes than in those not having

the disease. Of older adults with diabetes, falling is more common among those who have diabetes complications [6]. Among older adults with chronic kidney disease requiring dialysis (including but not limited to those with diabetes), the incidence of falls has been estimated to be 1.2 to 1.6 per patient-year (pt-yr) [7–9].

In the community, more than 50% of falls occur in the home. Approximately 15% of falls in the hospital setting lead to serious injury, and are associated with a longer length of stay and increased admission to long-stay nursing facilities. Fall rates are higher for those residing in long-stay nursing facilities, with an incidence rate of over 1% per pt-yr [10].

29.3.2   Complications of falls

Serious complications of falls include death, injury, a long period of being down and unable to get up following a fall, loss of independence, and fear of falling.

Fractures and other serious injuries are a feared outcome of falling. Some 10% of falls in the older adult population result in non-fatal injury. Falling is the most common cause of hospital admission for trauma in the older adult population, with falls being responsible for 87% of all fractures and over 95% of all hip fractures [11].

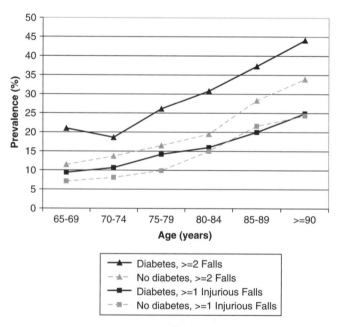

Figure 29.1   Prevalence of falls by diabetes status and age. Weighted percentages derived using the Health and Retirement Study (HRS) respondent population weights to adjust for the complex sampling design of the HRS survey (these data are from the 2004 wave of the HRS).

A long period of being immobile on the floor or ground after a fall and prior to discovery can result in dehydration, rhabdomyolysis and aspiration pneumonia.

The loss of independence – including the need for placement in a long-stay nursing facility – is another feared outcome for older adults. Indeed, over 50% of older adults who have a hip fracture are unable to live independently thereafter.

The fear of falling, and attempts to decrease the likelihood of falling, can lead to a cascade of events: restriction of activities, including both social participation and physical activities; deconditioning; decline in functional status; and, finally, placement in a long-stay nursing facility.

Older adults with diabetes are at risk for worse consequences from falls, due to a variety of causes, including an increased risk of fracture.

29.4 Pathophysiology of, and risk factors for, falling

29.4.1 Multifactorial in Aetiology

As a geriatric condition or geriatric syndrome, falling typically has a complex aetiology; that is, falling is the result of the "...accumulated effects of impairments in multiple systems" [12]. Risk factors for falling may be classified as intrinsic versus extrinsic [13]:

- Intrinsic, or personal, causes include age-related changes, chronic diseases, acute illnesses, medications and mobility.

- Extrinsic causes are those in the environment and include items such as room design, lighting, walking surfaces, stairs, and obstructions and impediments.

29.4.2 The role of diabetes

Research studies continue to disclose the complex relationship between diabetes and falling. Diabetes as a disease – and its management, complications and comorbid conditions – interacts with ongoing age-related functional decline in leading to falls in the older adult population [14]. As diabetes progresses in the older adult, diabetes complications and impairments accumulate in multiple systems. Diabetes becomes a major contributor to – and interacts with – many of the risk factors for falling, and so plays a substantial and multi-faceted role in the pathophysiology underlying falling (Table 29.1).

Table 29.1 Risk factors for falling in older adults with diabetes.

- Hyperglycaemia, hypoglycaemia
- Multisensory impairment: vision, hearing, vestibular, proprioceptive
- Dehydration, fluid overload/oedema
- Postural hypotension
- Neuropathy, autonomic and peripheral
- Foot disorders
- Balance, mobility, and gait disorders
- Cognitive impairment
- Depression
- Comorbid diseases and conditions: cardiovascular, cerebrovascular, peripheral vascular, anaemia, incontinence, sleep disorders, arthritis, etc.
- Medications, especially centrally acting and psychoactive drugs and cardiovascular agents
- Polypharmacy

29.4.3 Hyperglycaemia and hypoglycaemia

Hyperglycaemia can cause vision impairment, dizziness, increased urination due to osmotic diuresis, and dehydration, each of which can lead to falls. *Hypoglycaemia* can cause confusion and imbalance, also resulting in falls. Lower haemoglobin A_{1c} levels, reflecting lower blood glucose levels, have been associated with falling in frail older adults [15]. Older adults with diabetes may have a decreased ability to perceive the onset and occurrence of both hyperglycaemia and hypoglycaemia, and thus fail to take appropriate corrective actions. There are no randomized controlled trials indicating the degree of glycaemic control that is most appropriate and beneficial for vulnerable older adults, nor is there any evidence for the level of glycaemic control that decreases the risk of falling.

29.4.4 Sensory impairment

Sensory impairment contributes to falling by causing older adults to become disoriented in their physical environment. Diabetes is directly responsible for several serious sensory impairments, which interact with and exacerbate other sensory impairments common in older adults resulting from physiologic changes of aging and comorbid conditions.

Vision

Eye diseases prevalent in the older adult population include refractive error (e.g. far-sightedness), cataracts, glaucoma and macular degeneration. Diabetes causes diabetic retinopathy and is a risk factor for cataracts and glaucoma.

Impairment in vision in older adults is associated with limitations in mobility, in activities of daily living, and in the instrumental activities of daily living. The impairments in vision which most likely to lead to falls are those that most directly affect everyday functioning. Visual field loss, as compared to declines in visual acuity, stereoacuity and contrast sensitivity, is the component of vision most associated with an increased risk for falls [16–19].

Vision difficulties can be a factor in patient medication errors, especially in the setting of polypharmacy, and so also indirectly contribute to falling. Older adults needing to read glucometer results and fill insulin syringes are at particular risk.

Hearing

Hearing impairment is common in older adults, and diabetes has been shown to be associated with early development of sensorineural hearing loss [20]. Hearing impairment, by distorting environmental input about an individual's position in space, may contribute to falls. It may be synergistic with vision impairment in causing functional decline.

Vestibular

A loss of vestibular function leads to disorders of balance, especially with changes in the body position.

Proprioceptive

Proprioceptive impairment, with diabetic neuropathy being a significant cause (see below), leads to disorientation with ambulation. Older adults are at greatest risk for falling in those circumstances when proprioceptive input is most relied upon, for example, when walking on uneven surfaces or in dark or poorly lit areas.

29.4.5 Alterations in fluid status

Older adults with diabetes are particularly vulnerable to alterations in fluid status, which may be due to a variety of causes, including physiological changes of aging (e.g. decreased thirst), comorbid diseases (e.g.

congestive heart failure) and medications (e.g. diuretics). Hyperglycaemia resulting from poorly controlled diabetes can cause an osmotic diuresis leading to dehydration. Both, diabetic nephropathy and its treatment affect the fluid status of older adults, thereby increasing the complexity of their medication regimens and predisposing them to falls. Predialysis systolic blood pressure levels have been correlated with falls in dialysis patients. Other associations with falls in the dialysis population include advancing age, increased comorbidity, medications (especially antidepressants), a previous history of falling and the use of assistive devices [8, 9].

29.4.6 Postural hypotension

Diabetes contributes to, or is associated with, multiple aetiologies of postural instability including:

- Age-related physiological changes, such as diastolic dysfunction, vascular stiffness and decreased renal salt and water conservation.

- Postprandial and exercise-induced hypotension.

- Autonomic insufficiency, both central and peripheral.

- Cardiac disease, including myocardial ischaemia and arrhythmia.

- Infection.

- Dehydration.

- Medications, including alpha-receptor blockers, diuretics, beta-receptor blockers, vasodilators and other antihypertensives, opiates and sedative-hypnotics, antipsychotics and phosphodiesterase-5 inhibitors.

29.4.7 Neuropathy

- *Autonomic:* Diabetic autonomic neuropathy can cause hypotension, particularly postural hypotension and diarrhoea, and may have a role in muscle weakness.

- *Peripheral:* Diabetic peripheral neuropathy is a significant cause of balance and gait disorders and of falls in the older adult population. Motor neuropathy contributes to formation of calluses, hammer-toes and other deformities of the feet. Sensory neuropathy causes loss of sensation, paraethesias and chronic pain, and can ultimately lead to a lack of coordination of gait and to the development and poor healing of foot ulcers.

29.4.8 Foot disorders

Disorders of the feet and ankles, resulting from the neuropathic and vascular complications of diabetes, include loss of sensation, pain, wounds and amputation. These disorders can lead to a reduced walking speed, balance difficulties and falling. Toe strength plays a critical role in maintaining balance when the body's centre of gravity is displaced, and weakness or amputation decreases the body's ability to avoid or break a fall [21, 22].

29.4.9 Balance, mobility and gait disorders

Older adults with diabetes have reduced self-reported physical functioning, and also have a decreased performance on standard physical performance measures of balance and mobility [23, 24]. Vision, hearing and vestibular impairments; changes in fluid status; postural instability; neuropathy; and foot problems all contribute to disorders in balance, mobility and gait in this population. These disorders interact with musculoskeletal diseases such as osteoarthritis to contribute to: (i) difficulty and dependency in transferring and in mobility functions; and (ii) falling.

29.4.10 Cognitive impairment and depression

Diabetes is postulated to have an aetiology in Alzheimer's disease as well as vascular dementia. Diabetes is also strongly associated with depression, and both cognitive impairment and depression can lead to impairments in judgement and problem-solving. Depression causes impairment in concentration, while advancing dementia causes apraxia, and impairments in these executive functions predispose to falling. Impairment in immediate recall may be especially predictive of fall risk. Both severity of cognitive impairment and change in cognitive function (i.e. a recent decline in cognitive status) are associated with falling.

29.4.11 Diabetes complications and comorbid diseases and conditions

Multiple diabetes complications and comorbid diseases and conditions are associated with falling. Microvascular complications causing falls include diabetic retinopathy, nephropathy and neuropathy. Macrovascular complications causing falls include coronary artery disease (myocardial ischaemia, congestive heart failure, arrhythmia), cerebrovascular disease (transient ischaemic attacks, strokes) and peripheral vascular disease (claudication, foot ulceration, amputation). The comorbid condition most associated with falling in older adults with diabetes is previous stroke.

Anaemia of chronic disease, anaemia resulting from chronic kidney disease and anaemia associated with the use of angiotensin-converting enzyme (ACE) inhibitors (in susceptible individuals) may complicate diabetes in older adults.

Urinary incontinence, the need for frequent toileting (due to hyperglycaemia or diuretic use) and dependency in toileting all can be associated with falls. Diabetes is a leading aetiology for neurogenic bladder and overflow incontinence. Urge incontinence precipitates the need for rapid access to toileting; functional incontinence occurs when the older adult is unable to toilet in an expeditious manner. In trying to toilet to avoid an accident, older adults can increase their risk for falling.

29.4.12 Other diseases and conditions

Diseases not necessarily related to diabetes that increase fall risk include sleep disorders (associated with obesity and the metabolic syndrome), restless leg syndrome, other autonomic and peripheral neuropathies and arthritis disorders.

29.4.13 Overall health status

Older adults who report fair or poor health or a decline in health over the previous year have been shown to be more likely to fall [25].

29.4.14 Medications

Multiple medications – either individually or in combination with other medications and conditions – predispose older adults to falling. Central nervous system and cardiovascular drug classes are particularly problematic [26, 27].

At-risk medications include the following:

- opiates

- sedative-hypnotics and anxiolytics (especially benzodiazepines)

- antidepressants (especially tricyclic antidepressants; selective serotonin reuptake inhibitors are associated with falls to a lesser extent)

- anticonvulsants

- anticholinesterase inhibitors

- antipsychotics

- antiparkinsonian agents

- muscle relaxants

- diuretics

- vasodilators

- alpha-blockers

- beta-blockers

- other antihypertensives

- anti-arrhythmics (especially class 1A anti-arrhythmics)

- diabetes medications (especially those with pronounced hypoglycaemic effects such as insulin and the sulphonylureas)

- medications to treat erectile dysfunction (e.g. phosphodiesterase-5 inhibitors), and

- all medications with anticholinergic effects.

The antipsychotics are well known for their risk for falls, especially for older adults in institutional settings. This drug class is also problematic for its effects on glucose and lipid metabolism, worsening the metabolic syndrome and so exacerbating both diabetes and vascular disease.

Findings from the United Kingdom Prospective Diabetes Study showed that a tight control of blood glucose levels was associated with twice as many episodes of hypoglycaemia. Medications with pronounced hypoglycaemic effects, such as insulin and the sulphonylureas, can be especially challenging in this regard [14, 15, 28].

Combinations of certain medications increase the risk of fall for older adults (e.g. multiple agents having psychoactive effects or anticholinergic side effects). Certain drug-drug interactions (e.g. when one agent is a benzodiazepine) result from alterations in hepatic metabolism or renal excretion, perhaps as a consequence of diabetic nephropathy. *Polypharmacy* is well-documented as a risk for falling, with research studies having demonstrated an increased number of falls for those taking more than four different drugs concurrently [29, 30].

29.5 Risk factors for fall injury

Injury resulting from a fall is a function of the force of the fall, and of the part of the body impacted in the fall. Falls from greater height (e.g. a stairway or a bed using bedrails in the upright position), an inability to break a fall (e.g. an inability to reach for and hold onto a handrail or piece of furniture) and landing on a hard surface all increase the force of a fall. Older adults have slowed reaction times and impaired protective responses, and so may be unable to avoid injury as a consequence of falling. The physical impact of falls may be increased in older adults having a lower body mass index, and who have decreased musculature and subcutaneous tissues. Fracture is more likely with certain types of fall; for example, falling sideways on the femur is more likely to lead to hip fracture, while falling on an outstretched hand may lead to wrist fractures.

Older adults with diabetes may have worse consequences from falls, due not only to slow wound healing that can delay recovery but also to an increased risk of fractures with falling. Diabetes is a risk factor for osteoporosis and for osteoporotic fractures resulting from falls. The Study of Osteoporotic Fractures found that postmenopausal women with diabetes had an increased risk for falling and for hip and proximal humerus fractures with falling [31, 32]. The Women's Health Initiative found that postmenopausal women with diabetes had an increased risk for fractures overall and increased risks of hip, foot and spine fractures separately, despite having a higher bone mineral density [33]. These findings may reflect differences in the structure of bone.

Older adults with diabetes frequently have comorbid cardiac and vascular diseases warranting anticoagulation which, itself, can lead to an increase in injuries as a result of falling.

29.6 Evaluation of older adults with diabetes who fall

29.6.1 Screening

Older adults with diabetes should be screened yearly for falls. Those having two or more falls in the previous year, a single fall and an associated gait or balance disorder, or an injurious fall should be further evaluated. The aims of screening and evaluation are to identify potentially reversible or modifiable causes and conditions for falling, and to develop a management plan to limit falls and fall injuries. The evaluation of older adults with diabetes who fall is not substantially different from the evaluation of those without diabetes who fall. Rather, older adults with diabetes can have a greater burden of comorbid conditions predisposing to falls and a greater potential for worse consequences from falling [34–36].

29.6.2 History

Pertinent history includes the circumstances surrounding the fall(s) and associated medical and social conditions, and should be obtained from the patient and, if appropriate and possible, from caregivers. Older adults with diabetes should be questioned specifically about glycaemic management and diabetes complications. History-taking should cover:

- The circumstances of the fall(s), including location, time of day, activity associated with the fall, etc.

- Associated symptoms, including presyncope (and syncope), light-headedness, dizziness, confusion, palpitations, hypoglycaemic symptoms, etc.

- Any history of previous falls, including their frequency and pattern.

- Details of high-risk behaviours, such as certain home repairs, outdoor activities, etc.

- Environmental hazards [37].

- The status of the patient's diabetes and its management, including frequency and degree of hyperglycaemia and hypoglycaemia, current management and interventions, diabetes complications, etc.

- The presence of comorbid diseases and conditions, including heart disease (coronary artery disease, congestive heart failure, arrhythmia), anaemia, seizure disorder, stroke, Parkinson's disease and other movement disorders, cognitive impairment, neuropathy, depression/anxiety, sensory impairment, arthritis, etc.

- The patient's overall cognitive status and any recent change in cognition (e.g. delirium).

- The presence of other geriatric conditions and symptoms (e.g. incontinence, nocturia) and their relation to falls.

- Details of current medications, including over-the-counter products. Recent changes in the medication regimen, including any new medications, should be investigated. The use of high-risk medications should prompt questioning about the presence of any side effects and their severity. Similarly, the use of anticoagulants should prompt questioning about compliance, bleeding episodes, etc. An overall assessment of polypharmacy should be made.

- The pattern of alcohol use.

- The patient's functional status, including impairments in activities of daily living (ADLs), instrumental activities of daily living (IADLs) and mobility.

- Details of recent transitions which can be associated with an increased risk for falling (e.g. acute illness, discharge from a hospital or nursing facility, new medications).

- The availability and level of family and social support.

29.6.3 Physical examination

The physical examination should be directed by the patient's history, and include targeted assessment of cardiovascular, neurological and musculoskeletal systems. The examination should include a search for physical findings that indicate the state of diabetes and its complications:

- Vital signs, including orthostatic pulse and blood pressure. Vital signs should be measured, first, after the patient has been supine for 5 min; next, immediately upon standing; and last, after standing for 2 min. A 20 mmHg drop in systolic pressure in either standing position indicates orthostatic hypotension [36].

- Head and neck examination, including assessment of vision, hearing, the thyroid gland and carotid arteries.

- Cardiac examination, including evaluation for arrhythmia and assessment of volume status (dehydration, oedema).

- Neurological examination to assess cognitive status, sensory function (proprioception), muscle strength, cerebellar function, tremor, as well as balance, movement and gait difficulties. The evaluation of sensory function should include the extent and severity of sensory loss due to diabetic neuropathy. A timed 'Get-Up and Go' test may be considered to evaluate mobility and the ability to stand from a seated position [38, 39]. Older adults using assistive devices should be evaluated for their correct use.

- Musculoskeletal examination to assess joints for range of motion and presence of arthritic changes.

- Foot examination, including the evaluation of ulcerations, deformities and painful lesions.

29.6.4 Laboratory evaluation and radiological imaging

Laboratory testing and imaging should be directed by the results of the history and physical examination. Glucose monitoring and HbA$_{1c}$ level are important as indicators of glycaemic control in diabetes management. The following may also be considered, depending on the particularities of the fall syndrome: complete blood count; electrolytes; renal function; thyroid-stimulating hormone; vitamin B$_{12}$; electrocardiogram; brain imaging; and bone density scan. Indications for imaging of the brain include a history of head injury and focal deficits on neurological examination.

29.6.5 Assessment of older adults in hospital or nursing facility settings

Older adults with diabetes are more likely to be hospitalized and to reside in long-stay nursing facilities than those without diabetes, and represent 'special' populations when evaluating falls. These patients should be initially assessed and then regularly monitored for acute cognitive changes (e.g. delirium) which might increase fall risk during hospitalization. Similarly, older adults with diabetes in institutional settings are at risk for nosocomially acquired dehydration and infection (e.g. pneumonia, urinary tract infection), and so should be monitored for these conditions, which contribute to falls if not diagnosed. Older adults with difficulty or dependency in transferring and toileting are at risk for falls when attempting these tasks, especially when without assistance.

29.7 Management of older adults with diabetes who fall

The goals of management for older adults with diabetes who fall are to prevent future falls, to prevent fall-related injuries, to maintain independence, and to address the fear of falling [34–36].

Management strategies for this population come with a number of inherent challenges. Because falls have multiple possible causes and, therefore, multiple possible interventions (Table 29.2), effective fall management requires targeting interventions to individual patients and their environments. The typical older adult with diabetes has a multifactorial aetiology for falling, necessitating multicomponent intervention strategies. For each patient, the benefits of each intervention must be weighed against its burdens and risks. Many interventions are time- and effort-demanding for older adults and their caregivers. Some interventions require ongoing monitoring and optimization (e.g. glycaemic and hypertension medication regimens, correct use of assistive devices). The benefits of some interventions can be time-limited in nature (e.g. physical therapy). Interventions frequently entail the physician coordinating care with other providers, such as physical therapists, occupational therapists and social workers. Older adults with diabetes who fall almost always have multiple comorbid diseases and conditions; fall management interventions can conflict with evidence-based guidelines for diabetes and those comorbidities [40]. Finally, in some health care systems and settings, physician reimbursement may be geared toward diagnosis and the management of diseases and not toward prevention – which is the primary focus of fall management interventions.

29.7.1 Glycaemic status

It appears that no conclusive studies have been conducted to determine the optimal level of glycaemic control for the frail or vulnerable older adult population; neither is any evidence-derived algorithm available to stratify older adults for glycaemic control based on their medical and functional status. Falling is one important consideration in the context of the overall health of individuals in deciding on targets for diabetes management. For older adults with diabetes who fall, the optimal level of glycaemic control should be determined on an individual basis. Those with recurrent falls especially need to avoid hypoglycaemia. Medications with potent hypoglycaemic effects (e.g. insulin, sulphonylureas) should be used cautiously, particularly in those older adults who are especially vulnerable, who live alone, who have cognitive impairment, or who have previously demonstrated inconsistent eating patterns (e.g. missing meals).

Table 29.2 Management interventions for older adults with diabetes who fall.

- Avoid hyperglycaemia and hypoglycaemia.
- Ophthalmology consultation. Treatment of diabetic retinopathy, cataracts, glaucoma, macular degeneration, etc. Corrective lenses. Environmental modifications.
- Audiology consultation. Hearing aids and other assistive devices.
- Address underlying causes of postural imbalance. Eliminate or decrease medication doses. Compression stockings. Liberalize fluid, salt, and caffeine restrictions.
- Referral to podiatry. Appropriate footwear.
- Address underlying causes of postural imbalance, movement disorders, and impairments in gait or balance. Referral to physical and occupational therapy. Strength/resistance training; range of motion exercises. Gait and balance training. Postural awareness exercises. Appropriate assistive devices.
- Regular assessment of diabetes comorbid conditions for progression and change in impact on mobility and risk for falls. Continual optimization of management of comorbidities. Treatment/management of depression and cognitive impairment.
- Minimize medications that are centrally acting and/or that have psychoactive and anticholinergic side effects. Minimize polypharmacy. Consider vitamin D supplementation.
- Review benefits and risks of anticoagulation.
- Consider treatment of osteoporosis.
- Home safety assessment and environmental interventions.

29.7.2 Sensory impairments

Vision and hearing impairments should be further assessed (e.g. ophthalmology and audiology consultations) and managed with the appropriate interventions (e.g. cataract surgery, laser therapy for diabetic retinopathy) and assistive devices (corrective lenses, hearing aids). Environmental modifications for older adults with diabetes who have vision impairment include lighting in the home and glare reduction. Mobility training for the visually impaired can also be considered.

29.7.3 Alterations in fluid balance and postural hypotension

Management interventions should be directed to correcting or treating the underlying causes. Diuretics, vasodilators, alpha-blockers and other antihypertensive medications should be used with caution (and at the lowest dose that provides benefit) in older adults who fall. Other interventions that may be considered include use of compression stockings and the liberalization of fluid, salt and caffeine restrictions. Older adults and their caregivers should be educated about the risk of falling with postural changes.

29.7.4 Neuropathy and foot disorders

Older adults with diabetes should be referred to podiatry when appropriate. Footwear that minimizes balance and gait difficulties (e.g. low heel, thin sole) should be selected.

29.7.5 Balance, mobility and gait disorders

Older adults with movement disorders or impairments in balance or gait can be referred for physical and/or occupational therapy. Physical therapists can assess impaired arm or leg strength and/or range of motion and recommend strength/resistance training or range of motion exercises. Therapists can also provide balance and gait training. Older adults may benefit from postural awareness exercises, such as tai chi or yoga. Appropriate assistive devices, such as canes and walkers, which provide a wider base of support, should be prescribed and assessed for their correct use.

29.7.6 Comorbid diseases and conditions

Diabetes comorbid diseases and conditions should be regularly evaluated for their progression and changing impact on mobility and risk for falls (e.g. progression of coronary artery disease, increasing frequency of urinary incontinence). Management should be continually optimized to lessen the risk for falls, with providers periodically screening for depression and cognitive impairment. Effective depression treatment can improve attention and concentration deficits that can lead to falls, but many agents have side effects that can increase fall risk. The management of cognitive impairment includes minimizing offending medications and providing a supportive environment. Older adults with cognitive impairment should be prescribed assistive devices appropriate to their cognitive ability.

29.7.7 Medications

Medications that are centrally acting and have psychoactive effects should be assessed for their overall benefit versus their risk for falls. Medications with anticholinergic effects should be similarly evaluated. Any medications implicated in postural hypotension or in balance, mobility or gait disorders should be discontinued, if possible.

Polypharmacy should be addressed, with the aim of eliminating medications or reducing their dosage, especially those that are risk factors for falls. Consideration should be given to eliminating medications that have benefit but are of low priority in an individual patient's treatment plans (e.g. ACE inhibitors or beta-blockers in patients with advanced cancer). The resulting medication regimens should be examined for drug–drug interactions and for the optimal dosing of medications (e.g. spreading antihypertensive medications throughout the day, taking certain medications at bedtime). Finally, ongoing medication reconciliation is required, with continual attention to optimal dosing, the potential for medication interactions, and the correct use of medications by older patients. The results of several studies have indicated that vitamin D supplementation decreases the risk for falls, most likely by its beneficial effects on muscle function [41, 42]. However, to be effective and safe the total daily dosing should be 800–2000 IU and accompanied by an adequate calcium supplementation [43].

29.7.8 Fall-related injury

Older adults with certain cardiac and vascular diabetes comorbidities may be candidates for anticoagulation. A discussion with patients and their caregivers should address the anticoagulation's benefits and its risks for fall-related injury (e.g. intracranial bleeding). Of note,

anticoagulation in this population is the subject of ongoing research; physicians and other providers should examine research study population samples and outcomes to determine if these are applicable to their own patient populations and settings. Older adults continuing on anticoagulants should be regularly reassessed for fall risk.

The treatment of osteoporosis can decrease the incidence of fall-related fractures. However, medications currently indicated for osteoporosis can have problematic side effects in older adults with diabetes: calcium binds many medications, making dosing regimens difficult for older adults with polypharmacy; bisphosphonates are contraindicated in individuals with upper gastrointestinal disease, such as diabetic gastroparesis; and oestrogen increases the incidence of cardiovascular and thromboembolic events and so is contraindicated in those with known disease. Hip protectors – a non-pharmacological intervention – have poor adherence rates, and the evidence for their ability to prevent hip fractures is conflicting. One recent study with good adherence rates failed to show any benefit in a long-stay nursing facility population [44]. One final intervention to consider is routine weight-bearing exercise.

29.7.9 Environmental interventions

Home safety assessment and recommended environmental interventions should target each older adult's particular fall risks, with emphasis placed on the circumstances of previous falls. Older adults in new or unfamiliar settings may require additional care and attention.

Lighting should be optimized, especially for older adults with vision impairment. Lighting at night must be adequate to enable safe night-time toileting. Contrasts can be used to highlight steps and stairways; high gloss and high glare flooring should be avoided.

Caregivers should attend to barriers at floor level, including slippery floors, carpeting and throw rugs, electric cords and obstructions, and impediments such as furniture and clutter. Older adults – especially those with impairments in mobility and transferring – often use the furniture as a support; consequently, any furniture should be stable and of the correct height and without sharp edges. Railings and grab bars can be placed in the home to assist with mobility and to help the older adult avoid or break a fall.

The *bathroom* is a high risk environment for falling, with bathroom floor mats a particular hazard. Older adults are at risk for falls when getting into and out of the bath and shower, and may be aided by the use of shower chairs and the judicious placement of grab bars. Individuals with urge incontinence, frequent urination, nocturia or difficulty or dependency in toileting, may also benefit from grab bars and night lighting.

29.7.10 Hospital or nursing facility settings

Older adults with diabetes in hospital and nursing facility settings have unique fall risks. Providers should avoid prescribing medications and other interventions in the hospital that can precipitate or worsen acute cognitive changes (e.g. delirium) and thereby increase the risk for falling. Likewise, polypharmacy and the use of psychotropic medications and medications that lead to dehydration should be minimized in long-stay nursing facilities. In both settings, it is important to coordinate the patient's medication regimens with other parts of their daily schedules. For example, those receiving hypoglycaemic agents need to receive their meals on time; the dosing of antihypertensives should also take into account the possibility of postprandial hypotension.

Physical restraints should be avoided. Bedrails in the upright position may act as physical restraints and lead to falls from a greater height than otherwise. Low beds and bedside mattresses are alternatives that decrease the risk of fall-related injury. Other preventive measures should focus on transfers and on toileting (e.g. frequent toileting for patients undergoing diuretic treatment). In general, caregivers should search for the least restrictive means by which older adults can maintain independence in a safe fashion (e.g. correct use of assistive devices, assistance in transferring).

One critical component to reducing falls and fall-related injuries in institutional settings is the ongoing education of nursing staff and other care providers.

29.8 Patient safety and quality of care

The impact of falls on morbidity, disability, loss of independence and mortality in the older adult population is recognized by health policy decision makers. Falls and fall-related injuries are an ongoing focus of regulatory agencies, initiatives and guidelines aimed at improving patient safety and the quality of care in hospital, long-term care and outpatient settings (e.g. Joint Commission on the Accreditation of Healthcare Organizations (JCAHO) in the United States). The Assessing Care of the Vulnerable Elders (ACOVE) initiative developed the Vulnerable Elders Survey (VES-13), a clinical measure of vulnerability whose goal was to identify older adults at risk for functional decline or death [45]. The ACOVE initiative has since developed quality indicators for a number of diseases and conditions prevalent among vulnerable older adults, including diabetes and falls [46, 47]. The complexity underlying falling in the older adult population with diabetes presents a challenge for guidelines and quality indicators to improve outcomes at the population level and yet remain flexible to accommodate the needs of individual patients.

References

1. Centers for Disease Control and Prevention. (2008) Costs of Falls Among Older Adults. Available at: http://www.cdc.gov/ncipc/factsheets/fallcost.htm.
2. Stevens, J.A., Corso, P.S., Finkelstein, E.A. and Miller, T.R. (2006) The costs of fatal and non-fatal falls among older adults. *Inj Prev*, 12, 290–5.
3. King, M.B. (2003) Falls. In: Hazzard, W.R., Blass, J.P., Halter, J.B., Ouslander, J.G. and Tinetti, M.E. (eds) *Principles of Geriatric Medicine and Gerontology*. 5th edition. McGraw-Hill, New York, pp. 1517–29.
4. Rubenstein, L.Z. and Josephson, K. R. (2002) The epidemiology of falls and syncope. *Clin Geriatr Med*, 18, 141–58.
5. Cigolle, C. T., Lee, P. G., Tian, Z. and Blaum, C. S. (2008) Geriatric conditions and diabetes: The Health and Retirement Study. *Journal of the American Geriatrics Society*, 56 (s1), s186–7.
6. Wallace, C., Reiber, G. E., Lemaster, J., Smith, D. G., Sullivan, K., Hayes, S. and Vath, C. (2002) Incidence of falls, risk factors for falls, and fall-related fractures in individuals with diabetes and a prior foot ulcer. *Diabetes Care*, 25, 1983–6.
7. Cook, W. L. and Jassal, S. V. (2005) Prevalence of falls among seniors maintained on hemodialysis. *Int Urol Nephrol*, 37, 649–52.
8. Cook, W. L., Tomlinson, G., Donaldson, M., Markowitz, S. N., Naglie, G., Sobolev, B. and Jassal, S. V. (2006) Falls and fall-related injuries in older dialysis patients. *Clin J Am Soc Nephrol*, 1, 1197–204.
9. Desmet, C., Beguin, C., Swine, C. and Jadoul, M. (2005) Falls in hemodialysis patients: prospective study of incidence, risk factors, and complications. *Am J Kidney Dis*, 45, 148–53.

10. Ray, W. A., Taylor, J. A., Brown, A. K., Gideon, P., Hall, K., Arbogast, P. and Meredith, S. (2005) Prevention of fall-related injuries in long-term care: a randomized controlled trial of staff education. *Arch Intern Med*, 165, 2293–8.

11. Fife, D. and Barancik, J. I. (1985) Northeastern Ohio Trauma Study III: incidence of fractures. *Ann Emerg Med*, 14, 244–8.

12. Tinetti, M. E., Inouye, S. K., Gill, T. M. and Doucette, J. T. (1995) Shared risk factors for falls, incontinence, and functional dependence. Unifying the approach to geriatric syndromes. *JAMA*, 273, 1348–53.

13. King, M. B. and Tinetti, M. E. (1995) Falls in community-dwelling older persons. *J Am Geriatr Soc*, 43, 1146–54.

14. Volpato, S., Leveille, S. G., Blaum, C., Fried, L. P. and Guralnik, J. M. (2005) Risk factors for falls in older disabled women with diabetes: the women's health and aging study. *J Gerontol A Biol Sci Med Sci*, 60, 1539–45.

15. Nelson, J. M., Dufraux, K. and Cook, P. F. (2007) The relationship between glycemic control and falls in older adults. *J Am Geriatr Soc*, 55, 2041–4.

16. Adler, A. I., Stratton, I. M., Neil, H. A., Yudkin, J. S., Matthews, D. R., Cull, C. A., Wright, A. D., Turner, R. C. and Holman, R. R. (2000) Association of systolic blood pressure with macrovascular and microvascular complications of type 2 diabetes (UKPDS 36): prospective observational study. *Br Med J*, 321, 412–19.

17. Coleman, A.L., Cummings, S.R., Yu, F., Kodjebacheva, G., Ensrud, K. E., Gutierrez, P., Stone, K. L., Cauley, J. A., Pedula, K. L., Hochberg, M.C. and Mangione, C.M. (2007) Binocular visual-field loss increases the risk of future falls in older white women. *J Am Geriatr Soc*, 55, 357–64.

18. Freeman, E. E., Munoz, B., Rubin, G. and West, S. K. (2007) Visual field loss increases the risk of falls in older adults: the Salisbury eye evaluation. *Invest Ophthalmol Vis Sci*, 48, 4445–50.

19. Stratton, I. M., Adler, A. I., Neil, H. A., Matthews, D. R., Manley, S. E., Cull, C. A., Hadden, D., Turner, R. C. and Holman, R. R. (2000) Association of glycaemia with macrovascular and microvascular complications of type 2 diabetes (UKPDS 35): prospective observational study. *Be Med J*, 321, 405–12.

20. Vaughan, N., James, K., McDermott, D., Griest, S. and Fausti, S. (2006) A 5-year prospective study of diabetes and hearing loss in a veteran population. *Otol Neurotol*, 27, 37–43.

21. Menz, H. B., Lord, S. R., St George, R. and Fitzpatrick, R. C. (2004) Walking stability and sensorimotor function in older people with diabetic peripheral neuropathy. *Arch Phys Med Rehabil*, 85, 245–52.

22. Menz, H. B., Morris, M. E. and Lord, S. R. (2006) Foot and ankle risk factors for falls in older people: a prospective study. *J Gerontol A Biol Sci Med Sci*, 61, 866–70.

23. Volpato, S., Blaum, C., Resnick, H., Ferrucci, L., Fried, L. P. and Guralnik, J. M. (2002) Comorbidities and impairments explaining the association between diabetes and lower extremity disability: The Women's Health and Aging Study. *Diabetes Care*, 25, 678–83.

24. Volpato, S., Ferrucci, L., Blaum, C., Ostir, G., Cappola, A., Fried, L. P., Fellin, R. and Guralnik, J. M. (2003) Progression of lower-extremity disability in older women with diabetes: the Women's Health and Aging Study. *Diabetes Care*, 26, 70–5.

25. Gill, T., Taylor, A. W. and Pengelly, A. (2005) A population-based survey of factors relating to the prevalence of falls in older people. *Gerontology*, 51, 340–5.

26. Leipzig, R. M., Cumming, R. G. and Tinetti, M. E. (1999a) Drugs and falls in older people: a systematic review and meta-analysis: I. Psychotropic drugs. *J Am Geriatr Soc*, 47, 30–9.

27. Leipzig, R. M., Cumming, R. G. and Tinetti, M. E. (1999b) Drugs and falls in older people: a systematic review and meta-analysis: II. Cardiac and analgesic drugs. *J Am Geriatr Soc*, 47, 40–50.

28. UK Prospective Diabetes Study (UKPDS) Group (1998) Intensive blood-glucose control with sulphonylureas or insulin compared with conventional treatment and risk of complications in patients with type 2 diabetes (UKPDS 33). *Lancet*, 352, 837–53.

29. Campbell, A. J., Borrie, M. J. and Spears, G. F. (1989) Risk factors for falls in a community-based prospective study of people 70 years and older. *J Gerontol*, 44, M112–17.

30. Cumming, R.G. (1998) Epidemiology of medication-related falls and fractures in the elderly. *Drugs Aging*, 12, 43–53.

31. Schwartz, A. V., Hillier, T. A., Sellmeyer, D. E., Resnick, H. E., Gregg, E., Ensrud, K. E., Schreiner, P. J., Margolis, K. L., Cauley, J. A., Nevitt, M. C., Black, D. M. and Cummings, S. R. (2002) Older women with diabetes have a higher risk of falls: a prospective study. *Diabetes Care*, 25, 1749–54.

32. Schwartz, A. V., Sellmeyer, D. E., Ensrud, K. E., Cauley, J. A., Tabor, H. K., Schreiner, P. J., Jamal, S. A., Black, D. M. and Cummings, S. R. (2001) Older women with diabetes have an increased risk of fracture: a prospective study. *J Clin Endocrinol Metab*, 86, 32–8.

33. Bonds, D. E., Larson, J. C., Schwartz, A. V., Strotmeyer, E. S., Robbins, J., Rodriguez, B. L., Johnson, K. C. and Margolis, K. L. (2006) Risk of fracture in

women with type 2 diabetes: the Women's Health Initiative Observational Study. *J Clin Endocrinol Metab*, 91, 3404–10.

34. American Geriatrics Society, British Geriatrics Society and Prevention, American Academy Of Orthopaedic Surgeons Panel On Falls Prevention. (2001) Guideline for the prevention of falls in older persons. *J Am Geriatr Soc*, 49, 664–72.

35. Gillespie, L. D., Gillespie, W. J., Robertson, M. C., Lamb, S. E., Cumming, R. G. and Rowe, B. H. (2003) Interventions for preventing falls in elderly people. *Cochrane Database Syst Rev*, CD000340.

36. Tinetti, M.E. (2003) Clinical practice. Preventing falls in elderly persons. *N Engl J Med*, 348, 42–9.

37. Cumming, R. G., Thomas, M., Szonyi, G., Salkeld, G., O'Neill, E., Westbury, C. and Frampton, G. (1999) Home visits by an occupational therapist for assessment and modification of environmental hazards: a randomized trial of falls prevention. *J Am Geriatr Soc*, 47, 1397–402.

38. Mathias, S., Nayak, U. S. and Isaacs, B. (1986) Balance in elderly patients: the 'get-up and go' test. *Arch Phys Med Rehabil*, 67, 387–9.

39. Podsiadlo, D. and Richardson, S. (1991) The timed 'Up and Go': a test of basic functional mobility for frail elderly persons. *J Am Geriatr Soc*, 39, 142–8.

40. Boyd, C. M., Darer, J., Boult, C., Fried, L. P., Boult, L. and Wu, A. W. (2005) Clinical practice guidelines and quality of care for older patients with multiple co-morbid diseases: implications for pay for performance. *JAMA*, 294, 716–24.

41. Bischoff-Ferrari, H. A., Dawson-Hughes, B., Willett, W. C., Staehelin, H. B., Bazemore, M. G., Zee, R. Y.

and Wong, J. B. (2004) Effect of Vitamin D on falls: a meta-analysis. *JAMA*, 291, 1999–2006.

42. Bischoff-Ferrari, H. A., Orav, E. J. and Dawson-Hughes, B. (2006) Effect of cholecalciferol plus calcium on falling in ambulatory older men and women: a 3-year randomized controlled trial. *Arch Intern Med*, 166, 424–30.

43. Broe, K. E., Chen, T. C., Weinberg, J., Bischoff-Ferrari, H. A., Holick, M. F. and Kiel, D. P. (2007) A higher dose of vitamin d reduces the risk of falls in nursing home residents: a randomized, multiple-dose study. *J Am Geriatr Soc*, 55, 234–9.

44. Kiel, D. P., Magaziner, J., Zimmerman, S., Ball, L., Barton, B. A., Brown, K. M., Stone, J. P., Dewkett, D. and Birge, S. J. (2007) Efficacy of a hip protector to prevent hip fracture in nursing home residents: the HIP PRO randomized controlled trial. *JAMA*, 298, 413–22.

45. Saliba, D., Elliott, M., Rubenstein, L. Z., Solomon, D. H., Young, R. T., Kamberg, C. J., Roth, C., Maclean, C. H., Shekelle, P. G., Sloss, E. M. and Wenger, N. S. (2001) The Vulnerable Elders Survey: a tool for identifying vulnerable older people in the community. *J Am Geriatr Soc*, 49, 1691–9.

46. Rubenstein, L. Z., Powers, C. M. and MacLean, C. H. (2001) Quality indicators for the management and prevention of falls and mobility problems in vulnerable elders. *Ann Intern Med*, 135, 686–93.

47. Shekelle, P. and Vijan, S. (2007) Quality indicators for the care of diabetes mellitus in vulnerable elders. *J Am Geriatr Soc*, 55 (Suppl. 2), S312–17.

SECTION VI

Optimizing Diabetes Care in Older People

The Role of Specialist Nurses and Other Members of the Multidisciplinary Team (MDT)

Carolin D. Taylor and Timothy J. Hendra

Robert Hadfield Wing, Northern General Hospital, Department of Geriatric Medicine, Sheffield, UK

Key messages

- Multidisciplinary assessment of the older person with diabetes should include formal evaluation of cognition, mood and functional status.
- Liaison between the multidisciplinary team and the formal/informal carers is important in order to review treatment goals, the risk of hypoglycaemia, and the need for rehabilitation in particular as the older person with diabetes ages and becomes frail.
- The roles and scope of practice of Specialist Nurses and other members of the multidisciplinary team in the UK is evolving to include prescribing and other duties previously undertaken by medical staff.

30.1 Introduction

Older people with diabetes have a high prevalence of recognized and unrecognized cognitive dysfunction, depression and functional disability [1]. This presents particular challenges for the multidisciplinary team (MDT) that has to employ additional skills to those used when caring for younger adults with less comorbidity. The aims of the MDT in caring for an older person with diabetes embrace those for a younger adult but include, in addition, the need to take particular account of these comorbidities in the context of normal ageing and the need for informal and formal carer support (Table 30.1). As well as education and evaluating the factors that will influence diabetes management, the team may need to screen the person for mood, cognitive dysfunction and functional status, which could in turn influence the patient's treatment concordance and ability to cope with hypoglycaemia. The person's present and future reliance on formal and informal carers will affect the risk/benefit assessment of different therapy options, as well as treatment goals and the strategy for review.

When managing younger adults, the diabetes MDT often makes referrals to other agencies such as vascular surgeons and ophthalmologists. However, for the older person with diabetes the list of potential comorbidities and interactions with other specialist MDTs is greater, with the additional need to recognize when rehabilitation may be needed.

Diabetes in Old Age. Third Edition. Edited by Alan J. Sinclair
© 2009 John Wiley & Sons, Ltd

Table 30.1 The aims of multidisciplinary care for older people.

1	Development of a personalized care plan for the management of the person's diabetes that takes account of their other comorbidities.
2	Screening, prevention and treatment of acute and chronic diabetes complications.
3	Rapid identification and referral of the person with diabetes to other agencies for the management of non-diabetes related problems, including rehabilitation when necessary.
4	Maintenance of well-being of the person with diabetes with their continued residence at home in the community wherever possible.
5	Effective working with other specialist teams caring for older people.
6	Recognition of the need to change the management of a person's diabetes with normal ageing.
7	Education and effective support for the formal and informal carers of older people with diabetes.

30.2 The relationship of the diabetes MDT with other services for older people

The diabetes MDT will need to establish effective links with other teams who may care for the same person (Figure 30.1). These people may be dependent upon formal and informal carers for support in order to live independently in the community. As they approach the end of life they often become frail and unsteady, with an increased risk of falling that may be exacerbated by hypoglycaemia or poor diabetes control. Falls in the older person with diabetes are also associated with reduced muscle strength and greater risk of fracture [2–5]. Due to mood and cognitive problems, elderly people with diabetes in the UK may present to Old Age Psychiatry Team in the community as well as hospital, and also be supported by community psychiatric nurses.

Other teams that may be caring for the same person may include palliative care, heart failure and cardiac rehabilitation, as well community matrons and intermediate care teams. It is important that the diabetes MDT can link effectively with other teams and know when to step forward and coordinate care, or take a back seat, when diabetes is not the person's main problem.

A recent study from the UK has also demonstrated the value of inter-agency collaboration between the diabetes service and ambulance services for people with severe hypoglycaemia. In this study, ambulance crews who have been trained by Diabetes Specialist Nurses (DSNs) prospectively referred people who had been treated successfully at home for an acute hypoglycaemic episode and who were safe not to be admitted, to the local DSN team. All people referred were contacted by telephone, and the majority (79%) also attended a clinic appointment where their symptoms and treatment were reviewed. The people in this study were aged 25 to 92 years, and 50% of them were aged >60 years [6].

30.3 The changing role of the MDT in service delivery

The role of the MDT has been changing rapidly over recent years as professional boundaries have become less distinct and care has become firmly person-based, with service changes aimed at reducing constraints associated with the primary/secondary care interface. Within the team the roles of the DSN – and to a lesser extent of the pharmacist – may evolve further in the UK as a consequence of their ability to act as independent and supplementary prescribers, respectively.

Many changes in service delivery are, however, driven in the main to achieve biomedical targets of glycaemic, blood pressure and lipid control, as well preventive screening of the eyes and feet. In pursuit of these goals, people are submitted to ever-increasing polypharmacy that invariably leads to problems with concordance and the potential for treatment-limiting side effects such as hypoglycaemia. Some of the unmeasured benefits of multidisciplinary care may be lost – those of spending time with the person to evaluate their knowledge deficiencies, providing information and encouraging health-related behaviours that may result in the achievement of biomedical targets, without the need for a quickly written prescription. General practitioners in the UK recognize that their efforts often do not meet their patients' expectations and that the MDT may provide the tailored approach to care, encompassing their need to meet targets and improve patient adherence/compliance with their advice [7].

30.4 The 'Patient'

Patient empowerment and role in deciding their own management and treatment goals are well established as the centre of MDT functioning. The majority of

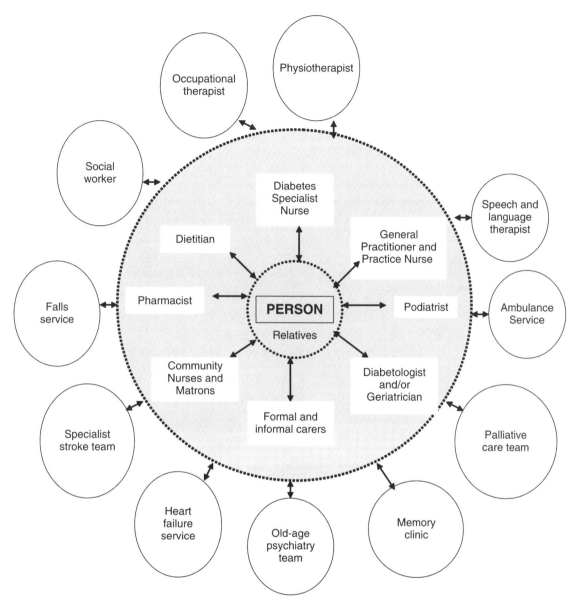

Figure 30.1 The relationships of the diabetes multidisciplinary team (MDT).

younger adults are cognitively intact and have capacity to participate in these decisions. However, many older people have a limited capacity for decision making as a result of dementia, mood abnormalities or cerebrovascular disease. The effect of these diseases on the ability of the person to make a decision may be exacerbated by hypo- and hyperglycaemia, and may fluctuate in severity. These issues are the centre of the Mental Capacity Act in the UK, which clarifies the roles of relatives and friends in supporting older people who lack

capacity, as well as the position of Advance Directives in guiding care for someone who lacks capacity.

For those people who lack or who have limited capacity, the MDT should liaise with relatives, friends and perhaps formal and informal carers to identify risks of hypoglycaemia due to over-medication or inconsistent food intake, as well as the person's ability to recognize and cope with this problem. The information supplied should influence the choice of treatment, glycaemic targets and any monitoring in the community.

30.5   The roles of the individual team members

30.5.1   The diabetes specialist nurse or diabetes educator

The diabetes specialist nurse (DSN) in the past has had two main roles (see Table 30.2). Principally, in terms of the time involved, DSNs delivered or supported care by giving advice either face to face or over the telephone to people, as well as to other health care professionals. Previously, the role of the DSN in educating people,

relatives and friends, and formal carers often took second place to the immediate demands of the service, but is no less important. To these roles may now be added that of delivering nurse-led diabetes clinics as a consequence of their ability to prescribe, thereby allowing the additional scope to manage aspects of patient care that hitherto were the sole prerogative of medical staff.

Hospital-based DSNs have traditionally concentrated upon giving lifestyle advice, support and medicines management, either face to face or over the telephone. There is evidence that their role improves glycaemic control and reduces hospital length of stay

Table 30.2   Key roles for the multidisciplinary team (MDT).

	Team member	Role
1	Diabetes Specialist Nurse (DSN) or Diabetes Educator (Hospital or community nurse with additional qualifications in diabetes)	• Education for patients and carers • Advice on diabetes medicines management • Delivering specialist diabetes clinics • Diabetes related prescribing to protocol/algorithm • Education and advice for health care professionals
2	Nurses other than DSNs	• Management of non-diabetes problems • Non-diabetes prescribing to protocol/algorithm
3	Dietician	• Assessment of nutritional status • Advice on healthy eating • Advice to older people with malnutrition • Diabetes-related dietary advice
4	Podiatrist	• Education for self-examination of feet and appropriate footwear • Advice for age-related foot problems • Screening, prevention and treatment of diabetes-related foot problems
5	Community Pharmacist	• Educational support • Recognition of iatrogenic problems • Medication review clinics (UK) • Diabetes related prescribing to protocol/algorithm (USA and UK)
6	Doctor	• Advice on diabetes medicines management • Delivering specialist diabetes clinics • Service development and clinical governance • Audit

[8–10]. DSNs employed specifically to manage older adults with diabetes, either in the acute setting or community, play a vital role in meeting the changing needs of this increasing population.

Recently, changes in the United Kingdom have allowed DSNs to become independent prescribers; provided that the medicines are within their area of competence, independent prescribers may prescribe any licensed medicine and some controlled drugs. Hospital-based DSN prescribers have been shown to reduce medication errors and to have a beneficial effect on length of stay [11].

In the USA, Diabetes Managed Care Programs can be delivered by specially trained nurses and pharmacists, using detailed protocols and algorithms under the supervision of a diabetologist. In both middle-class populations and populations of mixed ethnic backgrounds, the American Diabetes Association process and outcome measures are more likely to be met in people receiving nurse-directed care compared to those receiving usual care from busy physicians [12–14]. Whereas, physicians are not good at completing guidelines due to time constraints, trained nurses are good at sticking to protocols and have more time to provide lifestyle advice and preventive care. In the USA there is a clear trend for preventive care to be delivered by non-physician clinicians [15], and this has been reinforced by the results of a recent study which showed that nurse-directed diabetes care in a US county public health clinic reduced urgent hospital visits and admissions for preventable diabetes-related causes compared to usual care [16].

30.5.2 Nurses other than DSNs

The ability of nurses to prescribe according to protocol has led to the development of nurse-led clinics in many specialties in the UK. For people with diabetes at high risk of vascular disease, nurse-led clinics employing a systematic approach to blood pressure control with a pre-set drug protocol can provide adequate surveillance and achieve blood pressure targets with reduction in cardiovascular risk [17, 18]. It is possible that the beneficial effect was related to both improved compliance as well to a greater number of treatment changes; however, the challenge is to translate these studies into consistent practice in the long term.

30.5.3 The dietician

Within the MDT, dieticians have a traditional role of providing healthy eating guidelines or advice on diet,

more recently specifically around carbohydrate counting. In the older person it may be much more important to assess overall nutritional status, especially following, for example, a cerebrovascular accident when the person's ability to eat may be severely affected. The dietician can advise on a balanced diet and/or recommend dietary supplements to ensure adequate nutritional intake to both stabilize glycaemia and prevent potential complications of malnutrition, such as pressure ulcers (see Table 30.2).

30.5.4 The podiatrist

Good footcare is important for all older people, whether or not they have diabetes. Ageing is associated with a thinning of the skin and loss of elasticity and well as degenerative joint problems. With appropriate advice from a chiropodist/podiatrist, growing old need not be associated with discomfort, pain and poor mobility due to some common foot problems. Podiatry services also play a significant role in improving the quality of life and reducing the long-term complications associated with diabetes. As a consequence, their role in preventing diabetic amputations can save the UK National Health Service an average of £80 000 per person. Podiatrists have a role in the treatment of hard skin and callus, as well providing nail care. They can teach older people how to care for and examine their feet regularly, to look for changes in colour, swelling, skin damage, redness and discharge. In addition, they can provide advice on footwear.

30.5.5 The community pharmacist

Elderly people often approach community pharmacists for help and advice with non-diabetes-related problems. These interactions provide the opportunity for diabetes-related advice about lifestyle, the use of existing medications, and the need to consult other members of the MDT, as well for the purchase of new over-the-counter medications or devices. In addition, a community-based pharmacist may be the first to recognize new adverse reactions to medications and, in particular, any previously unrecognized hypoglyaemia. In the UK, pharmacists may also participate in primary care medication review clinics.

In the USA pharmacists can contribute to interdisciplinary health management programmes where their interventions include education and comprehensive medication management through collaborative practice agreements with physicians. This allows them to initiate, adjust or discontinue pharmacotherapy, to order investigations and to make podiatry referrals. In this situation, pharmacists have been shown to be effective in meeting biomedical targets of glycated haemoglobin levels and lipids, as well as improving adherence to preventive care measures such as annual eye and foot inspections [19].

30.5.6   The doctor

Traditionally, the role of the doctor was often to discuss management plans with the MDT at a weekly meeting at a fixed time and place. However, in the UK the duties and responsibilities of some diabetologists, geriatricians and GPs are changing significantly, such that it is usually impractical and unnecessary for them to be personally involved in discussing the management of the majority of people cared for by the MDT. The doctor's clinical role as part of the MDT often cannot be restricted to a fixed time with the need to be available to discuss problems with other MDT members as issues arise and decisions need to be made on a daily basis. A doctor's roles of leadership and clinical responsibility today often require a flexible pattern of working that allows him/her to respond quickly and to support other team members as the need arises.

The doctors' role frequently involves being responsible for governance of the diabetes service that incorporates the implementation of clinical protocols, auditing the processes of care and the achievement of clinical and managerial outcomes by the MDT. In the past, the doctor would sometimes personally receive most of the referrals of people with diabetes to the MDT, but today most MDTs in the UK have a single point of contact that bypasses the doctor and allows other team members to deal with issues quickly, rather than waiting for the person's details to be passed on.

Many GPs in the UK have little experience, and are understandably wary, of initiating insulin in the community for people with type 2 diabetes. Despite this there is increasing pressure from commissioners, as well as expectations from people with diabetes, for this treatment to be started outside of hospital. Many elderly people with diabetes will be unable to attend a hospital clinic or GP surgery, and will expect the service to come to them. The DSN has a unique role in this situation in terms of being able to support a district or GP surgery nurse in educating the patient and supervising treatment in the early stages. Once the patient is stabilized on insulin, and the community services have developed confidence with monitoring and reviewing glycaemic targets, then the DSN can

withdraw while remaining a point of reference for unexpected difficulties.

30.6   The role of the MDT in specific situations

30.6.1   Age-related frailty

Frail elderly people sometimes have relatively small meals or eat at times that are different to when they were younger. This may be due to the increased time it takes to prepare food or to a lack of nutritional drive, but is frequently due to unrecognized depression or cognitive impairment. It is important for the diabetes MDT to recognize when a previously fit older person with diabetes is becoming frail, as this may be unknown to other agencies and it may become the role of the diabetes team to assess the patient's mood, cognition and functional ability, or to make a referral to another agency to perform these assessments. Frequently the onset of frailty is insidious, and with it comes a significantly increased risk of hypoglycaemia, both in terms of the incidence of low blood sugar levels and an inability of the person to manage the problem – if he or she recognizes the symptoms. The occurrence of falls should indicate a need to urgently review the person's glycaemic control and targets, as well as to make the appropriate referral to a falls team or for rehabilitation.

The onset of frailty – with or without altered mood or cognitive function – frequently necessitates the need for additional support at home from either family or formal/informal carers, or perhaps the relocation of a person to sheltered housing or a care home. With the change in circumstances it is useful for the relatives, carers and or warden to have a contact number for the diabetes team at times of crisis, or if the person is 'off colour' and there is concern that this could be related to diabetes *per se*, or due to another problem such as a chest/urinary infection that is being treated by the primary care physician and may affect the person's food intake or diabetes control.

Sometimes, the presence of diabetes with the need to manage increasing hyperglycaemia, or to avoid recurrent hypoglycaemia, may be seen as a 'tipping point' for a previously independent frail person with diabetes to be admitted to a care home. In this situation the DSN may be able to offer alternative options for managing the person's diabetes, or provide additional support for formal and informal carers as well as their primary care physician, sufficient for a package of care in the community to be sustained. As a rule, the issues associated with managing diabetes should never be the reason for admission to a care home *per se*.

30.6.2 Care home residents

In the UK there are widespread concerns about the quality of diabetes care in residential and nursing homes that encompass the training needs of the formal carers and lack of structured review. Many care home residents are frail, with physical and cognitive impairments that make them vulnerable to poor nutrition and neglect [20]. Weight loss and protein-calorie under-nutrition are common, and will adversely affect diabetes care. Very often, diabetes and its complications are not the only chronic disease process present, yet the optimal treatment of blood glucose levels may significantly improve a resident's quality of life. The diabetes MDT can act as a point of reference for the referral of diabetes-related problems, as well as ensuring that the formal carers have access to education and support.

30.6.3 Terminal illness

People with diabetes approaching the end of their lives due to cancer, cardiac failure or other incurable disease, frequently present a challenge to health care professionals. Often, the management of diabetes in this situation is haphazard and left to clinical staff who do not have any particular expertise in diabetes management. A study from Cheltenham in the UK found that there was variability in diabetes monitoring, and little record of discussion with the person or family in this situation. A significant number of people continued to have their blood glucose monitored up until the day they died [21]. In another study conducted in Australia, the results emphasized the lack of evidence-based guidelines for managing diabetes in the context of palliative care, and recommended their development as well as the importance of increased collaboration between the diabetes MDT and palliative care specialists [22].

30.6.4 People from wide ethnic backgrounds

There is concern that people from non-Caucasian ethnic backgrounds have specific needs that pose particular challenges to the diabetes MDT. The issues of greater deprivation and social isolation, as well as dietary needs and cultural beliefs, may be of particular relevance to older people with diabetes, many of whom may neither speak nor understand English. This problem has been studied specifically in younger adults, but not in older people.

In the United Kingdom Asian Study Group an intervention of enhanced care using Asian link workers and extra community DSN sessions was associated with reductions in blood pressure and total cholesterol, but there was no significant effect on glycaemic control [23].

30.7 Summary

DSNs and the diabetes MDT need to work effectively with other specialist teams caring for older people with multiple pathology and comorbidities as well as diabetes.

The roles of the DSN and MDT differ when caring for the older person with diabetes compared to the younger adult in relation to the need to routinely assess cognitive function, mood and functional ability when setting treatment goals and assessing hypoglycaemic risk.

Although DSNs have always had a major role in education and prevention, in the UK the development of extended practice – and prescribing in particular – means that they may take on more tasks previously performed by medical staff, including the routine management of glycaemic control and cardiovascular risk factors, including hypertension and dyslipidaemia.

The basis for caring for the older person with diabetes remains thorough assessment, appropriate treatment goals, and structured care that accommodates changes in the person's cognitive and functional ability, while referring them for rehabilitation when necessary.

References

1. Munshi M, Grande L, Hayes M, Ayres D, Suhl E, Capelson R, Lin S, Milberg W and Weinger K. Cognitive dysfunction is associated with poor diabetes control in older adults. Diabetes Care 2006; 29: 1794–9.
2. Park SW, Goodpaster BH, Strotmeyer ES, Kuller LH, Broudeau R, Kammerer C, de Rekeneire N, Harris TB, Schwatz AV, Tylavsky FA, Cho Y-W and Newman AB. Accelerated loss of skeletal muscle strength in older adults with type 2 diabetes; the health aging and body composition study. Diabetes Care 2007; 30: 1507–12.

3. Schwartz AV, Hillier TA, Sellmeyer DE, Resnick HE, Gregg E, Ensrud KE, Schreiner PJ, Margolis KL, Cauley JA, Nevitt MC, Black DM and Cummings SR. Older women with diabetes have a higher risk of falls: a prospective study. Diabetes Care 2002; 25: 1749–54.

4. Bonds DE, Larson JC, Schwartz AV, Strotmeyer ES, Robbins J, Rodriguez BL, Johnson KC and Margolis KL. Risk of fracture in women with type 2 diabetes: the Women's Health Initiative Observational Study. J Clin Endocrinol Metab 2006; 91: 3404–10.

5. Lipscombe LL, Jamal SA, Booth GL and Hawker GA. The risk of hip fractures in older individuals with diabetes: a population-based study. Diabetes Care 2007: 30: 835–41.

6. Walker A, James C, Bannister M and Jobes E. Evaluation of a diabetes referral pathway for the management of hypoglycaemia following emergency contact with the ambulance service to a diabetes specialist nurse team. Emerg Med J 2006; 23: 449–51.

7. Wens J, Vermeire E, Royen PV, Sabbe B and Denekens J. GPs perspectives of type 2 diabetes people' adherence to treatment: A qualitative analysis of barriers and solutions. BMC Fam Pract 2005; 6: 20

8. Koproski J, Pretto Z and Poretsky L. Effects of an intervention by a diabetes team in hospitalised people with diabetes. Diabetes Care 1997; 20: 1553–55.

9. Thompson DM, Kozak SE and Sheps S. Insulin adjustment by a nurse educator improves glucose control in insulin-requiring diabetic people: a randomised trial. Can Med Assoc J 1999; 161: 959–62.

10. Wong FKY, Mok MPH, Chan T and Tsang MW. Nurse follow up of people with diabetes: randomized controlled trial. J Adv Nur 2005; 50: 391–402.

11. Courtenay M, Carey N, James J, Hills M and Roland J. An evaluation of a specialist nurse prescriber on diabetes in-person service delivery. Pract Diab Int 2007; 24: 69–74.

12. Aubert RE, Herman WH, Waters J, Moore W, Sutton D, Peterson BL, Bailey C and Koplan JP. Nurse case management to improve glycaemic control in diabetic people in a health maintenance organization: a randomized trial. Ann Intern Med 1998; 129: 605–12.

13. Taylor CB, Miller NH, Reilly KR, Greenwald G, Cunning D, Deeter A and Abascal L. Evaluation of a nurse care management system to improve outcomes in people with complicated diabetes. Diabetes Care 2007; 26: 1058–63.

14. Davidson MB. Effect of nurse-directed diabetes care in a minority population. Diabetes Care 2003, 26, 2281–7.

15. Druss BG, Marcus SC, Olfson M, Tanielian T and Pincus HA. Trends in care by non-physician clinicians in the United States, N Engl J Med 2003; 348: 130–7.

16. Davidson MB, Ansari A and Karlan VJ. Effect of a nurse-directed diabetes management program on urgent care/emergency room visits and hospitalisations in a minority population. Diabetes Care 2007; 30: 224–7.

17. Singh PK, Beach P, Iqbal N, Buch HN and Singh BM. Nurse-led management of uncontrolled hypertension in those with diabetes and high vascular risk. Pract Diab Int 2007; 24: 92–6.

18. Denver EA, Barnard M, Woolfson RG and Earle KA. Management of uncontrolled hypertension in nurse-led clinic compared with conventional care for people with type 2 diabetes. Diabetes Care 2003; 26: 2256–60.

19. Brooks AD, Rihani RS and Derus CL. Pharmacist membership in a medical group's diabetes health management program. Am J Health-Syst Pharm 2007; 64: 617–21.

20. Morley JE and Silver AJ, Nutritional issues in nursing home care. Ann Intern Med 1995; 123: 850–9.

21. McCoubrie R, Jeffrey D, Paton C and Dawes L. Managing diabetes mellitus in people with advanced cancer: a case note audit and guidelines. Eur J Cancer Care 2005; 14: 244–8.

22. Quinn K, Hudson P and Dunning T. Diabetes management in people receiving palliative care. J Pain Symptom Manage 2006; 32: 275–86.

23. O'Hare JP, Raymond NT, Mughal S, Dodd L, Hanif W, Ahmad Y, Mishra K, Jones A, Kumar S, Szczepura A, Hillhouse EW and Barnett AH. UKADS Study Group. Evaluation of delivery of enhanced diabetes care to people of South Asian ethnicity: the United Kingdom Asian Diabetes Study. Diabet Med 2004; 21: 1357–65.

31

Diabetes Education in the Elderly

Charles Fox and Anne Kilvert

Diabetes Centre, Northampton General Hospital, Northampton, UK

Key messages

- As with younger people, diabetes education is an essential intervention to enhance care in the elderly.
- In its simplest form, diabetes education is a learning process that requires a positive attitude in older people, with regular reinforcement and engagement.
- Group education is increasingly regarded as a more effective method of educating people with diabetes.
- In order for diabetes education in the elderly to be effective, several patient-related and professional-related barriers need to be overcome.

31.1   Introduction

Although today, diabetes education is regarded as central to diabetes care, very little published evidence is available to demonstrate its effectiveness. The National Institute for Health and Clinical Excellence (NICE) provides 'Guidance in the use of patient education models in diabetes' [1], which includes the following statement:

> "The paucity of high-quality trials of the effectiveness of patient-education models for diabetes, particularly those for people with type 2 diabetes, reveals a need for more research. Further research should

involve RCTs with designs based on explicit hypotheses and educational theory, and include a range of outcomes evaluated after long follow-up intervals. Studies should aim to determine the characteristics, in terms of type, length and frequency of intervention, team composition and setting, that would maximise the impact of patient education in both the short and longer term. Such studies should also include qualitative evaluation of the educational intervention itself, and research to identify the characteristics of education that are most important for different stages of the disease, and that best match different cultural and social needs."

As a result of the renewed focus on education, a number of courses have been developed in various formats, but DAFNE, X-PERT and DESMOND are among the few which have been validated.

Even less has been published on the specific challenge of education for the elderly. The joint Diabetes UK and Department of Health Report from the Patient Education Working Group ('Structured Education in Diabetes' [2]) identifies several groups, where there is an education gap. This includes children, adolescents and their carers, pregnant women, and vulnerable groups such as those with learning disabilities and limited learning and language skills. There is no mention in this exhaustive document of the special educational needs of elderly people. Much of the present comment on the specific needs of the older person is derived from the personal observations of people who have delivered educational courses to people of all ages. The main focus will be on type 2 diabetes,

Diabetes in Old Age. Third Edition. Edited by Alan J. Sinclair
© 2009 John Wiley & Sons, Ltd

although the aspects of type 1 diabetes that are particularly relevant to the elderly will also be discussed.

31.2 Principles of adult diabetes education

Successful education for adults is a process of learning (by the adult) rather than teaching (by the expert). These principles apply as much to diabetes as any other form of learning. We quote the Joslin Clinic principles for diabetes education as an example of person-centred diabetes care from a leading US diabetes centre with a longstanding reputation for patient education. The Joslin Clinic was founded by Elliott Joslin (1869–1962), the first doctor in the USA to specialize in diabetes, and an advocate for patient education. The Joslin Clinic is a leader in promoting diabetes self-management education.

31.2.1 The Joslin Clinic principles

- The person with diabetes is the centre of her/his health care team.

- People with diabetes live multifaceted lives with competing demands that influence their diabetes self-care.

- People living with diabetes make complex self-care decisions every day.

- Family and other support systems strongly influence diabetes self-care.

- People with diabetes learn ideas and concepts that they perceive as important.

- Learning occurs when the individuals are engaged.

- Learning is a process that requires reinforcement and flexibility.

Patients and professionals interested in interactive education should log onto the Joslin Clinic website (www.joslin.org). This is an active, simple to access website for diabetes information with a lively discussion board. It has an American flavour – that is, upbeat and honest about feelings.

"Around lunch time today I was feeling kind of icky and yucky and hi blood sugary, so I took two hours off work and grabbed my pocket camera and hit the trail along the beaches between False Creek and Wreck Beach here in Vancouver. Now I feel a lot better. The fresh air and activity and mental exercise of taking a few pictures makes a big difference to me when I am in need of perking up. Eat fish, lean chicken and low GI carbs, and walk 10,000 steps a day. Works for me."

Older people may need some encouragement to enter the website, but they can join the army of 'silver surfers' who know their way round the internet.

31.3 How should education be delivered?

31.3.1 Evidence for effectiveness of group education

Traditionally, education has been delivered in a one-to-one, didactic fashion, with the agenda determined by the experienced health care professional. However, there is increasing evidence for the effectiveness of group education, with the agenda determined by the participants as a 'discovery learning' process.

The strongest evidence for group education comes from two European studies conducted by Trento *et al.* in Italy [3] and by Kultzer *et al.* Germany [4].

In Turin, Italy, Marina Trento and colleagues set up a programme in 1998 to test the effectiveness and feasibility of a carefully designed long-term group education programme [3]. A total of 112 people with type 2 diabetes was randomly allocated to either group or individual education. The groups were approximately the same age (60 years), with a mean known duration of diabetes of 9.5 years. The groups met every three months, and each session was facilitated by an educationalist and a physician. The educational objectives were to:

- reach a desirable body weight

- learn to shop for food (reading labels for content, energy values, etc.)

- choose an appropriate quality and quantity of food, both at home and when eating out

- increase physical activity, when feasible

- take medication properly and regularly

- know the meaning of the main laboratory tests of metabolic control

- recognize early symptoms of, and be able to react to, hypoglycaemia

- take appropriate action in case of intercurrent illnesses

- care for the feet and buy appropriate footwear

- regularly attend clinic and screening checks for complications.

Each session was structured into four phases: (1) welcome and introduction to the subject; (2) interactive learning; (3) discussion of patient experiences; and (4) conclusions with directions for 'homework' and medical consultation with the physician, if necessary.

During phase 1, patients were given sealed envelopes containing the results of blood tests, but these were only discussed collectively if the patients so desired. During phases 2 and 3, various hands-on activities, group work, problem-solving exercises, real-life simulations and role play were carried out. In order to induce positive group dynamics, the facilitators worked with each patient to identify and share problems and successes with other group members. This helped the group dynamics, and any examples of unhelpful behaviour were not criticised but rather used as a source of positive learning for the group. The control group received traditional one-to-one consultations and education sessions.

The groups were maintained over five years and, while the control group showed a steady and expected rise in HbA_{1c} level over time, those patients taking part in group care maintained a steady HbA_{1c} level (Table 31.1).

In Bamberg, Germany, Bernhard Kulzer and colleagues [4] compared three different treatment/education programmes to evaluate the didactic versus self-management approach as well as the group effect:

- Group A received a didactic intervention focused on teaching knowledge, skills and information about the correct treatment of diabetes. This was delivered as four, 90-min sessions in a group setting.

- Group B took part in a self-management/empowerment programme focused on emotional, cognitive and motivational aspects of behaviour change to promote lifestyle modifications, especially with regards to eating and exercise. This consisted of 12, 90-min sessions in a group setting.

- Group C was also a self-management/empowerment programme with the same curriculum as group B, but delivered as 12 sessions – six individual and six in a group.

The groups were assessed for glycaemic control, knowledge, psychological well-being and self-care behaviour at 3 and 15 months after the intervention. While knowledge was seen to improve equally in all groups, HbA_{1c} levels were unchanged in the didactic group but fell by 0.7% at 3 months in both self-management groups. This fall was not sustained in group C, but was maintained at 15 months in group B. Both psychological well-being and self-care behaviour were significantly higher in the self-management groups, but there was no added benefit from the individual sessions. The authors concluded that self management training had a significantly higher medium-term efficacy, and that group sessions were more effective than an individual approach

31.3.2 Comparison of one-to-one and group education

The group effect can be very powerful, particularly if it is well facilitated. This outweighs the obvious drawbacks of having to coordinate group sessions (see Table 31.1). Group discussions allow patients and their carers to share experiences and feelings, and to identify with stories that others bring to the group. Discussion with others in the same situation often reinforces the educational message. However, people with specific disabilities may have difficulty coping with the group setting.

The advantages and disadvantages of individual and group education are compared in Table 31.2.

31.4 Empowerment in diabetes care

It is now widely accepted that the only realistic way to achieve good control of diabetes is to enable the person with diabetes to make their own decisions. This is an integral part of the Department of Health philosophy, and underpins the National Service Framework for Diabetes [5]. Standard 3 states that: "All children, young people and adults with diabetes will receive a service which encourages partnership in decision-making, supports them in managing their diabetes and helps them to adopt and maintain a healthy lifestyle. This will be reflected in an agreed and shared care plan in an appropriate format and language. Where appropriate, parents and carers should be fully engaged in this process." The NSF Standards document goes on to specify how empowerment should be promoted:

- The provision of information, education and psychological support that facilitates self-management

Table 31.1 Biochemical and clinical variables at baseline and year 5 in patients followed by group care (n = 42) and control subjects (n = 42).

	Baseline	Year 5	Change from baseline	P-value[a]
Knowledge of diabetes[b]				
Group	15.5	27.9	12.4	<0.001
Control	21.4	18.0	−3.4	
Problem-solving ability[b]				
Group	11.4	17.0	5.6	<0.001
Control	12.3	10.0	−2.3	
Quality of life[b]				
Group	67.4	43.7	−23.7	<0.001
Control	70	89.2	19.2	
HbA_{1c} (%)				
Group	7.4	7.3	0	<0.001
Control	7.4	9.0	1.6	

[a]Difference between group care and control subjects.
[b]Details of the measures used are provided in Ref. [3].

Table 31.2 Comparison of one-to-one and group education.

	One to one	Group
Timing	Easy to organize	Requires coordination
Location	No special requirements	Limited by space and accessibility
Format	Tailored to individual	Determined by group – different perspectives
Adaptability	Easy to adjust for patient disability	May be unsuitable for those with physical or mental disability
Agenda	Individualized and may be limited	Enriched by group
Educator training	Adult education skills	Group education skills
Added benefit	Intimacy, personalized	Group experience reinforces learning
Efficiency	Limited by available time	More time available for learning
Patient's anticipation	Security/safety	Social anxiety of group exposure

is therefore the cornerstone of diabetes care. People with diabetes need the knowledge, skills and motivation to assess their risks, to understand what they will gain from changing their behaviour or lifestyle and to act on that understanding by engaging in appropriate behaviours. Other beneficial factors include:

- A family and social environment that supports behaviour change: families and communities provide both practical support and a framework for the individual's beliefs.
- The tools to support behaviour, for example, affordable healthier food options both at home and in the workplace.
- Active involvement in negotiating, agreeing and owning goals.
- Knowledge to understand the consequences of different choices and to enable action.

Self-management can only be successful if the person feels empowered to make their own decisions. The empowerment model was developed in the US by Anderson and Funnell [6], and is one of many approaches designed to encourage the individual to work out their own management plan and implement their own decisions. Traditional diabetes care is often disempowering, as it instructs people on the changes they need to make in order to achieve good control, without giving them the opportunity to identify the changes they would choose for themselves. People may feel pressurized to agree to changes to keep the health professional happy, but if they do not perceive a personal benefit, they will not generate the motivation to change.

The structure of UK health care is weighted in favour of the professionals. Clinics are arranged around the convenience of doctors, and the people are routinely kept waiting. In secondary care, the consultation may be with an unfamiliar health care professional, who sees their role as an advice-giver. In primary care, the hard-pressed practice nurse may feel obliged to focus on NHS targets, rather than the expectations and needs of the individual patient. The following items are examples of common practice, though many health care professionals try very hard to provide patient-centred care:

- Primary Care
  - Focus on annual review and targets
  - Computer screen demanding attention of health care professional
  - Template rather than patient-focussed
  - Pressure to achieve Quality and Outcomes Framework (QOF) points

- Secondary Care
  - Large clinics and waiting rooms
  - Multiple health care professionals
  - Poor continuity of care
  - 'Clinical' environment
  - Lack of privacy

- Access
  - Appointments centred on convenience of the organization
  - Travel and parking

31.4.1 Who should be empowered?

All people who are capable of making their own decisions about self-management should be encouraged to set their own goals, and to decide how these are to be achieved. The priorities may not necessarily be those of the health care professional. This approach is embodied in the Care Planning process, which is being introduced by the Department of Health for all people with long term-conditions.

31.4.2 The principles of care planning for diabetes and other long-term conditions

Care planning is underpinned by the principles of patient-centredness and partnership working [7]. It is an ongoing process of two-way communication, negotiation and joint decision-making, in which both the person with diabetes and the health care professional make an equal contribution to the consultation. It differs from the 'paternalistic' or 'health care professional-centred' model of consulting, traditionally applied in acute settings.

The *Disease-Illness model* has been proposed as a means of achieving this [8]. This emphasizes the importance of the health care professional's perspective of disease and pathology, but suggests that these should always be considered in parallel with – and in equal importance to – the patient's individual experiences of their condition (see Figure 31.1). This specifically includes eliciting the individual's ideas, concerns and expectations of their condition and treatments.

31.4.3 Care planning model

A Diabetes Care Planning Working Group was set up by the Department of Health and Diabetes UK to facilitate this process in the UK. The group developed a model for effective care planning which should be incorporated into routine diabetes care [7]. This draws on research in clinical practice, psychology and education to set out a process of negotiation and shared decision making between the health care professional and the person with diabetes. Family members or carers should be involved in this process, if possible (Figure 31.2).

The components of the model include:

- The individual's story and the professional's story

- Possible topics for discussion

- Learning about diabetes

- Managing diabetes

- Living with diabetes

- Other health and social issues

- Sharing and discussing information and negotiating the agenda

- Action planning

- Documentation

Each of these topics is discussed in detail in the Department of Health/Diabetes UK booklet.

31.4.4 Empowerment in the elderly

While there is good evidence for the effectiveness of the empowerment approach in general diabetes care, its value in the elderly cannot be assumed. This has been evaluated in a group of 148 Cuban subjects aged >60 years who participated in a 5-year study of Continuing Interactive Education (CIE), which followed on from the established basic diabetes information course [9]. Sixty interactive meetings, each lasting for approximately 90 minutes and ranging in format from group discussions to cultural activities, meals out and formal

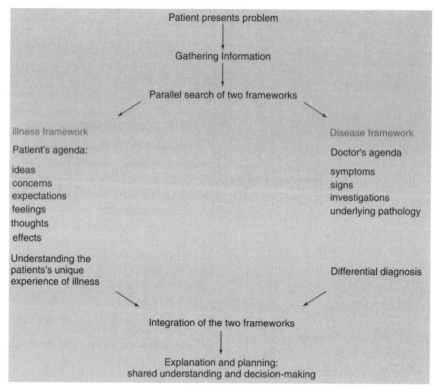

Figure 31.1 Parallel history-taking in care planning.

conferences, were held at monthly intervals over a 5-year period. The aim was to empower patients by encouraging skills and perceptions required to cope with diabetes, rather than to provide clinical information. Participants were invited to select the topics for discussion and to work in several small groups (up to 15 people) to identify problems and arrive at solutions. The health care professionals acted as facilitators, but not as information givers. The small groups then united to exchange ideas and enrich discussion.

A comparison of results pre-programme and 5 years later showed significant reductions in HbA_{1c} level (from 12.4 to 7.9%; p<0.02), body weight and medication requirements, together with an increased adherence to self-care strategies (e.g. diet, exercise, footcare) and a reduction in the number of diabetes-related conditions requiring emergency services and hospital admission. There was a significant increase in knowledge and skills scores (p < 0.001), and the prevalence of depression fell from 69% to 24%. Although the study lacked a control group, it demonstrated clearly that this method was effective in encouraging diabetes self-management in older people.

Not all older people are able to benefit from such educational techniques, and Garcia and Suarez excluded those with deafness, psychiatric disease and other conditions, such as stroke, which may interfere with their ability to comprehend. Elderly people need to be assessed to identify factors which may interfere with their capacity for empowerment.

31.4.5 Barriers to empowerment in the elderly

Such barriers might derive from the older person themselves, or from the professionals working with or caring for them. There is a tendency to treat older people as dependents who are not capable of making their own decisions:

- Barriers from the elderly person
  - confused/forgetful
  - hearing or visual impairment
  - reluctance to make decisions for themselves – "You just tell me what to do"
  - ingrained respect for authority – "I will do what you tell me"
  - may be less assertive/afraid to ask

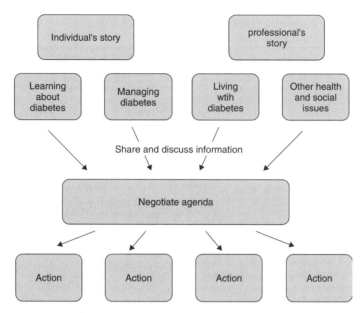

Figure 31.2 The care-planning process.

○ may believe that nothing can be done to improve the situation

○ may be happy to maintain the status quo; an informed decision not to change

○ may not be in a position to make decisions (e.g. residential homes) – no control over food intake

• Barriers from professionals

○ ageism – assumption that the individual cannot make their own decisions

○ protection – "keep things simple" – "I'll tell you what to do"

○ Elderspeak (see below)

31.4.6 Elderspeak

The concept of Elderspeak was taken up in 1991 by Susan Kemper [10], Professor in Psychology and Gerontology at the University of Kansas. Professor Kemper published widely in the field of language and ageing, and set out to develop speech modifications to improve communication with the elderly, which she called 'Elderspeak'. However, the term Elderspeak has come to describe adjustments well-meaning people make when addressing someone who is old. These may be both helpful and unhelpful and include:

• Using a 'singsong' voice, changing pitch and tone, exaggerating words

• Simplifying the length and complexity of sentences

• Speaking louder and more slowly

• Using limited vocabulary

• Repeating or paraphrasing what has just been said

• Using terms of endearment out of context (e.g. 'honey', 'sweetie', 'dearie', 'pop')

• Referring to a person in the plural – "Are we ready for our bath?"

• Using patronizing statements that sound like questions – "You would rather wear blue socks, wouldn't you?"

Elderspeak is commonly heard in nursing homes, hospitals and other settings where frail elders are found. It may be used indiscriminately with anyone who looks old or dependent, and stereotypes the person at the receiving end. It may also be heard in everyday places such as banks and supermarkets, where the old person is clearly able to function normally.

Elderspeak may be harmful as it implies that the older person is not competent, and therefore any communication problems are their fault. This language pattern affects an older person's evaluation of their own abilities, reinforces negative stereotypes about aging, and also erodes their self-confidence. Thus, the use of Elderspeak may promote the very problem it is trying to avoid.

Table 31.3 Meeting patient expectations in the consultation: Results from UK patients compared with European mean.

Patient scores	Mean ($n = 625$)	Range	UK participants ($n = 81$)
Reported consultation length (min)	16.0	12.4–20.1	12.4
Patient enablement score (1–12)	5.5	3.9–6.1	3.9
Preference for involvement (%)	82.6	74.6–87.7	87.7
Evaluation of involvement (%)	70.6	55.6–81.6	55.6

Nevertheless, some important positive messages have emerged from studies of Elderspeak; namely that older people will understand you better if you: (i) use short sentences; (ii) simplify – but be explicit; and (iii) repeat and paraphrase.

The topic of Elderspeak is reviewed in an excellent article available as a PDF file [11].

31.4.7 What do older people feel about empowerment?

There is a feeling that older people are socialized to expect a doctor or nurse to give them advice, which they will then carry out to the letter.

For example, Wensing *et al.* [12] investigated the factors associated with patient enablement – defined as the ability to cope with life and illness – in 625 elderly patients (aged ≥ 70 years) in seven European countries. Enhancing enablement is regarded as an important part of health care, and relies on effective communication between the patient and the clinician. However, patient characteristics may influence their contribution to decision-making in the consultation and elderly people may be less assertive, thereby reducing their involvement in their own care. The study investigated the link between enablement, the patient's evaluation of their involvement in the consultation, and their preference for involvement following a visit to their primary care physician.

Immediately after the consultation, patients were asked to complete validated questionnaires to assess enablement, evaluation of involvement and preference for involvement. Enablement was scored on a scale of 1 to 12 (high = more enablement). The mean age of the participants was 77 years and 63% had a chronic disease. The results showed the enablement score to be higher in those patients who reported a more positive evaluation of their involvement, and this was increased if they expressed a high preference for involvement. Thus, improving elderly patients' evaluations of involvement may help to enhance enablement, but the patient preference for involvement is variable and unpredictable, and so needs to be explored with the individual.

It was of interest to see that the 81 patients recruited from the UK reported the shortest consultation time, lowest enablement score, highest preference for involvement and lowest evaluation of involvement (Table 31.3), which suggested that the UK might lag behind their European counterparts in meeting the patients needs and expectations.

31.5 The development of structured education: What to teach people about diabetes

In the US, the NIH/US National Library of Health programme for diabetes education delivers essential information first, followed by more complex lifestyle and 'special situations' advice. The programme provides an interactive web-based tutorial for people with diabetes: www.nlm.nih.gov/medlineplus/tutorials/diabetesintroduction/, and is based on three stages:

- Basic "survival skills"
  ○ Dealing with hypoglycaemic episodes ('hypos')
  ○ Dealing with high blood sugar levels
  ○ Selecting the right food
  ○ How to take tablets or insulin for diabetes
  ○ How to test and record blood glucose levels

- Home management
  ○ How to adjust insulin/food before exercise
  ○ How to handle 'sick' days
  ○ Foot care
  ○ How to watch for complications and associated conditions, e.g. blood pressure, cholesterol

- Lifestyle changes
  ○ Eating out
  ○ Alcohol

○ How to modify insulin, depending on raised blood glucose level

○ Varying meal times and changes in routine

○ Importance of exercise

In the UK, many groups have developed local education courses for type 2 diabetes, but only two have been validated and published in peer review journals:

- DESMOND (Diabetes Education and Self Management, Ongoing and Newly Diagnosed) was developed by a large collaborative of health care professionals and patients and designed to become a national programme.

- X-PERT was designed in Burnley by Trudi Deakin, a specialist dietician and. following initial success. it is now being rolled out nationally.

31.5.1   DESMOND

DESMOND was set up to fill a gap identified by the National Institute for Health and Clinical Excellence (NICE), who found very little evidence of effective structured education for type 2 diabetes in the UK [13]. A large collaborative of psychologists, primary and secondary care physicians, specialist and practice nurses, dieticians, educators, managers and people with diabetes met to address this void. Their vision was to develop a national educational programme, based on patient-centred principles. To quote verbatim from the informative website (www.desmond-project.org.uk/):

> "The educators or facilitators delivering the programme are healthcare professionals working in the community - mainly practice nurses, diabetes specialist nurses or dieticians. Resources include patient support material especially written or produced for the programme and meeting its empowering philosophy. Participants are not 'taught' in a formal way, but are rather supported to discover and work out knowledge, and to allow this to inform the goals and plans they make for themselves."

The principles of DESMOND

- Each individual is responsible for the day-to-day management of their diabetes.

- People make decisions to achieve best quality of life.

- Barriers to self-management lie in the individual's personal world.

- Consequences of self-management decisions impact solely on the patient, their family and carers.

- Acquiring new information is not easy.

DESMOND acknowledges that day-to-day, minute-by-minute decisions (e.g. food choices, physical activity, medication-taking, monitoring, etc.) which affect outcomes are made by the patient themselves. The person with diabetes is thus responsible for managing their own condition

The DESMOND randomized controlled trial

Following a successful pilot study conducted in 17 UK centres, the effectiveness of the DESMOND programme was investigated in a randomized controlled trial [14]. A total of 834 patients with newly diagnosed type 2 diabetes was recruited from 203 general practices and randomized either to the control group, who received a total of 6 h of one-to-one education from a practice nurse, or to the DESMOND programme.

The DESMOND curriculum, which was designed to be accessible to a wide range of people with diabetes, was as follows:

- Tell your story

- Professional story – normal physiology

- What is diabetes?

- Diet – done as games, choices

- Sugars

- Fats

- Monitoring

- Physical activity

- Complications

- Goal setting – be specific

The programme could be provided either as a single 6-h session or in two 3-h sessions. The aim was to incorporate it into routine diabetes care, delivered in the community. The DESMOND educators received intensive training both in adult education techniques and facilitation of group learning, and adopted a non-didactic approach, so that learning was elicited rather than taught. Participants were encouraged to focus on lifestyle changes, such as food choices, physical activity, and on their personal risk factors. They were then invited to choose a specific, achievable goal of behaviour change to work on.

Measures of biomedical, lifestyle and psychosocial status – including depression – were made at baseline and 4, 8 and 12 months. All participants had recently discovered that they had type 2 diabetes, and therefore made lifestyle changes in response to whatever advice they had received. As one might expect, this led to a marked fall in HbA$_{1c}$ level over the first 12 months in both groups, mirroring the findings of the UK Prospective Diabetes Study [15]. No significant changes were found in biochemical measures, but there was a significant fall in body weight at all three time intervals in the intervention group (overall p = 0.025), even though weight reduction was not a specific target of the programme. There was also an unexpected positive effect in the DESMOND group on abstinence from smoking after 6 and 12 months, with an odds ratio of 3.56.

Four distinct health beliefs about diabetes were measured in the DESMOND trial, and all showed consistent and significant improvements (p < 0.001) in the intervention group, who had a greater understanding of their illness, including its seriousness and permanence with more confidence about their ability to affect the course of their disease. The DESMOND group also had lower depression scores at 12 months (p = 0.032), though there was no difference found in measures of diabetes-specific emotional distress.

The DESMOND trial showed that a structured education programme for patients with newly diagnosed type 2 diabetes would lead to sustained benefits in health beliefs and depression, but did not demonstrate any difference in HbA$_{1c}$ level in the first year. Thus, the programme could be introduced widely across primary care.

The DESMOND educators observed that older patients contributed to the group and brought valuable experience, but that they may have needed a different approach at times (see adaptations for the elderly).

31.5.2 Case study

Ken, aged 64, had recently been found to have type 2 diabetes and recorded his impressions of the DESMOND programme:

"It was very interesting that a group of people who were all recently diagnosed as type 2 diabetic were sitting together as a group with two very knowledgeable nurses who were talking to us about diabetes. These were very much group sessions and we were all given the opportunity to talk about experiences and discuss issues and all sort of things were put up on a flip chart about people's feelings about different aspects of diabetes.

Each person had a slightly different experience so these things were coming up – there were things you had probably experienced yourself but hadn't really thought about, and a picture developed of attitudes. Towards the end of the course, the flip chart was reproduced and we went through it all again. It was interesting to find how people had changed. One lady when she came on the course said she felt like a leper, which I found surprising, but at the end of the course that had gone and she was feeling far more positive.

Someone would make a comment, which would trigger something else, which without the previous comment may not have come out. I think with things like diabetes, you do need to talk about it. And to be able to do that with people in similar circumstances - to hear what they feel and what their experience had been, helped towards this positive attitude that came out at the end of the course.

I don't believe that you would get the same level of information from your GP or practice nurse as you wouldn't have the amount of time with them. To be able to have two half-day sessions with two knowledgeable people that could answer questions and talk about different issues was very reassuring and supported everything you had learnt from your practice nurse, your GP and websites and what have you and I believe that everybody when they left that course felt very, very positive about it."

31.5.3 X-PERT programme

The X-PERT programme [16] was developed as a patient-centred, group-based, self-management programme based on theories of empowerment [6] and discovery learning [17]. The effectiveness of the programme, as measured by clinical, lifestyle and psychosocial outcomes was demonstrated in a randomized controlled trial.

For this, 157 participants were invited to attend six weekly 2-h sessions in groups of 16 people with diabetes and four to eight carers. The programme (see Table 31.4) aimed to develop skills and build confidence to enable people to make informed decisions about their diabetes self-care. Separate sessions were held for Urdu-speaking participants, with a translator present. The 157 controls were offered one-to-one sessions with a dietician (30 min), practice nurse (15 min) and a GP (10 min). The mean age of participants was 61 years in each group, and the mean duration of known diabetes was 6.7 years. Some 14 months later, the

Table 31.4 The content of the X-PERT programme.

Topic	Description
Week 1: What is Diabetes?	Explore what happens to food when we eat it; self-monitoring of diabetes; diabetes treatments; feelings about living with diabetes. Dispel myths by using visual educational materials.
Week 2: Weight Management	Examine the 'balance of good health' model and use food models to distinguish between food containing protein, fat and carbohydrate. Inform about sensible eating whilst exploring barriers in doing so. Advise about the benefits of exercise and give practical examples including information about local exercise-on-prescription schemes.
Week 3: Carbohydrate Awareness	Perform a group task, developed to show the effect of quantity and quality of carbohydrate food on blood glucose levels. Use ping-pong ball models and laminated food pictures to dispel the myths surrounding glucose, sucrose and starch.
Week 4: Supermarket Tour	Address some common confusion surrounding dietary fat, sugar and food labelling. Encourage a diet that is enjoyable, variable and balanced whilst dispelling the concept of 'good' and 'bad' foods.
Week 5: Complications & Prevention	Discuss how to reduce the risk of developing longer-term complications through lifestyle changes, treatment and regular monitoring. Use visual educational aids to explore medical conditions in layman terms such as nephropathy, retinopathy, arteriosclerosis, neuropathy and blood pressure.
Week 6: Evaluation & Question time	Play "Living with diabetes", a board game to bring the X-PERT programme to a close in a relaxed manner, reinforcing the main messages whilst encouraging participants to reflect on how much they have learnt.
Goal Setting: Last 20 minutes each week	The final 20–30 minutes each week involves the goal setting component of the empowerment model. Participants obtain and examine their health results, the implications of them and acceptable ranges. If participants make an informed decision to work on improving any of their health results, they work through the five step empowerment model. Psychosocial aspects of diabetes i.e. fitting diabetes into life rather than fitting life into living with diabetes. An important aspect of the empowerment model is to respect the decisions made by some of the participants not to goal-set.
Patient Manual	Resource manual given to participants at the beginning of the course. Background reading, health results and goal setting material added each week as appropriate.

intervention group had improved control (HbA$_{1c}$ – 0.6% versus + 0.1%, p<0.001) and a greater reduction in body weight and waist circumference. The X-PERT participants were less likely to have increased their medication, and more likely to be exercising and performing footcare self-management. They were 'much more satisfied' with their diabetes treatment compared to those receiving individual appointments (p < 0.04), and had a higher total empowerment score (p < 0.04), but there was no significant difference in their overall quality of life.

Following the success of the trial, the X-PERT programme now has a written curriculum, visual aids, a 'train the trainers' course, an evaluation scheme and a quality assurance programme, and is being rolled out to other centres.

31.5.4 Comment on educational content

Local health care commissioners are responsible for funding educational and self-management programmes for people with diabetes. DESMOND and X-PERT are two examples of validated structured education programmes which fulfil NICE guidelines, and have subsequently been rolled out widely in the UK. Most elderly patients will benefit from this type of programme, but if cognitive problems are suspected then any existing course must be modified along the lines described in the following section.

31.6 Adaptations of educational principles for the elderly

While the general principles for adult education are well established, special consideration needs to be given to elderly people and the factors which may limit their ability to deal with new information and the need for change. Older people are often aware that their ability to take in new ideas may be limited, and this may reduce their self-confidence. They should be encouraged to become actively involved in working out what they can do and, whenever possible, given the opportunity to practice skills. Diabetes may be perceived as a small and relatively unimportant part of their life and they may feel reluctant to make changes. Many older people expect to be told what to do, and find it disconcerting to be invited to make their own decisions.

Information needs to be personalized, with the pace of delivery and specificity adapted for the individual. Language should be basic but not patronizing, with the information selected so that people learn what they need to know, rather than everything there is to know about diabetes. Avoid trying to put over more than one concept at a time. It is important to establish the meal pattern and the extent to which the person has control over what they eat before exploring options for change.

Stereotypes of the elderly are usually negative, and this in itself may reduce self-confidence and hence the learning ability of the older person. Any assessment must try to overcome the negative, while being realistic.

31.6.1 Do the elderly have special needs in diabetes education?

There is an assumption that old people will have special educational needs, in particular concerning difficulties with understanding and in concentrating on abstract concepts such as the pathophysiology of diabetes. In addition, people with diabetes could be at greater risk of cognitive impairment than those without diabetes, which could affect their ability to care for their diabetes. These questions were addressed by Sinclair *et al.* [18], who studied 369 patients with diabetes over the age of 65 years and compared their cognitive function with a carefully matched group of non-diabetics. The odds ratios (95% CI) for normal cognitive test results in subjects with diabetes, after adjusting for all significant variables, was 0.74. Diabetic subjects with a Mini Mental State Examination (MMSE) score <23 had the following associations (all with $p < 0.001$):

- A reduced involvement in diabetes self-care.

- Less diabetes monitoring.

- A reduced ADL (activities of daily living) ability.

- A higher risk of hospitalisation in the previous year.

- An increased need for assistance in personal care.

The specific educational needs of the elderly have been addressed in a study conducted in Germany [19], where education has been an intrinsic part of diabetes care for many years. A group from Jena recognized that many elderly patients were not keeping up with the routine education programme (Treatment and Teaching Programme; TTP), mainly because of impaired neuropsychological function. Thus, a programme was devised for elderly patients with poor cognitive function, which took account of their reduced life expectancy. The aim was to enhance the patient's quality of life by maintaining autonomy and independence. The course was designed to emphasize individual therapeutic goals and to highlight catabolic symptoms, acute complications and depression. A total of 102 patients was included in the study, and cognitive function was assessed by multiple tests. Sixty-eight patients, who were found to have cognitive impairment (IQ score <91), were randomized to take part either in a standard TTP programme or in the geriatric DICOF TTP. This adaptation places less emphasis on theoretical knowledge, such as pathophysiology or blood glucose self-monitoring and detailed carbohydrate counting, and leaves room for intensive training in the practical matters of insulin injection, coping with hypoglycaemia and urine glucose testing. A key feature of the programme is repetition to reinforce key topics. The DICOF TTP takes 5 days to complete, and there are nine education units:

- Unit 1: What is diabetes?

- Unit 2: Urine/blood glucose self-monitoring

- Unit 3: Insulin injection – group and one-to-one education

- Units 4, 6 and 7: Nutrition

- Unit 5: Hypoglycaemia

- Units 8 and 9: Late complications – group and one-to-one education

Each session is facilitated by a trained educator and an interested physician.

At the follow-up examination 6 months later, there were no differences in HbA_{1c} levels, but the DICOF group showed improvements over the standard group in the following areas:

- better self-management (insulin injections and self-monitoring)

- greater satisfaction with the education programme

- higher quality of life

- reduced fear of hypoglycaemia.

Thus, although it is difficult to produce hard evidence for customized education programmes for the elderly, the Jena group have proved the effectiveness of their carefully designed education package.

31.7 Assessment of the educational needs of the individual

31.7.1 Timing of assessment

- The first health care professional (HCP) to speak with the newly diagnosed person is the best placed to make an initial assessment of their response to the news of the diagnosis and their ability to take in new information. This should include an assessment of physical (e.g. vision, hearing) and cognitive function and potential to work within a group.

31.7.2 Nature of assessment

The assessment should be considered from two perspectives:

1. The HCP assessment of patient and carers:
   - Physical: restrictions which may impact on ability to work within a group (e.g.. deafness, reduced vision, cognition, mobility).
   - Psychological: factors which may impair ability to take in new information (e.g. depression, low self-confidence, level of independence, flexibility, passivity).
   - Social: factors which may limit ability to meet targets (e.g. isolation, exercise capacity, realistic targets for control).

2. The patient's (and their carer's) assessment of the process:
   - Their expectations of what the system may provide.
   - Preconceived ideas and beliefs, readiness to make changes.
   - Perception of their mortality/morbidity.
   - Physical restrictions.

The assessor should decide whether the elderly person would benefit from group education, perhaps with specific additional support, whether they need special treatment such as one-to-one education, or whether the education needs to be provided to carers rather than to the elderly patient themselves.

31.8 Specific cases

31.8.1 Insulin refusal

Many people of all ages find the prospect of taking insulin daunting and have to be convinced that it is really necessary. This is particularly true if the reason for recommending insulin is to achieve an HbA_{1c} target in an asymptomatic patient, rather than to relieve symptoms of hyperglycaemia. The major barriers to taking insulin are the fear of self-injecting and anxiety about hypoglycaemia. Most people have heard of someone who has terrible trouble with 'hypos', and assume that it is an inevitable consequence of taking insulin.

Elderly people are often reluctant to accept insulin injections, and feel it is should not be necessary in someone of their age. They are less convinced by the arguments of long-term risk reduction and are not disposed to make changes unless they see a clear and immediate benefit, such as a relief of the symptoms of hyperglycaemia. It is incumbent on health care professionals to try to assess the actual benefit of insulin in the context of comorbidities and life expectancy before recommending a change.

Exploration of the individual barriers to insulin and the reasons for refusal should help identify solutions, which could be:

- intensified educational support during the initiation stages

- administration by district nurse or a carer, either temporarily or in the long term; and/or

- the selection of a suitable insulin delivery device.

In some circumstances the person may remain unconvinced and decide to accept the risk associated with poor glycaemic control.

31.8.2 Choice of insulin

The insulin regimen should be discussed and chosen in the context of the ability of the elderly person to make day-to-day decisions about dose and activity. Those with a regular routine of food intake and activity may prefer a twice-daily mixture which can be adjusted to suit a regular meal pattern. For people with erratic eating habits or variable activity levels, a decision should be made about the individual's ability to vary the insulin dose. Although, in general, elderly people may not take well to the decision making associated with a basal bolus regimen, some are happy to take it on. Those who cannot make their own decisions, but who may not be able to keep to a regular routine, are better treated with a simple insulin regimen such as once- or twice-daily background insulin. In this situation, the aim should be to control symptomatic hyperglycaemia and avoid hypos, rather than to achieve a specific HbA$_{1c}$ target.

For those unfamiliar with blood glucose monitoring there is even more to learn, and this technique should be taught before insulin is introduced, unless the need for insulin is urgent. The pace of the education should be dictated by the individual, with repetition and reinforcement of information [18].

Insulin administration devices should be chosen after an assessment of the patient's dexterity and visual impairment. The Innolet device is particularly useful for those with poor vision or reduced dexterity, but unfortunately this may limit the choice of insulin as only Mixtard 30, Insulatard and Detemir are available in this format.

31.8.3 Hypoglycaemia

Elderly people are at particular risk from hypoglycaemia as the consequences are potentially more severe, with increased vulnerability to confusion, cognitive impairment and neurological deficit. Hypoglycaemic episodes may be acute and severe, sometimes presenting as a stroke, but they may also be mild and recurrent. The signs of mild hypoglycaemia can be more difficult to recognize, as the only manifestation may be confusion and cognitive impairment, which is often attributed to other causes. Although most people are alert to the possibility of hypoglycaemia in somebody taking insulin, sulphonylureas also carry a significant risk of hypoglycaemia, particularly if their food intake is reduced or their renal function deteriorates. Many elderly people receiving oral therapy will not be monitoring their blood glucose, and the problem may only come to light when the person is admitted to hospital with cognitive or neurological impairment and blood glucose monitoring reveals persistently low levels.

Elderly people with longstanding type 1 diabetes can be a particularly difficult group. They have often kept tight control of their blood glucose levels over many years, which is why they have lived to a great age. They may accept hypoglycaemia as an inevitable consequence of tight control. However, increasing frailty and forgetfulness may make decisions about food and insulin more erratic, and it is not uncommon to see big swings in the blood glucose level, with the potential for severe hypoglycaemia. This can be very difficult to correct, as the strategy of avoiding high and low levels by use of intermediate and long-acting insulin does not work well in this insulin-deficient group. Written advice on insulin adjustment, depending on the blood glucose level may help. Carers may be educated to support decision making, but the results are often unsatisfactory, particularly for people in institutional care.

31.8.4 Coping with illness

'Sick day' rules can be complicated, and elderly people often become confused as a consequence of intercurrent infection and so may not be able to implement advice. Dehydration can lead to a rapid deterioration in renal function, and this carries a risk of life-threatening lactic acidosis for those taking metformin. As an acute intercurrent illness (e.g. gastroenteritis) is likely to be an infrequent event and verbal advice may have been forgotten, written guidelines should be provided for both patients and carers. These should be simple and should recommend frequent monitoring of the blood glucose during the illness, seeking medical advice if the results are outside a specified range. Specific indications for urgent medical treatment, such as vomiting, breathlessness, confusion or altered conscious level, should be listed.

31.8.5 Polypharmacy

Many people with diabetes are now advised to take large numbers of medications to reduce cardiovascular risk. There is evidence to demonstrate that people are more likely to adhere to treatment if they understand and accept the reasons for taking it, and this underpins the self-management philosophy of programmes such as DESMOND and X-PERT. Complicated regimens may be confusing to elderly people, although there are various practical ways of simplifying things, for example daily dosing boxes. The role of the local pharmacist is crucial to the success of such methods.

31.9 Conclusions

The general principles of diabetes education for adults apply equally to the elderly population. However, the specific needs of the elderly – taking into account attitudes and disabilities – need to be assessed so that modifications may be made to meet their individual needs.

31.10 Acknowledgments

The authors thank many experienced diabetes educators in the planning of this chapter, and in particular Penny Meade, the community diabetes facilitator at Northampton Diabetes Centre, and Kathryn Sutton, senior dietician at the Ipswich Diabetes Centre, who provided thoughtful and concrete suggestions.

References

1. National Institute for Health and Clinical Excellence (NICE) (2003) *Guidance on the use of patient-education models for diabetes.* Technology Appraisal 60. NICE, London.
2. Structured Patient Education in Diabetes – Report from the Patient Education Working Group. (2005) Department of Health and Diabetes UK, London. DH 4113197.
3. Trento M, Passero P, Borgo E *et al.* (2004) A 5-year randomized controlled study of learning, problem solving ability, and quality of life modifications in people with type 2 diabetes managed by group care. Diabetes Care 27: 670–5.
4. Kulzer B, Hermanns N, Reinecker H *et al.* (2007) Effects of self-management training in Type 2 diabetes: a randomised, prospective trial. Diabet Med 24: 415–23.
5. *National Service Framework for Diabetes: Standards.* (2001) Department of Health, London (www.doh.gov.uk/nsf/diabetes).
6. Anderson RM and Funnell MM. (2005) *The Art of Empowerment*, 2nd edition. American Diabetes Association, Alexandria, USA.
7. Care Planning in Diabetes. (2006) Report from the joint Department of Health and Diabetes UK Care Planning Working Group. www.diabetes.nhs.uk/downloads/care_planning_in_diabetes_report.pdf
8. Stewart M and Roter D. (1989) *Communicating with medical patients.* Sage, Newbury Park, CA.
9. Garcia R and Suarez R. (1997) Diabetes education in the elderly: a 5-year follow-up of an interactive approach. Patient Education and Counseling 29: 87–97.
10. Kemper S. (2003) Elderspeak. Acoustical Society of America Journal 113: 2295–5.
11. Williams K, Kemper S and Hummert ML. (2004) Enhancing communication with older adults: Overcoming Elderspeak. Journal of Gerontological Nursing, 30: 1–8.
12. Wensing M, Wetzel S, Hemsen J and Baker R (2007) Do elderly patients feel more enabled if they had been actively involved in primary care consultations? Patient Education and Counseling 68: 265–9.
13. Skinner TC, Carey ME, Cradock S *et al.* (2006) Diabetes education and self-management for ongoing and newly diagnosed (DESMOND): Process modelling of pilot study. Patient Education and Counseling 64: 369–77.
14. Davies MJ, Heller S, Skinner TC *et al.* (2008) Effectiveness of the diabetes education and self management for ongoing and newly diagnosed (DESMOND) programme for people with newly diagnosed type 2 diabetes: cluster randomised controlled trial. Br Med J 336: 491–5.
15. United Kingdom Prospective Diabetes Study (UKPDS) Group. (1995) UKPDS 13: relative efficacy of randomly allocated diet, sulphonylurea, insulin or metformin in patients with newly diagnosed non-insulin dependent diabetes followed for three years. Br Med J 310: 83–8.
16. Deakin TA, Cade JE, Williams R and Greenwood DC (2006) Structured patient education: the Diabetes X-Pert programme makes a difference. Diab Med 23: 944–54.
17. Brunner J. (1966) *Toward a Theory of Instruction.* Harvard University Press, Cambridge, MA.
18. Sinclair AJ, Girling AJ and Bayer AJ (2000) Cognitive dysfunction in older subjects with diabetes mellitus: impact of diabetes self-management and use of care services. All Wales Research in Elderly (AWARE) Study. Diabetes Res Clin Pract 50: 203–12.
19. Braun, U., Muller, A., Muller, R. *et al.* (2004) Structured treatment and teaching of patients with Type 2 diabetes mellitus and impaired cognitive function – the DICOF trial. Diabetic Medicine 21: 999–1006.

32

Supporting the Family and Informal Carers

Antony Bayer[1] and Alan Sinclair[2]

[1]*Department of Geriatric Medicine, Academic Centre, Cardiff University, Llandough Hospital, Vale of Glamorgan, UK*
[2]*Bedfordshire and Hertfordshire Postgraduate Medical School, University of Bedfordshire, Luton, UK*

Key messages

- Informal carers (caregivers) are the primary source of everyday advice, emotional support and practical help for many older people with diabetes.
- A supportive environment for carers must be provided that allows them to receive educational advice about diabetes and its management, and creates opportunities for greater involvement in treatment decisions.
- The effects of caring on the carer in terms of physical, emotional, social and economic well-being must not be overlooked

32.1 Introduction

Most people with diabetes live at home with support from family and friends. Many of these patients would not regard themselves as requiring care, and most close relatives would not regard themselves as carers. Nevertheless, in reality, nearly all of the 2 million or so older people with diabetes in the United Kingdom will look to their family and friends for advice and practical and emotional support in managing their diabetes and

its complications and in adopting and maintaining a healthy lifestyle.

There is a significant literature on the role of family carers in childhood (type 1) diabetes [1, 2], where it is taken for granted that parents will play an active role in positively influencing management and make efforts to ensure that glucose control is optimal. Numerous studies have examined the value of psycho-educational interventions and family support on health outcomes of children and young people with insulin-dependent diabetes, and have shown that family-based interventions can be effective in improving diabetes knowledge, promoting adherence to management regimens and achieving better diabetic control and increasing quality of life and emotional health [3, 4].

In contrast to this active research and clinical interest in carers of young people with diabetes, there is much less acknowledgement from health professionals and policy makers of the important role of family and informal carers in delivering and monitoring optimal diabetes care for older adults. In the UK, the Diabetes National Service Framework (NSF) [5] emphasizes the importance of empowering people to control day-to-day management of their diabetes and does mention that "...where appropriate, ... carers should be fully engaged in this process". Carers are also mentioned as needing to be alert to the dangers of diabetic emergencies, but no consideration is given to how this should be achieved or that caring relatives and friends may have needs and wants of their own.

This does not seem to reflect adequately the qualitative research that was undertaken to inform the development of the NSF [6]. Whilst only carers of children were included in the focus groups and in-depth interviews, the older patients who were interviewed stated that they wanted partners and carers to be with them at the time they were told their diagnosis – both for emotional support and to be able to learn together about the condition and how to deal with it. They also suggested that partners or other carers should be given more opportunities for learning about diabetes. This was not only because carers required the information to help look after the person, but also because the adjustments related to living with diabetes affected both those with diabetes and the people with whom they share their lives. It was therefore suggested that carers should be invited to attend routine and other appointments with the service user and to ask questions, as required.

It is encouraging that the updated guideline on management of type 2 diabetes from the National Institute for Health and Clinical Excellence [7] acknowledges that diabetes is "...predominantly managed by the person with the diabetes and/or by their carer as part of their daily life", and that, if the patient agrees, families and carers should have the opportunity to be involved in decisions about treatment and care and they should also be given the information and support that they need. A key priority for implementation is that structured education should be offered "...to every person with diabetes and/or their carer at and around the time of diagnosis and with reinforcement and review on an annual basis". Yet, the UK National Director for Diabetes published a document in 2007 that claims to "...set out how services are changing to meet the needs of patients and how they need to change in the future" [8]. This states that the average patient with diabetes will spend three hours a year with a professional and the remaining 8757 hours caring for themselves. That family or friends might play any role at all is not considered.

In practice, the involvement of non-professionals in various aspects of care of older people with diabetes is commonplace. In an observational study of patients aged ≥70 years participating in a study of type 2 diabetes in primary care, between 22% and 50% of their family members reported helping with various aspects of diabetes-specific care [9]. In the present authors' study of older patients attending hospital-based diabetes clinics – about half of whom were taking insulin therapy – nearly all reported that they regularly received help with day-to-day activities or looking after from someone else [10]. Thus, informal carers are the main source of support for older people with diabetes, helping with emotional adjustment to the diagnosis, adherence to diabetes regimens, management of complications and coping with everyday life [11–13]. Yet, service providers too often ignore the potential needs of the carer because the focus of concern is inevitably the needs of the care recipient [14].

32.2 Who are the carers?

Informal carers may be family members (e.g., spouse, sibling, child or grandchild), friends, neighbours, or members of a specific support system such as a church or social organization. The results of the carers module of the General Household Survey (GHS) of 2000 [15] reported that just over half (52%) of carers were looking after a parent (or parent-in-law) and 18% were caring for their spouse or partner. Two-thirds were caring for women, reflecting the predominance of women in the older age groups. The most common age group of carers was between 45 and 64 years (24%), although a significant proportion (12%) were themselves aged over 65 years.

Whilst there have been few reports that have focused specifically on the informal carers of older people with diabetes, in general these seem to reflect the findings of the broader carer literature [9, 16, 17].

Generally, one person takes on the lead carer role, with a secondary network of support provided by more distant relatives and friends. The role of primary carer is decided by generation (when available, spouses whether husband or wife take on most care), gender (typically the hierarchy of selection is wife, daughter, daughter-in-law and even granddaughter before sons), geography (those living with, or closest to the person) and competing responsibilities (employment, childcare and other family responsibilities). Widowhood becomes more common with increasing age, and so children inevitably then become more actively involved. Husbands rarely give direct help to wives who are carers, and women are more likely to have to give up their job to take on caring responsibilities [18, 19].

It is fairly clear that in many cases there is what is described as a 'caregiving trajectory', where the nature of caregiving varies over time [20] for most adults. This may be especially true in poorer communities with three phases usually identified: semi-care, care, and dying.

Ethnicity also plays an important role, with differences in the caring roles and expectations [21]. Due to patterns of migration, there are proportionally more older men requiring care within ethnic minorities and there is less acceptability of available formal care services and institutional care. Consequently, there is a greater care burden on families. In their study of South Asian carers, Townsend and Godfrey [22] found that caring is influenced by gender role stereotypes and filial responsibility. Spouse carers were less common and carers tended to be younger [23]. Sons took a more active responsibility for decision making, organizing care and assisting with instrumental activities of daily living, with daughters and daughters-in-law helping with personal care and housework. Often, daughters and daughters in law did not regard themselves as carers, but the support given to their relative was considered part of normal family responsibilities. The belief that ethnic minority families 'look after their own' and so do not require attention is not supported by evidence [24].

In many instances, adults within ethnic minority groups may be both patients with diabetes and have a caring role for younger people. For instance, in a study of 109 urban midlife African American women with type 2 diabetes, 60% were grandmothers who had higher levels of diabetes-related emotional stress and worse glycaemic control than those without grandmother status, and yet had higher quality of life scores than non-grandmothers [25].

The contribution of *children* to care should not be overlooked. In a study of child carers of adults with diabetes by Jacobson and Wood [26], one in five were looking after grandparents, having begun caring at a mean age of 11 years. Most provided care at least several times a week, ranging from calling to check on the adult or staying with them overnight, to performing glucose testing and giving medication and insulin injections. The youngest child administering insulin was aged 5 years. Nearly half of the children had no education about diabetes care, not even from the family member with diabetes.

32.3 What do carers do?

The term 'carer' relates to a broad spectrum of tasks, ranging from emotional support, to organizing help, to providing company, to doing household tasks and to help with intimate personal care. In the GHS [15], over two-thirds (71%) of carers provided practical help such as preparing a meal, shopping and doing laundry, 60% kept an eye on the person being cared for, and 55% provided company. Smaller proportions of carers provided more intimate forms of help. About one-quarter (26%) gave assistance with personal care such as washing, 22% administered medicines, and 35% provided physical help, for example with walking.

The availability of a close family member or friend to take on the role of carer, rather than need, seems to be the most important predictor of having someone involved in medical care [27], and not all recipients of care appreciate the level of involvement (too little or too much) that is provided [28].

The general carer research literature distinguishes between caring (the affective component) and caregiving (the behavioural component) [29]. 'Care providers' give hands-on-care (e.g. dressing, bathing, daily supervision, cooking, managing finances, transportation) and 'care managers' arrange for others to provide care (e.g. organizing a nurse to attend daily to give medication or dress leg ulcers, a professional carer to attend to personal care and provision of meals, an accountant to manage finances and social care assistants to provide companionship and supervision during the day). Care providers are most often spouses (especially wives) and daughters/daughters-in-law, whilst care managers are most often husbands, adult children (especially sons), friends and other relatives. Care providers tend to be more burdened/stressed than care managers, but inevitably have less contact with professionals who might be able to provide practical and emotional support [30].

A study conducted by Murphy *et al.* [16] in a family practice in the United States looked specifically at the supportive family members of adults with type 2 diabetes (mean age 59 years) and identified two broad categories of family participation. As well as the conventional supportive family member (primary carer or helper) who provided supportive tasks in the care of the illness, there was often the 'family health monitor', an internal health expert usually consulted before any consultation with external resources, including the doctor.

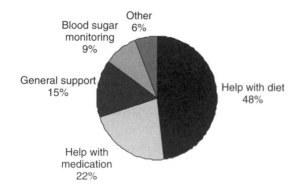

Figure 32.1 Helping activities provided by family members to adults with type 2 diabetes. (Adapted from Ref. [16]).

This person is described as fulfilling a unique executive function as an authoritative information resource and supervisor – acting to critically evaluate medical advice before family members incorporate the information into daily practice. Three-quarters of the patients identified such an individual within their family, and often this was not the same person as the primary carer. No relationship was shown between the presence or absence of a family health monitor and the level of metabolic control as measured by glycosolated haemoglobin (HbA$_{1c}$) level. This suggests a need for health professionals to recognize and involve family health monitors in the therapeutic team, so that they may impact more positively on management.

The study by Murphy *et al.* also identified the most frequent helping tasks undertaken by the primary carer (Figure 32.1). By far the most common activity was helping the person with diabetes with their diet. This included food selection and preparation ('helps buy the right foods', 'cooks properly'), reminders about proper diet ('keeps after me about diet', 'watches diet') and support for dietary restrictions ('cooperates at meals', 'hides sugar'). Help with medications was both general ('keeps track of medications') and specific ('buys medicine', 'reads directions on medicine bottles'). General support was defined as 'encouragement' or 'talking to me'. Other helping activities included financial support, reminders about medical appointments, assistance with hygiene and exercise.

In the primary care-based study conducted by Silliman *et al.* [9], it was reported that between 6% and 17% of older patients with type 2 diabetes received regular help from family members with basic activities of daily living, and between 37% and 48% with instrumental activities of daily living. The most commonly

reported help given was 'keeping enough medication on hand' and 'following a diet'. Between 23% and 38% of family members also reported participating regularly in the patient's medical encounters, whilst 20–40% rarely or never discussed diabetes-related issues with the doctor. When they did go to appointments, family members usually talked to the doctor with the patient present, although the most common reason for wanting to talk was to get their own questions answered. Prognosis was discussed less frequently with family members than were test results, treatment issues and preventive strategies. Carer needs were almost never considered. Predictors of participation in the patient's medical encounters included older age and a greater physical impairment of patients and increased involvement in diabetes-related and general care.

Among carers of community-living elderly patients attending hospital-based diabetes clinics in Birmingham [10], up to 90% reported providing help with instrumental activities of daily living, such as shopping, housework, preparing meals, finances and transport, and up to 25% help with personal care such as washing and bathing/showering, walking about outside, dressing/undressing, getting in and out of bed and toileting.

As would be expected, when patients are less physically functional, when family members are spouses, when they provide more assistance with basic care, and when they have a greater understanding of diabetes management issues, family members are more likely to provide assistance with diabetes-related care [9]. Cognitive impairment is also a strong predictor of a greater need for the involvement of carers in supervising medication, monitoring blood glucose and helping with personal care [31].

Using data from the Oldest Old Study, a nationally representative survey of people aged ≥70 years in the US, Langa *et al.* [32] determined the weekly hours of informal caregiving received by community-dwelling elderly individuals with and without a diagnosis of diabetes. Those without diabetes received an average of 6.1 h of informal care, those with diabetes taking no medications received 10.5 h, those with diabetes taking oral medications received 10.1 h, and those on insulin received 14.4 h of care (p<0.01). Disabilities related to heart disease, stroke and visual impairment were important predictors of a need for diabetes-related informal care.

32.4   What effect can caring have on the carer?

The responsibilities of the caring role can take their toll on the physical, emotional, social and economic well-being of the family and others closely involved in care provision [33–36]. Most published studies of the experience of significant others of persons with diabetes have been about adults with Type 1 diabetes. These show that relatives may harbour even higher levels of concern and worry about the illness and its effects than the patients themselves [37], with spouses reporting marital conflicts about diabetes management and disturbed sleep [38]. Furthermore, it has been reported that the diabetes self-management behaviour of husbands often deteriorated when conflict existed with their spouses [39].

A qualitative study conducted Stodberg *et al.* [40] of the 'lived experience' of being a close relative (significant other) of persons with type 1 diabetes identified four major themes: (i) living in concern about the other's health; (ii) striving to be involved; (iii) experiencing confidence; and (iv) handling the illness. Many of the carers said that they lived a normal life and had come to accept diabetes as a normal part of life. At the same time, they felt they needed to be constantly attentive to how the person with diabetes was feeling, and lived their life waiting for the complications to come. They felt sorrow when they watched the health of the patient deteriorate and, whilst they had found ways to handle the illness, many felt that they lacked adequate recognition and support from health care staff. When professionals took little notice of the significant others, carers felt humiliated and neglected, and uncertain as to how best they should care for the ill person. They had questions, but no one to direct them to.

The emotional burden of caring is a recurring topic in the caregiving literature [41]. Levels of low mood and anxiety and rates of likely depression (21%) were as high, or even higher, in partners of European-American and Latino patients with type 2 diabetes as they were in the patients, especially if the partner was female [42]. Psychological distress in either partner either increases or is positively correlated with marital discord, hostility and conflict which, in turn, decreases disease-related problem solving and marital satisfaction and can affect disease management and disease progression [43]. A study in Taiwan of the primary carers of elderly people with type 2 diabetes

that used the SF-36 questionnaire to measure aspects of health-related quality of life, found that the carers had a poorer mental but better physical well-being than the population norm [44]. A study of family caregivers of diabetes patients in Sudan, using the WHO 26-item quality of life measure, found that those who were younger, single, less-educated and caring for people with more recently diagnosed illness, were relatively vulnerable to the negative effects of caring [45]. This latter research group also published evidence that there was greater concordance between the impressions of family caregivers on the patient's quality of life in type 1 than type 2 diabetes, presumably because in those with type 1 diabetes it was easier to define the factors that adversely impacted on a patient's quality of life, such as diminished sexual desire or additional medical conditions [46].

Patients with complications of their diabetes are likely to require more care, and this will place an even greater burden on their carers. A small qualitative study found that the development of diabetic foot ulcers leads to both patients and carers experiencing a reduction in social activities, increased family tensions, lost time from work and a negative effect on general health [47]. Another study of patients with diabetic foot ulcers (mean age 60 years) and their carers from centres in the USA, UK and Europe found that patient and carer scores on the SF-36 were closely correlated, with healing associated with a large improvement in the subscale related to emotional difficulties of the carers [48]. Starting insulin treatment for selected elderly people with type 2 diabetes with poor glycaemic control on tablet therapy improved not only the patients' quality of life and mood, but also limited carer strain, as measured by the general health questionnaire [49].

A UK study estimated the annual average financial cost to working-age carers of looking after someone with type 2 diabetes to be £1300, but when earnings were actually lost the cost was almost £11000. Carers who lose earnings report higher levels of strain. Only one-third of carers reported receiving state benefits, and the shortfall between earnings lost and benefits received was substantial [50].

Not surprisingly, given that people who spend a lot of time together will share many lifestyle behaviours, non-genetically related partners of people with diabetes also have a greater than twofold increased risk of being diagnosed with diabetes themselves during their lifetime compared to controls, and one in five display evidence of glucose intolerance [51].

While there is increasing support for a link between caregiver burden and diabetes, this requires further testing. For example, in a longitudinal study of frail elderly subjects in Japan, which included use of the Japanese version of the Zarit Caregiver Burden Interview, diabetes did not appear to feature as an independent predictor of caregiver burden [52].

32.5　What do carers want?

Families and friends involved in caregiving speak of their need for recognition, information and advice to help them in their caring role, and adequate support services and respite when needed (Table 32.1). While many carers are eligible to receive formal care services, practical help from the family is often the preferred option. This is not due to dissatisfaction with formal services, but rather there is a general sense that while informal networks exist an atmosphere of normality can prevail [14].

A qualitative study by Hennessy et al. [17] of family members caring for elderly American Indians with diabetes investigated diabetes care management, the challenges faced and the support services needed. The focus group participants reported a number of concerns, including anxiety about home care management, coping with psychosocial issues such as depression or non-compliance, decision making and communication with other family members. The findings would seem relevant to most informal carers trying to help and support older people with diabetes in the community.

A need for more information is the most common request of carers [53]. Subject to the consent of the older person, carers want timely education and advice about the specific health problems of the person they are caring for, what they can do to help, and the services available. Good information enables carers to

Table 32.1　What do carers want?

- Respect and recognition as a partner in care
- Timely explanation and relevant information
- The right skills and expertise to manage and care
- Knowing the options and what help is available
- Practical support, especially the opportunity to take a break
- Appropriate and flexible services, available when they are wanted
- Adequate income

become partners in the provision of care, and supports them in best helping the person they are caring for. Conversely, without information, carers are more likely to suffer from stress and consequently be less able to continue to care.

In Hennessey's study there was a perceived lack of information about the nature and the expected course of diabetes (especially in those with comorbid conditions), trepidation in handling tasks such as postoperative amputation care or coping with dialysis machines, and fears concerning the occurrence of a diabetic crisis. All of the carers emphasized the importance of developing and implementing efficient caregiving routines and mastering care techniques for successful diabetes care management. They looked for expert guidance and support on how this might be best achieved, and the implementation of diabetes education programmes targeted at family caregivers was strongly recommended.

Although any information provided must include medical management of the disease, it is equally important that consideration be given to the social and practical management of diabetes within a family context. Thus, diabetes education programmes should also offer content on predictable psychosocial and behavioural problems encountered in diabetes care management with older adults, how these problems can be addressed within the family, and where help is available when family efforts have not been successful. Despite the increasing reliance on the internet for information provision, there still is little material on diabetes that is specifically targeted at carers.

The family members in the study conducted by Hennessy and colleagues also highlighted perceived gaps in the provision and continuity of formal care services, with carers stating that they often felt stranded without sufficient professional backup for care. One common complaint was a difficulty in knowing who to contact and of obtaining a prompt response. Whilst the appointment of a case-manager should, in theory, address this, some artificial boundary or restriction is all too-often cited as a reason to be unable to help, or carers are told that 'the case has been closed' and they must go back to the end of the queue. The lack of an adequate response from professionals is short-sighted, as problems may then escalate and lead to carer breakdown and avoidable hospital admission, or a need for permanent nursing home care. Levine [54] described her sense of isolation and frustration with formal care providers in a personal account, entitled 'The Loneliness of the Long-Term Caregiver', where she said that it often felt as if "...she was challenging Goliath with a tiny pebble. More often than not, Goliath just puts me on hold."

Everyday problems such as substandard housing, a lack of modern conveniences, lack of financial resources and reliance on others for transportation will exacerbate the burden on carers, as well as interfering with the ability to develop a routine for the cared-for person. A perceived absence of professional guidance or support in dealing with psychosocial problems will mean that carers have to devise their own strategies for dealing with behavioural or psychological aspects of care, such as attempting to coax, cajole, or coerce patients into compliance with care regimens [17].

The importance of coordinating the activities of all family carers who provide assistance with diabetes care is also emphasized, with primary carers expressing frustration when they are unable to inform and synchronize the caregiving efforts of those involved. Periodically holding a family meeting with or without the participation of healthcare providers can be as an effective intervention to resolve or significantly improve understanding of diabetes care requirements [17].

32.6 What are the benefits of carer intervention?

In patients with chronic disease, adherence to medical treatment is increased when family relationships are supportive [55], and this can improve outcomes [56]. Certainly, patients who feel supported and 'cared for' report a greater sense of well-being [57], fewer depressive symptoms [58] and better general health [59]. However, family members seem to view diabetes as a more serious illness than those with the condition [60], and this lack of concordance can lead to conflict. Certainly, if patients perceive care as controlling and limiting it may have a negative impact, conceptualized as 'miscarried helping' in relation to adolescents with diabetes and their parents [61]. It is important that any carer input does not undermine patient autonomy [13, 62].

There is some (albeit limited) research evidence that the involvement of family and friends in diabetes care can improve metabolic control and the management of complications. A systematic review of prospective intervention trials of social support on health outcomes in primary and outpatient care for type 2 diabetes identified six trials of adequate quality for review [63]. Most carried evidence in support of the idea that social support is influential on self-care and outcomes.

Table 32.2 Potential benefits of networking and supported informal care.

- Provision of additional social and emotional support
- Increased availability and access to relevant health care information
- Sharing of Good Clinical Practice
- Promotion of improved health care behaviours among both patients and carers
- Increased mobilization of community-based diabetes resources
- Provide better opportunities for integrated diabetes education
- Promotes leadership qualities
- Improved blood glucose management

However, only three of the studies involved spouses, family or friends, and the mean age of the patients involved was only 59.3 years. During a 6-week educational programme with older patients with diabetes, those with participating spouses, compared to those without, showed a greater improvement in diabetes knowledge and metabolic control [64]. In contrast, the participation of family and friends in diabetes education group sessions for Native Americans had no effect on metabolic control in women with type 2 diabetes [65]. Indeed, social support may have different effects for men and women. In the study conducted by Wing *et al.* [66], support from the spouse (in the same educational programme) acted positively on weight loss for obese women with type 2 diabetes, while participating without the spouse worked out better for men.

In the observational study by Silliman [9], patients receiving more assistance from family members were more likely to report that they were taking their medications as prescribed, that they were following their diabetes diets, and that there was some correlation between family member assistance and random glucose levels.

There may be potential benefits of closer networking and greater support for carers, and these have been listed in Table 32.2.

References

1. Burroughs, T.E., Harris, M.A., Pontious, S.L., *et al.* (1997) Research on social support in adolescents with IDDM: a critical review. *The Diabetes Educator*, **23**, 438–48.

2. Lowes, L. and Lyne, P. (1999) A normal lifestyle: parental stress and coping in childhood diabetes. *British Journal of Nursing*, **8**, 133–9.

3. Armour, T.A., Norris, S.L., Jack Jr, L., *et al* (2005) The effectiveness of family interventions in people with diabetes mellitus: a systematic review. *Diabetic Medicine*, **22**, 1295–305.

4. Keogh, K.M., White, P., Smith, S.M., *et al.* (2007) Changing illness perceptions in patients with poorly controlled type 2 diabetes, a randomised controlled trial of a family-based intervention: protocol and pilot study. *BMC Family Practice*, **8**, 36.

5. Department of Health (2001) *Diabetes National Service Framework (NSF)*. Department of Health, London.

6. Hiscock, J., Legard, R. and Snape, D. (2001) *Listening to Diabetes Service Users: Qualitative Findings for the Diabetes National Service Framework*. Department of Health, London.

7. National Institute of Health and Clinical Excellence (NICE). (2007) *Type 2 diabetes (update): national clinical guideline for the management in primary and secondary care*. NICE, London.

8. Roberts, S. (2007) *Working Together for better diabetes care*. Department of Health, London.

9. Silliman, R.A., Bhatti, S., Khan, A., *et al.* (1996) The care of older persons with diabetes mellitus: families and primary care physicians. *Journal of the American Geriatrics Society*, **44**, 1314–21.

10. Sinclair, A.J. and Bayer, A.J. (2002) Informal carers of older adults with diabetes from different ethnic backgrounds. Report to British Diabetic Association and NHS Executive, West Midlands, UK.

11. Pibernik-Okanovic, M., Rogli, G., Prasek, M., *et al.* (1996). Emotional adjustment and metabolic control in newly diagnosed diabetic persons. *Diabetes Research and Clinical Practice*, **34**, 99–105.

12. Toljamo, M. and Hentinen, M. (2001) Adherence to self-care and social support. *Journal of Clinical Nursing*, **10**, 618–27.

13. Trief, P.M., Wade, M.J., Pine, D., *et al.* (2003) A comparison of health-related quality of life of elderly and younger insulin-treated adults with diabetes. *Age and Ageing*, **32**, 613–18.

14. McGarry, J. and Arthur, A. (2001) Informal caring in late life: a qualitative study of the experiences of older carers. *Journal of Advanced Nursing*, **33**, 182–9.

15. Maher, J. and Green, H. (2002) *Carers 2000*. Office of National Statistics, London.

16. Murphy, D.J., Williamson, P.S. and Nease, D.E. (1994) Supportive family members of diabetic adults. *Family Practice Research Journal*, **14**, 323–31.

17. Hennessy, C.H., John, R. and Anderson, L.A. (1999) Diabetes education needs of family members caring for American Indian elders. *The Diabetes Educator*, **25**, 747–54.

18. Parker, G. (1985) *With due care and attention: a review of research on informal care*. Family Policy Studies Centre, London.

19. Twigg, J., Atkins, K. and Perring, C. (1990) *Carers and services. A Review of research*. Her Majesty's Stationery Office, London.

20. Robles-Silva, L. (2008) The caregiving trajectory among poor and chronically ill people. *Qual Health Res*; **18** (3), 358–68.

21. Adamson, J. and Donovan, J. (2005) 'Normal disruption': South Asian and African/Caribbean relatives caring for an older family member in the UK. *Social Science and Medicine*, **60**, 37–48.

22. Godfrey, M. and Townsend, J. (2001) *Caring for an Elder with Dementia: the Experience of Asian Caregivers and Barriers to the Take-up of Support Services*. Nuffield Institute for Health, Leeds.

23. Pinquart, M. and Sörensen, S. (2005) Ethnic differences in stressors, resources, and psychological outcomes of family caregiving: a meta-analysis. *The Gerontologist*, **45**, 90–106.

24. Katbamna, S., Ahmad, W., Bhakta, P., *et al.* (2004). Do they look after their own? Informal support for South Asian carers. *Health and Social Care in the Community*, **12**, 398–406.

25. Balukonis J, Melkus GD and Chyun D (2008) Grandparenthood status and health outcomes in midlife African American women with type 2 diabetes. *Ethn Dis*; **18** (2), 141–6.

26. Jacobson, S. and Wood, F.G. (2004) Contributions of children to the care of adults with diabetes. *The Diabetes Educator*, **30**, 820–6.

27. Sayers, S.L., White, T., Zubritsky, C., *et al.* (2006). Family involvement in the care of healthy medical outpatients. *Family Practice*, **23**, 317–24.

28. Connell, C.M. (1991). Psychosocial contexts of diabetes and older adulthood: reciprocal effects. *The Diabetes Educator*, **17**, 364–71.

29. Pearlin, L.I., Mullan, J.T., Semple, S.J., *et al.* (1990). Caregiving and the stress process: an overview of concepts and their measures. *The Gerontologist*, **30**, 583–94.

30. Archbold, P.F. (1983). Impact of parent-caring on women. *Family Relations*, **32**, 39–45.

31. Sinclair, A.J., Girling, A.J. and Bayer, A.J. (2000) Cognitive dysfunction in older subjects with diabetes mellitus: impact on diabetes self-management and use of care services. *Diabetes Research and Clinical Practice*, **50**, 203–12.

32. Langa, K.M., Vijan, S., Hayward, R.A., *et al.* (2002). Informal caregiving for diabetes and diabetic complications among elderly Americans. *Journal of Gerontology*

Series B Psychological Sciences and Social Sciences, **57**, S177–86.

33. McKinlay, J.B., Crawford, S.L. and Tennstedt, S.L. (1995) The everyday impacts of providing informal care to dependent elders and their consequences for the care recipients. *Journal of Aging and Health*, **7**, 497–528.

34. Faison, K.J., Faria, S.H. and Frank, D. (1999) Caregivers of chronically ill elderly: perceived burden. *Journal of Community Health Nursing*, **16**, 243–53.

35. Ekwall, A.K., Sivberg, B. and Hallberg, I.R. (2005) Loneliness as a predictor of quality of life among older caregivers. *Journal of Advanced Nursing*, **49**, 23–32.

36. Lee, S., Kawachi, I. and Grodstein, F. (2004) Does caregiving stress affect cognitive function in older women? *The Journal of Nervous and Mental Disease*, **192**, 51–7.

37. Jørgensen, H.V., Pedersen-Bjergaard, U., Rasmussen, A.K., *et al.* (2003). The impact of severe hypoglycemia and impaired awareness of hypoglycemia on relatives of patients with type 1 diabetes. *Diabetes Care*, **26**, 1106–9.

38. Gonder-Frederick, L., Cox, D., Kovatchev, B., *et al.* (1997). The psychosocial impact of severe hypoglycemic episodes on spouses of patients with IDDM. *Diabetes Care*, **20**, 1543–6.

39. Trief, P.M., Ploutz-Snyder, R., Britton, K.D., *et al.* (2004). The relationship between marital quality and adherence to the diabetes care regimen. *Annals of Behavioral Medicine*, **27**, 148–54.

40. Stödberg, R., Sunvisson, H. and Ahlström, G. (2007) Lived experience of significant others of persons with diabetes. *Journal of Clinical Nursing*, **16**, 215–22.

41. Chappel, N.L. and Reid, R.C. (2002) Burden and well-being among caregivers: examining the distinction. *Gerontologist*, **42**, 772–80.

42. Fisher, L., Chesla, C.A., Skaff, M.M., *et al.* (2002) Depression and anxiety among partners of European-American and Latino patients with type 2 diabetes. *Diabetes Care*, **25**, 1564–70.

43. Fisher, L. (2006) Research on the family and chronic disease among adults: Major trends and directions. *Families, Systems, and Health*, **24**, 373–80.

44. Li, T.C., Lee, Y.D., Lin, C.C., *et al.* (2004) Quality of life of primary caregivers of elderly with cerebrovascular disease or diabetes hospitalized for acute care: assessment of well-being and functioning using the SF-36 health questionnaire. *Quality of Life Research*, **13**, 1081–8.

45. Awadalla, A.W., Ohaeri, J.U., Al-Awadi, S.A., *et al* (2006) Diabetes mellitus patients' family caregivers' subjective quality of life. *Journal of the National Medical Association* **98**, 727–36.

46. Awadalla AW, Ohaeri JU, Tawfiq AM and Al-Awadi SA (2006) Subjective quality of life of outpatients with diabetes: comparison with family caregivers' impressions and control group. *J Natl Med Assoc* **98** (5), 737–45.

47. Brod, M. (1998) Quality of life issues in patients with diabetes and lower extremity ulcers: patients and caregivers. *Quality of Life Research*, **7**, 365–72.

48. Nabuurs-Franssen, M.H., Huijberts, M.S.P., Nieuwenhuijzen Kruseman, A.C., *et al.* (2005) Health-related quality of life of diabetic foot ulcers patients and their caregivers. *Diabetologia*, **48**, 1906–10.

49. Reza, M., Taylor, C.D., Towse, K., *et al* (2002) Insulin improves well-being for selected elderly type 2 diabetic subjects. *Diabetes Research and Clinical Practice*, **55**, 201–7.

50. Holmes, J., Gear, E., Bottomley, J., *et al* (2003). Do people with type 2 diabetes and their carers lose income? (T2ARDIS-4). *Health Policy*, **64**, 291–6.

51. Khan, A., Lasker, S.S. and Chowdhury, T.A. (2003) Are spouses of patients with type 2 diabetes at increased risk of developing diabetes? *Diabetes Care*, **26**, 710–12.

52. Hirakawa Y, Kuzuya M, Masuda Y, Enoki H and Iguchi A (2008) Influence of diabetes mellitus on caregiver burden in home care: a report based on the Nagoya Longitudinal Study of the Frail Elderly (NLS-FE). *Geriatr Gerontol Int*; **8** (1), 41–7.

53. Bayer, A. (2004) Telling older patients and their families what they want to know. *Reviews in Clinical Gerontology*, **13**, 1–4.

54. Levine, C. (1999) The loneliness of the long-term caregiver. *New England Journal of Medicine*, **340**, 1587–90.

55. DiMatteo, M.R. (2004) Social support and patient adherence to medical treatment: a meta-analysis. *Health Psychology*, **23**, 207–18.

56. Fisher, L. and Weihs, K.L. (2000) Can addressing family relationships improve outcomes in chronic disease? *Journal of Family Practice*. **49**, 561–6.

57. Karlsen, B., Idsoe, T., Dirdal, I., *et al.* (2004). Effects of a group-based counselling programme on diabetes-related stress, coping, psychological well-being and metabolic control in adults with type 1 or type 2 diabetes. *Patient Education and Counselling*, **53**, 299–308.

58. Weihs, K., Fisher, L. and Baird, M. (2002) Families, health, and behavior. *Families, Systems, and Health*, **20**, 7–46.

59. Goodall, T.A. and Halford, W.K. (1991) Self-management of diabetes mellitus: a critical review. *Health Psychology*, **10**, 1–8.

60. White, P., Smith, S.M. and O'Dowd, T. (2007). Living with type 2 diabetes: a family perspective. *Diabetic Medicine*, **24**, 796–801.

61. Harris, M.A. (2006) The family's involvement in diabetes care and the problem of 'miscarried helping'. *European Endocrine Review*, 1–3. Available at: www.touchbriefings.com/pdf/1711/Harris.pdf. Accessed 21 December 2007.

62. Boehm, S., Schlenk, E.A., Funnell, M.M., *et al.* (1997) Predictors of adherence to nutrition recommendations in people with non-insulin-dependent diabetes mellitus. *The Diabetes Educator*, **23**, 157–65.

63. van Dam, H.A., van der Horst, F.G., Knoops, L., *et al.* (2005) Social support in diabetes: a systematic review of controlled intervention studies. *Patient Education and Counselling*, **59**, 1–12.

64. Gilden, J.L., Hendryx, M.S., Clar, S., *et al.* (1992). Diabetes support groups improve health care of older diabetic patients. *Journal of the American Geriatrics Society*, **40**, 147–50.

65. Gilliland, S.S., Azen, S.P., Perez, G.E., *et al* (2002). Strong in body and spirit: lifestyle intervention for Native American adults with diabetes in New Mexico. *Diabetes Care*, **25**, 78–83.

66. Wing, R.R., Marcus, M.D., Epstein, L.H., *et al.* (1991) A family-based approach to the treatment of obese type II diabetic patients. *Journal of Consulting and Clinical Psychology*, **59**, 156–62.

33

Diabetes Mellitus Care Models for Older People

I The European Perspective
Isabelle Bourdel-Marchasson
Geriatric Department, Hôpital Xavier Arnozan, CHU of Bordeaux, Pessac cedex, UMR 5536 CNRS/Université Victor Segalen Bordeaux 2, Bordeaux, France
II The United States Perspective
John E. Morley
GRECC, VA Medical Center and Division of Geriatric Medicine, Saint Louis University School of Medicine, St Louis, MO, USA

I The European Perspective

Key messages

- The increasing numbers of older subjects with diabetes will lead to a further public health burden associated with corresponding socioeconomic burden.
- Relatively little research data are available in the area of quality of life and health status in older people with diabetes.
- Enhancing diabetes care for older people requires well-designed and focused diabetes audits and the evaluation of differing models of care.

33.1 Introduction

Today, European countries are facing an increasing rate of obesity and sedentary lifestyle among their populations. In conjunction with an increasing life expectancy, this will inevitably result in a higher prevalence of diabetes, particularly among older people. At the beginning of the twenty-first century, approximately 50% of all French or British diabetic subjects receiving treatment were aged >65 years, and 25% were aged >75 years [1, 2]. Similar proportions among the diabetes population were identified in the Netherlands during the same time period, with some 50% of people with type 2 diabetes aged >70 years [3]. This change in the proportion of people with diabetes has numerous implications, most notably the problems of associated costs and the quality of care. In France, in 2004, the mean annual health insurance reimbursement for diabetes was €5910 per person, this value having increased slightly during the past 10 years. Yet, the growth in the proportion of diabetic subjects in any age group was estimated at 6% per year, leading to expanding health care costs [4]. Direct medical expenses were also found to be higher in subjects aged >70 years than in younger subjects in the Netherlands

(€2080 per year in those aged >70 years versus €1040 in those aged <50 years) [5].

The efficiency of current diabetes care models in the prevention of complications requires assessment especially in the elderly. Indeed, the lack of evidence in the field of geriatric diabetes – and particularly in those aged >75 years – makes the provision of clinical guidance a difficult proposition. Assuming that one-quarter of the diabetic population may be aged >75 years in Europe, major efforts towards efficiency analysis are now required in different European countries.

33.2 Current clinical guidelines in Europe

When the European Diabetes Working Party for Older People (2001–2004) developed evidence-based clinical guidelines dedicated to the elderly, they were in fact designed to complement the existing guidelines of the International Diabetes Federation (IDF, European Region), and the European Association for the Study of Diabetes (EASD) [6]. The founding statement was the promotion of overall well-being and normal life expectancy, and in particular the maintenance of an optimal level of physical and cognitive function. The right of older diabetic patients to have access, with confidence, to skilled care was also proposed. However, the position of prevention of diabetes – whether secondary or tertiary – must be clarified for each elderly patient in a similar manner as for younger patients.

33.2.1 The screening of diabetes in the elderly

The early detection of diabetes in the elderly could improve the efficiency of prevention of diabetes-induced disabilities. Undiagnosed diabetes could involve one-third of elderly diabetic people, although this proportion seems to vary widely according to the country of origin. For example, among British institutions one study estimated that 16.9% of residents had undiagnosed diabetes compared to 12.1% with known diabetes [7]. In contrast, among a French community-based population, the proportion of undiagnosed diabetes was only 1.4%, compared to 8.2% with known diabetes [8]. Moreover, undiagnosed diabetes does not necessarily mean that the condition is 'mild', as both microvascular and macrovascular complications are invariably present at the time of diagnosis. In the French community

study described above [7], the proportion of diabetic patients with a HbA_{1c} level >8% was similar in both known or unknown diabetes (respectively 19.6% and 16.1%). The criteria for screening include the presence of symptoms of hyperglycaemia, or the presence of conditions that are frequently associated with diabetes. Unfortunately, however, diabetes is frequently asymptomatic or the symptoms are non-specific, such as fatigue, weight loss and mood changes. As a result, diabetes screening should also be instigated when other geriatric problems emerge such as falls, incontinence, mental alterations and pain [6]. According to the European guidelines mentioned above, the frequency of screening for diabetes in those subjects with one or more risk factors should be at two-yearly intervals for those aged 65–74 years, and annually for those aged ≥75 years. The Desktop Guide to Type 2 Diabetes Mellitus, as approved by the IDF (European Region), has recommended that an oral glucose tolerance test (OGTT) be conducted particularly in the elderly, when the fasting plasma glucose (FPG) is normal but the suspicion is high, or there is a high risk of diabetes.

33.2.2 Healthy ageing, frailty and pathological ageing

Whilst much ethical discussion has arisen – and continues to arise – regarding the problem of prevention in the frail elderly, it I important first to clarify the target population for intensive multifactorial and expensive prevention programmes. Furthermore, such intervention might be problematic in frail elders, in which frailty represents the state between full autonomy or successful ageing and irreversible functional dependency, or pathological ageing. Yet, while this definition is imprecise the potential clinical criteria are both numerous and interrelated [9]. Indeed, diabetes could itself be considered as a frailty factor due to the multifaceted association between diabetes and disability [10]. Frailty is therefore not necessarily associated with a high mortality risk since, beyond frailty guidelines for the care of subjects with irreversible functional dependency are lacking. Indeed, in this later category, prevention is likely to be of a tertiary nature, with emphasis placed on daily living and the quality of life.

33.2.3 Construction of targets for diabetes control

In European countries, few diabetes care guidelines have addressed the issue of control in elderly diabetic patients. Targets for control and preventive actions could be derived from the categorization according to frailty criteria. According to the European Diabetes Working Party for Older People, in older patients with single system involvement (i.e. free of other major co-morbidities), a target HbA$_{1c}$ level of 6.5–7.5% should be aimed for [6]. However, the precise target agreed will depend on any existing cardiovascular risk, the presence of microvascular complications, and the ability of the individual to self-manage. For those subjects who are dependent, suffering from multisystem disease, living in care home residency (including those with dementia), and those patients in whom the hypoglycaemia risk is high and symptom control and avoidance of metabolic decompensation paramount, the target HbA$_{1c}$ range should be >7.5% to 8.5% [6]. Thus, targets for control are highly dependent on a benefit:risk ratio assessment, which itself may be related to iatrogenic problems and difficulties in self-management. The most recent French guidelines for diabetes treatment have recommended the identification of three types of elderly subject: (i) in the case of end of life and a necessity for comfort, insulin treatment should be used; (ii) in the case of poly-pathology, target of 8% should be preferred; and (iii) in the case of patients with a single system involvement, the extrapolation of data obtained in younger subjects seems reasonable, with a recommendation of starting treatment with reduced dosages, the use of Cockcroft formulae and respect of contraindications [11]. The clinical guide for the elderly diabetic patient care among a French-speaking group for study of diabetes in the elderly, has incorporated the same strategy for control target determination as did the European guide in 2004 [12].

33.2.4 Therapeutic education

Access to adequate support service – and particularly to therapeutic education – are considered the rights of elderly diabetic patients. It has been shown that an 8-week education programme utilizing telemedicine could be applied to elderly subjects (mean $\pm$ SD age 73.3 $\pm$ 6.9 years), and could also increase the subjects' quality of life [13]. The provision of diabetes education could be limited due to sensorial, cognitive and mobility impairments. Moreover, the expectations and beliefs of older people could also be altered, thus complicating the communication process. Therefore, it is recommended that, besides educational needs, any significant barrier to the receipt of education should

also be identified [6]. Caregivers, whether professional or familial, should receive diabetic education, and for this purpose a number of dietetic guidelines for caregivers have been derived. In France, for example, a mini-guide for caregivers of subjects with different health problems (including diabetes) is currently available (at no cost) from the AFSSA (the French agency for the health security of food).

33.2.5 The rationale for Comprehensive Geriatric Assessment (CGE) in frail elderly diabetic subjects

There are several arguments for performing an extended CGE in elderly diabetic patients. In general, the CGE is recommended in frail elderly, with diabetes being considered a frailty factor, much like cancer [9]. A CGE offers procedures to address the needs of frail subjects, with the aim of increasing their quality of life and preventing any worsening of their functional dependency. The CGE targets multidisciplinary domains and approaches, including medical, social and psychological fields. Indeed, diabetic subjects are prone to have social difficulties that interfere with both diabetes risk and diabetes care. The CGE also provides a good opportunity for controlling polypharmacy and preventing adverse drug reactions and interactions. On the other hand, it might be considered a waste of time and money to perform the CGE in either vigorous people or in those with irreversible functional and mental dependency. Prior to the CGE, the identification of frail subjects is therefore necessary, and consequently frailty criteria have been proposed (Table 33.1) [6, 9, 12]. In clinical practice, the CGE could take on different frameworks related to the level of complexity of the patient's situation. The minimum staff requirement to perform a CGE includes a physician, a nurse and a social worker, although the team is greatly and advantageously enriched by the presence of a psychologist, a rehabilitation therapist, a dietician and a dental surgeon. Access to basic biochemistry and haematological analyses and X-ray examinations is also required.

33.2.6 Specificity of institutions

Today, an increasing number of older people are living in geriatric institutions. A recent meta-analysis has shown that main risk factors for admission were impairment of at least two basic activities of daily living, cognitive impairment, social isolation and low income, and prior hospitalization or nursing home residence

Table 33.1 The criteria for frailty screening [6, 9, 12].

Category	Criteria
Age	Continuous effect after age 65 years
Morbidity	Stroke
	Chronic and disabling disease
	Cancer
	Absence of terminal illness
	Diabetes
	Polypharmacy and complex drug regimens
Functional impairment	Need for help with shopping, cooking and housekeeping
	Mobility impairment
	Slow gait speed
	Sensorial impairment
Geriatric syndromes	Delirium
	Under-nutrition
	Falls
	Incontinence
	Pressure ulcer
	Increased susceptibility to adverse drug events
Mental health	Depression
	Dementia from mild to moderate (severe excluded)
Nursing	Restraints
	Bed-ridden
General	Poor subjective health
Social	Socioeconomic problems
	Familial difficulties

[14]. In a geriatric setting, the prevalence of diabetes will most likely be higher than in the community, due largely to the role of diabetes in the disablement process in elderly. Thus, specific guidelines for care home residency have been proposed [6].

The baseline concerns were a lack in specialist follow-up, an inadequate dietary care, a lack of individualized diabetes care plans, and a lack of any educational and training programmes for the care home staff. Until now, no significant intervention study of any type has been conducted to assess the benefit of metabolic control and educational strategy in institutionalized elderly diabetic patients. However, the European guidelines recommended an early detection of diabetes in elderly [6], where the field is not primary prevention but rather the diagnosis of diabetes at an early stage. This could lead to early dietary intervention and perhaps then delay the use of an hypoglycaemic agent. Diabetes-related symptoms, such as hyperosmolar conditions, could be prevented. In 1999, the British Diabetic Association (now known as Diabetes UK) proposed the introduction of specific guidelines for care homes [15].

These recommendations state that each resident should be screened for the presence of diabetes, at admission to the home, and then annually. An individualized care plan should subsequently be implemented with a blood glucose control target, a dietary plan, a suggested body weight and a nursing plan. Any diabetic resident should then undergo an annual review, and have access to the following services: ophthalmology, diabetes foot clinic, dietetic and diabetes specialist team (nurse and physician).

33.2.7 Physician and staff training to diabetes care

There are moves in hand to increase the level of diabetes education and training among health care staff. It is thus recommended to enhance initial teaching and postgraduate training to address these new and increasing needs of skilled prevention and care. The initiation of insulin therapy necessitates a large degree of competency. In the elderly (notably among the frail elderly) and in institutions, the rate of insulin therapy use is particularly high and recommended, which again emphasizes the importance of training in this area. It has been suggested that, in each geriatric institution, diabetes education and training courses for staff should be available [6].

33.3 Care organization

Today, in the field of diabetes care, professional networks are now either currently in operation or are under development. In France, the national association of regional networks for diabetes care (ANCRED) includes professionals and patients with the aim of providing to patients the best care they need, where they live. Such networks were constructed to help the application of current guidelines. Despite this, the specific needs of vulnerable elders are addressed very little, which again echoes the minimal portion of the guidelines that is dedicated to the elderly.

Thus, the European guidelines [6] have proposed a framework for a management system of diabetes in the elderly, with the aim of implementing guidelines in clinical practice. Such management systems should

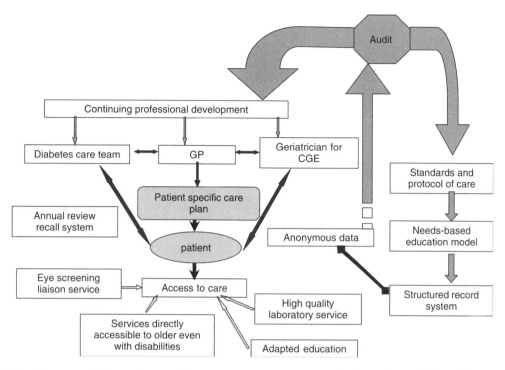

Figure 33.1 Recommendations for a diabetes management system dedicated to elderly diabetic subjects. GP = General practitioner; CGE = Comprehensive Gerontological Evaluation.

function in networks and provide training and measures through planned audits of application and effects. In the elderly, the criteria for quality of care should include the rates of disability and institutionalization (Figure 33.1).

33.4 Call for audit of quality of care

The European Diabetes Working Party for Older People in 2004 called for audits of care in elderly diabetic populations. The level of evidence for guidelines in this population is particularly low, and observational studies are required to assess the quality of care with reference to current guidelines, and to follow the effects on such quality of care. Although quality of care audits in the general population with reference to current guidelines have been widely performed in Europe, very little attention has been paid to the oldest subjects. Some target points for audits in diabetes care for older people are listed in Table 33.2.

ENTRED 2001 was an observational study of a representative sample of 10 000 French diabetic patients constructed on the basis of anti-diabetic drug

Table 33.2 Audit of Quality of care for older diabetic people.

Target point	Rationale
Assessment of criteria for diabetes care according to current guidelines for the young	Acquisition of baseline data on quality of care
Description of subjects according to frailty criteria and diabetes complications	Designing prevention procedures according to subjects' health status all along the audit process
Description of actual care networks around older subjects	Improving quality of care in continuous management based on available resources
Assessment of functional outcome	Assessment of performance at patient level
Including professionals of care in the audit process	Optimizing feedback from/to the professionals

reimbursement from the National Health Service [16]. As mentioned above, one-quarter of these patients were aged >75 years. Subjects and their general practitioners were asked to complete a questionnaire and, for each patient, reimbursements of medical consultations and biological analysis were recorded. The response rate to self-questionnaires was low in older subjects compared to younger, with a linear shape decrease from 50% in those aged <65 years to 25% in those aged >85 years. This audit showed a low referral to specialists in the older subjects, and also a lower level of follow-up. A lack of any HbA_{1c} measurement was found in 11% of subjects aged >75 years, in 6% in those aged 65–74 years, and in 7% in those aged <64 years. A global analysis showed that the care of subjects aged >65 years displayed a tertiary prevention pattern.

An audit of quality of care performed in diabetes centres in Italy showed that the application of current guidelines was different according to centres, and that this was the most important cause of variation [17]. In Italy, the aim of the IMPLEMEG study was to assess the efficiency of different strategies for the implementation of diabetes care guidelines [18]. However, investigations of the effect of age and comorbidity on care choices were not planned. This issue seems an interesting point to explore, and it has indeed been shown that age and comorbidity reduced the rate of intensification of therapy [19]. In fact, in this latter study no reference to the CGE was made, and the quality of care audit was based on guidelines for the general diabetic population in a secondary prevention perspective, which was unlikely to have been adapted to all of the oldest patients.

The quality of care provided to elderly people with diabetes living in long-term care facilities is generally insufficient, and worse than that provided to people living in their own home, although this may of course be true for any chronic condition [20]. In a French audit of a group of geriatric care homes, various procedures of medical follow-up were performed as recommended in only 25–50% of residents. Among those items, HbA_{1c} was tested at least three times each year in 25% of residents, while another 25% had no HbA_{1c} measurement at all, 40% had no weight measurement, and 47% had no blood pressure recorded within the past 18 months. The level of HbA_{1c} was poorly controlled (>8.5%) in 20% of the people, which was close to the estimate of 17% found in a British study [21]. The other items included blood pressure and weight monitoring, while annual eye, foot, cardiovascular, renal and dental examinations were also performed to an insufficient degree.

33.5 Perspectives

The future outlook suggests that there is a need to increase the evidence base in geriatric diabetes, and also to ensure that the guidelines provide sound and robust assistance in delivering high-quality diabetes care. The first step in this direction would seem to be the establishment of pragmatic guidelines that are specific to elderly subjects, but with special attention being paid to frail or dependent subjects. In addition, these guidelines should be periodically reassessed on the basis of both cohort follow-up studies and on investigations of both feasibility and cost-effectiveness. A minimum data set has been recently established via Gerontonet, a European network for the study of health care among older people. This comprised a short CGE which was particularly fitted to diabetic subjects [22]. In old patients, end points such as quality of life and disability-free expectancy should be preferred, rather than survival.

II The United States Perspective

Key messages
* The prevalence of diabetes mellitus in older people within the United States has doubled over the past 25 years.
* Both, metformin and thiazolidinediones, are increasingly used in the United States to treat older people with type 2 diabetes.

33.6 Introduction

In the United States, 12.2 million persons aged >60 years have diabetes mellitus and thus, over half of all diabetics are aged >60 years. Currently, over half a million new cases of diabetes mellitus are diagnosed each year in persons aged over 60 years, with the mean age of onset of the condition being 51.9 years. The prevalence of diabetes mellitus in persons aged >65 years doubled between 1980 and 2005 (Table 33.3). The rate of increase in diabetes mellitus has been greater than the rate of increase in obesity. On an ethnic basis, diabetes is almost twice as common in Blacks than Whites, and 60% more common in Hispanics, while older males are more likely to be diabetic than are females. Among persons with diabetes mellitus aged 65–79 years, the average duration of the condition is 9.6 years. Moreover, diabetes is the seventh leading cause of death in persons aged >65 years.

Diabetic complications are more common in older persons (Table 33.4). For example, Rosenthal *et al.* [23] found that nephropathy and retinopathy occurred

Table 33.3 The changing prevalence of diabetes mellitus in the United States, between 1980 and 2005.

Year	Prevalence (%)	
	Aged 65–74 years	Aged 75+ years
1980	9.1	8.9
1985	10.2	10.0
1990	9.9	8.6
1995	11.1	10.6
2000	15.4	13.0
2005	18.5	15.6

Table 33.4 Complications in older persons with diabetes mellitus.

Complication	Prevalence (per 1000)	
	Aged 65–74 years	Aged 75+ years
Mobility impairment	662	783
Cardiovascular disease	480	580
Visual impairment	226	271
Peripheral arterial disease	8	12
Ulcers	8	10
End-stage renal disease	4	4
Neuropathy	4	4

after 5 years in older diabetics compared to 15 years in younger diabetics. Cardiovascular disease is present in 58% of diabetics aged >75 years, while mobility is impaired in 78.3% and visual impairment occurs in 27.1% of diabetics aged >65 years. Amputations occur commonly in diabetics aged ≥65 years; each year, 3.4 subjects in 1000 have above-knee amputations, 3.3 in 1000 below-knee amputations, and one in 1000 a foot amputation.

In two national studies examining the prevalence of diabetes mellitus in nursing homes [24, 25], one study reported a value of 24.6%, and the other 26.4%, which was similar to the value of 23.8% seen in the general population aged >60 years. The present author's unpublished data have suggested that the prevalence of diabetes mellitus may be closer to 30% in nursing homes when diagnoses are carefully made, instead of relying on the physicians' diagnoses. This is in keeping with the prevalence of undiagnosed diabetes mellitus in the community. Typically, those people with diabetes mellitus who are resident in nursing homes receive more medications (mean 10.3) than those non-resident (mean 8.4).

33.7 Specific issues in older diabetics

Cognitive problems are extremely common in older diabetics [26], and clearly this is, in part, associated with an increase in vascular dementia secondary to the increase in atherosclerosis. In addition, hyperinsulinaemia is associated with an increase in Alzheimer's disease, possibly because the insulin-degrading enzyme also degrades amyloid-beta peptide in the brain. Both, hyperglycaemia and hypoglycaemia are associated with memory disturbances; indeed, it was recently shown that hypertriglyceridaemia causes a direct decrease in memory capability [27]. Cognitive disturbances in persons with diabetes lead to compliance issues, and for these reasons it is suggested that all older diabetics have their cognitive function regularly checked, using a tool such as the Saint Louis University Mental Status Test [28].

Depression is more common among older diabetics than among other older persons, and is largely associated with an increase in hospitalizations and mortality [23]. Depression is also a cause of worse compliance in older persons.

Falls are a major cause of injuries in older persons, with injurious falls being more common among older diabetics than among others living in the community [29]. Among people with diabetes, falls tend to be more common when the HbA_{1c} level is <7% [30]; the causes of such falls include hypoglycaemia, orthostasis, syncope, medications, peripheral neuropathy, myopathies, balance problems, foot abnormalities, impaired vision and impaired executive function leading to problems with dual tasking (a failure to be able to 'walk and talk'). Therapy with statins may be an important cause of falls in older diabetics.

Pressure ulcers are more common and heal more slowly in older persons with diabetes mellitus [31, 32], possibly due to zinc deficiency, to tissue glycation and vascular impairment. Zinc deficiency is common in diabetics as people with diabetes mellitus have an impaired absorption of zinc and consequent hyperzincuria [33].

People with type 2 diabetes mellitus tend to have an increase in numbers of fractures, despite having an increase in their bone mineral density (BMD) [34]. *Thiazolidinediones* tend to reduce BMD, with the result being a greater incidence of fracture [35].

Hyperglycaemia results in a hyperosmolar diuresis that is associated with nocturia and sleep disturbances, as well as incontinence. In many cases, however, good diabetic control can decrease nocturia and incontinence.

Diabetics tend to have an accelerated loss of muscle mass (sarcopenia) that occurs with ageing. This may be due to a greater prevalence of hypogonadism in older diabetic males [36]. Diabetics may also show increases

Table 33.5 Special issues in the care of the older diabetic patient.

- Cognitive impairment
- Vascular dementia
- Alzheimer's disease
- Hypoglycaemia
- Hyperglycaemia
- Hypertriglyceridaemia
- Depression
- Falls
- Fractures
- Sarcopenia
- Disability
- Pressure ulcers
- Nocturia
- Sleep disturbances
- Incontinence
- Tuberculosis
- Recurrent urinary tract infection
- Hypogonadism

in cytokine levels, and this leads to an accelerated muscle loss [37]. Insulin resistance leads to an increased fat accumulation in muscle and decreased muscle power, while atherosclerosis leads to peripheral vascular disease and muscle anoxia. Sarcopenia results in increased functional impairment in older diabetics [38].

High glucose levels represent an excellent medium for the growth of bacteria and fungi; consequently, older diabetics are highly prone to recurrent tuberculosis, to suffer fungal infections and have recurrent urinary tract infections.

Some of the special issues that must be considered in the older diabetic patient are listed in Table 33.5.

33.8 Management of diabetes

The treatment of older diabetics tends to be relatively aggressive in the United States where, in nursing homes, many patients will have serum HbA_{1c} levels <7% [39]. Among the older diabetic community there is also a greater use of medications in persons aged >65 years (88%) compared to those aged 18–44 years (71.7%).

In older diabetics, weight loss has been shown to be associated with increased mortality [40], although in various institutions it has been shown that neither diabetic diets nor the restriction of sweets improves diabetic control [41, 42].

In the Diabetes Prevention Program, a lifestyle modification with a focus on exercise was most effective in preventing diabetes in the 60–85-year-old group (3.3 per 100 persons-years) compared to that in the 45–59-year olds (4.9 per 100 persons-years) and the 25–44-year olds (6.3 per 100 persons-years) [43]. Metformin, on the other hand, was less effective with advancing age [43].

Between 1990 and 2001 there was a 2.9-fold increase in the use of oral anti-diabetic drugs in the United States, due mainly to the introduction of metformin in 1995, followed by the thiazolidinediones. By 2007, the thiazolidinediones accounted for 6.3 million prescriptions compared to 1.4 million for glyburide. A subsequent meta-analysis suggested that rosiglitizone was associated with increased cardiovascular disease, and this led to a rapid decrease in the drug's prescriptions. Although, in 2007 the long-acting insulin gla-insulin (lantus) was the second best selling anti-diabetic drug in the United States, during the same year the total sales of the first of the dipeptidyl peptidase IV (DPP-IV) inhibitors reached US$ 471 million.

The anti-diabetic drugs most commonly used in the United States are listed in Table 33.6. Long-acting insulin, which is now commonly administered as a basal insulin in older persons, can be used with or without other oral anti-diabetic drugs or shorter-acting insulins. Metformin is generally not used in the United States in persons aged >80 years, as the majority of such patients will have some degree of impaired renal function. As calculated by the Cockcroft–Gault equation, metformin also causes anorexia and weight loss [44].

Although *pioglitazone* is still commonly used in 'old-old' patients, its potential effects to enhance the loss of bone have limited its use in this population. The oedema associated with rosiglitazone has also markedly limited its use, while both exenatide and pramilentide – both of which cause weight loss – are rarely used in older persons because of their potential interaction with the anorexia of aging [45].

The use of *sitagliptin*, a DPP-IV inhibitor, which increases the incretin, glucagon-like peptide, is rapidly increasing. Interestingly, there has also been some use – albeit minimal – of the two alpha-1-glucosidase inhibitors which also increase glucagon-like peptide [46, 47].

33.9 Conclusions

Overall in the United States, diabetes mellitus is relatively aggressively treated, especially in institutionalized older persons. The National Health Objectives for 2010 require: (i) a dilated eye examination in 75% of cases; (ii) a foot examination in 75%; (iii) the measurement of plasma glucose daily in 60%; and (iv) an annual assessment of serum HbA_{1c} level in 50% of cases. Among those persons aged >65 years by the year 2000, almost 72% had undergone a dilated eye examination and 55% a foot examination. The self-monitoring of blood glucose in persons aged 65–74 years was 43%, while HbA_{1c} levels were monitored in 15.9%. Moreover, the proportions were even less than in those subjects aged >75 years. Based on the NHANES data, the mean serum HbA_{1c} level in persons aged >65 years with diabetes was reduced from 7.49% (i.e. <7% in 36.2% of cases) in 1999–2000 to 6.72% (<7% in 68.3% of cases) in 2003–2004 [48]. The management of hypertension and lipids was also improved. Despite these findings, the results of some recent studies have proposed that the excessive control of diabetes mellitus might in fact be deleterious, which suggests that the care of older diabetics may be approaching optimal levels in the United States.

Table 33.6 Drugs used to treat diabetes mellitus in older persons in the United States.

	Insulins	Sulphonylureas	Metformin	α-Glucosidase inhibitors	Thiazolidenediones	DPP-IV inhibitors
Target	Muscle/fat	Beta cell	Liver	Gut/beta cell	Muscle/fat	Beta cell
HbA_{1c}	>2%	1–2%	1–2%	0.5–1%	0.5–2%	0.5–1%
Effect on fasting	Positive	Positive	Positive	Moderate	Positive	Moderate
Postprandial effect	Positive	Moderate	Moderate	Positive	Moderate	Positive
Weight change	Increase	Increase	Decrease	Decrease	Increase	No change
Cost (US$)	30–450	10–15	30–60	40–80	80–100	200

Acknowledgments

The author acknowledges that the statistics on diabetes in the United States were abstracted from www.cdc.gov in June, 2008.

References

1. *Diabetes in the UK* (2004) Diabetes, UK, London.
2. Névanen S, Tambekou J, Fosse S, Simon D, Weill A, Varroud-Vial M, *et al.* Caractéristiques et état de santé des personnes diabétiques âgées et leur prise en charge médicale, étude Entred 2001. Bulletin Epidemiologique Hebdomadaire 2005; 12–13: 51–2.
3. Ubink-Veltmaat LJ, Bilo HJ, Groenier KH, Houweling ST, Rischen RO and Meyboom-de Jong B. Prevalence, incidence and mortality of type 2 diabetes mellitus revisited: a prospective population-based study in The Netherlands (ZODIAC-1). European Journal of Epidemiology 2003; 18 (8): 793–800.
4. Vallier N, Weill A, Salanave B, Bourrel R, Cayla M, Suarez C, *et al.* Cost of thirty long-term diseases for beneficiaries of the French general health insurance scheme in 2004. Pratiques et Organisation des Soins 2006; 37 (4): 267–83.
5. Redekop WK, Koopmanschap MA, Rutten GE, Wolfenbuttel BH, Stolk RP and Niessen LW. Resource consumption and costs in Dutch patients with type 2 diabetes mellitus. Results from 29 general practices. Diabet Med. 2002; 19 (3): 246–53.
6. European Diabetes Working Party for Older People (2004) Clinical Guidelines for Type 2 Diabetes Mellitus. Available from: http://www.eugms.org/index.php (accessed 1 November 2007).
7. Sinclair AJ, Gadsby R, Penfold S, Croxson SC and Bayer AJ. Prevalence of diabetes in care home residents. Diabetes Care 2001; 24 (6): 1066–8.
8. Bourdel-Marchasson I, Helmer C, Barberger-Gateau P, Peuchant E, Fevrier B, Ritchie K, *et al.* Characteristics of undiagnosed diabetes in community-dwelling French elderly: the 3C study. Diabetes Research and Clinical Practice 2007; 76 (2): 257–64.
9. Bourdel-Marchasson I and Berrut G. Caring the elderly diabetic patient with respect to concepts of successful aging and frailty. Diabetes Metab. 2005; 31 (Spec. No. 2): 13–19.
10. Bourdel-Marchasson I, Helmer C, Fagot-Campagna A, Dehail P and Joseph PA. Disability and quality of life in elderly people with diabetes. Diabetes Metab. 2007; 33 (Suppl. 1): S66–74.
11. Traitement médicamenteux du diabète de type 2. Recommandation de bonne pratique [Medical treatment of type 2 diabetes. Recommendations for good practice]. Diabetes Metab. 2007; 33 (1Pt 2): 1S7–25.
12. French-speaking group for study of diabetes in the elderly. (2008) Guide pour la prise en charge du diabétique âgé [Clinical guide for elderly diabetic patient care]. Médecine des Maladies Métaboliques 2008; 2 (Hors série): 1–53.
13. Chan WM, Woo J, Hui E, Lau WW, Lai JC and Lee D. A community model for care of elderly people with diabetes via telemedicine. Appl Nurs Res. 2005; 18 (2): 77–81.
14. Gaugler JE, Duval S, Anderson KA and Kane RL. Predicting nursing home admission in the U.S: a meta-analysis. BMC Geriatrics. 2007; 7: 13.
15. British Diabetic Association. (1999) Guidelines of Practice for Residents with Diabetes in Care Homes. Available from: www.diabetes.org.uk/Documents/ Reports/guideline_residents.pdf. (accessed 1 November 2007).
16. Institut National de veille sanitaire. (2005) ENTRED study. Representative sample of French diabetic people. Available from: http://www.invs.sante.fr/ recherche/index2.asp?txtQuery=Entred (accessed 1 November 2007).
17. Petrelli A, Saitto C, Arca M and Perucci CA. Diabetes management by hospital-affiliated diabetes centres in Lazio, Italy. European Journal of Public Health 2004; 14 (2): 120–2.
18. Perria C. Strategies for the introduction and implementation of a guideline for the treatment of type 2 diabetics by general practitioners (GPs) of the Lazio region of Italy (IMPLEMEG study): protocol for a cluster randomised controlled trial [ISRCTN80116232]. BMC Health Services Research 2004; 4 (1): 13.
19. Chaudhury SI, Berlowitz DR and Concato J. Do age and comorbidity affect intensity of pharmacological therapy for poorly controlled diabetes mellitus? Journal of the American Geriatrics Society 2005; 53 (7): 1214–16.
20. Fahey T, Montgomery AA, Barnes J and Protheroe J. Quality of care for elderly residents in nursing homes and elderly people living at home: controlled observational study. Br Med J (Clinical Research Ed.) 2003; 326 (7389): 580.
21. Taylor CD and Hendra TJ. The prevalence of diabetes mellitus and quality of diabetic care in residential and nursing homes. A postal survey. Age and Ageing 2000; 29 (5): 447–50.
22. Sinclair AJ. Towards a minimum data set for intervention studies in type 2 diabetes in older people. Journal of Nutrition, Health and Aging 2007; 11 (3): 289–93; discussion 92–3.

23. Rosenthal MJ, Fajardo M, Gilmore S, *et al.* Hospitalization and mortality of diabetes in older adults. A 3-year prospective study. Diabetes Care 1998; 21: 231–5.

24. Resnick HE, Heineman J, Stone R and Shorr RI. (2008) Diabetes in U.S. Nursing Homes, 2004. Diabetes Care, 31, 287–8.

25. Travis SS, Buchanan RJ, Wang S and Kim M. Analyses of nursing home residents with diabetes at admission. J Am Med Dir Assoc. 2004, 5, 320–7.

26. Biessels GJ, Deary IM and Ryan CM. Cognition and diabetes: a lifespan perspective. Lancet Neurol. 2008, 7, 184–90.

27. Farr SA, Yamada KA, Butterfield DA, *et al.* Obesity and hypertriglyceridemia produce cognitive impairment. Endocrinology 2008, 149, 2628–36.

28. Tariq SH, Tumosa N, Chibnall JT, *et al.* Comparison of the Saint Louis University mental status examination and the mini-mental state examination for detecting dementia and mild neurocognitive disorder – a pilot study. Am J Geriatr Psychiatr. 2006, 14, 900–10.

29. Miller DK, Lui LY, Perry HM, III, *et al.* Reported and measured physical functioning in older inner-city diabetic African Americans. J Gerontol A Biol Sci Med Sci. 1999, 54, M230–6.

30. Nelson JM, Dufraux K and Cook PF. The relationship between glycemic control and falls in older adults. J Am Geriatr Soc. 2007, 55, 2041–4.

31. Brandeis GH, Ooi WL, Hossain M, *et al.* A longitudinal study of risk factors associated with the formation of pressure ulcers in nursing homes. J Am Geriatr Soc. 1994, 42, 388–93.

32. Berlowitz DR, Brandeis GH, Morris JN, *et al.* Deriving a risk-adjustment model for pressure ulcer development using the Minimum Data Set. J Am Geriatr Soc. 2001, 49, 866–71.

33. Neiwoehner CB, Allen JI, Boosalis M, *et al.* Role of zinc supplementation in type II diabetes mellitus. Am J Med. 1986, 81, 63–8.

34. Dobnig H, Piswanger-Solkner JC, Roth M, *et al.* Type 2 diabetes mellitus in nursing home patients: effects on bone turnover, bone mass, and fracture risk. J Clin Endocrniol Metab. 2006, 91, 3355–63.

35. Meier C, Kraenzlin ME, Bodmer M, *et al.* Use of thiazolidinediones and fracture risk. Arch Intern Med. 2008, 168, 820–5.

36. Tripathy D, Dhindsa S, Garg R, *et al.* Hypogonadotropic hypogonadism in erectile dysfunction associated with type 2 diabetes mellitus: a common defect? Metab Syndr Relat Disord. 2003, 1, 75–80.

37. Kim MJ, Rolland Y, Cepeda O, *et al.* Diabetes mellitus in older men. Aging Male 2006, 9, 139–47.

38. Morley JE, Kim MJ, Haren MT, *et al.* Frailty and the aging male. Aging Male 2005, 8, 135–40.

39. Joseph J, Koka M and Aronow WS. Prevalence of a hemoglobin A1c less than 7.0%, of a blood pressure less than 130/80mmHg, and of a serum low-density lipoprotein cholesterol less than 100mg/dL in older patients with diabetes mellitus in an academic nursing home. J Am Med Dir Assoc. 2008, 9, 51–4.

40. Wedick NM, Barrett-Connor E, Knoke JD and Wingard DL. The relationship between weight loss and all-cause mortality in older men and women with and without diabetes mellitus: the Rancho Bernardo study. J Am Geriatr Soc. 2002, 50, 1810–15.

41. Tariq SH, Karcic E, Thomas DR, *et al.* The use of a no-concentrated-sweets diet in the management of type 2 diabetes in the nursing homes. J Am Diet Assoc. 2001, 101, 1463–6.

42. Coulston AM, Mandelbaum D and Reaven GM. Dietary management of nursing home residents with non-insulin-dependent diabetes mellitus. Am J Clin Nutr. 1990, 51, 67–71.

43. Drandall J, Schade D, *et al.* and the Diabetes Prevention Program Research Group. The influence of age on the effects of lifestyle modification and metformin in prevention of diabetes. J Gerontol A Biol Sci Med Sci., 2006, 61, 1075–81.

44. Lee A and Morley JE. Metformin decreases food consumption and induces weight loss in subjects with obesity with type II non-insulin-dependent diabetes. Obes Res. 1998, 6, 47–53.

45. Rolland Y, Kim MJ, Gammack JK, *et al.* Office management of weight loss in older persons. Am J Med. 2006, 119, 1019–26.

46. Lee A, Patrick P, Wishart J, *et al.* The effects of miglitol on glucagon-like peptide-1 secretion and appetite sensations in obese type 2 diabetics. Diabetes Obes Metab. 2002, 4, 329–35.

47. DeLeon MJ, Chandurkar V, Albert SG and Mooradian AD. Glucagon-like peptide-1 response to acarbose in elderly type 2 diabetic subjects. Diabetes Res Clin Pract. 2002, 56, 101–6.

48. Hoerger TJ, Segel JE, Gregg EW and Saaddine JB. Is glycemic control improving in the U.S. adults? Diabetes Care 2008, 31, 81–6.

34

Further Initiatives to Enhance Diabetes Care in Older People

Alan Sinclair

Bedfordshire and Hertfordshire Postgraduate Medical School, University of Bedfordshire, Luton, UK

Key Messages

- Improving diabetes care for older people is a major challenge for modern-day clinicians, and involves achieving high-quality care and standards across all clinical domains.
- Inpatient diabetes care is a relatively understudied area of research. However, the application of sound principles of assessment and prevention can do much to alleviate inpatient problems and improve discharge outcomes.
- The development of a robust minimum dataset for patients with diabetes will increase the likelihood of consistency of outcome data, and provide a more meaningful interpretation of the results of clinical trials.

34.1 Introduction

One of the greatest challenges that the medical profession faces in the twenty-first century is the epidemic relating to obesity and the marked rise in type 2 diabetes. All members of the profession must honour their own commitment to strive for excellence in medical care, and diabetes in ageing subjects poses one of the more distinct of these challenges.

Thoroughness and vigilance are prime qualities that are needed in managing older people with diabetes, especially in the areas of assessment and treatment [1]. This may be particularly important in older patients with diabetes who may have considerable (but often undetected) impaired lower-extremity function. The wide spectrum of vascular complications, acute metabolic decompensation, adverse effects of medication, and the effects of the condition on nutrition and lifestyle behaviour, may all create varying levels of impairment and/or disability. These changes may have adverse rebound effects on vulnerability to other comorbidities, independence and quality of life. Advancing age itself – even in the absence of specific diagnosed conditions – is associated with disability, suggesting that disease prevention or amelioration would only be partially effective.

Each disability has the potential to disadvantage individuals considerably (handicap), such as failure to enjoy outside entertainment and leisure activities, and an inability to go shopping. Yet, handicap is not an inevitable occurrence, as many factors such as the reversibility of the intrinsic impairment, the presence of other medical comorbidities, mood, and even social support and financial status, can have dramatic effects on the level of impact of the disability.

Whilst the need for specific rehabilitation programmes for diabetes-related disability requires justification, those clinicians managing older subjects will require a detailed knowledge of any assessments and available therapies via a multidisciplinary environment.

Diabetes in Old Age. Third Edition. Edited by Alan J. Sinclair
© 2009 John Wiley & Sons, Ltd

Also required is an ability to set not only the goals and a realistic time frame for rehabilitation, but also what aides and appliances are available to achieve this. In a similar manner to educational programmes, encouraging subjects to take an active part in rehabilitation can, in the present author's experience, foster autonomy, improve self-esteem and coping skills and also reduce anxiety and depression.

Although this is complex area, several research groups have undertaken studies which take us forward to understanding the nature of the disabling process, and are continuing to pave the way for re-enablement in diabetes [2, 3]. Whilst the 'multifactorial' nature of this process may prevent straightforward interventions from being effective, there is a need for a greater understanding of the role of glycaemic control, and larger-scale randomized controlled trials need to be conducted to assist in this exploration.

In addition, there is a need to stimulate the interest of clinical and laboratory research groups to provide the evidence that can justify particular therapeutic interventions and promote specific patterns of care characterized by three themes: (i) a major emphasis on the quality of life and well-being of each patient; (ii) early and effective interventions; and (iii) a commitment to improve, or at least maintain, functional status.

Acquiring unique knowledge and skills in *geriatric diabetes* enhances diabetes care for the vulnerable directly, and often indirectly by influencing attitudes (avoiding ageism and a reductionist approach) to care. This book has been devoted to this goal.

The following two areas are distinct – but complementary – themes which have significant potential to improve diabetes care for older people:

- Improving inpatient diabetes care

- The use of a diabetes minimum dataset (MDS) to enhance care.

34.2 Improving inpatient diabetes care

Older adults with diabetes have a two- to fourfold increase in the risk of hospitalization, while factors such as a high likelihood of significant preadmission medical comorbidities and disability often result in poor clinical outcomes and a prolonged length of stay. Major vascular episodes such as a stroke or myocardial infarction are common causes of admission in older patients with diabetes. The diagnosis of diabetes is often made for the first time at admission into hospital, since some 40% of older adults presenting with hyperglycaemia have no previous history of diabetes. In this situation it is imperative that the treatment of diabetes is not delayed, as mortality may be significant within the first two days of admission.

Older adults pose several additional problems of diabetes care relating to the time of admission, their inpatient stay, and the predischarge and discharge phases. Preventive strategies in the community to reduce hospitalization include the prompt treatment of urinary and chest and skin infections, the opportunistic screening for diabetes in housebound elderly and care home residents [4], where early treatment will reduce metabolic decompensation, and the early recognition of depressive illness [5].

In the following section, further commentary on inpatient diabetes care will be provided to complement the detailed and comprehensive information on acute hospital admissions in Chapter 24. These studies have formed the basis of a contribution to a UK document on emergency and inpatient diabetes care [6]. The basic aims of inpatient care are listed in Table 34.1.

34.2.1 Admission

Decompensation due to ketoacidosis is often rapid in onset, whilst hyperglycaemic non-ketotic coma may

Table 34.1 Inpatient care of older adults with diabetes: the aims of care.

- Treat infection promptly and aim to stabilize glycaemia within 48 h of admission.

- To exclude nutritional impairment and ensure dietary planning: consider enteral feeding early for those with critical illness or postoperative cases.

- To undertake a full functional assessment, including the assessment of mood, cognition, gait and socioeconomic factors.

- To diagnose all cases of diabetes in those presenting with acute hyperglycaemia: use both a fasting glucose and an oral glucose tolerance test where necessary, and be prepared to repeat at time of discharge.

- Ensure that a comprehensive predischarge assessment is carried out to minimize readmission and increase the overall quality of diabetes care.

- Maintain dignity and equity of care in all hospital departments at all times.

follow an insidious course of several days, associated with signs of dehydration, reduced consciousness and other signs of hyperosmolality. Thiazide diuretics, calcium-channel blockers and steroids have each been associated with precipitating hyperglycaemic crises in elderly patients.

Hyperglycaemic emergencies require prompt treatment in order to reduce disabling morbidity and premature death. The residents of care homes are particularly vulnerable, with admission due to metabolic decompensation carrying a high mortality rate, presumably due to multiple comorbidities and a delay in admission. Treatment involves adequate rehydration, intravenous insulin and also antibiotics where infection is considered an underlying precipitating factor. In severe cases, there should be no hesitation in transferring patients to a critical care unit for intensive monitoring.

34.2.2 Postoperative care

In order to minimize thromboembolic complications, infection rates and prolonged hospitalization, postoperative diabetes care should be supervised where possible by the diabetes team with a focus on skin and wound care by employing pressure-relieving support mattresses, a tailored nutritional therapy that ensures adequate calories and protein intake to offset the effects of surgery and catabolism, and early mobilization to enhance lower-limb functional recovery. The glycaemic targets should be set at HbA_{1c} <7.5%, fasting glucose <8.0 mmol l^{-1}, and random levels of <9 mmol l^{-1}, to reduce infection rates, enhance wound repair and avoid metabolic decompensation. The consideration for insulin therapy should be an early decision.

34.2.3 Nutritional and feeding issues

Nutritional impairment – if untreated – leads to increased mortality, a greater length of hospital stay, additional drug therapy, and a higher infection rate due to a depressed immune function. This in essence reflects a 'failure to thrive' state, and is often complicated by both water and electrolyte disturbances. Older people with diabetes thus require an early assessment of nutrient needs by a qualified hospital dietician, consideration for influenza vaccination (depending on the time of year), and a programme of nursing and medical care which minimizes dehydration, pressure sore development and pain.

At the time of admission, signs of malnutrition [body mass index (BMI) <18.5 and >10% weight loss in the previous three months] are present in as many as 25% of cases, with this situation being more prevalent in those aged ≥80 years. All older adults require a nutritional assessment to be made within 48 h of admission, with signs of anorexia in particularly being sought. Currently, a suitable instrument for this, which is recommended by NICE and BAPEN, is the Malnutrition Universal Screening Tool (MUST) [7]. This approach does not require the measurement of both height and weight, and has been correlated with clinical outcome.

34.2.4 Tube-feeding

Older adults often have a significant reduced caloric intake due to acute illness, to the effects of multiple drugs, and to cognitive impairment. Dysphagia – both temporary and neurologically induced (e.g. by a stroke) – requires enteral tube feeding via a nasogastric tube or percutaneous endoscopic gastrostomy (PEG). Patients will benefit from a well-planned enteral formula (high concentrations of fructose, fibre and monounsaturated fatty acids), which has been shown to optimize the patient's nutritional status and reduce postprandial glucose excursions. A daily dietary provision should be at least 25–35 kcal kg^{-1} body weight, and this should reduce the likelihood of hypoglycaemia in those receiving insulin. Tube-feeding for many older adults is affected by changes in mental performance or mood status, and may prove to be a barrier to successful compliance.

34.2.5 Inpatient functional assessment

In view of the increased likelihood of disability in those with diabetes who are aged ≥80 years, patients require not only an assessment of lower-limb strength (to exclude proximal myopathy) but also a foot examination to assess their neurovascular status. Observation of the patient's gait is essential to identify any remedial problems and to plan muscle-strengthening exercises: this process promotes the maintenance of mobility, reduces the falls rate, and may also lessen urinary incontinence – which may be present in up to 30% of older patients with diabetes.

In addition, in view of the high incidence of depression (a significant predictor of admission into hospital of older people with diabetes) and cognitive impairment, all older people require an evaluation for the presence of these conditions. This can be carried out using a Geriatric Depression Score (GDS) [8], and a

Mini-Mental State Examination score [9] or a 2-minute Clock Test [10]. Each of these tests may identify issues which require further specialist investigation and treatment.

34.2.6 Predischarge and discharge

At the predischarge period, a close liaison with the family and/or carers – including referral to social services – is recommended. Clear nutritional instructions and meal planning guidelines should be provided by an experienced nutritional health professional. A predischarge visit by a specialist diabetes nurse is of paramount importance.

A clear *medication schedule* is essential, documenting clearly what changes to treatment have taken place. This is necessary because hospitalization is known to increase the postdischarge rate of hypoglycaemia, presumably due to inpatient discontinuance of usual therapy (e.g. a sulphonylurea), followed by the reinstitution of therapy which may create misunderstandings among health professional staff, patients and families.

Those older adults with diabetes who require subsequent admission (or return) to a care home should receive a preadmission comprehensive geriatric assessment. Here, the patient's further nutritional needs are assessed, the feeding regimens planned, drug schedules rationalized, and specialist diabetes follow-up arranged as appropriate. Liaison with Primary Care is essential in these circumstances.

34.3 The use of a diabetes minimum dataset (MDS) to enhance care

As a means of enhancing the validity and consistency of data collected during clinical trials with older subjects, a geriatric minimum dataset has been developed [11]. This approach ensures that the essential data are collected to allow a more informed interpretation of outcome data. It is reasonable to conclude that this approach may be valid in different disease areas, where a more uniform approach to research is required.

In the field of type 2 diabetes, a minimum data set might serve four primary purposes:

- To provide a standardized method of assessment and outcome measures for conducting large-scale intervention studies with a randomized controlled design.

- To enable valid comparisons of research findings in different populations of patients.

- To allow a more detailed analysis of the validity, reliability and sensitivity of existing measures, and to promote the development of new measures suitable for studies in older people.

- By systematic review procedures and meta-analyses of studies using a recognized minimum data set, there will be an increased likelihood of demonstrating both clinical and cost-effectiveness of a range of interventions.

Several diabetes datasets have also been developed and published. The European Commission were recently involved in the design of the DIABCARD, which consists of diabetes-related data and administrative data [12] and forms part of an initiative towards having European healthcards (EU/G7 healthcards). The DIABCARD has the advantage of being compatible with other datasets being developed, such as the German Diabetes Passport, V8. The Australian government have produced a summary core dataset for diabetes which is primarily clinically orientated [13]. This has 37 items for collection, ranging from demographics through to procedure coding, and is designed to bring about a degree of national consistency in recording information about people with diabetes. In 2003, a Scottish Diabetes Core Dataset was prepared for the collection of data about people with diabetes in primary care [14]. This was a very comprehensive dataset (over 50 separate items, many of which have subcategories), but has already required an extension due to new clinical contract arrangements for general practitioners in the United Kingdom [15].

34.3.1 Use of a MDS in a clinic (outpatient department): the first-stage appraisal process

In the frailty model of diabetes [16], a framework was developed that provides further assistance with clinical decisions, and allows the scope for establishing minimum core assessment criteria. Previously, it has been recommended that the annual review process should now include an assessment of basic measures of activities of daily life (ADL) function, such as a Barthel test; tests of cognitive function, such as the Mini-Mental State Examination (MMSE) or Clock Test; a screen for depression, such as the Geriatric Depression Score; and an assessment of gait and balance, which can be simply estimated by the timed 'Get Up and Go' test (for details of all tests, see Ref. [16]). This integrated process of comprehensive geriatric assessment can suitably be applied to diabetes, and allows investigators to create the culture of defining criteria not only in an academic scenario but also in a clinical setting.

Several clinical intervention models have been proposed [17] which might also serve as a template for determining the items of a diabetes MDS for intervention research. These were developed for frail subjects with diabetes, and designed to detect early vascular complications, optimize functional status and improve well-being – the very 'hallmarks' of assessing diabetes interventions. The models proposed were the metabolic model, vascular model and the rehabilitation model. The latter two would require a major input from multidisciplinary (MD) staff.

Both, assessment and outcome criteria have previously been published for diabetic residents of care homes in the United Kingdom [18, 19]. In the British Diabetic Association Report, at assessment, 11 items were recommended which comprised a clinical data and medication list, BMI, blood pressure (BP), fundoscopy, feet examination, urine/blood tests and a dietary plan. The outcome data related to HbA$_{1c}$, lipids and BP, nutritional status, frequency and severity of hypoglycaemia, frequency and outcome of hospital admissions, vascular complication rate, change in level of dependency and mental function, and quality of life/mobility measures. These can be extrapolated easily to intervention studies in older people with type 2 diabetes, depending on the nature of the intervention, for example, a drug intervention or care model approach.

The Minimum Data Set/Resident Assessment Instrument (MDS/RAI) was developed in response to a series of scandals relating to the quality of care in long-term facilities in the United States [20]. This is a computerized system designed to be used by nursing staff in the development of care plans. It has 17 domains in the assessment phase and 18 separate resident assessment protocols dealing with issues such as acute confusional states, visual function, mood, falls, nutritional status, and so on. While not directly categorizing by disease, these items have direct relevance to residents with diabetes.

A set of European-wide Clinical Guidelines [21] indicated assessment tools which could form part of the basis of defining a MDS based on functional status. The latter item is one of the principal assessment/outcome criteria for interventional studies in older people with diabetes. The others relate to the assessment of subjects at the time of clinical trial entry, to outcome data relating to the quality of life, health economic data

and metabolic control, with the other dimensions of the MDS relating to the organization and delivery of care and patient-centred outcomes/informal carer issues [22]. In some cases, these might also be used as prospective and longitudinal outcome data.

By a strict appraisal of the evidence-base for studies in geriatric diabetes, the European Guidelines was also able to define up to 30 new research areas for future study. These areas naturally influence the components of a minimum data set, thus emphasizing the need for flexibility and adaptation as a key property of a modern research MDS. With this background, multiple potential areas for research by a randomized controlled design (RCT) in geriatric diabetes begin to emerge. As an example, a priority list of research trials in older subjects with type 2 diabetes might include:

- Benefits of lifestyle intervention and/or therapeutic approaches (e.g. ACE-inhibitor, insulin sensitizer, etc.) in reducing the incidence of type 2 diabetes in hypertension or other cardiovascular risk factors.

- Outcome of intensive treatment with oral agents and/or insulin in reducing primary macrovascular and microvascular outcomes, and mortality.

- Benefits (vascular/mortality outcome data; cost-effectiveness) of statin and/or fibrate therapy in proven cardiovascular disease.

- Benefits of prolonged comprehensive geriatric assessment programmes (CGA) (>12 months) in determining clinical outcomes and longevity.

- Does lowering blood pressure reduce the risk of dementia in type 2 diabetes and hypertension?

- Value of educational approaches in the prevention of diabetic foot disease in terms of behaviour and knowledge, frequency of ulceration and amputation, quality of life and patient satisfaction.

- Value of both clinical and educational approaches in reducing the severity of hospital admission and metabolic decompensation, infections, and pain outcomes in diabetic residents of care homes.

34.3.2 A minimum data set for intervention trials in type 2 diabetes: defining the purpose and content

The chosen will ideally need to satisfy four principal criteria:

1. Each item should be directly applicable and have clinically relevance to the patient with type 2 diabetes.

2. As far as possible, all functional, quality of life and patient-centred outcomes should have been validated in older populations.

3. Each item should retain validity over time, making it suitable for prospective study designs.

4. Each item within the dataset should be precise, unambiguous and acceptable to all major research stakeholders.

An agreed MDS-Diabetes would need to be considered as the minimum dataset that research organizations (whether public or private) should use to collect consistent and standardized (unified) information about the value of interventions. In addition, a Clinical MDS-Diabetes (as mentioned above) can be established from this, so that health care organizations can adopt these items for benchmarking and quality assurance purposes. It can also be used by health care staff as part of the clinical audit process. By providing this standardized framework, clinical services and networks providing diabetes care to older people can be evaluated critically from a quality perspective, and modifications of the dataset can be used for Commissioning purposes both in primary and secondary care settings. Future evidenced-based decision making will also be enhanced as these datasets become uniformly employed.

An analysis of studies involving older subjects with diabetes from the electronic databases of Medline, EMBASE and CINAHL, suggests that the spectrum on outcome measurement is often not extensive, with common repeating sequences such as body weight, HbA_{1c}, stroke rate, cardiovascular event rate and adverse event rate. However, many studies lack depth of enquiry by restricting the number of variables examined; this – combined with the recruitment of poorly documented subjects – can limit the effectiveness of any well-designed minimum data set. This must be borne in mind in collaborative efforts when developing a final MDS.

For studies in diabetes, the extensive list of items provided in Table 34.2 should be considered as important elements of this disorder (disease)-specific MDS, although some further selection will be necessary.

Outcome variables which measure the effectiveness of differing models of care are not generally available for studies in diabetes. They are, however, likely

Table 34.2 The possible components of a diabetes MDS.

Metabolic and laboratory
- Waist–hip ratio and waist circumference/BMI
- Glycosylated haemoglobin (HbA_{1c})
- Fasting glucose
- Postprandial glucose
- Fasting insulin
- Full lipid profile, including LDL- and HDL-cholesterol
- Blood pressure
- Serum creatinine
- Microalbuminuria
- Uric acid, C-reactive protein and interleukin-6, tumour necrosis factor-alpha

Quality of life
- Euro-QOL
- ADDQOL Senior

Patient-centred outcomes
- Hypoglycaemia rate
- Hospital admission rate
- Satisfaction with treatment: DSTQ
- Self-rated health and Health status: SF-36
- Pain control
- Carer Strain Index

Other diabetes-specific data items
- Cardiovascular event rate, stroke rate, fatal and non-fatal
- Myocardial infarction (MI) for macrovascular and hypertension intervention studies
- Any diabetes-related end-point, including erectile dysfunction

Cost-effectiveness/health economics
- No diabetes-specific data sets identified

to require items relating to mortality, inpatient care, quality of life and health economic analysis.

It is also anticipated that data collection will need to include guidance on minimum criteria for enrolment in the clinical trial relating to referral criteria, demographics and the precise assessment of diabetes-related complications and current treatments. This may require additional effort to define minimum datasets for patient demographics, patient categories by diagnosis including patients in hospital, outpatient clinics, and those in care homes, treatment categories and vascular complications at entry to the trial.

34.4 Conclusions

In order for progress to be made, an international agreement is required to collect this specified minimum dataset in future clinical trials. This requires cooperation between all key organizations involved in diabetes care and those involved in the specialist care of older people. A consensus on the final list of items and format of the dataset is overdue and is now required.

Diabetes in the elderly represents an exciting phase of research because the special issues involved in the effective management and realization of important gaps in care provision are being increasingly recognized [23]. Moreover, today an increasing number of major clinical trials involve older subjects, thereby providing the data to support specific interventions, even among the aged.

References

1. Sinclair AJ. Special considerations in older adults with diabetes: meeting the challenge. Diabetes Spectr 2006, 19: 229–33.
2. Gregg EW, Beckles GL, Williamson DF, Leveille SG, Langlois JA, Engelgau MM and Narayan KM. Diabetes and physical disability among older U.S. adults. Diabetes Care 2000; 23 (9): 1272–7.
3. Volpato S, Blaum C, Resnick H, Ferrucci L, Fried LP and Guralnik JM. Comorbidities and impairments explaining the association between diabetes and lower extremity disability: The Women's Health and Aging Study. Diabetes Care 2002; 25 (4): 678–83.
4. Sinclair AJ and Gadsby R. Diabetes in Care Homes. In: A.J. Sinclair and P. Finucane (eds), *Diabetes in Old Age*, 2nd edition. John Wiley & Sons, Chichester, 2001; pp. 241–252.
5. Rosenthal MJ, Fajardo M, Gilmore S, Morley JE and Naliboff BD. Hospitalisation and mortality of diabetes in older adults. A 3-year prospective study. Diabetes Care 1998; 21 (2): 231–5.
6. National Diabetes Support Team (2008) Improving emergency and inpatient care for people with diabetes. Available from NDST@prolog.uk.com.
7. Stratton RJ, King CL, Stroud MA, Jackson AA and Elia M. 'Malnutrition Universal Screening Test' predicts mortality and length of hospital stay in acutely ill elderly. Br J Nutr 2006; 95 (2): 325–30.
8. Burke WJ, Roccaforte WH and Wengel SP. The short form of the Geriatric Depression Scale: a comparison with the 30-item form. J Geriatr Psychiatry Neurol 1991; 4 (3): 173–8.
9. Folstein MF, Folstein SE and McHugh PR. Mini-mental state. A practical method for grading the cognitive state of patients for the clinician. J Psychiatr Res 1975; 12 (3): 189–98.
10. Shulman KI. Clock-drawing: is it the ideal cognitive screening test? Int J Geriatr Psychiatry 2000; 15 (6): 548–61.
11. Abellan Van Kan G, Sinclair A, Andrieu S, Olde Rikkert M, Gambassi G and Vellas B. The Geriatric Minimum Data Set for Clinical Trials (GMDS). J Nutr Health Aging 2008; 12 (3): 197–200.
12. The DIABCARD Data Set. (2001) Version 4.0 EU/G7 Administrative and Emergency Data. Contact: diabcard@gsf.de.
13. National Health Data Committee (now HDSC), Australian Institute of Health and Welfare. (2003) *The Diabetes (Clinical) Data Set Specifications* 2003. ISBN 1 74024 287 4.
14. Scottish Executive, Edinburgh. (2003) Scottish Diabetes Core Dataset December 2003. SCI Diabetes Collaboration and SCIMP. Available at: www.diabetesinscotland.org and www.ceppc.org/scimp.
15. Quality Outcomes Framework, 2008/9. Department of Health. Available at: www.dh.gov.uk.
16. Sinclair AJ. Towards a minimum data set for intervention studies in type 2 diabetes in older people. J Nutr Health Aging 2007; 11 (3): 289–93.
17. Sinclair AJ. Diabetes in old age – changing concepts in the secondary care arena. J Roy Coll Phys (Lond) 2000; 34 (3): 240–4.
18. British Diabetic Association. (1999) *Guidelines of practice for residents with diabetes in care homes.* British Diabetic Association, London.
19. Sinclair AJ, Turnbull CJ and Croxson SCM. Document of Diabetes Care for Residential and Nursing Homes. Postgrad Med J 1997; 73: 611–612.
20. Hawes C, Morris J, Phillips C, Fries B, Murphy K and Mor V. Development of the nursing home Residents Assessment Instrument in the USA. Age Ageing 1997; 27 (Suppl. 2): 19–25.
21. European Diabetes Working Party for Older People 2001–2004: Clinical guidelines for type 2 diabetes mellitus [article online]. Available from www.eugms.org.
22. Sinclair AJ, Turnbull CJ and Croxson SCM. Document of care for older people with diabetes. Postgrad Med J 1996; 72: 334–8.
23. Sinclair AJ. Aging and diabetes. (2004) In: *International Textbook of Diabetes Mellitus*, 3rd edition. R.A. De Fronzo, E. Ferrannini, H. Keen and P. Zimmet (eds). John Wiley & Sons, Chichester, UK, pp. 1579–97.

Index

Note: Page references in *italics* refer to Figures; those in **bold** refer to Tables

---

Index compiled by Alison Musker